Targeting the STAT Pathway in Cancer

Targeting the STAT Pathway in Cancer

Edited by Finn McFarland

hayle medical

New York

Hayle Medical,
750 Third Avenue, 9th Floor,
New York, NY 10017, USA

Visit us on the World Wide Web at:
www.haylemedical.com

ISBN: 978-1-64647-523-0

Cataloging-in-Publication Data

Targeting the STAT pathway in cancer / edited by Finn McFarland.
p. cm.
Includes bibliographical references and index.
ISBN 978-1-64647-523-0
1. Cancer. 2. Cancer--Diagnosis. 3. Metastasis. 4. Cancer of unknown primary origin.
I. McFarland, Finn.
RC261 .T37 2023
616.994--dc23

Table of Contents

Preface

The world is advancing at a fast pace like never before. Therefore, the need is to keep up with the latest developments. This book was an idea that came to fruition when the specialists in the area realized the need to coordinate together and document essential themes in the subject. That's when I was requested to be the editor. Editing this book has been an honour as it brings together diverse authors researching on different streams of the field. The book collates essential materials contributed by veterans in the area which can be utilized by students and researchers alike.

The JAK-STAT signal pathway refers to a cytokine-stimulated signal transduction pathway which plays an important role in numerous biological processes which include cell proliferation, differentiation, apoptosis and immune regulation. The signal transducer and activator of transcription (STAT) pathway is linked upstream with the Janus kinase (JAK) family of proteins. It is also capable of integrating inputs from several signaling pathways. Each member of the family performs a distinct role in signal transduction and is critical in mediating cellular responses to various types of cytokines. STAT family members particularly STAT3 and STAT5 have been associated with the progression of cancer. Persistent STAT3 and STAT5 activation is known to stimulate chronic inflammation, which makes healthy cells more susceptible to carcinogenesis. STAT3 is significantly linked to immune evasion and tumor growth. Several mechanisms appear to play a role in the activation of STAT5 proteins in human cancer, comprising miRNA- and hormone-regulated TFs, gene amplification, epigenetic alterations, aberrant growth factor signaling and altered proteolytic pathways. This book contains some path-breaking studies on the STAT pathway. It will serve as a valuable source of reference for graduate and postgraduate students.

Each chapter is a sole-standing publication that reflects each author´s interpretation. Thus, the book displays a multi-facetted picture of our current understanding of application, resources and aspects of the field. I would like to thank the contributors of this book and my family for their endless support.

Editor

1

ADAM17 Activity and IL-6 Trans-Signaling in Inflammation and Cancer

Neele Schumacher and Stefan Rose-John *

Biochemical Institute, University of Kiel, 24118 Kiel, Germany; nschumacher@biochem.uni-kiel.de
* Correspondence: rosejohn@biochem.uni-kiel.de

Abstract: All ligands of the epidermal growth factor receptor (EGF-R) are transmembrane proteins, which need to be proteolytically cleaved in order to be systemically active. The major protease responsible for this cleavage is the membrane metalloprotease ADAM17, which also has been implicated in cleavage of TNFα and interleukin-6 (IL-6) receptor. It has been recently shown that in the absence of ADAM17, the main protease for EGF-R ligand processing, colon cancer formation is largely abrogated. Intriguingly, colon cancer formation depends on EGF-R activity on myeloid cells rather than on intestinal epithelial cells. A major activity of EGF-R on myeloid cells is the stimulation of IL-6 synthesis. Subsequently, IL-6 together with the ADAM17 shed soluble IL-6 receptor acts on intestinal epithelial cells via IL-6 trans-signaling to induce colon cancer formation, which can be blocked by the inhibitor of IL-6 trans-signaling, sgp130Fc. Blockade of IL-6 trans-signaling therefore offers a new therapeutic window downstream of the EGF-R for the treatment of colon cancer and possibly of other EGF-R related neoplastic diseases.

Keywords: ADAM17; interleukin-6; trans-signaling; epidermal growth factor receptor (EGF-R); shedding; metalloprotease; tumor necrosis factor alpha (TNFα); inflammation associated cancer; colon cancer; lung cancer

---

1. Introduction

IL-6 is a four-helical cytokine with pleiotropic activities, which is synthesized by many cell types upon appropriate stimulation and which can act on many cell types during several disease states such as inflammation and cancer [1]. IL-6 exerts its function through binding to the alpha-receptor Interleukin-6 receptor (IL-6R). The complex of IL-6 and IL-6R binds to the beta-receptor glycoprotein 130 (gp130) and induces dimerization of gp130 [2]. This dimerized gp130 leads to an activation of the tyrosine kinase Janus kinase 1 (JAK1), which is constitutively associated with the cytoplasmic portion of gp130. JAK1 phosphorylates tyrosine residues within the cytoplasmic portion of gp130. This leads to the recruitment of the adapter protein and phosphatase SHP2 that initiates MAP kinase and PI3 kinase signaling [3]. Furthermore, phosphorylated tyrosine residues recruit the cytoplasmic transcription factors STAT1 and STAT3, which thereupon become phosphorylated, dimerize, and translocate into the nucleus, where they bind to DNA and stimulate the transcription of gp130 target genes [3]. One of the earliest gp130 target genes is the gene coding for SOCS3. The SOCS3 protein is recruited to the membrane proximal tyrosine residue within the gp130 cytoplasmic tail where it inhibits the activity of JAK1. Therefore, SOCS3 is a negative feedback inhibitor of gp130 signaling [3]. Recently, it was shown that gp130 activation leads to the phosphorylation and activation of the YAP pathway (Figure 1). This pathway was shown to be important in the development of colon cancer [4,5].

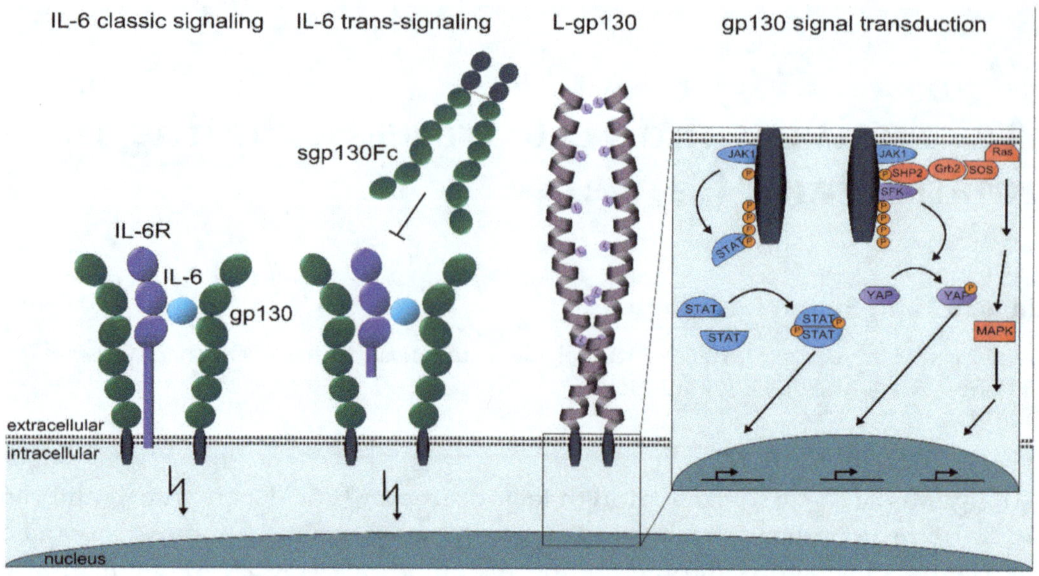

Figure 1. Modes of IL-6 signaling. IL-6 can signal via the membrane-bound IL-6R, which, however, is only expressed on some cell types. Alternatively, IL-6 can bind to the soluble IL-6R (sIL-6R) and the complex of IL-6/sIL-6R can stimulate virtually all cells in the body since gp130 is ubiquitously expressed. In an artificial model of cell-autonomous gp130 stimulation, the extracellular portion of gp130 has been exchanged for a leucine zipper, leading to constitutive gp130 signaling in the absence of any ligand [6]. The insert shows the main intracellular signaling pathways stimulated by gp130 activation.

While gp130 is expressed on all cells in the body, IL-6R is only expressed on some cells including hepatocytes, some leukocytes and some epithelial cells. Since IL-6 shows only measurable binding to the IL-6R but not to gp130, it follows that IL-6 can only act on cells, which express the IL-6R [2,7]. Interestingly, the membrane-bound IL-6R can be cleaved from the cell membrane by A disintegrin and metalloproteinases (ADAMs), resulting in a soluble form of the receptor [8–10]. The soluble IL-6R (sIL-6R) can still bind its ligand IL-6 and the complex of IL-6 and sIL-6R can bind to gp130 and induce dimerization of signaling. This mode of signaling has been called IL-6 trans-signaling [11]. Since gp130 is ubiquitously expressed, IL-6 trans-signaling can lead to the stimulation of virtually every cell in the body (Figure 1) [12]. However, there are few proteases described that can cleave membrane-bound IL-6R thus enabling IL-6 trans-signaling. Besides, the closely related ADAM proteases ADAM10 and ADAM17, meprin metalloproteases were reported to release the soluble form of the IL-6R [13–16].

Moreover, since on most cells gp130 is expressed at higher levels than IL-6R, stimulation by IL-6 leads to the stimulation of only some gp130 molecules whereas stimulation with the IL-6/sIL-6R complex leads to the activation and stimulation of all gp130 proteins resulting in a higher signal amplitude as a consequence of IL-6 trans-signaling as compared with IL-6 signaling via the membrane-bound IL-6R. IL-6 upon binding to the IL-6R is rapidly internalized in contrast to the IL-6/sIL-6R complex, which is internalized only with low efficacy [17]. This resulted in significantly longer stimulation mediated by the IL-6/sIL-6R complex as compared to IL-6 alone [17]. This property of IL-6 trans-signaling might be important for several cellular or tissue responses, which can only be induced by IL-6 trans-signaling but not by IL-6 classic signaling via the membrane-bound IL-6R [18].

Importantly, IL-6 trans-signaling can be specifically blocked by the extracellular portion of gp130 fused to the Fc-portion of a human IgG1 antibody (sgp130Fc) [1,19]. This blockade of IL-6 trans-signaling does not affect activities of IL-6 via the membrane-bound IL-6R. In transgenic mice overexpressing the sgp130Fc, IL-6 trans-signaling is completely blocked. These mice have been widely used to define the role of IL-6 classic signaling and IL-6 trans-signaling in many mouse models of human diseases (Figure 1) [1,12,20].

In healthy individuals, IL-6 levels are in the range between 1 and 5 pg/mL, but they can increase by many orders of magnitude during inflammatory states or upon infection. Plasma IL-6 levels of up to several μg/mL have been reported in patients with septic shock [21]. Interestingly, the level of sIL-6R in the blood of healthy individuals is in the range of 40–80 ng/mL, more than 1000 times higher than IL-6 [20]. A soluble form of gp130, which is generated by differential splicing [22] is found in the plasma of healthy individuals at approximately 400 ng/mL [20]. IL-6 binds to the IL-6R with an affinity of about 1 nM, whereas the complex of IL-6 and sIL-6R binds to gp130 with an affinity of 10 pM. Therefore, IL-6 released into the circulation will bind to sIL-6R and thereafter be trapped by sgp130. Thus, sIL-6R and sgp130 form a buffer for IL-6 [23]. The important function of the IL-6 buffer was underlined by studies on the coding single nucleotide polymorphism (SNP; rs2228145) in the human IL-6R that results in the alteration of Asp358 into Ala358. These amino acid residues are in close proximity of the proteolytic cleavage site of the IL-6R [16]. Interestingly, the IL-6R with Ala358 is a better protease substrate and is shed more efficiently leading to significantly increased plasma levels of sIL-6R [24]. Patients with the Ala358 variant of the IL-6R not only show about 2-fold elevated levels of sIL-6R [25], but they are also protected from inflammatory diseases such as congestive heart disease, abdominal aneurism, and rheumatoid arthritis [26–28]. Moreover, patients with the rs2228145 SNP showed a significant lower risk of Crohn's disease and ulcerative colitis as compared to control individuals [29]. Furthermore, growth rates of abdominal aortic aneurisms in patients were smaller with the Ala358 variant of the IL-6R [30]. These results can be explained by a higher capacity of the IL-6 buffer in the blood, which is caused by the higher circulating sIL-6R levels [20,23].

IL-6 is synthesized and secreted by many cell types and the cytokine also acts on many cell types. IL-6 transgenic animals and IL-6 knock-out animals have been generated to define the major activities of this cytokine [31–37]. In order to explore cell-specific activities of IL-6, we generated a constitutively active gp130 construct. To this end, we replaced the entire extracellular portion of gp130 by a leucine zipper of the c-jun oncogene. Such an arrangement had been used to generate constitutively active cytokine receptor complexes [38]. Transfection of various cell types with the leucine zipper dimerized gp130 molecule, which we called L-gp130, was shown to lead to phosphorylation of STAT3 and to long-term growth of IL-6 dependent cells. Moreover, mouse embryonic stem cells transfected with the L-gp130 cDNA construct remained undifferentiated even in the absence of exogenously supplied LIF, indicating that cell autonomous gp130 activation had been achieved [6]. Interestingly, these data also supported the view that sustained gp130 signaling could not be completely switched off by the induction of the negative feed-back inhibitor protein SOCS3 (Figure 1) [6]. Recently, we inserted the L-gp130 cDNA construct into the ROSA26 locus of the mouse. In these mice, by breeding to an appropriate cre transgenic mouse, the L-gp130 molecule can be switched on constitutively in a cell autonomous manner. Activating gp130 in B-cells or in the entire hematopoietic system resulted in B-cell lymphomas and plasma cell disorders with full penetrance [39]. These mice will be useful in the future to study many more cell-specific activities of IL-6 without confounding activities of other cells or tissues.

ADAM17 is a membrane-bound metalloprotease, which was originally identified as the protease responsible for cleavage of the membrane-bound cytokine TNFα [40,41]. Upon gene deletion of ADAM17, it turned out that this protease is essential for life and it is also responsible for cleavage of ligands of the EGF-R [42]. In the following years, it was found that ADAM17 is also responsible for cleavage of the membrane-bound IL-6R [43] and for around 80 additional transmembrane protein substrates [44,45]. Conditional deletion of ADAM17 [46] and analysis of hypomorphic ADAM17$^{ex/ex}$ mice [47] revealed important roles of the protease in immune regulation and homeostasis of many different tissues [44], including the central nervous system [45]. ADAM17 is expressed in most types of tissues but the cell surface activity of ADAM17 seems to be tightly regulated [44]. It turned out that intracellular trafficking of ADAM17 through the Golgi to the plasma membrane requires the presence of iRhoms, which are members of the intramembrane rhomboid proteases and which have lost protease activity in the course of evolution [48]. In the absence of iRhom1 or iRhom2, ADAM17 mRNA is expressed but the protein does not reach the cell surface [49,50]. Moreover, an additional protein, FRMD8 or iTAP, which binds to iRhom2 is involved in the activation of the ADAM17 protease via phosphorylation [51,52]. An additional mechanism of ADAM17 activation is the cell surface exposure of phosphatidylserine, which binds to a cationic phosphatidylserine-binding motif within the membrane-proximal domain of ADAM17 [53]. This mechanism explains the profound activation of ADAM17 by all inducers of apoptosis analyzed thus far [54].

Since ADAM17 orchestrates at least three major signaling pathways—namely TNFα, IL-6R, and EGF-R signaling—it is not surprising that the regulation of protease activity is under tight control. Moreover, the involvement of ADAM17 in fundamental pathophysiologic processes such as inflammation and cancer can be envisaged. Of note, the importance of ADAM17 has been largely overlooked by all transcriptomics based studies since the mRNA expression of ADAM17 does not show major changes between organs as well as in health and disease [44,45]. The role of ADAM17 and IL-6 trans-signaling in inflammation and cancer will therefore be reviewed in the following paragraphs (Figure 2).

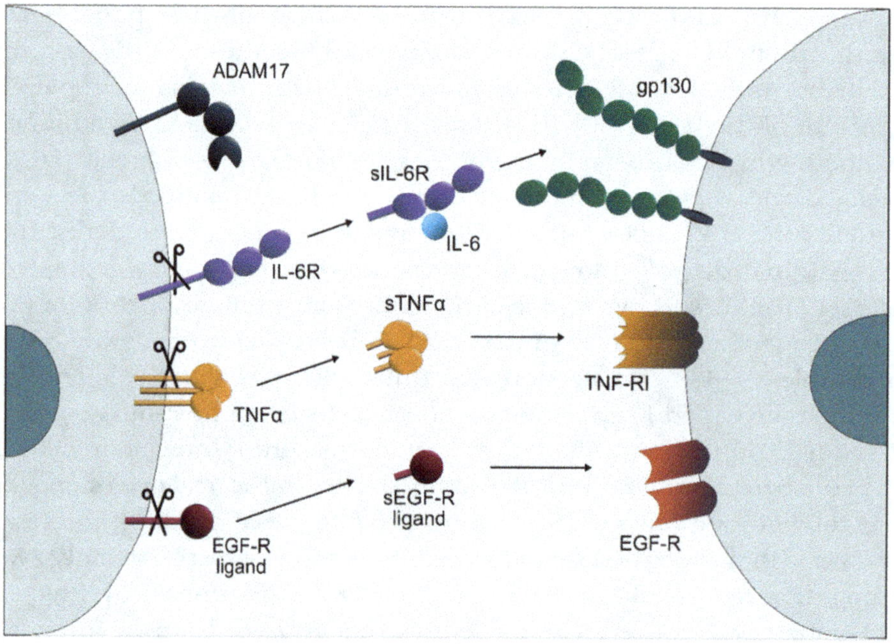

Figure 2. ADAM17 is a membrane-bound metalloprotease, which cleaves more than 80 substrates [44,45]. Major substrates of ADAM17 are IL-6R, TNFα, and ligands of the EGF-R. Cleavage of the IL-6R is a prerequisite of the pro-inflammatory IL-6 trans-signaling pathway via the sIL-6R. Cleavage of TNFα and the formation of soluble TNFα (sTNFα) leads to the stimulation of the pro-inflammatory TNFα receptor 1 (TNF-R_I). Cleavage of ligands of the EGF-R is needed for the systemic activity of the ligands and therefore for the full stimulation of the EGF-R [47].

2. Results

2.1. *IL-6 Trans-Signaling and ADAM17 in Inflammation*

IL-6 is essential for the induction, progression and resolution of local and systemic inflammatory responses that activate acute phase reaction, promote tissue damage and development of autoimmune reactions, and plays a pivotal role in transition from innate to adaptive immune responses [55].

IL-6 knock-out mice are protected from development of experimental autoimmune encephalomyelitis (EAE), the mouse model of human multiple sclerosis [56–58] and mouse models of rheumatoid arthritis [59,60]. These mice also fail to efficiently control bacterial and viral infections with vaccinia virus, *Listeria monocytogenes* and *Mycobacterium tuberculosis* [31,61]. Similar to IL-6-deficient mice, IL-6R knock-out mice display a deficit in acute phase response, compromised wound healing, and reduced cellular infiltration during inflammation [62]. While acute phase reactions and defense against bacteria is mediated via membrane-bound IL-6R [63] delayed macrophage invasion in mouse models of inflammation was dependent on the availability of sIL-6R [64–66].

The cellular origin of sIL-6R was longtime unknown. Since it is evident that increased sIL-6R levels correlate with infiltrated leukocytes in various inflammatory pathologies like arthritic joints [67] and acute inflammation [64] macrophages were considered as a main source of sIL-6R. Furthermore, IL-6 stimulates polarization and proliferation of M2 macrophages via induction of IL-4R expression as shown in mouse models of obesity [68,69].

T cell responses can also be governed by both forms of IL-6 activities. Whereas T_{reg} development during experimental airway inflammation is controlled via membrane-bound IL-6R [70], IL-6 trans-signaling orchestrates T cell recruitment in an experimental peritoneal inflammation model [71]. Recently, it was found that TGFß, together with IL-6, drives the initial differentiation from naïve T-cells to pathogenic IL-17-producing T-cells (T_H17 cells), which are key factors for induction of tissue damage in a variety of chronic inflammatory and autoimmune diseases [72,73]. Due to its complex role in immune modulation, it is essential to understand how IL-6 contributes to the respective pathology.

2.1.1. Rheumatoid Arthritis

The first successful biologics-based therapy of rheumatoid arthritis patients was developed in the early 1990s by Marc Feldman and Ravinder Maini at the Charing Cross Hospital, London, UK and made use of antibodies neutralizing TNFα [74]. These TNFα antibodies had originally been prepared for clinical trials in human sepsis, which, however, entirely failed [75,76]. The first clinical trial with TNFα antibodies, which only involved few rheumatoid arthritis patients, was highly successful and led finally to the development of several TNFα-blocking drugs, which by now changed the perception of rheumatoid arthritis from a vastly debilitating disease to a largely manageable condition [76,77].

A decade ago, blocking IL-6R signaling with anti-IL-6R antibodies was approved for treatment of rheumatoid arthritis [78]. Beforehand, mouse models of rheumatoid arthritis had shown that IL-6 signaling drives disease progression by stimulating synovial hyperplasia, preservation of joint inflammation, and damage of underlying cartilage and bone [79–81]. All these disease symptoms are largely regulated by STAT3. Interestingly, it turned out that monotherapy with anti-IL-6R antibodies was superior to treatment of patients with the TNFα antibody adalimumab [82,83].

Mice which carry a Y757F mutation in the cytoplasmic tail of gp130 are unable to initiate the SHP2–MAP kinase–PI3 kinase axis because Y757 of gp130 is the docking site of SHP2 [84,85]. These mice can still activate the STAT1/STAT3 pathway [86,87]. Furthermore, these mice do not show negative regulation by SOCS3 since also this protein requires phosphorylated Y757 for its negative feedback activity [88,89]. These so-called $gp130^{F/F}$ mice therefore show increased STAT1/STAT3, but no SHP2–MAP kinase–PI3 kinase signaling [86]. Besides enhanced autoantibody production against DNA, amplified cell infiltration into the joints and enhanced osteoclast activation, $gp130^{F/F}$ mice develop arthritis-like symptoms within one year of age, thus resembling human rheumatoid arthritis [87]. Furthermore, clonal deletion of activated T cells was altered and these chronically activated T cells showed persistent IL-6-induced STAT3 and JAK1 phosphorylation indicating that IL-6 signaling in T cells plays a critical role in disease progression of rheumatoid arthritis [87]. In contrast, a dominant-negative STAT3 mutant with reduced STAT3 activity exhibits diminished cell infiltration into the joints, pannus formation, and cartilage damage in experimental arthritis in mice [90].

IL-6 signaling initiates a range of degenerative and inflammatory processes during rheumatoid arthritis. In vitro experiments suggested a possible effect of IL-6 and its soluble receptor on synovial fibroblasts proliferation [91] and survival [92]. Furthermore, IL-6 trans-signaling promotes the generation of osteoclasts [93–95] and bone resorption by stimulating the expression of receptor activator of nuclear factor kappa κ B (NFκB) (RANK) ligand (RANKL), which stimulates RANK expressed on osteoclast precursors leading to differentiation to bone-resorbing osteoclasts [96]. Binding of RANKL to RANK activates downstream signaling pathways like NFκB, MAPK, JNK, and Akt, which consequently stimulate the expression of osteoclastic transcription factors in osteoclast precursors. The study of Feng et al. [97] showed that IL-6 trans-signaling attenuated RANKL-induced ERK and JNK activation suggesting that IL-6 trans-signaling differentially regulates RANKL-induced osteoclastogenesis.

Enhanced proliferation and activation of synovial fibroblasts and osteoclasts leads to irreversible destruction of cartilage and bone of the affected joint. The majority of these processes could be abrogated by blocking IL-6 trans signaling, which coordinated leukocyte infiltration and severity of joint damage [79,98,99].

Interestingly, EGF-R inhibition reduced the severity of experimental arthritis, most likely due to reduction of synovial fibroblasts proliferation, cytokine production, and reduction of osteoclastogenesis [100]. Furthermore, iRhom2-dependent trafficking of the IL-6R sheddase ADAM17 and its activity on myeloid cells was shown to be involved in development of experimental arthritis in mice [101]. Since ADAM17 mediates the release of TNFα, sIL-6R, and EGF-R ligands, its activity is likely to play an important role in the development of rheumatoid arthritis (see below).

2.1.2. Acute Inflammation

Rapid infiltration of neutrophils followed by replacement of mononuclear leukocytes is crucial for proper resolution of an acute inflammatory situation. IL-6 signaling via its soluble receptor regulates expression of CXC and CC chemokines that are needed for the switch of initial neutrophil influx to attraction of monocytes. In this context, IL-6 controls neutrophil infiltration by suppressing neutrophil-attracting chemokines and directs their apoptosis [64,102]. These effects were shown to be dependent on STAT3 activity [103]. The switch from neutrophil to monocytic cells could be abrogated by blocking IL-6 trans-signaling with the sgp130Fc protein in an acute peritonitis model [64,104] and in an air pouch model of acute inflammation in mice [65]. Furthermore, it was described that depletion of infiltrating neutrophils reduced the amount of sIL-6R in a model of local and acute inflammation. Thus, it was reasoned that in local and acute inflammation processes, neutrophils were a major source of sIL-6R [54]. This led us to investigate if proteolysis by ADAM17 is needed for the local release of sIL-6R and resolution of an acute inflammation. Contrary to our expectations, local ADAM17 activity was not critical for proper cell infiltration in acute inflammation in mice since the sIL-6R was infiltrating from the circulation in an ADAM17-independent process. These studies, however, confirmed the critical role of IL-6 trans-signaling in local and acute inflammation [105].

Initial recruitment of neutrophils and IL-6 secretion during acute peritonitis was described to be dependent on IFNγ. Defective IL-6 secretion into the site of inflammation in IFN$\gamma^{-/-}$ mice could be restored by treatment with recombinant IFNγ and IL-1ß, but not with IFNγ alone [102]. IL-6 trans-signaling was furthermore shown to be critical for transition between innate and acquired immune responses. T cell recruitment was impaired in IL-6$^{-/-}$ mice in a mouse model of peritonitis due to reduced chemokine expression which was mediated by STAT3 activation [71].

Unresolved inflammation leads inevitably to chronic fibrotic tissue damage. IL-6$^{-/-}$ mice were protected from the development of fibrosis in recurrent inflammatory activation of peritonitis. In this particular model, IL-6 was needed for survival and expansion of Th1 cells, which were shown to be crucial for STAT1 activation in stromal cells [106]. Recently, it was shown that IL-6-mediated STAT1 phosphorylation, which reflects the effector characteristics of CD4^{+} T cells, is critically regulated by the tyrosine phosphatases PTPN2 and PTPN22. These two phosphatases were described to limit STAT1-mediated IL-6 signaling in both activated and memory CD4^{+} T cells thus modulating the expression of genes associated with particular immune responses [107].

2.1.3. Sepsis

Mice with gp130-dependent STAT3 hyperactivation (gp130$^{F/F}$) were hypersensitive to LPS-induced endotoxic shock. Overall survival of these mice was reduced accompanied by increased IL-6 expression and neutrophil influx into the peritoneal cavity. Both, genetic ablation of IL-6 in gp130$^{F/F}$ or wildtype mice and specific inhibition of IL-6 trans-signaling led to an increased overall survival of LPS-induced endotoxic shock, suggesting that IL-6 signaling via the sIL-6R triggers the proinflammatory actions of IL-6 during LPS-induced endotoxic shock [108].

In a large animal study with 120 mice, the effect of total IL-6 blockade or selective inhibition of IL-6 trans-signaling on survival of sepsis induced by cecal ligation puncture was compared. Interestingly, inhibition of IL-6 trans-signaling via sgp130Fc was far superior to global IL-6 signaling blockade with an IL-6 neutralizing antibody. In this model, mice treated with sgp130Fc showed an up to 100% survival rate, an intact acute phase response, and less intestinal epithelial cell apoptosis, whereas no benefit was seen upon global IL-6 signaling blockade [109]. This enhanced therapeutic efficacy of inhibiting only the IL-6 trans-signaling pathway might be due to regenerative effects of IL-6 via the classic signaling pathway that was left intact when only IL-6 trans-signaling was blocked [12,110].

Deficiency of ADAM17 in inflammatory mouse models was shown to greatly diminish inflammatory responses [46,111,112]. When myeloid cells lacked ADAM17, mice showed slightly better survival rate after cecal ligation puncture. Blood and peritoneal bacteria levels, as well as inflammatory cytokine and chemokine plasma concentrations, were reduced in myeloid ADAM17-deficient mice, while increased neutrophil influx was observed [113]. This was possibly due to reduced proteolysis of the chemokine receptor CXCR2 or L-selectin [114,115].

2.1.4. Inflammatory Bowel Disease

IL-6 has been described as a T cell activation factor and shown to induce T cell proliferation and survival [116,117]. This ability has been linked to the pathology of several models of chronic inflammatory disease [87,118]. In several animal models of intestinal inflammation, the disease could be alleviated by specific blockade of IL-6 trans-signaling with sgp130Fc. Blockade of IL-6 trans-signaling led to beneficial T-cell apoptosis in the colon of mice with chronic intestinal inflammation [118], since an enhanced T-cell resistance against apoptosis may contribute to disease perpetuation in Crohn's disease [119]. In a murine model of intestinal inflammation using SAMP1/Yit mice, which is considered to be similar to inflammatory bowel disease in humans, treatment with sgp130Fc improved inflammation, as validated by less destruction of the epithelial layer and by less inflammatory infiltrates in the lamina propria of the small intestine [120]. In patients with inflammatory bowel disease, treatment with the IL-6R neutralizing antibody Tocilizumab suggested a clinical benefit [121], but this treatment has not been approved by the FDA. It is possible that, like in the murine cecal ligation puncture model of sepsis, specific blockade of IL-6 trans-signaling with sgp130Fc might be superior to global IL-6 blockade due to regenerative effects of IL-6 via the classic signaling pathway [12,110]. Of note, the sgp130Fc protein under the WHO name Olamkicept is currently tested in phase II clinical trials in patients with inflammatory bowel disease [20].

2.1.5. Lung Pathophysiology: Emphysema, Asthma, and Idiopathic Pulmonary Fibrosis

Proinflammatory actions of IL-6 are implicated in the pathogenesis of lung emphysema and patients with COPD [122]. Analysis in mice revealed that development of emphysema was reliant on IL-6. In contrast to wt mice, $gp130^{F/F}$ mice showed spontaneous development of lung emphysema at 6 months of age due to alveolar cell apoptosis, which was abrogated by genetic deletion of IL-6. Treatment of wt mice with cigarette smoke increased emphysema-associated lung volume increase, which was not seen in IL-6-deficient animals [123]. In both models, in the spontaneous development of lung emphysema seen in $gp130^{F/F}$ mice and in cigarette smoke treated wildtype mice, treatment with sgp130Fc abrogated alveolar cell apoptosis and disease pathogenesis. This study furthermore revealed a possible connection of IL-6 trans-signaling and the mTOR pathway. After blockade of the serine/threonine kinase mTOR with rapamycin, IL-6 mediated lung pathologies were significantly reduced [124].

IL-6 was claimed to be important for the maintenance of the balance of effector T cells and regulatory T cells in lung pathogenesis. In a mouse model of asthma, IL-6 trans-signaling rather supported Th2 cytokine production, whereas classic IL-6 signaling was needed for the development of

FoxP3$^+$ regulatory T cells in the lung [70]. A recent study revealed an IL-6 trans-signaling specific gene signature in patients with asthma, which was accompanied by an increase in submucosal T cell and macrophage infiltration. Stimulation of primary human bronchial epithelial with both IL-6 and sIL-6R induced genes associated with airway remodeling such as matrix metalloproteinases and reduced expression of genes associated with epithelial barrier function such as ß-catenin. The gene signature found in this study was hypothesized to be helpful in determining patient subsets with high submucosal-inflammation and poor asthma control [125].

Idiopathic pulmonary fibrosis (IPF) characterizes a heterogeneous, chronic, and irreversible disorder in which deposition of collagen results in the loss of lung function. Although it is unsure if pulmonary fibrosis is the result of an unresolved inflammatory process the role of inflammatory cytokines is discussed. A study of cytokine levels in serum of patients with IPF revealed that IL-6 and IL-8 were increased in individuals with exacerbated disease state and that these increased levels correlated with a worse outcome [126]. This deleterious impact of IL-6 on the development of lung fibrosis was analyzed in different mouse models. In adenosine deaminase-deficient mice, which develop pulmonary inflammation and remodeling as well as in bleomycin-induced lung injury, IL-6 was shown to drive cellular infiltration and collagen deposition in the lungs [127,128]. A role for IL-6 trans-signaling in IPF was suggested as elevated sIL-6R levels were found in the lungs of patients with IPF and of mice with bleomycin-induced pulmonary fibrosis. Neutralization of IL-6 trans-signaling with sgp130Fc led to reduction of pulmonary inflammation, diminished myofibroblast accumulation and improved respiratory functions [129]. The development of pulmonary fibrosis in mice and differentiation of lung fibroblasts to collagen-producing myofibroblasts involves STAT3 activation by TGFß or IL-6 trans-signaling [130]. It was suggested that increased STAT3 activity in fibroblasts from IPF patients led to reduced apoptosis and thus contributes to the persistence of these cells [131,132].

2.2. *IL-6 Trans-Signaling and ADAM17 in Cancer*

It is widely accepted that inflammatory cytokine signaling plays key roles at many stages of tumorigenesis and supports malignant cell proliferation and metastasis [133]. Intestinal inflammation in several different animal models was efficiently blocked by a blockade of IL-6 trans-signaling [118,120] using sgp130Fc. On the other hand, intestinal inflammation was exacerbated by the application of Hyper-IL-6, a fusion protein of IL-6 and sIL-6R, which is a strong stimulator of IL-6 trans-signaling [134]. Therefore, it was reasonable to assume that inflammation associated cancer might also be driven by IL-6 trans-signaling [135].

2.2.1. Colorectal Cancer

When mice were treated with a low dose of the mutagen azoxymethane (AOM) followed by consecutive cycles of orally administered dextran sulfate sodium (DSS), they developed small visible lesions around day 20, followed by the appearance of large tumors until day 80 [136]. When analyzing RAG-1 knockout mice, which are defective in B-cell and T-cell receptor recombination and therefore lack B- and T-lymphocytes and hence are severely immune-deficient, it became clear that these animals did not develop large tumors indicating that lymphocytes are involved in the regulation of tumor growth [136]. Colon samples from different time points after AOM/DSS treatment demonstrated massive IL-6 and sIL-6R accumulation from day 21 onwards. Treatment of the mice with a neutralizing antibody against IL-6R drastically reduced the tumor score [136]. Interestingly, also selective blockade of IL-6 trans-signaling by injection of the sgp130Fc protein effectively suppressed colon carcinogenesis, suggesting that IL-6 trans-signaling by inducing STAT3 phosphorylation and expression of the anti-apoptotic proteins bcl-xl and bcl-2 was responsible for growth of epithelial tumor cells [136]. In human colon tumor tissues, it was shown that the expression and activity of ADAM17 was significantly increased as compared with normal tissue, underlining an important role of ADAM17 in mediating the IL-6 trans-signaling response via the sIL-6R [137]. In a different intestinal tumor model, mice repeatedly treated only with 9 DSS but not with AOM developed intestinal tumors after 18 weeks. The incidence and number of tumors was drastically reduced when the mice were treated with the sgp130Fc protein. Interestingly, it was shown that lamina propria macrophages via induction of ADAM17 were important for the generation of sIL-6R and therefore for the induction of IL-6 trans-signaling [138].

When IL-6$^{-/-}$ mice were compared to wt mice in their susceptibility to inflammatory colon cancer in the AOM/DSS model, it turned out that IL-6$^{-/-}$ mice had less tumors but more inflammation in the intestine, arguing for a role of IL-6 in the intestinal regeneration response. [110]. Indeed, it was shown in the same study that deletion of STAT3 in the intestinal epithelium led to more severe DSS colitis with pronounced colonic ulcerations and body weight loss, indicating that the IL-6 response in the intestinal epithelial cells was important for regeneration [110]. These data were further corroborated by a parallel study in which the authors used transgenic mice expressing in intestinal epithelial cells a constitutively active form of gp130 dimerized by a leucine zipper [6], which led to cell-autonomous STAT3 activation. These mice were largely resistant to DSS-induced colitis [139]. The above data suggested a role of IL-6 in the regeneration of the intestine. Indeed, treatment of mice with recombinant IL-6 protected the animals from DSS-induced colitis whereas treatment with a neutralizing IL-6 antibody aggravated DSS-induced colitis [140,141].

Inflammatory hepatocellular adenomas often harbor mutations in the gp130 gene, which leads to ligand independent activation of gp130 [142]. Transgenic mice, which express constitutively active gp130 transgene developed aberrant proliferation of intestinal epithelial cells. Interestingly, it was observed that the YAP and Notch signaling pathway were activated by the constitutively active gp130 mutant [5]. Furthermore, it was reported by the same authors that loss of APC in mice and in human patients led to the activation of Src, YAP, Notch, and STAT3. The presence of the activated gp130 transgene in intestinal epithelial cells accelerated the development of colorectal cancer and depended on the activities of Src family and JAK kinases [4].

Mice with a complete deletion of the ADAM17 gene are not viable [42]. Although, ADAM17 floxed mice are available [46], it was not completely clear in which cell types we wanted to delete the ADAM17 in order to show a decisive role of the protease, since many cells including macrophages can be the source of the sIL-6R in vivo [2]. We therefore made use of ADAM17 hypomorphic ADAM17$^{ex/ex}$ mice, which we had engineered to only express about 5% of ADAM17 protein levels in all cells [47]. ADAM17 hypomorphic ADAM17$^{ex/ex}$ mice were shown to be hypersensitive to DSS-induced colitis due to a failure to induce EGF-R signaling, which was needed for intestinal regeneration. EGF-R activation could be compensated by treatment of the mice with recombinant ligands of the EGF-R, which compensated for the lack of cleavage of these membrane-bound proteins [47]. We therefore applied a colon cancer model to ADAM17$^{ex/ex}$ mice. In APC$^{min/+}$ mice, a heterozygous germ line truncation in the APC gene results in the formation of intestinal tumors after spontaneous loss of heterozygosity of the remaining APC wt allele [143,144]. Strikingly, in the absence of ADAM17 activity, almost no intestinal tumors were detected and the few remaining tumors were only of low-grade dysplasia whereas in the presence of ADAM17, also high-grade dysplasias and invasive carcinomas were detected [144]. Surprisingly, we failed to detect significantly elevated levels of phosphorylated EGF-R on intestine sections of wt and ADAM17$^{ex/ex}$ mice (Figure 3) [144].

Elevated activity of the EGF-R has been associated with an increased risk of colon carcinogenesis [144,145]. Recently, it was reported that in patients, EGF-R was expressed on myeloid cells within intestinal tumors and that in mice, EGF-R on myeloid cells but not on intestinal epithelial cells promoted colitis associated cancer in the AOM/DSS model and tumorigenesis in the APC$^{min/+}$ model and protects from colitis in an independent fashion [141]. Moreover, EGF-R activation in myeloid cells led to strongly increased synthesis and secretion of IL-6 [141].

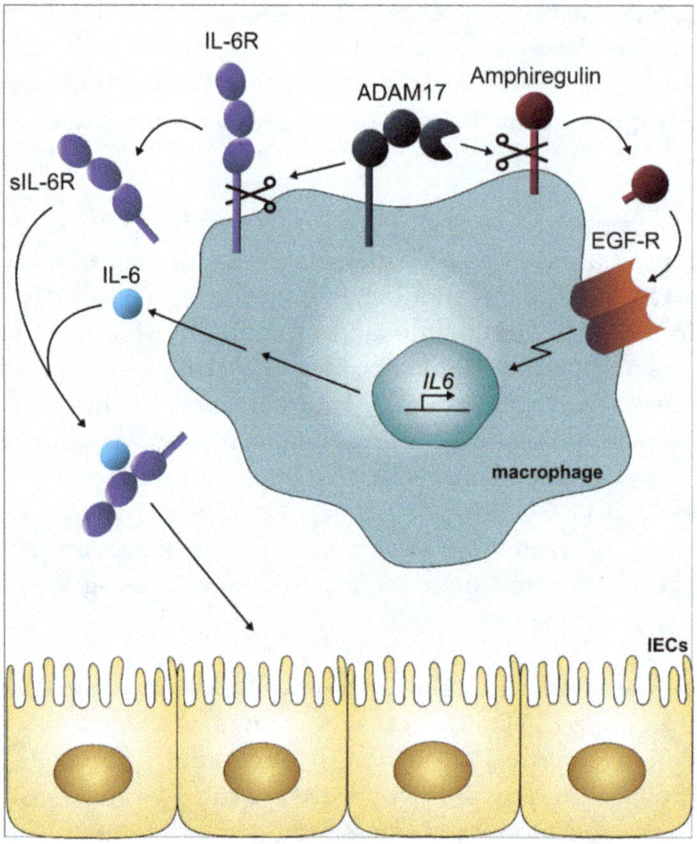

Figure 3. Involvement of ADAM17 in the formation of colon cancer. Under inflammatory conditions, ADAM17 cleaves the membrane-bound EGF-R ligand amphiregulin, leading to the stimulation of the EGF-R on macrophages. This EGF-R stimulation on macrophages leads to increased IL-6 synthesis via transcriptional stimulation. Moreover, activation of ADAM17 under inflammatory conditions leads to cleavage of the membrane-bound IL-6R on macrophages to generate soluble IL-6R (sIL-6R). IL-6 in complex with sIL-6R leads to stimulation of intestinal epithelial cells (IECs) via IL-6 trans-signaling resulting in colon cancer formation [144].

ADAM17 on myeloid cells can lead to the shedding of ligands of the EGF-R such as amphiregulin and to the shedding of the IL-6R [10]. We therefore speculated that IL-6 trans-signaling initiated by the EGF-R mediated IL-6 secretion and the ADAM17-mediated IL-6R shedding might contribute to colon cancer formation in the $APC^{min/+}$ model. We therefore crossed $APC^{min/+}$ mice with either $IL\text{-}6^{-/-}$ mice or mice, which were transgenic for sgp130Fc and in which IL-6 trans-signaling was blocked [19,65]. Indeed, tumorigenesis was strongly reduced to the same extent in $IL\text{-}6^{-/-}$ mice and sgp130Fc transgenic mice indicating that IL-6 trans-signaling strongly contributed to tumor formation in the $APC^{min/+}$ model [144]. Furthermore, in a chemical colon cancer model, in which mice were repeatedly treated with AOM but not with DSS, sgp130Fc transgenic mice were protected from colon cancer [144]. We concluded from these data that in colon cancer, IL-6 trans-signaling apparently acted downstream of the EGF-R and blockade of IL-6 trans-signaling might represent a novel therapeutic window for patients resistant to anti-EGF-R antibodies (Figure 3) [146].

2.2.2. Pancreatic Cancer

In the $Kras^{G12D}$ pancreatic cancer model, strong non-cell-autonomous STAT3 activation in tumor cells was observed [147]. IL-6 mRNA levels were significantly increased in tumor tissue. The cellular source of IL-6 was infiltrating immune cells, mainly F4/80-positive macrophages. When the pancreatic $Kras^{G12D}$ mice were crossed with $IL\text{-}6^{-/-}$ mice or sgp130Fc transgenic mice. $IL\text{-}6^{-/-}$ mice had fewer and predominantly low grade pancreatic intraepithelial neoplasias. Interestingly, blocking IL-6 trans-signaling had a similar effect as deletion of the IL-6 gene since sgp130Fc transgenic mice also showed strongly reduced tumor numbers. This decrease in tumor development was paralleled by a marked reduction of STAT3 phosphorylation [147]. It was speculated that the concept of non-cell-autonomous STAT3 activation of tumor cells brought about by IL-6 trans-signaling was a general phenomenon, which might also be applied to other neoplasias and cancer diseases [147].

2.2.3. Liver Cancer

During liver regeneration, quiescent hepatocytes regain their ability to enter the cell cycle. Importantly, IL-6 [148] and in particular IL-6 trans-signaling has been found to be required for liver regeneration [149]. Accordingly, in IL-6/sIL-6R double transgenic mice, permanent hepatocyte proliferation and formation of adenomas was observed, indicating a possible role of IL-6 trans-signaling for hepatocellular neoplasia [150,151]. Treatment of mice with diethylnitrosamine is used as one of the standard models for liver cancer [152]. In this model, it has been recognized that IL-6 deficient mice develop substantially less tumors as compared to wt mice [153]. When sgp130Fc transgenic mice were treated with diethylnitrosamine, it turned out that myeloid cell derived sIL-6R increased upon treatment and liver tumor development the animals was largely blocked [154]. We concluded from these experiments that IL-6 trans-signaling but not IL-6 classic signaling was involved in the development of hepatocellular carcinoma, at least in the diethylnitrosamine model [154].

2.2.4. Lung Cancer

As mentioned above, gp130 signal transduction is mediated by the SHP2–MAP kinase–PI3 kinase axis. In addition, STAT1 and STAT3 become recruited to the cytoplasmic tail of gp130, are phosphorylated by JAK1, and dimerize and travel to the nucleus to act as transcription factors [3]. Mice, which carry a Y757F mutation in the cytoplasmic tail of gp130 are unable to initiate the SHP2–MAP kinase–PI3 kinase axis because Y757 of gp130 is the docking site of SHP2. These mice can still activate the STAT1/STAT3 pathway [86]. Furthermore, these mice do not show negative regulation by SOCS3 since also this protein requires phosphorylated Y757 for its negative feedback activity [86]. These so-called gp130$^{F/F}$ mice therefore show increased STAT1/STAT3 but no SHP2–MAP kinase–PI3 kinase signaling [86].

The gp130$^{F/F}$ mouse model has been widely used to explore a range of gp130 mediated disease states. The more pronounced gp130/STAT1/STAT3 response seen in these mice has been used to analyze novel therapeutic strategies for inflammatory diseases. Gp130$^{F/F}$ mice are more sensitive than wt mice towards endotoxin. It was found that genetic ablation of IL-6, antibody-mediated inhibition of the IL-6R or blockade of IL-6 trans-signaling by the sgp130Fc protein completely protected gp130$^{F/F}$ mice from endotoxin hypersensitivity [108]. Gp130$^{F/F}$ mice spontaneously develop lung emphysema, which could be prevented by blocking IL-6 trans-signaling [124]. When floxed Kras^{G12D} mice were treated via intranasal inhalation with adenovirus, which encoded cre recombinase 6 weeks prior to analysis, massive lung cancer development was observed, which was much more pronounced in gp130$^{F/F}$ mice as compared to wt mice [155]. Ablation of IL-6 or STAT3 suppressed the extent of lung cancer in this model [155]. Furthermore, we could demonstrate that specific inhibition of IL-6 trans-signaling by the sgp130Fc protein significantly ameliorated lung cancer pathogenesis [155].

Since IL-6 trans-signaling depends on the proteolysis of the membrane-bound IL-6R by the metalloprotease ADAM17, we asked whether in the absence of ADAM17 activity, lung tumor formation in the Kras^{G12D} mouse model would be blocked. When ADAM17$^{ex/ex}$ mice were crossed with Kras^{G12D} mice, tumor formation in the lung was largely inhibited [156]. Interestingly, the cytoplasmic portion of ADAM17 was phosphorylated in Kras^{G12D} mice but not in wt mice [156]. Phosphorylation of the cytoplasmic portion of ADAM17 has been shown to lead to activation of the enzyme [157]. Interestingly, in Kras^{G12D} mice, the levels of sIL-6R were significantly elevated, whereas in compound ADAM17$^{ex/ex}$: Kras^{G12D} mice, sIL-6R levels were comparable to wt mice. No changes in soluble TNFα levels were observed [156]. Moreover, in a xenograft model with ADAM17-deleted A549 cells, tumor formation was abrogated as compared to unedited A549 cells [156]. Along the same line, pharmacologic inhibition of ADAM17 activity also led to decreased tumor formation in Kras^{G12D} mice together with decreased sIL-6R levels [156]. Moreover, in a nicotine-derived nitrosamine ketone model of tobacco-related lung cancer, genetic or pharmacologic blockade of ADAM17 led to a significant reduction of lung lesions and concomitant reduced sIL-6R levels [158]. Together, these data indicated that ADAM17 via IL-6 trans-signaling was a prerequisite of lung tumor formation in these animal models.

3. Conclusions and Outlook

ADAM17 activation orchestrates three major signal transduction pathways, namely IL-6 trans-signaling, stimulation of the TNFα signaling pathway via TNF-R_I and the EGF-R pathway via cleavage of EGF-R ligands such as amphiregulin, TGFα, or Hb-EGF. Apparently, in many inflammatory diseases as well as in colon cancer and lung cancer, the IL-6 trans-signaling pathway plays a dominant role as compared to the TNFα signaling pathway (Table 1).

Table 1. Efficacy of IL-6 trans-signaling blockade by sgp130Fc in preclinical models of inflammation and inflammation associated cancer.

Disease Model	Outcome of the Study
Intestinal inflammation [118,138]	Suppression of colitis activity
Acute inflammation [54,64,65]	Blockade of inflammatory processes
Atherosclerosis [159]	Regression of advanced atherosclerosis
Rheumatoid arthritis [79,98,99]	Improvement of established arthritis
Sepsis [108,109]	Up to 100% survival in different sepsis models
Pancreatitis-lung failure [160]	100% survival of severe acute pancreatitis
Lung emphysema [124]	Improvement by blockade of alveolar cell apoptosis
Abdominal aortic aneurism [30]	Improved survival in two animal models
Colon cancer [110,136–138,144]	Blockade of tumor formation
Pancreatic cancer [147]	Inhibition of pancreatic neoplasia progression
Liver cancer [154]	Protection from tumor formation
Lung cancer [156,158]	Amelioration of lung cancer pathogenesis

The dependence of IL-6 trans-signaling via the generation of IL-6 and sIL-6R by the EGF-R on macrophages demonstrates the existence of a possible novel therapeutic window for the treatment of colon cancer and lung cancer, which might be important in view of the fact that EGF-R antibodies including cetuximab or pantuximab are only useful in patients in whom there are no activating KRAS mutations [161,162]. Even in such patients without KRAS mutations, who show an initial response, almost invariably resistance against EGF-R blockade is seen [163]. In all of these cases, blockade of the IL-6 trans-signaling pathway might offer an additional and alternative treatment option. This treatment option, however, will need to be verified in future human studies.

Author Contributions: N.S. and S.R.-J. wrote and edited the review article.

Abbreviations

ADAM	a disintegrin and metalloprotease
AOM	azoxymethane
APC	adenomatous polyposis coli protein
COPD	chronic obstructive pulmonary disease
DSS	dextransulfate sodium
EAE	experimental autoimmune encephalomyelitis

EGF	epidermal growth factor
FDA	US food and drug administration
FoxP3	forkhead box protein 3
FRMD	FERM domain containing protein, identical to iTAP
Gp130	glycoprotein 130 kDa
IECs	intestinal epithelial cells
IFN	interferon
IL-6	Interleukin-6
IL-6R	Interleukin-6 receptor
iRhom	inactive rhomboid protease
iTAP	iRhom Tail-Associated Protein identical to FRMD8
JAK	Janus kinase
JNK	c-Jun N-terminal kinase
Kras	oncogene first identified in Kirsten RAt Sarcoma virus
MAP	mitogen-activated protein
mTOR	mechanistic target of rapamycin
NFκB	nuclear factor kappa-light-chain-enhancer
Notch	cell signaling receptor present in most animals
PTPN	tyrosine phosphatase
RANK	Receptor Activator of NFκB
RANKL	ligand of RANK
ROSA26	reverse oriented splice acceptor, Clone 26
SHP2	protein-tyrosine phosphatase shp2
SOCS	suppressor of cytokine signaling
Src	proto-oncogene tyrosine-protein kinase
STAT	signal transducer and activator of transcription
TNF	tumor necrosis factor
WHO	world health organization
YAP	proto-oncogene yes associated protein.

References

1. Jones, S.A.; Scheller, J.; Rose-John, S. Therapeutic strategies for the clinical blockade of IL-6/gp130 signaling. *J. Clin. Invest.* **2011**, *121*, 3375–3383. [CrossRef]
2. Rose-John, S. IL-6 Trans-Signaling via the Soluble IL-6 Receptor: Importance for the Pro-Inflammatory Activities of IL-6. *Int. J. Biol. Sci.* **2012**, *8*, 1237–1247. [CrossRef] [PubMed]
3. Schaper, F.; Rose-John, S. Interleukin-6: Biology, signaling and strategies of blockade. *Cytokine Growth Factor Rev.* **2015**, *26*, 475–487. [CrossRef] [PubMed]
4. Taniguchi, K.; Moroishi, T.; De Jong, P.R.; Krawczyk, M.; Grebbin, B.M.; Luo, H.; Xu, R.H.; Golob-Schwarzl, N.; Schweiger, C.; Wang, K.; et al. YAP–IL-6ST autoregulatory loop activated on APC loss controls colonic tumorigenesis. *Proc. Natl. Acad. Sci. USA* **2017**, *114*, 1643–1648. [CrossRef] [PubMed]
5. Taniguchi, K.; Wu, L.W.; Grivennikov, S.I.; De Jong, P.R.; Lian, I.; Yu, F.X.; Wang, K.; Ho, S.B.; Boland, B.S.; Chang, J.T.; et al. A gp130–Src–YAP module links inflammation to epithelial regeneration. *Nature* **2015**, *519*, 57–62. [CrossRef] [PubMed]
6. Stuhlmann-Laeisz, C.; Lang, S.; Chalaris, A.; Krzysztof, P.; Enge, S.; Eichler, J.; Klingmüller, U.; Samuel, M.; Ernst, M.; Rose-John, S.; et al. Forced Dimerization of gp130 Leads to Constitutive STAT3 Activation, Cytokine-independent Growth, and Blockade of Differentiation of Embryonic Stem Cells. *Mol. Biol. Cell* **2006**, *17*, 2986–2995. [CrossRef] [PubMed]
7. Rose-John, S. Interleukin-6 family cytokines. *Cold Spring Harb. Perspect. Biol.* **2018**, *10*. [CrossRef] [PubMed]
8. Mülberg, J.; Schooltink, H.; Stoyan, T.; Günther, M.; Graeve, L.; Buse, G.; Mackiewicz, A.; Heinrich, P.C.; Rose-John, S. The soluble interleukin-6 receptor is generated by shedding. *Eur. J. Immunol.* **1993**, *23*, 473–480. [CrossRef]
9. Yan, I.; Schwarz, J.; Lücke, K.; Schumacher, N.; Schumacher, V.; Schmidt, S.; Rabe, B.; Saftig, P.; Donners, M.; Rose-John, S.; et al. Adam17 controls IL-6 signaling by cleavage of the murine IL-6Rα from the cell surface of leukocytes during inflammatory responses. *J. Leukoc. Biol.* **2016**, *99*, 749–760. [CrossRef]

10. Schumacher, N.; Meyer, D.; Mauermann, A.; Von Der Heyde, J.; Wolf, J.; Schwarz, J.; Knittler, K.; Murphy, G.; Michalek, M.; Garbers, C.; et al. Shedding of Endogenous Interleukin-6 Receptor (IL-6R) Is Governed by A Disintegrin and Metalloproteinase (ADAM) Proteases while a Full-length IL-6R Isoform Localizes to Circulating Microvesicles. *J. Biol. Chem.* **2015**, *290*, 26059–26071. [CrossRef]
11. Rose-John, S.; Heinrich, P.C. Soluble receptors for cytokines and growth factors: Generation and biological function. *Biochem. J.* **1994**, *300*, 281–290. [CrossRef] [PubMed]
12. Scheller, J.; Chalaris, A.; Schmidt-Arras, D.; Rose-John, S. The pro-and anti-inflammatory properties of the cytokine interleukin-6. *Biochim. Biophys. Acta* **2011**, *1813*, 878–888. [CrossRef] [PubMed]
13. Arnold, P.; Boll, I.; Rothaug, M.; Schumacher, N.; Schmidt, F.; Wichert, R.; Schneppenheim, J.; Lokau, J.; Pickhinke, U.; Koudelka, T.; et al. Meprin Metalloproteases Generate Biologically Active Soluble Interleukin-6 Receptor to Induce Trans-Signaling. *Sci. Rep.* **2017**, *7*, 44053. [CrossRef] [PubMed]
14. Garbers, C.; Jänner, N.; Chalaris, A.; Moss, M.L.; Floss, D.M.; Meyer, D.; Koch-Nolte, F.; Rose-John, S.; Scheller, J. Species Specificity of ADAM10 and ADAM17 Proteins in Interleukin-6 (IL-6) Trans-signaling and Novel Role of ADAM10 in Inducible IL-6 Receptor Shedding. *J. Biol. Chem.* **2011**, *286*, 14804–14811. [CrossRef]
15. Riethmueller, S.; Ehlers, J.C.; Lokau, J.; Düsterhöft, S.; Knittler, K.; Dombrowsky, G.; Grötzinger, J.; Rabe, B.; Rose-John, S.; Garbers, C. Cleavage Site Localization Differentially Controls Interleukin-6 Receptor Proteolysis by ADAM10 and ADAM17. *Sci. Rep.* **2016**, *6*, 25550. [CrossRef]
16. Riethmueller, S.; Somasundaram, P.; Ehlers, J.C.; Hung, C.W.; Flynn, C.M.; Lokau, J.; Agthe, M.; Düsterhöft, S.; Zhu, Y.; Grötzinger, J.; et al. Proteolytic origin of the soluble human IL-6R in vivo and a decisive role of n-glycosylation. *PLoS Biol.* **2017**, *15*, e2000080. [CrossRef]
17. Peters, M.; Blinn, G.; Solem, F.; Fischer, M.; Zum Büschenfelde, K.H.M.; Rose-John, S. In vivo and in vitro activities of the gp130-stimulating designer cytokine Hyper-IL-6. *J. Immunol.* **1998**, *161*, 3575–3581.
18. Schmidt-Arras, D.; Rose-John, S. IL-6 pathway in the liver: From physiopathology to therapy. *J. Hepatol.* **2016**, *64*, 1403–1415. [CrossRef]
19. Jostock, T.; Müllberg, J.; Özbek, S.; Atreya, R.; Blinn, G.; Voltz, N.; Fischer, M.; Neurath, M.F.; Rose-John, S. Soluble gp130 is the natural inhibitor of soluble interleukin-6 receptor transsignaling responses. *Eur. J. Biochem.* **2001**, *268*, 160–167. [CrossRef]
20. Garbers, C.; Heink, S.; Korn, T.; Rose-John, S. Interleukin-6: Designing specific therapeutics for a complex cytokine. *Nat. Rev. Drug Discov.* **2018**, *17*, 395–412. [CrossRef]
21. Waage, A. The complex pattern of cytokines in serum from patients with meningococcal septic shock. Association between interleukin 6, interleukin 1, and fatal outcome. *J. Exp. Med.* **1989**, *169*, 333–338. [CrossRef] [PubMed]
22. Wolf, J.; Waetzig, G.H.; Chalaris, A.; Reinheimer, T.M.; Wege, H.; Rose-John, S.; Garbers, C. Different Soluble Forms of the Interleukin-6 Family Signal Transducer gp130 Fine-tune the Blockade of Interleukin-6 Trans-signaling. *J. Biol. Chem.* **2016**, *291*, 16186–16196. [CrossRef] [PubMed]
23. Scheller, J.; Rose-John, S. The interleukin 6 pathway and atherosclerosis. *Lancet* **2012**, *380*, 338. [CrossRef]
24. Garbers, C.; Monhasery, N.; Aparicio-Siegmund, S.; Lokau, J.; Baran, P.; Nowell, M.A.; Jones, S.A.; Rose-John, S.; Scheller, J. The interleukin-6 receptor Asp358Ala single nucleotide polymorphism rs2228145 confers increased proteolytic conversion rates by ADAM proteases. *Biochim. Biophys. Acta* **2014**, *1842*, 1485–1494. [CrossRef] [PubMed]
25. Aparicio-Siegmund, S.; Garbers, Y.; Flynn, C.M.; Waetzig, G.H.; Gouni-Berthold, I.; Krone, W.; Berthold, H.K.; Laudes, M.; Rose-John, S.; Garbers, C. The IL-6-neutralizing sIL-6R-sgp130 buffer system is disturbed in patients with type 2 diabetes. *Am. J. Physiol. Endocrinol. Metab.* **2019**, *317*, 411–420. [CrossRef] [PubMed]
26. Ferreira, R.C.; Freitag, D.F.; Cutler, A.J.; Howson, J.M.M.; Rainbow, D.B.; Smyth, D.J.; Kaptoge, S.; Clarke, P.; Boreham, C.; Coulson, R.M.; et al. Functional IL6R 358Ala Allele Impairs Classical IL-6 Receptor Signaling and Influences Risk of Diverse Inflammatory Diseases. *PLoS Genet.* **2013**, *9*, e1003444. [CrossRef]
27. IL6R Genetics Consortium Emerging Risk Factors Collaboration; Sarwar, N.; Butterworth, A.S.; Freitag, D.F.; Gregson, J.; Willeit, P.; Gorman, D.N.; Gao, P.; Saleheen, D.; Rendon, A.; et al. Interleukin-6 receptor pathways in coronary heart disease: A collaborative meta-analysis of 82 studies. *Lancet* **2012**, *379*, 1205–1213. [PubMed]
28. Interleukin-6 Receptor Mendelian Randomisation Analysis (IL6R MR) Consortium; Sarwar, N.;

Butterworth, A.S.; Freitag, D.F.; Gregson, J.; Willeit, P.; Gorman, D.N.; Gao, P.; Saleheen, D.; Rendon, A.; et al. The interleukin-6 receptor as a target for prevention of coronary heart disease: A mendelian randomisation analysis. *Lancet* **2012**, *379*, 1214–1224.

29. Parisinos, C.A.; Serghiou, S.; Katsoulis, M.; George, M.J.; Patel, R.S.; Hemingway, H.; Hingorani, A.D. Variation in Interleukin 6 Receptor Gene Associates with Risk of Crohn's Disease and Ulcerative Colitis. *Gastroenterology* **2018**, *155*, 303–306. [CrossRef]
30. Paige, E.; Clement, M.; Lareyre, F.; Sweeting, M.; Raffort, J.; Grenier, C.; Finigan, A.; Harrison, J.; Peters, J.E.; Sun, B.B.; et al. Interleukin-6 receptor signaling and abdominal aortic aneurysm growth rates. *Circ. Genom. Precis. Med.* **2019**, *12*, e002413. [CrossRef]
31. Kopf, M.; Baumann, H.; Freer, G.; Freudenberg, M.; Lamers, M.; Kishimoto, T.; Zinkernagel, R.; Bluethmann, H.; Köhler, G. Impaired immune and acute-phase responses in interleukin-6-deficient mice. *Nature* **1994**, *368*, 339–342. [CrossRef] [PubMed]
32. Poli, V.; Balena, R.; Fattori, E.; Markatos, A.; Yamamoto, M.; Tanaka, H.; Ciliberto, G.; Rodan, G.; Costantini, F. Interleukin-6 deficient mice are protected from bone loss caused by estrogen depletion. *EMBO J.* **1994**, *13*, 1189–1196. [CrossRef] [PubMed]
33. Fattori, E.; Cappelletti, M.; Costa, P.; Sellitto, C.; Cantoni, L.; Carelli, M.; Faggioni, R.; Fantuzzi, G.; Ghezzi, P.; Poli, V. Defective inflammatory response in interleukin 6-deficient mice. *J. Exp. Med.* **1994**, *180*, 1243–1250. [CrossRef] [PubMed]
34. Suematsu, S.; Matsuda, T.; Aozasa, K.; Akira, S.; Nakano, N.; Ohno, S.; Miyazaki, J.; Yamamura, K.; Hirano, T.; Kishimoto, T. IgG1 plasmacytosis in interleukin 6 transgenic mice. *Proc. Natl. Acad. Sci. USA* **1989**, *86*, 7547–7551. [CrossRef] [PubMed]
35. Suematsu, S.; Matsusaka, T.; Matsuda, T.; Ohno, S.; Miyazaki, J.; Yamamura, K.; Hirano, T.; Kishimoto, T. Generation of plasmacytomas with the chromosomal translocation t (12;15) in interleukin 6 transgenic mice. *Proc. Natl. Acad. Sci. USA* **1992**, *89*, 232–235. [CrossRef]
36. Peters, M.; Jacobs, S.; Ehlers, M.; Vollmer, P.; Müllberg, J.; Wolf, E.; Brem, G.; Meyer zum Büschenfelde, K.H.; Rose-John, S. The function of the soluble interleukin 6 (IL-6) receptor in vivo: Sensitization of human soluble IL-6 receptor transgenic mice towards IL-6 and prolongation of the plasma half-life of IL-6. *J. Exp. Med.* **1996**, *183*, 1399–1406. [CrossRef]
37. Peters, M.; Schirmacher, P.; Goldschmitt, J.; Odenthal, M.; Peschel, C.; Fattori, E.; Ciliberto, G.; Dienes, H.P.; Meyer zum Büschenfelde, K.H.; Rose-John, S. Extramedullary Expansion of Hematopoietic Progenitor Cells in Interleukin (IL)-6–sIL-6R Double Transgenic Mice. *J. Exp. Med.* **1997**, *185*, 755–766. [CrossRef]
38. Herrman, J.M.; Patel, N.; Timans, J.C.; Kastelein, R.A. Functional Replacement of Cytokine Receptor Extracellular Domains by Leucine Zippers. *J. Biol. Chem.* **1996**, *271*, 30386–30391.
39. Scherger, A.K.; Al-Maarri, M.; Maurer, H.C.; Schick, M.; Maurer, S.; Ollinger, R.; Gonzalez-Menendez, I.; Martella, M.; Thaler, M.; Pechloff, K.; et al. Activated gp130 signaling selectively targets b cell differentiation to induce mature lymphoma and plasmacytoma. *JCI Insight* **2019**, *4*, e128435. [CrossRef]
40. Black, R.A.; Rauch, C.T.; Kozlosky, C.J.; Peschon, J.J.; Slack, J.L.; Wolfson, M.F.; Castner, B.J.; Stocking, K.L.; Reddy, P.; Srinivasan, S.; et al. A metalloproteinase disintegrin that releases tumour-necrosis factor-alpha from cells. *Nature* **1997**, *385*, 729–733. [CrossRef]
41. Moss, M.L.; Jin, S.L.; Milla, M.E.; Bickett, D.M.; Burkhart, W.; Carter, H.L.; Chen, W.J.; Clay, W.C.; Didsbury, J.R.; Hassler, D.; et al. Cloning of a disintegrin metalloproteinase that processes precursor tumour-necrosis factor-alpha. *Nature* **1997**, *385*, 733–736. [CrossRef] [PubMed]
42. Peschon, J.J. An Essential Role for Ectodomain Shedding in Mammalian Development. *Science* **1998**, *282*, 1281–1284. [CrossRef] [PubMed]
43. Matthews, V.; Schuster, B.; Schütze, S.; Bussmeyer, I.; Ludwig, A.; Hundhausen, C.; Sadowski, T.; Saftig, P.; Hartmann, D.; Kallen, K.J.; et al. Cellular Cholesterol Depletion Triggers Shedding of the Human Interleukin-6 Receptor by ADAM10 and ADAM17 (TACE). *J. Biol. Chem.* **2003**, *278*, 38829–38839. [CrossRef] [PubMed]
44. Scheller, J.; Chalaris, A.; Garbers, C.; Rose-John, S. ADAM17: A molecular switch to control inflammation and tissue regeneration. *Trends Immunol.* **2011**, *32*, 380–387. [CrossRef] [PubMed]
45. Zunke, F.; Rose-John, S. The shedding protease adam17: Physiology and pathophysiology. *Biochim. Biophys. Acta* **2017**, *1864*, 2059–2070. [CrossRef] [PubMed]

46. Horiuchi, K.; Kimura, T.; Miyamoto, T.; Takaishi, H.; Okada, Y.; Toyama, Y.; Blobel, C.P. Cutting Edge: TNF-α-Converting Enzyme (TACE/ADAM17) Inactivation in Mouse Myeloid Cells Prevents Lethality from Endotoxin Shock. *J. Immunol.* **2007**, *179*, 2686–2689. [CrossRef] [PubMed]
47. Chalaris, A.; Adam, N.; Sina, C.; Rosenstiel, P.; Lehmann-Koch, J.; Schirmacher, P.; Hartmann, D.; Cichy, J.; Gavrilova, O.; Schreiber, S.; et al. Critical role of the disintegrin metalloprotease ADAM17 for intestinal inflammation and regeneration in mice. *J. Exp. Med.* **2010**, *207*, 1617–1624. [CrossRef]
48. Dulloo, I.; Muliyil, S.; Freeman, M. The molecular, cellular and pathophysiological roles of iRhom pseudoproteases. *Open Biol.* **2019**, *9*, 190003. [CrossRef]
49. Adrain, C.; Freeman, M. New lives for old: Evolution of pseudoenzyme function illustrated by iRhoms. *Nat. Rev. Mol. Cell Biol.* **2012**, *13*, 489–498. [CrossRef]
50. McIlwain, D.R.; Lang, P.A.; Maretzky, T.; Hamada, K.; Ohishi, K.; Maney, S.K.; Berger, T.; Murthy, A.; Duncan, G.; Xu, H.C.; et al. iRhom2 regulation of TACE controls TNF-mediated protection against Listeria and responses to LPS. *Science* **2012**, *335*, 229–232. [CrossRef]
51. Künzel, U.; Grieve, A.G.; Meng, Y.; Sieber, B.; Cowley, S.A.; Freeman, M. FRMD8 promotes inflammatory and growth factor signalling by stabilising the iRhom/ADAM17 sheddase complex. *Elife* **2018**, *7*, e35012. [CrossRef] [PubMed]
52. Oikonomidi, I.; Burbridge, E.; Cavadas, M.; Sullivan, G.; Collis, B.; Naegele, H.; Clancy, D.; Brezinova, J.; Hu, T.; Bileck, A.; et al. Itap, a novel irhom interactor, controls tnf secretion by policing the stability of irhom/tace. *Elife* **2018**, *7*, e35032. [CrossRef] [PubMed]
53. Sommer, A.; Kordowski, F.; Büch, J.; Maretzky, T.; Evers, A.; Andrä, J.; Düsterhöft, S.; Michalek, M.; Lorenzen, I.; Somasundaram, P.; et al. Phosphatidylserine exposure is required for ADAM17 sheddase function. *Nat. Commun.* **2016**, *7*, 11523. [CrossRef] [PubMed]
54. Chalaris, A.; Rabe, B.; Paliga, K.; Lange, H.; Laskay, T.; Fielding, C.A.; Jones, S.A.; Rose-John, S.; Scheller, J. Apoptosis is a natural stimulus of IL6R shedding and contributes to the proinflammatory trans-signaling function of neutrophils. *Blood* **2007**, *110*, 1748–1755. [CrossRef]
55. Hunter, C.A.; Jones, S.A. IL-6 as a keystone cytokine in health and disease. *Nat. Immunol.* **2015**, *16*, 448–457. [CrossRef]
56. Samoilova, E.B.; Horton, J.L.; Hilliard, B.; Liu, T.S.; Chen, Y. IL-6-deficient mice are resistant to experimental autoimmune encephalomyelitis: Roles of IL-6 in the activation and differentiation of autoreactive T cells. *J. Immunol.* **1998**, *161*, 6480–6486.
57. Okuda, Y.; Sakoda, S.; Bernard, C.C.; Fujimura, H.; Saeki, Y.; Kishimoto, T.; Yanagihara, T. IL-6-deficient mice are resistant to the induction of experimental autoimmune encephalomyelitis provoked by myelin oligodendrocyte glycoprotein. *Int. Immunol.* **1998**, *10*, 703–708. [CrossRef]
58. Eugster, H.P.; Frei, K.; Kopf, M.; Lassmann, H.; Fontana, A.; Eugster, H. IL-6-deficient mice resist myelin oligodendrocyte glycoprotein-induced autoimmune encephalomyelitis. *Eur. J. Immunol.* **1998**, *28*, 2178–2187. [CrossRef]
59. Ohshima, S.; Saeki, Y.; Mima, T.; Sasai, M.; Nishioka, K.; Nomura, S.; Kopf, M.; Katada, Y.; Tanaka, T.; Suemura, M.; et al. Interleukin 6 plays a key role in the development of antigen-induced arthritis. *Proc. Natl. Acad. Sci. USA* **1998**, *95*, 8222–8226. [CrossRef]
60. Alonzi, T.; Fattori, E.; Lazzaro, D.; Costa, P.; Probert, L.; Kollias, G.; De Benedetti, F.; Poli, V.; Ciliberto, G. Interleukin 6 Is Required for the Development of Collagen-induced Arthritis. *J. Exp. Med.* **1998**, *187*, 461–468. [CrossRef]
61. Ladel, C.H.; Blum, C.; Dreher, A.; Reifenberg, K.; Kopf, M.; Kaufmann, S.H. Lethal tuberculosis in interleukin-6-deficient mutant mice. *Infect. Immun.* **1997**, *65*, 4843–4849. [PubMed]
62. McFarland-Mancini, M.M.; Funk, H.M.; Paluch, A.M.; Zhou, M.; Giridhar, P.V.; Mercer, C.A.; Kozma, S.C.; Drew, A.F. Differences in Wound Healing in Mice with Deficiency of IL-6 versus IL-6 Receptor. *J. Immunol.* **2010**, *184*, 7219–7228. [CrossRef] [PubMed]
63. Hoge, J.; Yan, I.; Jänner, N.; Schumacher, V.; Chalaris, A.; Steinmetz, O.M.; Engel, D.R.; Scheller, J.; Rose-John, S.; Mittrücker, H.W. IL-6 controls the innate immune response against listeria monocytogenes via classical IL-6 signaling. *J. Immunol.* **2013**, *190*, 703–711. [CrossRef] [PubMed]
64. Hurst, S.M.; Wilkinson, T.S.; McLoughlin, R.M.; Jones, S.; Horiuchi, S.; Yamamoto, N.; Rose-John, S.; Fuller, G.M.; Topley, N.; Jones, S.A. IL-6 and Its Soluble Receptor Orchestrate a Temporal Switch in the

Pattern of Leukocyte Recruitment Seen during Acute Inflammation. *Immunity* **2001**, *14*, 705–714. [CrossRef]
65. Rabe, B.; Chalaris, A.; May, U.; Waetzig, G.H.; Seegert, D.; Williams, A.S.; Jones, S.A.; Rose-John, S.; Scheller, J. Transgenic blockade of interleukin 6 transsignaling abrogates inflammation. *Blood* **2008**, *111*, 1021–1028. [CrossRef]
66. Kraakman, M.J.; Kammoun, H.L.; Allen, T.L.; Deswaerte, V.; Henstridge, D.C.; Estevez, E.; Matthews, V.B.; Neill, B.; White, D.A.; Murphy, A.J.; et al. Blocking IL-6 trans-Signaling Prevents High-Fat Diet-Induced Adipose Tissue Macrophage Recruitment but Does Not Improve Insulin Resistance. *Cell Metab.* **2015**, *21*, 403–416. [CrossRef]
67. Desgeorges, A.; Gabay, C.; Silacci, P.; Novick, D.; Roux-Lombard, P.; Grau, G.; Dayer, J.M.; Vischer, T.; Guerne, P.A. Concentrations and origins of soluble interleukin 6 receptor-alpha in serum and synovial fluid. *J. Rheumatol.* **1997**, *24*, 1510–1516.
68. Braune, J.; Weyer, U.; Hobusch, C.; Mauer, J.; Brüning, J.C.; Bechmann, I.; Gericke, M. IL-6 Regulates M2 Polarization and Local Proliferation of Adipose Tissue Macrophages in Obesity. *J. Immunol.* **2017**, *198*, 2927–2934. [CrossRef]
69. Mauer, J.; Chaurasia, B.; Goldau, J.; Vogt, M.C.; Ruud, J.; Nguyen, K.D.; Theurich, S.; Hausen, A.C.; Schmitz, J.; Brönneke, H.S.; et al. Signaling by IL-6 promotes alternative activation of macrophages to limit endotoxemia and obesity-associated resistance to insulin. *Nat. Immunol.* **2014**, *15*, 423–430. [CrossRef]
70. Doganci, A.; Eigenbrod, T.; Krug, N.; De Sanctis, G.T.; Hausding, M.; Erpenbeck, V.J.; Haddad, E.B.; Schmitt, E.; Bopp, T.; Kallen, K.J.; et al. The IL-6R alpha chain controls lung $CD4^+$ $CD25^+$ Treg development and function during allergic airway inflammation in vivo. *J. Clin. Invest.* **2005**, *115*, 313–325. [CrossRef]
71. McLoughlin, R.M.; Jenkins, B.J.; Grail, D.; Williams, A.S.; Fielding, C.A.; Parker, C.R.; Ernst, M.; Topley, N.; Jones, S.A. IL-6 trans-signaling via STAT3 directs T cell infiltration in acute inflammation. *Proc. Natl. Acad. Sci. USA* **2005**, *102*, 9589–9594. [CrossRef] [PubMed]
72. Veldhoen, M.; Hocking, R.J.; Atkins, C.J.; Locksley, R.M.; Stockinger, B. Tgfbeta in the context of an inflammatory cytokine milieu supports de novo differentiation of IL-17-producing T cells. *Immunity* **2006**, *24*, 179–189. [CrossRef] [PubMed]
73. Bettelli, E.; Carrier, Y.; Gao, W.; Korn, T.; Strom, T.B.; Oukka, M.; Weiner, H.L.; Kuchroo, V.K. Reciprocal developmental pathways for the generation of pathogenic effector TH17 and regulatory T cells. *Nature* **2006**, *441*, 235–238. [CrossRef] [PubMed]
74. Elliott, M.J.; Maini, R.N.; Feldmann, M.; Kalden, J.R.; Antoni, C.; Smolen, J.S.; Leeb, B.; Breedveld, F.C.; Macfarlane, J.D.; Bijl, H. Randomised double-blind comparison of chimeric monoclonal antibody to tumour necrosis factor alpha (cA2) versus placebo in rheumatoid arthritis. *Lancet* **1994**, *344*, 1105–1110. [CrossRef]
75. Grau, G.E.; Maennel, D.N. TNF inhibition and sepsis—Sounding a cautionary note. *Nat. Med.* **1997**, *3*, 1193–1195. [CrossRef]
76. Feldmann, M. Development of anti-TNF therapy for rheumatoid arthritis. *Nat. Rev. Immunol.* **2002**, *2*, 364–371. [CrossRef]
77. Aggarwal, B.B.; Gupta, S.C.; Kim, J.H. Historical perspectives on tumor necrosis factor and its superfamily: 25 years later, a golden journey. *Blood* **2012**, *119*, 651–665. [CrossRef]
78. Ogata, A.; Hirano, T.; Hishitani, Y.; Tanaka, T. Safety and Efficacy of Tocilizumab for the Treatment of Rheumatoid Arthritis. *Clin. Med. Insights Arthritis Musculoskelet. Disord.* **2012**, *5*. [CrossRef]
79. Nowell, M.A.; Williams, A.S.; Carty, S.A.; Scheller, J.; Hayes, A.J.; Jones, G.W.; Richards, P.J.; Slinn, S.; Ernst, M.; Jenkins, B.J.; et al. Therapeutic targeting of IL-6 trans signaling counteracts STAT3 control of experimental inflammatory arthritis. *J. Immunol.* **2009**, *182*, 613–622. [CrossRef]
80. Ivashkiv, L.B.; Hu, X. The JAK/STAT pathway in rheumatoid arthritis: Pathogenic or protective? *Arthritis Rheum.* **2003**, *48*, 2092–2096. [CrossRef]
81. Walker, J.G.; Smith, M.D. The Jak-STAT pathway in rheumatoid arthritis. *J. Rheumatol.* **2005**, *32*, 1650–1653. [PubMed]
82. Burmester, G.R.; Lin, Y.; Patel, R.; van Adelsberg, J.; Mangan, E.K.; Graham, N.M.; van Hoogstraten, H.; Bauer, D.; Ignacio Vargas, J.; Lee, E.B. Efficacy and safety of sarilumab monotherapy versus adalimumab monotherapy for the treatment of patients with active rheumatoid arthritis (monarch): A randomised, double-blind, parallel-group phase iii trial. *Ann. Rheum. Dis* **2017**, *76*, 840–847. [CrossRef] [PubMed]

83. Gabay, C.; Emery, P.; Van Vollenhoven, R.; Dikranian, A.; Alten, R.; Pavelka, K.; Klearman, M.; Musselman, D.; Agarwal, S.; Green, J.; et al. Tocilizumab monotherapy versus adalimumab monotherapy for treatment of rheumatoid arthritis (ADACTA): A randomised, double-blind, controlled phase 4 trial. *Lancet* **2013**, *381*, 1541–1550. [CrossRef]
84. Sengupta, T.K.; Talbot, E.S.; Scherle, P.A.; Ivashkiv, L.B. Rapid inhibition of interleukin-6 signaling and Stat3 activation mediated by mitogen-activated protein kinases. *Proc. Natl. Acad. Sci. USA* **1998**, *95*, 11107–11112. [CrossRef]
85. Jain, N.; Zhang, T.; Fong, S.L.; Lim, C.P.; Cao, X. Repression of Stat3 activity by activation of mitogen-activated protein kinase (MAPK). *Oncogene* **1998**, *17*, 3157–3167. [CrossRef]
86. Tebbutt, N.C.; Giraud, A.S.; Inglese, M.; Jenkins, B.; Waring, P.; Clay, F.J.; Malki, S.; Alderman, B.M.; Grail, D.; Hollande, F.; et al. Reciprocal regulation of gastrointestinal homeostasis by SHP2 and STAT-mediated trefoil gene activation in gp130 mutant mice. *Nat. Med.* **2002**, *8*, 1089–1097. [CrossRef]
87. Atsumi, T.; Ishihara, K.; Kamimura, D.; Ikushima, H.; Ohtani, T.; Hirota, S.; Kobayashi, H.; Park, S.J.; Saeki, Y.; Kitamura, Y.; et al. A Point Mutation of Tyr-759 in Interleukin 6 Family Cytokine Receptor Subunit gp130 Causes Autoimmune Arthritis. *J. Exp. Med.* **2002**, *196*, 979–990. [CrossRef]
88. Nicholson, S.E.; De Souza, D.; Fabri, L.J.; Corbin, J.; Willson, T.A.; Zhang, J.G.; Silva, A.; Asimakis, M.; Farley, A.; Nash, A.D.; et al. Suppressor of cytokine signaling-3 preferentially binds to the shp-2-binding site on the shared cytokine receptor subunit gp130. *Proc. Natl. Acad. Sci. USA* **2000**, *97*, 6493–6498. [CrossRef]
89. Schmitz, J.; Weissenbach, M.; Haan, S.; Heinrich, P.C.; Schaper, F. SOCS3 Exerts Its Inhibitory Function on Interleukin-6 Signal Transduction through the SHP2 Recruitment Site of gp130. *J. Biol. Chem.* **2000**, *275*, 12848–12856. [CrossRef]
90. Shouda, T.; Yoshida, T.; Hanada, T.; Wakioka, T.; Oishi, M.; Miyoshi, K.; Komiya, S.; Kosai, K.I.; Hanakawa, Y.; Hashimoto, K.; et al. Induction of the cytokine signal regulator SOCS3/CIS3 as a therapeutic strategy for treating inflammatory arthritis. *J. Clin. Invest.* **2001**, *108*, 1781–1788. [CrossRef]
91. Mihara, M.; Moriya, Y.; Kishimoto, T.; Ohsugi, Y. Interleukin-6 (IL-6) induces the proliferation of synovial fibroblastic cells in the presence of soluble IL-6 receptor. *Rheumatology* **1995**, *34*, 321–325. [CrossRef] [PubMed]
92. Krause, A.; Scaletta, N.; Ji, J.D.; Ivashkiv, L.B. Rheumatoid arthritis synoviocyte survival is dependent on Stat3. *J. Immunol.* **2002**, *169*, 6610–6616. [CrossRef] [PubMed]
93. Tamura, T.; Udagawa, N.; Takahashi, N.; Miyaura, C.; Tanaka, S.; Yamada, Y.; Koishihara, Y.; Ohsugi, Y.; Kumaki, K.; Taga, T. Soluble interleukin-6 receptor triggers osteoclast formation by interleukin. *Proc. Natl. Acad. Sci. USA* **1993**, *90*, 11924–11928. [CrossRef] [PubMed]
94. Udagawa, N. Interleukin (IL)-6 induction of osteoclast differentiation depends on IL-6 receptors expressed on osteoblastic cells but not on osteoclast progenitors. *J. Exp. Med.* **1995**, *182*, 1461–1468. [CrossRef] [PubMed]
95. Kotake, S.; Sato, K.; Kim, K.J.; Takahashi, N.; Udagawa, N.; Nakamura, I.; Yamaguchi, A.; Kishimoto, T.; Suda, T.; Kashiwazaki, S. Interleukin-6 and soluble interleukin-6 receptors in the synovial fluids from rheumatoid arthritis patients are responsible for osteoclast-like cell formation. *J. Bone Miner. Res.* **1996**, *11*, 88–95. [CrossRef]
96. Palmqvist, P.; Persson, E.; Conaway, H.H.; Lerner, U.H. IL-6, leukemia inhibitory factor, and oncostatin M stimulate bone resorption and regulate the expression of receptor activator of NF-kappa B ligand, osteoprotegerin, and receptor activator of NF-kappa B in mouse calvariae. *J. Immunol.* **2002**, *169*, 3353–3362. [CrossRef]
97. Feng, W.; Liu, H.; Luo, T.; Liu, D.; Du, J.; Sun, J.; Wang, W.; Han, X.; Yang, K.; Guo, J.; et al. Combination of IL-6 and sIL-6R differentially regulate varying levels of RANKL-induced osteoclastogenesis through NF-kappab, ERK and JNK signaling pathways. *Sci. Rep.* **2017**, *7*, 41411. [CrossRef] [PubMed]
98. Nowell, M.A.; Richards, P.J.; Horiuchi, S.; Yamamoto, N.; Rose-John, S.; Topley, N.; Williams, A.S.; Jones, S.A. Soluble IL-6 receptor governs IL-6 activity in experimental arthritis: Blockade of arthritis severity by soluble glycoprotein130. *J. Immunol.* **2003**, *171*, 3202–3209. [CrossRef]
99. Richards, P.J.; Nowell, M.A.; Horiuchi, S.; McLoughlin, R.M.; Fielding, C.A.; Grau, S.; Yamamoto, N.; Ehrmann, M.; Williams, A.S.; Topley, N.; et al. Functional characterization of a soluble gp130 isoform and its therapeutic capacity in an experimental model of inflammatory arthritis. *Arthritis Rheum.* **2006**, *54*, 1662–1672. [CrossRef]

100. Swanson, C.D.; Akama-Garren, E.H.; Stein, E.A.; Petralia, J.D.; Ruiz, P.J.; Edalati, A.; Lindstrom, T.M.; Robinson, W.H. Inhibition of epidermal growth factor receptor tyrosine kinase ameliorates collagen-induced arthritis. *J. Immunol.* **2012**, *188*, 3513–3521. [CrossRef]
101. Issuree, P.D.A.; Maretzky, T.; McIlwain, D.R.; Monette, S.; Qing, X.; Lang, P.A.; Swendeman, S.L.; Park-Min, K.H.; Binder, N.; Kalliolias, G.D.; et al. iRHOM2 is a critical pathogenic mediator of inflammatory arthritis. *J. Clin. Invest.* **2013**, *123*, 928–932. [CrossRef] [PubMed]
102. McLoughlin, R.M.; Witowski, J.; Robson, R.L.; Wilkinson, T.S.; Hurst, S.M.; Williams, A.S.; Williams, J.D.; Rose-John, S.; Jones, S.A.; Topley, N. Interplay between IFN-gamma and IL-6 signaling governs neutrophil trafficking and apoptosis during acute inflammation. *J. Clin. Invest.* **2003**, *112*, 598–607. [CrossRef] [PubMed]
103. Fielding, C.A.; McLoughlin, R.M.; McLeod, L.; Colmont, C.S.; Najdovska, M.; Grail, D.; Ernst, M.; Jones, S.A.; Topley, N.; Jenkins, B.J. IL-6 regulates neutrophil trafficking during acute inflammation via STAT3. *J. Immunol.* **2008**, *181*, 2189–2195. [CrossRef] [PubMed]
104. Romano, M.; Sironi, M.; Toniatti, C.; Polentarutti, N.; Fruscella, P.; Ghezzi, P.; Faggioni, R.; Luini, W.; Van Hinsbergh, V.; Sozzani, S.; et al. Role of IL-6 and Its Soluble Receptor in Induction of Chemokines and Leukocyte Recruitment. *Immunity* **1997**, *6*, 315–325. [CrossRef]
105. Schumacher, N.; Schmidt, S.; Schwarz, J.; Dohr, D.; Lokau, J.; Scheller, J.; Garbers, C.; Chalaris, A.; Rose-John, S.; Rabe, B. Circulating Soluble IL-6R but Not ADAM17 Activation Drives Mononuclear Cell Migration in Tissue Inflammation. *J. Immunol.* **2016**, *197*, 3705–3715. [CrossRef] [PubMed]
106. Fielding, C.A.; Jones, G.W.; McLoughlin, R.M.; McLeod, L.; Hammond, V.J.; Uceda, J.; Williams, A.S.; Lambie, M.; Foster, T.L.; Liao, C.T.; et al. Interleukin-6 signaling drives fibrosis in unresolved inflammation. *Immunity* **2014**, *40*, 40–50. [CrossRef] [PubMed]
107. Twohig, J.P.; Cardus Figueras, A.; Andrews, R.; Wiede, F.; Cossins, B.C.; Derrac Soria, A.; Lewis, M.J.; Townsend, M.J.; Millrine, D.; Li, J.; et al. Activation of naive $CD4^+$ T cells re-tunes stat1 signaling to deliver unique cytokine responses in memory $CD4^+$ T cells. *Nat. Immunol.* **2019**, *20*, 458–470. [CrossRef] [PubMed]
108. Greenhill, C.J.; Rose-John, S.; Lissilaa, R.; Ferlin, W.; Ernst, M.; Hertzog, P.J.; Mansell, A.; Jenkins, B.J. IL-6 trans-signaling modulates TLR4-dependent inflammatory responses via STAT3. *J. Immunol.* **2011**, *186*, 1199–1208. [CrossRef]
109. Barkhausen, T.; Tschernig, T.; Rosenstiel, P.; van Griensven, M.; Vonberg, R.P.; Dorsch, M.; Mueller-Heine, A.; Chalaris, A.; Scheller, J.; Rose-John, S.; et al. Selective blockade of interleukin-6 trans-signaling improves survival in a murine polymicrobial sepsis model. *Crit. Care Med.* **2011**, *39*, 1407–1413. [CrossRef]
110. Grivennikov, S.; Karin, E.; Terzic, J.; Mucida, D.; Yu, G.Y.; Vallabhapurapu, S.; Scheller, J.; Rose-John, S.; Cheroutre, H.; Eckmann, L.; et al. IL-6 and Stat3 Are Required for Survival of Intestinal Epithelial Cells and Development of Colitis-Associated Cancer. *Cancer Cell* **2009**, *15*, 103–113. [CrossRef]
111. Arndt, P.G.; Strahan, B.; Wang, Y.; Long, C.; Horiuchi, K.; Walcheck, B. Leukocyte ADAM17 Regulates Acute Pulmonary Inflammation. *PLoS ONE* **2011**, *6*, e19938. [CrossRef] [PubMed]
112. Nicolaou, A.; Zhao, Z.; Northoff, B.H.; Sass, K.; Herbst, A.; Kohlmaier, A.; Chalaris, A.; Wolfrum, C.; Weber, C.; Steffens, S.; et al. Adam17 Deficiency Promotes Atherosclerosis by Enhanced TNFR2 Signaling in Mice. *Arterioscler. Thromb. Vasc. Biol.* **2017**, *37*, 247–257. [CrossRef] [PubMed]
113. Mishra, H.K.; Johnson, T.J.; Seelig, D.M.; Walcheck, B. Targeting ADAM17 in leukocytes increases neutrophil recruitment and reduces bacterial spread during polymicrobial sepsis. *J. Leukoc. Biol.* **2016**, *100*, 999–1004. [CrossRef] [PubMed]
114. Mishra, H.K.; Long, C.; Bahaie, N.S.; Walcheck, B. Regulation of cxcr2 expression and function by a disintegrin and metalloprotease-17 (ADAM17). *J. Leukoc. Biol.* **2015**, *97*, 447–454. [CrossRef]
115. Tang, J.; Zarbock, A.; Gomez, I.; Wilson, C.L.; Lefort, C.T.; Stadtmann, A.; Bell, B.; Huang, L.C.; Ley, K.; Raines, E.W. ADAM17-dependent shedding limits early neutrophil influx but does not alter early monocyte recruitment to inflammatory sites. *Blood* **2011**, *118*, 786–794. [CrossRef]
116. Teague, T.K.; Schaefer, B.C.; Hildeman, D.; Bender, J.; Mitchell, T.; Kappler, J.W.; Marrack, P. Activation-Induced Inhibition of Interleukin 6–Mediated T Cell Survival and Signal Transducer and Activator of Transcription 1 Signaling. *J. Exp. Med.* **2000**, *191*, 915–926. [CrossRef]
117. Takeda, K.; Kaisho, T.; Yoshida, N.; Takeda, J.; Kishimoto, T.; Akira, S. Stat3 activation is responsible for IL-6-dependent T cell proliferation through preventing apoptosis: Generation and characterization of T cell-specific Stat3-deficient mice. *J. Immunol.* **1998** *161*, 4652–4660. [CrossRef]

118. Atreya, R.; Mudter, J.; Finotto, S.; Müllberg, J.; Jostock, T.; Wirtz, S.; Schütz, M.; Bartsch, B.; Holtmann, M.; Becker, C.; et al. Blockade of interleukin 6 trans signaling suppresses T-cell resistance against apoptosis in chronic intestinal inflammation: Evidence in Crohn disease and experimental colitis in vivo. *Nat. Med.* **2000**, *6*, 583–588. [CrossRef]

119. Ina, K.; Itoh, J.; Fukushima, K.; Kusugami, K.; Yamaguchi, T.; Kyokane, K.; Imada, A.; Binion, D.G.; Musso, A.; West, G.A.; et al. Resistance of Crohn's disease T cells to multiple apoptotic signals is associated with a Bcl-2/Bax mucosal imbalance. *J. Immunol.* **1999**, *163*, 1081–1090.

120. Mitsuyama, K.; Matsumoto, S.; Rose-John, S.; Suzuki, A.; Hara, T.; Tomiyasu, N.; Handa, K.; Tsuruta, O.; Funabashi, H.; Scheller, J.; et al. STAT3 activation via interleukin 6 trans-signalling contributes to ileitis in SAMP1/Yit mice. *Gut* **2006**, *55*, 1263–1269. [CrossRef]

121. Ito, H.; Takazoe, M.; Fukuda, Y.; Hibi, T.; Kusugami, K.; Andoh, A.; Matsumoto, T.; Yamamura, T.; Azuma, J.; Nishimoto, N.; et al. A pilot randomized trial of a human anti-interleukin-6 receptor monoclonal antibody in active Crohn's disease. *Gastroenterology* **2004**, *126*, 989–996. [CrossRef] [PubMed]

122. Papaioannou, A.I.; Mazioti, A.; Kiropoulos, T.; Tsilioni, I.; Koutsokera, A.; Tanou, K.; Nikoulis, D.J.; Georgoulias, P.; Zakynthinos, E.; Gourgoulianis, K.I.; et al. Systemic and airway inflammation and the presence of emphysema in patients with COPD. *Respir. Med.* **2010**, *104*, 275–282. [CrossRef] [PubMed]

123. Ruwanpura, S.M.; McLeod, L.; Miller, A.; Jones, J.; Bozinovski, S.; Vlahos, R.; Ernst, M.; Armes, J.; Bardin, P.G.; Anderson, G.P.; et al. Interleukin-6 promotes pulmonary emphysema associated with apoptosis in mice. *Am. J. Respir. Cell Mol. Biol.* **2011**, *45*, 720–730. [CrossRef] [PubMed]

124. Ruwanpura, S.M.; McLeod, L.; Dousha, L.F.; Seow, H.J.; Alhayyani, S.; Tate, M.D.; Deswaerte, V.; Brooks, G.D.; Bozinovski, S.; MacDonald, M.; et al. Therapeutic targeting of the IL-6 trans-signaling/mechanistic target of rapamycin complex 1 axis in pulmonary emphysema. *Am. J. Respir. Crit. Care Med.* **2016**, *194*, 1494–1505. [CrossRef]

125. Jevnikar, Z.; Östling, J.; Ax, E.; Calvén, J.; Thörn, K.; Israelsson, E.; Oberg, L.; Singhania, A.; Lau, L.C.; Ward, J.A.; et al. Epithelial IL-6 trans-signaling defines a new asthma phenotype with increased airway inflammation. *J. Allergy Clin. Immunol.* **2019**, *143*, 577–590. [CrossRef]

126. Papiris, S.A.; Tomos, I.P.; Karakatsani, A.; Spathis, A.; Korbila, I.; Analitis, A.; Kolilekas, L.; Kagouridis, K.; Loukides, S.; Karakitsos, P.; et al. High levels of IL-6 and IL-8 characterize early-on idiopathic pulmonary fibrosis acute exacerbations. *Cytokine* **2018**, *102*, 168–172. [CrossRef]

127. Pedroza, M.; Schneider, D.J.; Karmouty-Quintana, H.; Coote, J.; Shaw, S.; Corrigan, R.; Molina, J.G.; Alcorn, J.L.; Galas, D.; Gelinas, R.; et al. Interleukin-6 contributes to inflammation and remodeling in a model of adenosine mediated lung injury. *PLoS ONE* **2011**, *6*, e22667. [CrossRef]

128. Saito, F.; Tasaka, S.; Inoue, K.I.; Miyamoto, K.; Nakano, Y.; Ogawa, Y.; Yamada, W.; Shiraishi, Y.; Hasegawa, N.; Fujishima, S.; et al. Role of Interleukin-6 in Bleomycin-Induced Lung Inflammatory Changes in Mice. *Am. J. Respir. Cell Mol. Biol.* **2008**, *38*, 566–571. [CrossRef]

129. Le, T.T.T.; Karmouty-Quintana, H.; Melicoff, E.; Le, T.T.T.; Weng, T.; Chen, N.Y.; Pedroza, M.; Zhou, Y.; Davies, J.; Philip, K.; et al. Blockade of IL-6 Trans Signaling Attenuates Pulmonary Fibrosis. *J. Immunol.* **2014**, *193*, 3755–3768. [CrossRef]

130. Pedroza, M.; Le, T.T.; Lewis, K.; Karmouty-Quintana, H.; To, S.; George, A.T.; Blackburn, M.R.; Tweardy, D.J.; Agarwal, S.K. Stat-3 contributes to pulmonary fibrosis through epithelial injury and fibroblast-myofibroblast differentiation. *FASEB J.* **2016**, *30*, 129–140. [CrossRef]

131. Moodley, Y.P.; Scaffidi, A.K.; Misso, N.L.; Keerthisingam, C.; McAnulty, R.J.; Laurent, G.J.; Mutsaers, S.E.; Thompson, P.J.; Knight, D.A. Fibroblasts Isolated from Normal Lungs and Those with Idiopathic Pulmonary Fibrosis Differ in Interleukin-6/gp130-Mediated Cell Signaling and Proliferation. *Am. J. Pathol.* **2003**, *163*, 345–354. [CrossRef]

132. Pechkovsky, D.V.; Prele, C.M.; Wong, J.; Hogaboam, C.M.; McAnulty, R.J.; Laurent, G.J.; Zhang, S.S.M.; Selman, M.; Mutsaers, S.E.; Knight, D.A. STAT3-Mediated Signaling Dysregulates Lung Fibroblast-Myofibroblast Activation and Differentiation in UIP/IPF. *Am. J. Pathol.* **2012**, *180*, 1398–1412. [CrossRef] [PubMed]

133. Balkwill, F.; Mantovani, A.; Balkwill, F. Inflammation and cancer: Back to Virchow? *Lancet* **2001**, *357*, 539–545. [CrossRef]
134. Fischer, M.; Goldschmitt, J.; Peschel, C.; Brakenhoff, J.P.G.; Kallen, K.J.; Wollmer, A.; Grötzinger, J.; Rose-John, S. A bioactive designer cytokine for human hematopoietic progenitor cell expansion. *Nat. Biotechnol.* **1997**, *15*, 142–145. [CrossRef] [PubMed]
135. Mitsuyama, K.; Sata, M.; Rose-John, S. Interleukin-6 trans-signaling in inflammatory bowel disease. *Cytokine Growth Factor Rev.* **2006**, *17*, 451–461. [CrossRef] [PubMed]
136. Becker, C.; Fantini, M.; Schramm, C.; Lehr, H.; Wirtz, S.; Burg, J.; Strand, S.; Kiesslich, R.; Huber, S.; Galle, P.; et al. TGF-beta suppresses tumor progression in colon cancer by inhibition of IL-6 trans-signaling. *Immunity* **2004**, *21*, 491–501. [CrossRef] [PubMed]
137. Becker, C.; Fantini, M.C.; Wirtz, S.; Nikolaev, A.; Lehr, H.A.; Galle, P.R.; Rose-John, S.; Neurath, M.F. IL-6 signaling promotes tumor growth in colorectal cancer. *Cell Cycle* **2005**, *4*, 217–220. [CrossRef] [PubMed]
138. Matsumoto, S.; Hara, T.; Mitsuyama, K.; Yamamoto, M.; Tsuruta, O.; Sata, M.; Scheller, J.; Rose-John, S.; Kado, S.; Takada, T. Essential roles of IL-6 trans-signaling in colonic epithelial cells, induced by the IL-6/soluble-IL-6 receptor derived from lamina propria macrophages, on the development of colitis-associated premalignant cancer in a murine model. *J. Immunol.* **2010**, *184*, 1543–1551. [CrossRef]
139. Bollrath, J.; Phesse, T.J.; Von Burstin, V.A.; Putoczki, T.; Bennecke, M.; Bateman, T.; Nebelsiek, T.; Lundgren-May, T.; Canli, O.; Schwitalla, S.; et al. gp130-Mediated Stat3 Activation in Enterocytes Regulates Cell Survival and Cell-Cycle Progression during Colitis-Associated Tumorigenesis. *Cancer Cell* **2009**, *15*, 91–102. [CrossRef]
140. Spehlmann, M.E.; Manthey, C.F.; Dann, S.M.; Hanson, E.; Sandhu, S.S.; Liu, L.Y.; Abdelmalak, F.K.; Diamanti, M.A.; Retzlaff, K.; Scheller, J.; et al. Trp53 deficiency protects against acute intestinal inflammation. *J. Immunol.* **2013**, *191*, 837–847. [CrossRef]
141. Srivatsa, S.; Paul, M.C.; Cardone, C.; Holcmann, M.; Amberg, N.; Pathria, P.; Diamanti, M.A.; Linder, M.; Timelthaler, G.; Dienes, H.P.; et al. EGFR in Tumor-Associated Myeloid Cells Promotes Development of Colorectal Cancer in Mice and Associates with Outcomes of Patients. *Gastroenterology* **2017**, *153*, 178–190. [CrossRef] [PubMed]
142. Rebouissou, S.; Amessou, M.; Couchy, G.; Poussin, K.; Imbeaud, S.; Pilati, C.; Izard, T.; Balabaud, C.; Bioulac-Sage, P.; Zucman-Rossi, J. Frequent in-frame somatic deletions activate gp130 in inflammatory hepatocellular tumours. *Nature* **2009**, *457*, 200–204. [CrossRef] [PubMed]
143. Yamada, Y.; Mori, H. Multistep carcinogenesis of the colon in $Apc^{min/+}$ mouse. *Cancer Sci.* **2007**, *98*, 6–10. [CrossRef] [PubMed]
144. Schmidt, S.; Schumacher, N.; Schwarz, J.; Tangermann, S.; Kenner, L.; Schlederer, M.; Sibilia, M.; Linder, M.; Altendorf-Hofmann, A.; Knösel, T.; et al. ADAM17 is required for EGF-R–induced intestinal tumors via IL-6 trans-signaling. *J. Exp. Med.* **2018**, *215*, 1205–1225. [CrossRef] [PubMed]
145. Sibilia, M.; Kroismayr, R.; Lichtenberger, B.M.; Natarajan, A.; Hecking, M.; Holcmann, M. The epidermal growth factor receptor: From development to tumorigenesis. *Differentiation* **2007**, *75*, 770–787. [CrossRef]
146. Van Emburgh, B.O.; Sartore-Bianchi, A.; Di Nicolantonio, F.; Siena, S.; Bardelli, A. Acquired resistance to EGFR-targeted therapies in colorectal cancer. *Mol. Oncol.* **2014**, *8*, 1084–1094. [CrossRef]
147. Lesina, M.; Kurkowski, M.U.; Ludes, K.; Rose-John, S.; Treiber, M.; Klöppel, G.; Yoshimura, A.; Reindl, W.; Sipos, B.; Akira, S.; et al. Stat3/Socs3 Activation by IL-6 Transsignaling Promotes Progression of Pancreatic Intraepithelial Neoplasia and Development of Pancreatic Cancer. *Cancer Cell* **2011**, *19*, 456–469. [CrossRef]
148. Cressman, D.E.; Greenbaum, L.E.; DeAngelis, R.A.; Ciliberto, G.; Furth, E.E.; Poli, V.; Taub, R. Liver Failure and Defective Hepatocyte Regeneration in Interleukin-6-Deficient Mice. *Science* **1996**, *274*, 1379–1383. [CrossRef]
149. Peters, M.; Blinn, G.; Jostock, T.; Schirmacher, P.; Büschenfelde, K.M.Z.; Galle, P.R.; Rose–John, S. Combined interleukin 6 and soluble interleukin 6 receptor accelerates murine liver regeneration. *Gastroenterology* **2000**, *119*, 1663–1671. [CrossRef]
150. Schirmacher, P.; Peters, M.; Ciliberto, G.; Blessing, M.; Lotz, J.; Meyer zum Büschenfelde, K.H.; Rose-John, S. Hepatocellular Hyperplasia, Plasmacytoma Formation, and Extramedullary Hematopoiesis in Interleukin (IL)-6/Soluble IL-6 Receptor Double-Transgenic Mice. *Am. J. Pathol.* **1998**, *153*, 639–648. [CrossRef]

151. Maione, D.; Di Carlo, E.; Li, W.; Musiani, P.; Modesti, A.; Peters, M.; Rose-John, S.; Della Rocca, C.; Tripodi, M.; Lazzaro, D.; et al. Coexpression of IL-6 and soluble IL-6R causes nodular regenerative hyperplasia and adenomas of the liver. *EMBO J.* **1998**, *17*, 5588–5597. [CrossRef] [PubMed]
152. Maeda, S.; Kamata, H.; Luo, J.L.; Leffert, H.; Karin, M. Ikkbeta couples hepatocyte death to cytokine-driven compensatory proliferation that promotes chemical hepatocarcinogenesis. *Cell* **2005**, *121*, 977–990. [CrossRef] [PubMed]
153. Naugler, W.E.; Sakurai, T.; Kim, S.; Maeda, S.; Kim, K.; Elsharkawy, A.M.; Karin, M. Gender Disparity in Liver Cancer Due to Sex Differences in MyD88-Dependent IL-6 Production. *Science* **2007**, *317*, 121–124. [CrossRef] [PubMed]
154. Bergmann, J.; Muller, M.; Baumann, N.; Reichert, M.; Heneweer, C.; Bolik, J.; Lucke, K.; Gruber, S.; Carambia, A.; Boretius, S.; et al. IL-6 trans-signaling is essential for the development of hepatocellular carcinoma in mice. *Hepatology* **2017**, *65*, 89–103. [CrossRef] [PubMed]
155. Brooks, G.D.; McLeod, L.; Alhayyani, S.; Miller, A.; Russell, P.A.; Ferlin, W.; Rose-John, S.; Ruwanpura, S.; Jenkins, B. IL-6 trans-signaling promotes KRAS-driven lung carcinogenesis. *Cancer Res.* **2016**, *76*, 866–876. [CrossRef]
156. Saad, M.I.; Alhayyani, S.; McLeod, L.; Yu, L.; Alanazi, M.; Deswaerte, V.; Tang, K.; Jarde, T.; Smith, J.A.; Prodanovic, Z.; et al. ADAM17 selectively activates the IL-6 trans-signaling/erk mapk axis in kras-addicted lung cancer. *EMBO Mol. Med.* **2019**, *11*, e9976. [CrossRef]
157. Xu, P.; Derynck, R. Direct activation of tace-mediated ectodomain shedding by p38 map kinase regulates egf receptor-dependent cell proliferation. *Mol. Cell* **2009**, *37*, 551–566. [CrossRef]
158. Saad, M.I.; McLeod, L.; Yu, L.; Ebi, H.; Ruwanpura, S.; Sagi, I.; Rose-John, S.; Jenkins, B.J. The ADAM17 protease promotes tobacco smoke carcinogen-induced lung tumourigenesis. *Carcinogenesis* **2019**. [CrossRef]
159. Schuett, H.; Oestreich, R.; Waetzig, G.H.; Annema, W.; Luchtefeld, M.; Hillmer, A.; Bavendiek, U.; Von Felden, J.; Divchev, D.; Kempf, T.; et al. Transsignaling of Interleukin-6 Crucially Contributes to Atherosclerosis in Mice. *Arterioscler. Thromb. Vasc. Biol.* **2012**, *32*, 281–290. [CrossRef]
160. Zhang, H.; Neuhöfer, P.; Song, L.; Rabe, B.; Lesina, M.; Kurkowski, M.U.; Treiber, M.; Wartmann, T.; Regnér, S.; Thorlacius, H.; et al. IL-6 trans-signaling promotes pancreatitis-associated lung injury and lethality. *J. Clin. Invest.* **2013**, *123*, 1019–1031. [CrossRef]
161. Linardou, H.; Dahabreh, I.J.; Kanaloupiti, D.; Siannis, F.; Bafaloukos, D.; Kosmidis, P.; Papadimitriou, C.A.; Murray, S. Assessment of somatic k-RAS mutations as a mechanism associated with resistance to EGFR-targeted agents: A systematic review and meta-analysis of studies in advanced non-small-cell lung cancer and metastatic colorectal cancer. *Lancet Oncol.* **2008**, *9*, 962–972. [CrossRef]
162. Tobin, N.P.; Foukakis, T.; De Petris, L.; Bergh, J. The importance of molecular markers for diagnosis and selection of targeted treatments in patients with cancer. *J. Intern. Med.* **2015**, *278*, 545–570. [CrossRef] [PubMed]
163. Pietrantonio, F.; Vernieri, C.; Siravegna, G.; Mennitto, A.; Berenato, R.; Perrone, F.; Gloghini, A.; Tamborini, E.; Lonardi, S.; Morano, F.; et al. Heterogeneity of acquired resistance to anti-EGFR monoclonal antibodies in patients with metastatic colorectal cancer. *Clin. Cancer Res.* **2017**, *23*, 2414–2422. [CrossRef] [PubMed]

2

Structural Implications of STAT3 and STAT5 SH2 Domain Mutations

Elvin D. de Araujo [1,2], Anna Orlova [3], Heidi A. Neubauer [3], Dávid Bajusz [4], Hyuk-Soo Seo [5,6], Sirano Dhe-Paganon [5,6], György M. Keserű [4], Richard Moriggl [3] and Patrick T. Gunning [1,2,*]

1 Centre for Medicinal Chemistry, University of Toronto at Mississauga, Mississauga, ON L5L 1C6, Canada; e.dearaujo@mail.utoronto.ca

2 Department of Chemical & Physical Sciences, University of Toronto at Mississauga, Mississauga, ON L5L 1C6, Canada

3 Institute of Animal Breeding and Genetics, University of Veterinary Medicine, A-1210 Vienna, Austria; Anna.Orlova@vetmeduni.ac.at (A.O.); Heidi.Neubauer@vetmeduni.ac.at (H.A.N.); Richard.Moriggl@vetmeduni.ac.at (R.M.)

4 Medicinal Chemistry Research Group, Research Center for Natural Sciences, 1117 Budapest, Hungary; bajusz.david@ttk.mta.hu (D.B.); keseru.gyorgy@ttk.mta.hu (G.M.K.)

5 Department of Cancer Biology, Dana-Farber Cancer Institute, Department of Biological Chemistry & Molecular Pharmacology, Harvard Medical School, Boston, MA 02115, USA; hux@crystal.harvard.edu (H.-S.S.); dhepag@crystal.harvard.edu (S.D.-P.)

6 Department of Biological Chemistry, Department of Biological Chemistry & Molecular Pharmacology, Harvard Medical School, Boston, MA 02115, USA

* Correspondence: patrick.gunning@utoronto.ca

Abstract: Src Homology 2 (SH2) domains arose within metazoan signaling pathways and are involved in protein regulation of multiple pleiotropic cascades. In signal transducer and activator of transcription (STAT) proteins, SH2 domain interactions are critical for molecular activation and nuclear accumulation of phosphorylated STAT dimers to drive transcription. Sequencing analysis of patient samples has revealed the SH2 domain as a hotspot in the mutational landscape of STAT proteins although the functional impact for the vast majority of these mutations remains poorly characterized. Despite several well resolved structures for SH2 domain-containing proteins, structural data regarding the distinctive STAT-type SH2 domain is limited. Here, we review the unique features of STAT-type SH2 domains in the context of all currently reported STAT3 and STAT5 SH2 domain clinical mutations. The genetic volatility of specific regions in the SH2 domain can result in either activating or deactivating mutations at the same site in the domain, underscoring the delicate evolutionary balance of wild type STAT structural motifs in maintaining precise levels of cellular activity. Understanding the molecular and biophysical impact of these disease-associated mutations can uncover convergent mechanisms of action for mutations localized within the STAT SH2 domain to facilitate the development of targeted therapeutic interventions.

Keywords: STAT3; STAT5; SH2 domain; mutations; cancer; autosomal-dominant hyper IgE syndrome; inflammatory hepatocellular adenomas; T-cell large granular lymphocytic leukemia; T-cell prolymphocytic leukemia; growth hormone insensitivity syndrome

---

1. Introduction

Several key cellular pathways converge on the multidomain signal transducer and activator of transcription (STAT) proteins highlighting their importance in the development and progression of oncogenic and malignant diseases. Conventional STAT activation is initiated by cytokine or growth-factor interactions with extracellular receptors, stimulating SH2 domain-mediated recruitment of tyrosine kinases and STAT isoforms to the receptor cytoplasmic domains [1,2]. Nuclear translocation and accumulation of the resulting phosphorylated STAT dimers facilitates transcription of a wide array of gene products involved in proliferation and cellular survival including C-MYC [3], BCL-XL [3], MCL-1 [4], FOXP3 [5], BCL-2 [6], HIF [7], D-type cyclins [8], IGF-1 [9], and self-regulation of STAT3/STAT5 [10]. Normal STAT function is dependent on the SH2 domain which arbitrates homo- or hetero- STAT dimerization as well as multiple protein–protein interactions. As such, structurally altered SH2 domains exhibit considerable effects on STAT activity, leading to either hyperactivated or refractory STAT mutants. These critical roles in governing the transcriptional capacity, coupled with the relatively shallow binding surfaces elsewhere on the protein, resulted in the STAT SH2 domain dominating therapeutic interest for small molecule inhibitor development and intervention [11–15]. However, currently there are no clinical drug candidates directly targeting the STAT protein family. This is partially due to the limited structural data available on the STAT SH2 domains or their mutated disease-associated counterparts, and further compounded by observations that STAT SH2 domains are distinct from those found in other well characterized systems such as Src kinase. Here, we summarize structural features of STAT-type SH2 domains in the context of STAT3/STAT5 disease-associated mutations, and discuss their effects on protein activity, as well as potential new druggable pockets within the STAT SH2 domain.

2. Structure of STAT SH2 Domains

SH2 domains are modular units that arose within multicellular life, approximately 600 million years ago, and are therefore heavily tied to metazoan signal transduction [16]. There are 121 human SH2 domains that are classified into different groups based on their structural or phylogenetic characteristics [16]. Broadly, they have been classified into either STAT- or Src-type SH2 domains based on the presence of either an α-helix (STAT-type) or β-sheet (Src-type) at the C-terminus [17]. Alternatively, phylogenetic analysis has categorized SH2 domain-containing proteins into 38 different sub-families [16]. Functional activity-based screens have also been employed to stratify SH2 domain-containing proteins into four categories based on the identity of the fifth residue in the βD strand, which has been shown to be a critical determinant in phospho-peptide selectivity [18,19]. Despite different methods for classification, all SH2 domains contain conserved structural motifs that are canonical to the core function of phospho-Tyr (pY) peptide binding. These features represent an evolutionary compromise to preserving critical structural motifs while maintaining highly specific peptide recognition capacity.

The structure of an SH2 domain consists of a central anti-parallel β-sheet (with the three β-strands conventionally labeled βB-βD) interposed between two α-helices (αA and αB), often referred to as the αβββα motif [16]. The structure and nomenclature for the motifs of STAT SH2 domains is shown in Figure 1a,b. The β-sheet partitions the SH2 domain into two subpockets, referred to as the pY (phosphate-binding) and pY+3 (specificity) pocket [16]. The pY pocket is formed by the αA helix, the BC loop (region connecting βB-βC strands) and one face of the central β-sheet. The pY+3 pocket is created by the opposite face of the β-sheet as well as residues from the αB helix and CD and BC* loops (regions connecting βC-βD strands and αB-αC helices, respectively). Both the pY and pY+3 pockets are common targets for drug design due to well defined features and conserved residues. Within the pY+3 pocket, there are additional clefts that also have drug targeting potential. This includes the C-terminal region of the pY+3 pocket, also known as the evolutionary active region (EAR) [17]. The EAR contains an additional α-helix (αB′) in STAT-type SH2 domains, as opposed to the Src-type which harbors a β-sheet (βE and βF although each strand is not always observed). Additionally, there is a cluster of non-polar residues (referred to as the hydrophobic system [20]) at the base of the pY+3 pocket that assists in stabilizing the conformation of the β-sheet and maintaining the integrity of the overall SH2 domain. The αB, αB′, and BC* loop also participate in SH2-mediated STAT dimerization forming important cross-domain interactions. Therefore, residues in the pY+3 pocket can have a dual effect on STAT dimerization capacity and phospho-peptide binding. Conventional phospho-peptide binding occurs perpendicular to the β-sheet with the peptide adopting a binding mode as illustrated with STAT1 in Figure 1c. The phospho-Tyr interacts with conserved amino acids in the pY pocket, while the C-terminal residues stretch across the SH2 domain into the pY+3 pocket.

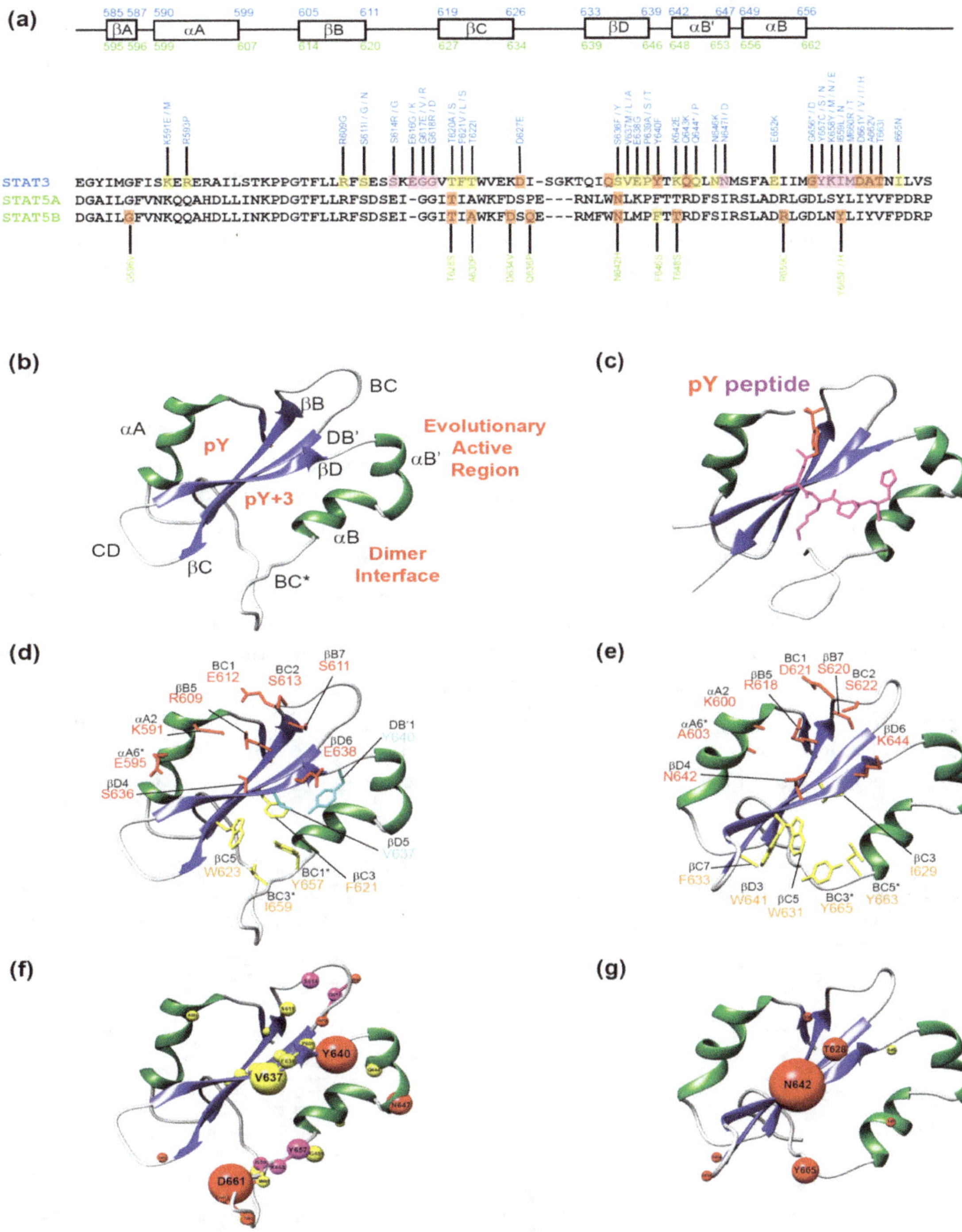

Figure 1. (**a**) Secondary structural motifs in STAT3 (blue) and STAT5 (green) with mutations annotated; (**b**) Structure of STAT3 SH2 domain; (**c**) Structure of pY-peptide-STAT1 SH2 domain. The pY residue is depicted in red with the C-terminal residues in violet; (**d**) Structure of STAT3 SH2 domain with Sheinerman residues (red), hydrophobic system residues (yellow) and the selectivity filter (cyan);

(**e**) Structure of STAT5B SH2 domain with the same color scheme as above; (**f**) STAT3 SH2 domain with all mutations highlighted in spheres. The volume of each sphere is proportional to frequency of cases identified. Red spheres indicate an activating mutation, yellow spheres indicate a destabilizing mutation and magenta spheres represent sites where both activating and refractory mutations are observed; (**g**) STAT5B SH2 domain with all mutations highlighted in spheres. The color scheme is the same as in (**f**). Protein structures were visualized using Chimera [21] with PDB codes: 4E68 [22] (STAT3), 6MBW (STAT5B) [23], 1YVL (STAT1) [24].

These residues are critical for maintaining proper binding interactions to facilitate protein dimerization, and specific mutations here can alter normal STAT function. An issue of particular relevance for drug discovery is protein flexibility, and indeed, STAT SH2 domains exhibit a particularly flexible behavior even in sub-microsecond timescales [23,25]. Notably, the accessible volume of the pY pocket varies dramatically. Also, crystal structures do not necessarily preserve even the main, targetable pockets in an accessible state. This further underlines the importance of accounting for protein dynamics in STAT-directed drug discovery efforts.

3. Disease-Associated Mutations in STAT3 and STAT5B SH2 Domains

Sequencing analysis of patient samples has identified multiple point mutations within the SH2 domain of STAT3 (Table 1) and STAT5B (Table 2) leading to variable effects on physiological activity. In mice, homozygous disruption of STAT3 is embryonically lethal [26], and correspondingly germline homozygous loss-of-function (LOF) mutations have not been identified in humans. Heterozygous loss of STAT3 can be tolerated to different extents and contributes to immunological deficiencies, most commonly autosomal-dominant Hyper IgE syndrome (AD-HIES) as a result of a reduced STAT3-mediated Th17 T-cell response [27–29]. Classical STAT3 function is implicated in Th17 T-cell lineage commitment, through upregulation of RORγt, promoting the release of IL-17 and IL-22. This stimulates transcription of genes associated with Th17 development. Loss of STAT3 function strongly diminishes Th17 T-cell expansion, thereby reducing the immunologic response leading to recurrent staphylococcal infections and exceedingly high levels of IgE that contribute to clinical presentations of eczema and eosinophilia.

Table 1. Disease-associated mutations in the STAT3 SH2 domain.

Mutation	Position	Location	Residue Relevance	Nucleotide Substitution	Cases	Pathology	Type	Ref
K591E	αA2	pY	Sheinerman	1771A>G	1	AD-HIES	Germline	[30]
K591M	αA2	pY	Sheinerman	1772A>T	1	AD-HIES	Germline	[31]
R593P	αA4	pY	-	1778G>C	1	AD-HIES	Germline	[32]
R609G	βB5	pY	Sheinerman& Signature	1825A>G	1	AD-HIES	Germline	[33]
S611G	βB7	pY	Sheinerman	1831A>G	2	AD-HIES	Germline	[34,35]
S611N	βB7	pY	& Signature Sheinerman	1832G>A	2	AD-HIES	Germline	[36,37]
S611I	βB7	pY	Sheinerman & Signature	1832G>T	1	AD-HIES	Germline	[38]
S614G	BC3	pY	Sheinerman	18040A>G	1	AD-HIES	Germline	[34]
S614R	BC3	pY	Sheinerman	1842C>G	1	T-LGLL	Somatic	[39–43]
					2	NK-LGLL		
					1	ALK$^-$ALCL		
					1	HSTL		

Table 1. *Cont.*

Mutation	Position	Location	Residue Relevance	Nucleotide Substitution	Cases	Pathology	Type	Ref
E616G	BC5	pY	BC loop	1847A>G	1	DLBCL, NOS	Somatic	[44]
E616K	BC5	pY	BC loop	1846G>A	1	NKTL	Somatic	[45]
G617E	BC6	pY	BC loop	1850G>A	1	AD-HIES	Germline	[46]
G617V	BC6	pY	BC loop	1850G>T	1	AD-HIES	Germline	[34]
G617R	BC6	pY	BC loop	1849G>A	1	DLBCL, NOS	Somatic	[44]
G618R	BC6	pY	BC loop	1852G>C	1	ALK$^-$ALCL	Somatic	[47,48]
					1	T-LGLL		
G618D	BC6	pY	BC loop	1853G>A	2	AD-HIES	Germline	[35,37]
T620A	βC2	pY	-	1858A>G	2	AD-HIES	Germline	[34,49]
T620S	βC2	pY	-	1859C>G	1	AD-HIES	Germline	[33]
F621V	βC3	pY+3	Hydro. Sys.	1861T>G	3	AD-HIES	Germline	[36,37,50]
F621L	βC3	pY+3	Hydro. Sys.	1863C>G	2	AD-HIES	Germline	[51,52]
F621S	βC3	pY+3	Hydro. Sys.	1862T>C	1	AD-HIES	Germline	[53]
T622I	βC4	pY	-	1865C>T	4	AD-HIES	Germline	[30,34,36]
D627E	CD1		-	1881C>A	1	ATLL	Somatic	[54]
S636F	βD4	pY	Sheinerman	1907C>T,	1	AD-HIES	Germline	[49]
S636Y	βD4	pY	Sheinerman	1907C>A	1	AD-HIES	Germline	[30]
V637M	βD5	pY+3	Sel. Filter	1909G>A	43	AD-HIES	Germline	[30,32–37,49,52,55,56]
V637L	βD5	pY+3	Sel. Filter	1909G>T	1	AD-HIES	Germline	[36]
V637A	βD5	pY+3	Sel. Filter	1910T>C	1	AD-HIES	Germline	[30]
E638G	βD6	pY	Sheinerman	1913A>G	4	AD-HIES	Germline	[49,51,57,58]
P639A	βD7	pY+3	-	1915C>G	1	AD-HIES	Germline	[37]
P639S	βD7	pY+3	-	1915C>T*	2	AD-HIES	Germline	[30,34]
P639T	βD7	pY+3	-	1915C>A	1	AD-HIES	Germline	[35]
Y640F	DB′1	pY+3	-	1919A>T	56	T-LGLL	Somatic	[43,44,47,48,57,59–69]
					2	IHT		
					3	CLPD-NKs		
					2	NK-LGLL		
					1	DLBCL, NOS		
					1	ANKL		
					1	NKTL		
					1	Sezary		
					3	HSTL		
K642E	αB′1	-	Dimer Inter	1924A>G	1	AD-HIES	Germline	[34]
Q643K	αB′2	-	Dimer Inter	1927C>A	1	T-LGLL	Somatic	[68]
Q644P	αB′3	-	Dimer Inter	1929A>C	3	AD-HIES	Germline	[52,70]
Q644del	αB′3	-	Dimer Inter	1930del CAG	2	AD-HIES	Germline	[35,36]
N646K	αB′5	pY+3	Dimer Inter	1938C>G	2	EOAD	Germline	[71]
N647D	αB′6	pY+3	Dimer Inter	1939A>G	8	AD-HIES	Germline	[36,72]
N647I	αB′6	pY+3	Dimer Inter	1940A>T	3	CLPD-NK	Somatic	[43,57,65,67]
					6	T-LGLL		
					1	HSTL		
E652K	αB3	pY+3	Dimer Inter	1954G>A	1	AD-HIES	Germline	[36]
G656D	αB7	pY+3	Dimer Inter	1967G>A	1	T-LGLL	Somatic	[73]
G656_Y657insF	αB7	pY+3	Hydro. Sys.	1968C>T; 1969_1970insTTT	1	IHCA	Somatic	[66]
Y657C	BC1*	pY+3	Hydro. Sys.	1970A>G	5	AD-HIES	Germline	[30,34,36,58]
Y657S	BC1*	pY+3	Hydro. Sys.	1970A>C	1	AD-HIES	Germline	[74]
Y657N	BC1*	pY+3	Hydro. Sys.	1969T>A	1	AD-HIES	Germline	[52]
Y657ins	BC1*	pY+3	Hydro. Sys.	-	1	TCL	Somatic	[47]
Y657dup	BC1*	pY+3	Hydro. Sys.	-	3	T-LGLL	Somatic	[48,65,72]

Table 1. *Cont.*

Mutation	Position	Location	Residue Relevance	Nucleotide Substitution	Cases	Pathology	Type	Ref
Y657_M660dup	BC1*	pY+3	Hydro. Sys.	1969T_1980G dup	1	IHCA	Somatic	[66]
K658M	BC2*	pY+3	Dimer Inter	1973A>T	2	T-LGLL	Somatic	[67,72]
K658N	BC2*	pY+3	Dimer Inter	1974G>T	1	T-LGLL EOAD	Somatic/Germline	[65,71]
K658Y	BC2*	pY+3	Dimer Inter	1972A>T; 1974G>T	1	IHCA	Somatic	[66]
K658E	BC2*	pY+3	Dimer Inter	1972A>G	1	AD-HIES	Germline	[75]
I659N	BC3*	pY+3	Hydro. Sys.	1976A>T	1	AD-HIES	Germline	[58]
I659L	BC3*	pY+3	Hydro. Sys.	1975A>C	2	T-LGLL	Somatic	[57,72]
M660R	BC4*	pY+3	Dimer Inter	1979T>G	1	AD-HIES	Germline	[55]
M660T	BC4*	pY+3	Dimer Inter	1978T>A	1	AD-HIES	Germline	[76]
D661I	BC5*	-	Dimer Inter	1981G>A; 1982A>T	1	CLPD-NK	Somatic	[67]
D661Y	BC5*	-	Dimer Inter	1981G>T	1	NK-LGL	Somatic	[41,47,48,60,63,65,67,68,72,77]
					56	T-LGL		
					1	HSTL		
					10	NKTL		
D661ins	BC5*	-	Dimer Inter	-	1	T-LGLL	Somatic	[47]
D661V	BC5*	-	Dimer Inter	1981A>T	10	T-LGLL	Somatic	[65,67]
D661H	BC5*	-	Dimer Inter	1981G>C	1	T-LGLL	Somatic	[65]
A662V	BC6*	-	Dimer Inter	1985C>T	1	ALK^{-}ALCL	Somatic	[78]
T663I	BC7*	-	Dimer Inter	1988, 1989>TT	2	DLBCL/B1	Germline	[44,75]
I665N	BC9*	-	Dimer Inter	1998T>A	2	AD-HIES	Germline	[34]
V667L	BC11*	-	Dimer Inter	1999C>G	1	NKTL	Somatic	[45]
S668F	BC12*	-	Dimer Inter	2003C>T	3	AD-HIES	Germline	[30,34,37]
S668Y	BC12*	-	Dimer Inter	2003C>A	1	AD-HIES	Germline	[34]

The final search date for mutations from medical case reports and literature was 30 August, 2019. Abbreviations: AD-HIES, autosomal-dominant Hyper IgE syndrome; ALK^{-}ALCL, anaplastic lymphoma kinase negative anaplastic large cell lymphoma; ANKL, aggressive natural killer cell leukemia; ATLL, adult T-cell leukemia lymphoma; EOAD, early onset autoimmune disease; CLPD-NKs, Chronic lymphoproliferative disorders of natural killer cells; DLBCL, NOS, Diffuse large B-cell lymphoma, not-otherwise-specified; NKTL, extranodal NK/T-cell lymphoma; HSTL, Hepatosplenic T-cell lymphoma; IHAC, inflammatory hepatocellular adenomas; IHT, inflammatory hepatocellular tumors; NK-LGLL, Natural killer cell large granular lymphocytic leukemia; T-LGLL, T-cell large granular lymphocytic leukemia; TCL, $\gamma\delta$-T-cell lymphoma.

Table 2. Disease-associated mutations in the STAT5B SH2 domain.

Mutation	Position	Location	Residue Relevance	Nucleotide Substitution	Cases	Pathology	Type	Ref.
G596V	βA2	-	-	1787G>T	1	APL	Somatic	[79]
T628S	βC2	pY	-	1883C>G	11	T-PLL	Somatic	[43,80,81]
					1	MEITL		
					3	HSTL		
					1	Eosinophilia		
A630P	βC4	pY	-	1888G>C	1	GHI	Germline *	[82]
D634V	βC8	pY	-	1901A>T	1	T-PLL	Somatic	[83]
Q636P	CD2	pY+3	-	1907A>C	1	MEITL	Somatic	[81]
N642H	βD4	pY	Sheinerman	1924A>C	39	MEITL	Somatic	[41,62,69,77,80,81,83–102]
					33	T-PLL		
					29	Eosinophilia		
					28	T-ALL		
					7	HSTL		
					11	LGLL		
					3	PCTL		
					3	Sézary		
					1	AAA		
					1	CNL		
					1	PTCL, NOS		
					1	AML		
F646S	DB′1	pY+3	-	1937T>C	1	GHI	Germline *	[103]
T648S	DB′3	pY+3	-	1942A>T	1	T-ALL	Somatic	[101]
R659C	αB′4	Dimer Inter	-	1975C>T	1	T-PLL	Somatic	[80]
Y665F	BC3*	Dimer Inter	Hydro. Sys.	1994A>T	6	T-PLL	Somatic	[43,80,101]
					3	HSTL		
					2	T-ALL		
					2	NKTL		
					5	LGLL		
Y665H	BC3*	Dimer Inter	Hydro. Sys.	1993T>C	2	T-PLL	Somatic	[80]

* Patients were homozygous for the point mutation. The final search date for mutations from medical case reports and literature was 30 August, 2019. Abbreviations: AAA, acquired aplastic anemia; AML, acute myeloid leukemia; APL, acute promyelocytic leukemia; CNL, chronic neutrophilic leukemia; GHI, growth hormone insensitivity; HSTL, hepatosplenic T-cell lymphoma; MEITL, monomorphic epitheliotropic intestinal T cell lymphoma; PCTL, primary cutaneous γδ T-cell lymphoma; PTCL-NOS, peripheral T-cell lymphoma not-other-specified; T-ALL, T-cell acute lymphoblastic leukemia; T-LGLL, T-cell large granular lymphocytic leukemia; T-PLL, T-cell prolymphocytic leukemia.

Comparatively, homozygous loss of both STAT5 gene products in mice is lethal late in embryonic development, due to the defective erythropoiesis and with loss of STAT5B manifesting with a myriad of physiological effects including sexual dimorphic body growth [104–106]. Clinical cases of patients with STAT5B LOF mutations on both alleles exhibit features similar to growth hormone insensitivity syndrome (GHIS). However, heterozygous human carriers of STAT5B LOF mutations generally do not present with any immunological deficiencies or growth complications, although there have been three germline dominant-negative heterozygous STAT5B mutations recently reported that result in postnatal growth impairment among other physiological symptoms [107]. Although these growth deficiencies are likely multifactorial in etiology, the growth hormone (GH)-growth hormone receptor (GHR) interactions that recruit JAK kinase and stimulate phosphorylation of STAT5B remain intact, suggesting a breakdown in corresponding STAT5B activity. STAT5B LOF patients often carry additional immunological burdens including reduced populations of several T-cell subtypes, suggesting multiple roles for STAT5 in T-cell differentiation [108].

Gain-of-function (GOF) germline mutations for STAT3 and STAT5 are rare and clinically diverse. STAT3 GOF mutations present with autoimmune responses, likely due to Th17 clonal expansion which also suppresses regulatory T-cell (Treg) formation. Clinical presentations of STAT3 GOF mutations also show parallels with STAT5 LOF mutations [28]. This is partially an effect of compensatory upregulation of SOCS3 (suppressor of cytokine signaling-3) which strongly inhibits hyperactivated STAT3, but by extension also dampens STAT5 and STAT1 activity. This potently reduces basal levels of STAT5 leading to growth immunodeficiencies.

Contrastingly, multiple de novo somatic GOF mutations arise in STAT3 and STAT5B leading to cancer pathogenesis, and such mutations have been implicated in both solid and liquid tumors. Hyperactivated STAT3 is identified in patients with diverse phenotypes and multiple somatic mutations have been associated with T-LGLL (T-cell large granular lymphocytic leukemia, 40–70% of all cases) and NK-LGLL (natural killer cell large granular lymphocytic leukemia, 30% of all cases), as well as different hepatocellular adenomas [40]. STAT5 is upregulated, directly and indirectly, through multiple mechanisms in several hematological malignancies leading to neoplastic transformation. For instance, in ~30% of acute myeloid leukemia (AML) cases, STAT5B is activated by mutated FLT3 (Fms-Like Tyrosine Kinase 3) [109]. Similarly, ~99% of all chronic myeloid leukemia (CML) cases, which result from the appearance of the Philadelphia chromosome, result in STAT5B hyperactivation [110]. B-cell cancers, such as B-ALL (B-cell acute lymphoid leukemia) and B-CLL (B-cell chronic lymphoid leukemia) are driven by upregulation of IL-7 and IL-22 which also simulate STAT5B [111–113]. Acute and chronic T-cell cancers have lower incidence, but a larger diversity, and are heavily implicated by STAT5B GOF driver mutations [84,114,115]. STAT GOF mutations generally stabilize protein structure thereby enhancing transcriptional output, leading to apoptosis-evading and survival phenotypes. LOF mutants generally distort secondary structure and contribute to either loss of activity or increased STAT degradation. Herein, we highlight the structural significance and mechanism of action of malignant STAT3/5B point mutations in the SH2 domain. Notably, STAT5A mutations are less frequently identified which is likely due to the differential roles of the protein isoforms. Although STAT5B has been characterized as a driver in several malignancies, STAT5A has been associated with tumor suppression [116,117]. STAT5A and STAT5B have similar SH2 domains (~93% amino acid similarity) with significant changes in the βD strand which likely contributes to varying peptide selectivity.

3.1. Mutations in the pY Pocket

As previously described, the pY pocket is formed by the αA helix, BC loop, and one face of the central β-sheet, and it harbors an overall positive electrostatic potential to stabilize binding with the electronegative phospho-Tyr side-chain (Figure 1). This region of the SH2 domain is characterized by strongly conserved residues that facilitate interactions with the phosphorylated peptide. It includes the SH2 domain signature sequence as well as a group of 8 phospho-Tyr interacting amino acids that have been collectively referred to as Sheinerman residues [20]. The SH2 domain signature sequence, FLXRXS (where X is a hydrophobic amino acid), corresponds to FLLRFS in all STAT proteins and is located on the βB strand. The eight Sheinerman residues correspond to the positions: αA2, αA6, βB5, βB7, BC1, BC2, βD4 and βD6 [20]. Critically, the βB5 residue is located within the SH2 domain signature sequence as an invariant Arg residue, which is conserved in 118 of 121 SH2 domain-containing proteins [16]. This indispensable Arg residue is the principal binding partner for phospho-Tyr with the side-chain guanidinium group participating in a bidentate ionic interaction with the phosphate. The side-chains of the αA2 (Arg/Lys in 118/121 SH2 domains), βB7 (Ser in 106/121 SH2 domains) and βD4 (His in 80/121 SH2 domains) residues also participate in direct interactions with the phospho-Tyr [16]. Notably, the αA2, βB7, and βD4 residues correspond to Lys591, Glu638, and Ser636 in STAT3 and Lys600, Ser620, and Asn642 in STAT5B. These interactions are highly important for phospho-peptide binding and are reported to contribute to >50% of Gibbs free energy of the protein–peptide interaction [16]. The high fidelity of these interactions ostensibly suggests that a mutation at these sites will have a dramatic effect on the activity or binding capacity of STAT3/5.

3.1.1. Mutations in Sheinerman Residues

Mutations identified at the αA2 site in STAT3 (Lys591Glu [30] and Lys591Met [31]) contribute to AD-HIES, a STAT3-deficient malignancy, due to removal of the positively-polarized Lys side-chain that directly coordinates the phospho-Tyr. Similarly, mutations at other critical residues in the pY pocket present with analogous clinical outcomes. Mutation of the invariant βB5 position (Arg609Gly [33]) in STAT3 leads to AD-HIES, presenting with reduced expression profiles of Th17 T-cells and high serum levels of IgE (11,300 IU/mL). Replacement of βD4 (Ser636Phe [49]) leads to strongly elevated IgE levels (17,407 IU/mL) with presentation of eczema, abscesses, and pneumonia, also characteristic of AD-HIES pathologies. Interestingly, a patient with a semi-conservative substitution (Ser636Tyr [30]) that retains H-bonding capacity at the βD4 position still presented with a reduced percentage of Th17 cells (0.31%) compared to healthy patients (>1%), highlighting the substantive role of changes in sterics at the phosphate binding positions. Examining the prevalence of mutations within the remaining Sheinerman residues shows infrequent mutations, such as STAT3 βB7 (in which Ser611Gly [34]/Asn [36] have been reported), which also lead to ablation of activity and AD-HIES. In cellulo studies with Ser611Asn indicate a reduced capacity for activation by phosphorylation consistent with altered phospho-Tyr binding [118]. Similarly, substitution at the Sheinerman βD6 position is also capable of triggering the AD-HIES phenotype. Notably, this βD6 (Glu638Gly [49,51]) mutation likely causes gross conformational changes in the β-sheet due to removal of a complete side-chain. Although mutations in the pY pocket of STAT3 tend to abolish peptide binding, specific mutations in the BC loop lead to either hyperactivation and LGL leukemias or protein dysfunction and AD-HIES. Since the BC loop is directly involved in multiple domain interactions including the pY and pY+3 pockets, mutations identified in this region will be discussed in detail in Section 3.3.

In STAT5, mutations at the conserved Sheinerman residues have not been identified apart from the βD4 position. In the majority of SH2 domain-containing proteins, the βD4 residue is a His, directly coordinating the phosphate, and mutagenesis of this residue abolishes peptide binding capacity [16]. As seen with STAT3 (Ser636Tyr), modification in sterics at this position greatly modulates phospho-Tyr peptide binding. In STAT5B, the βD4 residue is an Asn642, and the absence of a conserved His residue may represent an evolutionary response to tune down the basal activity of STAT5. Notably, this residue is most frequently mutated in STAT5B (Asn642His) and has been reported in multiple cancer phenotypes (>150 cases [41,62,69,77,80,81,83–102]), most commonly T-cell-prolymphocytic leukemia (T-PLL), monomorphic epitheliotropic intestinal T-cell lymphoma (MEITL), and T-cell acute lymphoblastic leukemia (T-ALL). Asn642His is an extremely aggressive oncodriver of T-cell neoplasia and previous studies have shown multiple T-cell subset organ infiltration and transformation in transgenic mice [23,119]. Recently, the crystal structure for the STAT5B Asn642His mutation was reported which suggested different SH2 domain conformations with either a neatly packed βD strand forming a tight central β-sheet or a more dissociated βD strand that provides greater access to the SH2 domain [23]. Additionally, different biophysical studies [23,41] have confirmed the substantial increase (~5–7 fold) in the affinity of pY containing peptides for mutated STAT5B (Asn642His) compared to wild type. This provides a molecular basis for the lower threshold of mutant STAT5B towards cytokine activation and the aggressive phenotype observed in patients. The Asn642His mutation is also predicted to lead to a more stable dimer interface and reduced dephosphorylation kinetics, prolonging the lifetime of the activation state [23].

3.1.2. Mutations Outside Sheinerman Residues

The mutational landscape of STAT3 and STAT5B within the pY pocket also extends to less conserved residues, predominantly on the βC strand. Mutations at βC4 have been identified in both STAT3 (Thr620Ser [33]/Ala [34,49]) and STAT5B (Thr628Ser). In STAT5B, this conservative mutation is commonly observed in T-PLL and T-ALL [86]. In vitro studies with STAT5B Asn642 variants have shown that bulkier substituents in the pY pocket reduce phospho-Tyr affinity [23]. Therefore, the loss of a single methylene group from Thr628 can better accommodate the cognate peptide yielding increased transcriptional activity. However, contrary effects are observed with Thr620Ser in STAT3, where this mutation, as well as Thr620Ala, both lead to reduced protein activity and AD-HIES. The contrasting effects of the same mutation at identical positions in STAT3 and STAT5B underscores the unique aspects of each structural motif, and more broadly, the potential for isoform specific drug targeting. Generally, STAT3 is less robust to molecular modifications with slight changes capable of strongly diminishing activity. This is unusual considering the melting temperature of isolated STAT3 (52.5 ± 0.7 °C) is higher than STAT5B (44.5 ± 0.3 °C) [120]. The total protein stability is likely the result of both structural and complex protein dynamics and requires further investigation. One destabilizing mutation has been observed in the pY pocket of STAT5B at the βC4 position (Ala630Pro [121]) which disrupts the β-sheet, reducing protein solubility and leading to misfolding and a clinical presentation of severe growth deficiency. Thus, destabilizing mutations are observed in STAT5B, but with a reduced frequency.

3.2. *Mutations in the pY+3 Pocket*

Adjacent to the pY pocket of the SH2 domain is the pY+3, or specificity pocket which interacts with C-terminal residues of the phospho-Tyr peptide. The βD strand is critical in facilitating these interactions, particularly the βD5 residue which controls accessibility to this pocket. In Src-type SH2 domains, additional interactions with the cognate phospho-peptide occur between residues in the evolutionary active region (EAR). This includes the βE and βF strands as well as the loops in between these structural elements. In STAT3 and STAT5, the EAR motif is comprised of an α-helix (αB′), and the corresponding interactions occur within the DB′ region (loop in between βD strand and αB′ helix), αB′, and αB helices. There is also a clustering of predominantly aromatic, hydrophobic residues at the base of the pY+3 pocket which has been referred to as the hydrophobic system (βC3, βC5, βD3, BC1*, and BC3*). In STAT3, this includes residues Phe621 (βC3), Trp623 (βC5), Tyr657 (BC1*), and Ile659 (BC3*) and in STAT5B, Ile629 (βC3), Trp631 (βC5), Phe633 (βC7), Trp641 (βD3), Leu663 (BC1*) and Tyr665 (BC3*). In STAT3, the hydrophobicity of this pocket is reduced by the presence of Gln635 and Lys626 at the βD3 and βC7 positions, respectively. The increased polarity leads to a reduced STAT3 preference for phospho-peptides with non-polar residues in the C-terminal positions compared to STAT5B. The SH2 dimerization interface is in close proximity to the pY+3 pocket and is formed by the BC* loop, αB′ helix and one face of the αB helix. As such, alterations in the pY+3 pocket directly affect the dimerization interface.

3.2.1. Mutations in the Hydrophobic System and βD Strand

The pY+3 pocket is a hotspot for STAT SH2 domain mutations. Generally, mutations that increase the polarity of this pocket result in protein destabilization and LOF. This was demonstrated in Epstein–Barr virus (EBV)-transformed B-cells expressing AD-HIES-associated STAT3 mutations. In these assays, the half-life of wild type STAT3 (25 ± 2 h) was shown to be substantially reduced by polar mutations at βD5 (Val637Met = 5.3 ± 4.5 h) and BC1* (Tyr657Cys = 5.5 ± 4.1 h) [122]. Conversely, STAT3 mutant Tyr640Phe (DB′1), which is a commonly identified mutation in solid and liquid tumors, leads to constitutive activation across several cell lines (hepatic epithelial cells, lung carcinomas, fibroblasts, etc.) through enhanced stability of STAT3 dimerization, nuclear accumulation and increased transcriptional activity following IFNγ stimulation [44,47,48,59–62,65–69]. In wild type STAT3, Tyr640 points directly into the hydrophobic system. Increasing hydrophobicity, through removal of the hydroxyl group tightens the packing of the pocket and enhances the activation potential. The STAT3 Tyr640Phe mutation has been identified in over >110 cancer cases in the COSMIC database and is most frequently observed in patients with T-LGLL. An analogous mutation is observed at the BC3* site in STAT5B where the second most frequent mutation (Tyr665Phe) results in STAT5B hyperactivation and has also been observed in patients with T-LGLL.

Within the hydrophobic system, the presence of aromaticity for π-π stacking interactions from key residue side-chains is strongly favored over non-aromatic Van der Waals interactions. This is especially seen at the βC3 position with patients harboring Phe621Val [36,37,50]/Leu [51,52]/Ser [53] mutations resulting in STAT3-deficient AD-HIES. In cellulo mutagenesis studies with the Phe621Val mutation have elucidated impaired STAT3 phosphorylation, resulting in defective DNA binding capacity. This strong requirement for aromaticity is also observed in STAT5B, where Tyr665His leads to a hyperactive mutant, since it retains the aromaticity of the imidazole ring to interact with Trp631 (βC5), despite the increase in side-chain polarity.

In addition to the hydrophobic system, the βD strand is critical for controlling pocket accessibility. This is primarily governed by the residue at the βD5 position in SH2 domains and corresponds to Val637 in STAT3. This residue serves as a selectivity filter, interacting with C-terminal amino acids of the phospho-Tyr peptide. In Src kinase, the βD5 residue corresponds to a Tyr and the aromatic ring is sandwiched between the Glu (pY+1 residue) and Ile (pY+3 residue) of the phospho-peptide [18]. In other SH2 domain-containing kinases, the βD5 residue interacts with all three C-terminal amino acids of the pY-peptide. Given the critical nature of this site, it is not unexpected that mutations strongly impair STAT3 activity. STAT3 Val637Met has been identified in a number of patient samples (>40 cases) and is associated with AD-HIES due to impaired response to cytokine activation and transcriptional activity. The importance of Val637Met [30,33,34,36,49,56] is further underscored by insensitivity to 100-fold increases in IL-6 to simulate phosphorylation. This inability to recognize specific phospho-peptides contributes to the defective STAT pathway observed in AD-HIES. As a crucial selectivity filter, even semi-conservative mutations Val637Leu [36] and Val637Ala [30] have also been shown to be disruptive to STAT3 activity and result in AD-HIES. Although STAT3 Val637Met may be a result of reduced protein stability [122], circular dichroism spectra for STAT3 Val637Ala suggest that this substitution does not cause large structural perturbations. Alternatively, this substitution likely reduces phospho-peptide binding in the pY+3 pocket [123]. The βD7 position also assists in the orientation of the βD5 residue, and mutation of the rigid Pro639 to 639Ala [37]/Ser [30,34]/Thr [35] also results in AD-HIES.

3.2.2. Mutations in the Dimerization Interface

In comparison to pY and pY+3 pockets of the SH2 domain, the dimerization interface represents a delicate balance in carefully regulating STAT activity. This region is littered with disease-causing mutations and slight changes to sterics or electronics at the αB, αB′, or BC* loop propagate their effects exponentially and lead to highly contrasting effects. There are multiple examples of such mutations throughout the dimerization interface. For instance, at the αB′6 site, patients with STAT3 Asn647Asp [36,72] exhibit symptoms of AD-HIES, but the Asn647Ile [57,65,67] mutation results in STAT3 hyperactivation manifesting as chronic lymphoproliferative disorder of NK cells (CPLD-NK) and T-LGLL. Comparable to trends observed at the central pY+3 pocket, hydrophobic or aromatic substitutions at the interface stabilize STAT3 dimer formation and subsequent phosphorylation, while changes in polarity, or in this case, an electrostatic reversal, effectively abolish STAT3 activity. Analogous effects are also observed at the BC1*–BC6* positions. At BC1* and BC2*, Tyr657Ser [74]/Asn [52]/Cys [30,34,36,58] and Lys658Glu [75] lead to AD-HIES, whereas Tyr657ins [47], Tyr657dup [48,72] and Lys658Met [67,72]/Asn [65]/Tyr [66] elicit several types of T-cell cancers [124]. At the BC3* position, Ile659Leu [57,72] has been characterized in T-LGLL, whereas the recently identified Ile659Asn [58] mutation distorts STAT3 activity leading to AD-HIES. Only destabilizing (AD-HIES causing) mutations have been identified at BC4* (Met660Arg [55] and Met660Thr [76]) in STAT3. The BC5* position was found to be genetically volatile with mutations occurring as Asp661His [65]/Val [78]/Tyr [41,47,48,60,63,65,67,68,72,77]/Ile [67], with all mutations resulting in STAT3 activation and enhanced response to cytokines. Finally, the BC6* (Ala662) and BC8* (Asn664) positions are critical SH2 domain interface determinants, where mutagenesis experiments have created artificial disulfide linked STAT3-Ala662Cys-Asn664Cys dimers that are constitutively active in cellulo and induce malignant transformation [66]. This further reinforces the role of the BC* loop in maintaining the dimer interface to control STAT activity. Individually, these Cys-mutations are likely destabilizing, but their pairing allows for covalent tethering of the STAT3 monomers and active dimer formation.

Within STAT3, the disordered BC* loop tends to be the only site amenable to insertion/deletion mutations. Since different mutations in this BC* loop lead to either hyper- or refractory activity, likely the substitutions have some degree of compensatory effect that allow them to persist compared to other regions of the SH2 domain. Furthermore, the remaining motifs of the SH2 domain are highly structured and less likely to tolerate insertions or deletions.

The volatility shown by each of the residues in the BC* loop to trigger such extreme changes in STAT3 behavior underscores both the importance of this region to STAT activity, but also the necessity to understand the underlying molecular dynamics that result in such variability. This is particularly true for the BC5* residue which has no prescribed role in other SH2 domains. However, as seen above, its malignant capacity is revealed in >100 identified cases featuring a mosaic of mutations, according to the COSMIC database. Specifically, the STAT3 Asp661Tyr mutation represents one of the most frequently occurring mutation in the SH2 domain of STAT3 along with Tyr640Phe (>100 cases). Although the increases in hydrophobicity and aromaticity have been speculated as critical determinants for the aggressive nature of this mutation, the site-specific mechanism of activation remains unclear. Notably, both of these frequently cancer-associated mutation sites in STAT3 (Tyr640 and Asp661) are by default Phe and Ile respectively in STAT5B. This substitution to the STAT3 cancer-associated genotype in STAT5B suggests that the protein may be more optimized for protein dimerization. This is an interesting observation and further suggests a delicate evolutionary balance in STAT5B by potentially improving interactions at the dimerization interface while reducing activity through the lack of an efficient phosphate-coordinating βD4 residue (Asn642). The functional significance of these changes in STAT5B, compared to STAT3, has not been biophysically characterized and may also suggest that additional mechanisms are relevant to the disease-associated phenotype including changes to protein stability or transcriptional regulation.

3.3. Mutations in the Additional Regions of the SH2 Domain

Mutational hotspots in regions outside the pY and pY+3 pockets may highlight additional areas that are important for protein regulation and exploitable for drug targeting and understanding disease progression. There is a tight clustering of mutations in the BC loop of STAT3 on the periphery of the pY pocket. Similar to the dimerization interface, mutations at these residues can either enhance or reduce STAT activity. This region is in close proximity to the pY pocket, pY+3 pocket, dimerization interface, and STAT linker domain and likely serves as an important allosteric communication bridge for interdomain signaling. As such, interactions at this region of the BC loop require a complex balance of flexibility and rigidity. For instance, at the STAT3 BC3 position, a mutation at Ser614Arg [39–42] leads to hyperactivation and LGLL, whereas a Ser614Gly [34] results in LOF and AD-HIES. Increasing the positive electrostatic potential at this region generally leads to STAT hyperactivation and draws the BC loop closer into the pY pocket. Mutations found at neighboring sites BC5, BC6, and B7 delineate similar trends, where Glu616Lys [45], Glu616Gly [44], Gly617Arg [44], and Gly618Arg [47,48] are found in diffuse large B-cell lymphoma and NK-malignancies. Corresponding electronegative or bulky substitutions are associated with AD-HIES and dysfunctional STAT3 (Gly617Glu [46], Gly618Asp [35 37], and Gly617Val [34]).

There are additional mutations that are located across STAT5 and identified in single patient cases. Given the general robust nature of STAT5 to mutations, it is difficult to assess the oncogenic driving capacity of a single mutation, or whether the disease is multifactorial in etiology. For instance, a mutation in the short βA strand was identified within STAT5B as Gly596Val [79]. However, this mutation was identified in a chimeric protein of STAT5B and retinoic acid receptor-α (STAT5B-RARα), which is associated with acute promyelocytic leukemia (APL) and is also resistant to all-trans retinoic acid therapy. All-trans retinoic acid (ATRA) is capable of inducing remission in almost all APL cases, with several exceptions [125]. Since this is a rare subtype of APL, where the fusion protein was identified in a small minority of cases (<10), it is difficult to judge the importance of the mutation to the progression of the disease, although the residue is conserved across species. Notably, a STAT3-RARα fusion was also recently discovered in an APL patient with a similar ATRA-resistance profile [126]. Surprisingly, no STAT5A fusions have been discovered. It would be interesting to define if the dimerization mechanism of these RARα fusions is mediated through a partially intact SH2 domain or other dimerization domain of STAT. Other mutations in STAT5B are located in non-hotspots including Asp634Val (βC8), Gln636Pro (CD2), and Arg659Cys (αB4) and were identified in patients with T-PLL and MEITL. Similar to STAT3, these mutations are in close proximity to the dimerization interface and increase the hydrophobicity of the region, which can facilitate hyperactivation. It is interesting to note that T-PLL represents the disease with most hyperactive STAT3/5B and JAK3 mutations among all subgroups of largely untargeted orphan T-cell neoplasias, and future targeting efforts in this pathway will likely benefit these patients.

4. Conclusions

Disease associated mutations are more frequently identified in STAT3 compared to STAT5B, suggesting that STAT5B is more robust to the alterations in structural motifs, or that STAT3 has a more pronounced role in normal physiological functioning. However, it is clear that even slight alterations to electronics or sterics in the SH2 domain can dramatically alter STAT3 activity. In STAT3, the majority of mutations identified in the pY pocket impair protein function, with the most substantial effects observed upon mutation of conserved Sheinerman residues (Figure 1f). In STAT5B, pY mutations are generally activating with the Asn642His substitution occurring most frequently in aggressive T-cell cancers (Figure 1g). The pY+3 specificity pockets are characterized by multiple mutations with variable effects. Broadly, mutations that improve hydrophobicity or introduce aromaticity lead to hyperactivation, while increases in pY+3 pocket polarity or removal of aromatic substituents diminish STAT function. This trend is also observed at the SH2 domain dimerization interface which is a hot-spot for mutations, and different substitutions at a single position can result in severe loss- or gain-of-function. Finally, the BC loop may be a critical region for allosteric communication pathways throughout the protein and has been evolutionarily tuned for the precise interactions. As such, marginally reducing electronegativity or increasing electropositivity leads to hyper- and hypo-activation, respectively.

Currently, additional structural studies and molecular dynamics simulations are required for a better understanding of the molecular mechanisms of STAT3/5B mutations at different sites within the SH2 domain. Considering the conformational flexibility of the main binding sites with state-of-the-art computational methods, for example thermodynamic integration, should be more thoroughly exploited in further work. These can be used to propose alternative treatments or highlight therapeutic approaches. For instance, the relative instability of the wild type STAT3 protein is shown to be amplified by AD-HIES-causing mutations. The use of small molecules that can trigger stimulation of protein chaperones to rescue dysfunctional STAT3 mutants has been shown to be effective in cellulo [122]. Alternatively, hyperactivated STAT3 is only marginally more stable than the wild-type protein which may be exploited by degradation enhancing therapeutic strategies such as the use of PROTACs and hydrophobic tagging. These efforts can be extended to STAT5 as well as examining the Asn642His site, as this hot-spot mutation mimics SH2 domain superbinders and is excessively aggressive due to its prime role in the pY pocket. Collectively, these structural studies offer a predictive approach for understanding the molecular foundations of additional mutations identified in the SH2 domain, based on their location and alterations to pocket electronics and sterics.

Acknowledgments: The authors also thank Open Access Funding by the Austrian Science Fund (FWF).

References

1. Wingelhofer, B.; Neubauer, H.A.; Valent, P.; Han, X.; Constantinescu, S.N.; Gunning, P.T.; Müller, M.; Moriggl, R. Implications of STAT3 and STAT5 signaling on gene regulation and chromatin remodeling in hematopoietic cancer. *Leuk.* **2018**, *32*, 1713–1726. [CrossRef]
2. O'Shea, J.J.; Schwartz, D.M.; Villarino, A.V.; Gadina, M.; McInnes, I.B.; Laurence, A. The JAK-STAT pathway: Impact on human disease and therapeutic intervention. *Annu. Rev. Med.* **2015**, *66*, 311–328. [CrossRef] [PubMed]
3. Bromberg, J.F.; Wrzeszczynska, M.H.; Devgan, G.; Zhao, Y.; Pestell, R.G.; Albanese, C.; E Darnell, J. Stat3 as an Oncogene. *Cell* **1999**, *98*, 295–303. [CrossRef]
4. Tsutsui, M.; Yasuda, H.; Suto, H.; Imai, H.; Isobe, Y.; Sasaki, M.; Kojima, Y.; Oshimi, K.; Sugimoto, K. Frequent STAT3 activation is associated with Mcl-1 expression in nasal NK-cell lymphoma. *Int. J. Lab. Hematol.* **2010**, *32*, 419–426. [CrossRef] [PubMed]
5. Passerini, L.; Allan, S.E.; Battaglia, M.; Di Nunzio, S.; Alstad, A.N.; Levings, M.K.; Roncarolo, M.G.; Bacchetta, R. STAT5-signaling cytokines regulate the expression of FOXP3 in CD4+CD25+ regulatory T cells and CD4+ CD25- effector T cells. *Int. Immunol.* **2008**, *20*, 421–431. [CrossRef] [PubMed]
6. Mirmohammadsadegh, A.; Hassan, M.; Bardenheuer, W.; Marini, A.; Gustrau, A.; Nambiar, S.; Tannapfel, A.; Bojar, H.; Ruzicka, T.; Hengge, U.R. STAT5 Phosphorylation in Malignant Melanoma Is Important for Survival and Is Mediated Through SRC and JAK1 Kinases. *J. Investig. Dermatol.* **2006**, *126*, 2272–2280. [CrossRef] [PubMed]
7. Xu, Q.; Briggs, J.; Park, S.; Niu, G.; Kortylewski, M.; Zhang, S.; Gritsko, T.; Turkson, J.; Kay, H.; Semenza, G.L.; et al. Targeting Stat3 blocks both HIF-1 and VEGF expression induced by multiple oncogenic growth signaling pathways. *Oncogene* **2005**, *24*, 5552–5560. [CrossRef]
8. Matsumura, I.; Kitamura, T.; Wakao, H.; Tanaka, H.; Hashimoto, K.; Albanese, C.; Downward, J.; Pestell, R.G.; Kanakura, Y. Transcriptional regulation of the cyclin D1 promoter by STAT5: Its involvement in cytokine-dependent growth of hematopoietic cells. *EMBO J.* **1999**, *18*, 1367–1377. [CrossRef]
9. Baik, M.; Yu, J.H.; Hennighausen, L. Growth hormone-STAT5 regulation of growth, hepatocellular carcinoma, and liver metabolism. *Ann. New York Acad. Sci.* **2011**, *1229*, 29–37. [CrossRef]
10. Nichane, M.; Ren, X.; Bellefroid, E.J. Self-regulation of Stat3 activity coordinates cell-cycle progression and neural crest specification. *EMBO J.* **2010**, *29*, 55–67. [CrossRef]
11. Ali, A.M.; Gómez-Biagi, R.F.; Rosa, D.A.; Lai, P.-S.; Heaton, W.L.; Park, J.S.; Eiring, A.M.; Vellore, N.A.; De Araujo, E.D.; Ball, D.P.; et al. Disarming an Electrophilic Warhead: Retaining Potency in Tyrosine Kinase Inhibitor (TKI)-Resistant CML Lines While Circumventing Pharmacokinetic Liabilities. *ChemMedChem* **2016**, *11*, 850–861. [CrossRef] [PubMed]
12. De Araujo, E.D.; Manaswiyoungkul, P.; Erdogan, F.; Qadree, A.K.; Sina, D.; Tin, G.; Toutah, K.; Yuen, K.; Gunning, P.T.; Erodgan, F. A functional in vitro assay for screening inhibitors of STAT5B phosphorylation. *J. Pharm. Biomed. Anal.* **2019**, *162*, 60–65. [CrossRef] [PubMed]
13. Wingelhofer, B.; Maurer, B.; Heyes, E.C.; Cumaraswamy, A.A.; Berger-Becvar, A.; De Araujo, E.D.; Orlova, A.; Freund, P.; Ruge, F.; Park, J.; et al. Pharmacologic inhibition of STAT5 in acute myeloid leukemia. *Leuk.* **2018**, *32*, 1135–1146. [CrossRef] [PubMed]
14. Elumalai, N.; Berg, A.; Rubner, S.; Blechschmidt, L.; Song, C.; Natarajan, K.; Matysik, J.; Berg, T. Rational development of Stafib-2: A selective, nanomolar inhibitor of the transcription factor STAT5b. *Sci. Rep.* **2017**, *7*, 819. [CrossRef]
15. Haftchenary, S.; Luchman, H.A.; Jouk, A.O.; Veloso, A.J.; Page, B.D.G.; Cheng, X.R.; Dawson, S.S.; Grinshtein, N.; Shahani, V.M.; Kerman, K.; et al. Potent Targeting of the STAT3 Protein in Brain Cancer Stem Cells: A Promising Route for Treating Glioblastoma. *ACS Med. Chem. Lett.* **2013**, *4*, 1102–1107. [CrossRef]
16. Liu, B.A.; Engelmann, B.W.; Nash, P.D. The language of SH2 domain interactions defines phosphotyrosine-mediated signal transduction. *FEBS Lett.* **2012**, *586*, 2597–2605. [CrossRef]
17. Gao, Q.; Hua, J.; Kimura, R.; Headd, J.J.; Fu, X.-Y.; Chin, Y.E. Identification of the Linker-SH2 Domain of STAT as the Origin of the SH2 Domain Using Two-dimensional Structural Alignment. *Mol. Cell. Proteom.* **2004**, *3*, 704–714. [CrossRef]
18. Zhou, S. SH2 domains recognize specific phosphopeptide sequences. *Cell* **1993**, *72*, 767–778. [CrossRef]

19. Songyang, Z.; Cantley, L.C. Recognition and specificity in protein tyrosine kinase-mediated signalling. *Trends Biochem. Sci.* **1995**, *20*, 470–475. [CrossRef]
20. Gianti, E.; Zauhar, R.J. An SH2 domain model of STAT5 in complex with phospho-peptides define "STAT5 Binding Signatures. " *J. Comput. Mol. Des.* **2015**, *29*, 451–470. [CrossRef]
21. Pettersen, E.F.; Goddard, T.D.; Huang, C.C.; Couch, G.S.; Greenblatt, D.M.; Meng, E.C.; Ferrin, T.E. UCSF Chimera?A visualization system for exploratory research and analysis. *J. Comput. Chem.* **2004**, *25*, 1605–1612. [CrossRef] [PubMed]
22. Nkansah, E.; Shah, R.; Collie, G.W.; Parkinson, G.N.; Palmer, J.; Rahman, K.M.; Bui, T.T.; Drake, A.F.; Husby, J.; Neidle, S.; et al. Observation of unphosphorylated STAT3 core protein binding to targetdsDNA by PEMSA and X-ray crystallography. *FEBS Lett.* **2013**, *587*, 833–839. [CrossRef] [PubMed]
23. De Araujo, E.D.; Erdogan, F.; Neubauer, H.A.; Meneksedag-Erol, D.; Manaswiyoungkul, P.; Eram, M.S.; Seo, H.-S.; Qadree, A.K.; Israelian, J.; Orlova, A.; et al. Structural and functional consequences of the STAT5BN642H driver mutation. *Nat. Commun.* **2019**, *10*, 2517. [CrossRef] [PubMed]
24. Mao, X.; Ren, Z.; Parker, G.N.; Sondermann, H.; Pastorello, M.A.; Wang, W.; McMurray, J.S.; Demeler, B.; Darnell, J.E.; Chen, X. Structural Bases of Unphosphorylated STAT1 Association and Receptor Binding. *Mol. Cell* **2005**, *17*, 761–771. [CrossRef]
25. Langenfeld, F.; Guarracino, Y.; Arock, M.; Trouve, A.; Tchertanov, L. How Intrinsic Molecular Dynamics Control Intramolecular Communication in Signal Transducers and Activators of Transcription Factor STAT5. *PLoS ONE* **2015**, *10*, e0145142. [CrossRef]
26. Takeda, K.; Noguchi, K.; Shi, W.; Tanaka, T.; Matsumoto, M.; Yoshida, N.; Kishimoto, T.; Akira, S. Targeted disruption of the mouse Stat3 gene leads to early embryonic lethality. *Proc. Natl. Acad. Sci. USA* **1997**, *94*, 3801–3804. [CrossRef]
27. Purvis, H.A.; Anderson, A.E.; Young, D.A.; Isaacs, J.D.; Hilkens, C.M.U. A Negative Feedback Loop Mediated by STAT3 Limits Human Th17 Responses. *J. Immunol.* **2014**, *193*, 1142–1150. [CrossRef]
28. Haddad, E. STAT3: Too much may be worse than not enough! *Blood* **2015**, *125*, 583–584. [CrossRef]
29. Laurence, A.D.J.; Uhlig, H.H. When half a glass of STAT3 is just not enough. *Blood* **2016**, *128*, 3020–3021. [CrossRef]
30. Woellner, C.; Gertz, E.M.; Schäffer, A.A.; Lagos, M.; Perro, M.; Glocker, E.-O.; Pietrogrande, M.C.; Cossu, F.; Franco, J.L.; Matamoros, N.; et al. Mutations in STAT3 and diagnostic guidelines for hyper-IgE syndrome. *J. Allergy Clin. Immunol.* **2010**, *125*, 424–432. [CrossRef]
31. Robinson, W.S.; Arnold, S.R.; Michael, C.F.; Vickery, J.D.; Schoumacher, R.A.; Pivnick, E.K.; Ward, J.C.; Nagabhushanam, V.; Lew, D.B. Case report of a young child with disseminated histoplasmosis and review of hyper immunoglobulin e syndrome (HIES). *Clin. Mol. Allergy* **2011**, *9*, 14. [CrossRef] [PubMed]
32. Ma, C.S.; Avery, D.T.; Chan, A.; Batten, M.; Bustamante, J.; Boisson-Dupuis, S.; Arkwright, P.D.; Kreins, A.Y.; Averbuch, D.; Engelhard, D.; et al. Functional STAT3 deficiency compromises the generation of human T follicular helper cells. *Blood* **2012**, *119*, 3997–4008. [CrossRef] [PubMed]
33. Zhang, L.-Y.; Tian, W.; Shu, L.; Jiang, L.-P.; Zhan, Y.-Z.; Zhao, X.-D.; Cui, Y.-X.; Tang, X.-M.; Wu, D.-Q.; Yang, X.-Q.; et al. Clinical Features, STAT3 Gene Mutations and Th17 Cell Analysis in Nine Children with Hyper-IgE Syndrome in Mainland China. *Scand. J. Immunol.* **2013**, *78*, 258–265. [CrossRef] [PubMed]
34. Chandesris, M.O.; Melki, I.; Natividad, A.; Puel, A.; Fieschi, C.; Yun, L.; Thumerelle, C.; Oksenhendler, E.; Boutboul, D.; Thomas, C.; et al. Autosomal dominant STAT3 deficiency and hyper-IgE syndrome: Molecular, cellular, and clinical features from a French national survey. *Medicine (United States)* **2012**, *91*. [CrossRef] [PubMed]
35. Freeman, A.F.; Renner, E.D.; Henderson, C.; Langenbeck, A.; Olivier, K.N.; Hsu, A.P.; Hagl, B.; Boos, A.; Davis, J.; Marciano, B.E.; et al. Lung Parenchyma Surgery in Autosomal Dominant Hyper-IgE Syndrome. *J. Clin. Immunol.* **2013**, *33*, 896–902. [CrossRef] [PubMed]
36. Holland, S.M.; DeLeo, F.R.; Elloumi, H.Z.; Hsu, A.P.; Uzel, G.; Brodsky, N.; Freeman, A.F.; Demidowich, A.; Davis, J.; Turner, M.L.; et al. STAT3Mutations in the Hyper-IgE Syndrome. *New Engl. J. Med.* **2007**, *357*, 1608–1619. [CrossRef] [PubMed]
37. Heimall, J.; Davis, J.; Shaw, P.A.; Hsu, A.P.; Gu, W.; Welch, P.; Holland, S.M.; Freeman, A.F. Paucity of genotype-phenotype correlations in STAT3 mutation positive Hyper IgE Syndrome (HIES). *Clin. Immunol.* **2011**, *139*, 75–84. [CrossRef]

38. Moreira Varanese, I.; Seminario, A.; Diaz Balve, D.; Uriarte, I.; Belardinelli, G.; Gomez Racio, A.; di Giovanni, D.; Bezrodnik, L. New STAT3 mutation in a patient with Hyper IgE Syndrome (HIGES) without criteria in HIES STAT3 score. *Transl. Biomed.* **2010**, *1*. [CrossRef]
39. Qiu, Z.-Y.; Fan, L.; Wang, L.; Qiao, C.; Wu, Y.-J.; Zhou, J.-F.; Xu, W.; Li, J.-Y. STAT3 mutations are frequent in T-cell large granular lymphocytic leukemia with pure red cell aplasia. *J. Hematol. Oncol.* **2013**, *6*, 82. [CrossRef]
40. Yan, Y.; Olson, T.L.; Nyland, S.B.; Feith, D.J.; Loughran, T.P. Emergence of a STAT3 mutated NK clone in LGL leukemia. *Leuk. Res. Rep.* **2015**, *4*, 4–7. [CrossRef]
41. Kűcűk, C.; Jiang, B.; Hu, X.; Zhang, W.; Chan, J.K.C.; Xiao, W.; Lack, N.; Alkan, C.; Williams, J.C.; Avery, K.N.; et al. Activating mutations of STAT5B and STAT3 in lymphomas derived from $\gamma\delta$-T or NK cells. *Nat. Commun.* **2015**, *6*, 6025. [CrossRef] [PubMed]
42. Blombery, P.; Thompson, E.R.; Jones, K.; Arnau, G.M.; Lade, S.; Markham, J.F.; Li, J.; Deva, A.; Johnstone, R.W.; Khot, A.; et al. Whole exome sequencing reveals activating JAK1 and STAT3 mutations in breast implant-associated anaplastic large cell lymphoma anaplastic large cell lymphoma. *Haematol.* **2016**, *101*, e387–e390. [CrossRef] [PubMed]
43. McKinney, M.; Moffitt, A.B.; Gaulard, P.; Travert, M.; De Leval, L.; Nicolae, A.; Raffeld, M.; Jaffe, E.S.; Pittaluga, S.; Xi, L.; et al. The Genetic Basis of Hepatosplenic T-cell Lymphoma. *Cancer Discov.* **2017**, *7*, 369–379. [CrossRef] [PubMed]
44. Ohgami, R.S.; Ma, L.; Monabati, A.; Zehnder, J.L.; Arber, D.A. STAT3 mutations are present in aggressive B-cell lymphomas including a subset of diffuse large B-cell lymphomas with CD30 expression. *Haematol.* **2014**, *99*, e105–e107. [CrossRef] [PubMed]
45. Song, T.L.; Nairismägi, M.L.; Laurensia, Y.; Lim, J.Q.; Tan, J.; Li, Z.M.; Kizhakeyil, A.; Wijaya, G.C.; Huang, D.C.; Nagarajan, S.; et al. Oncogenic activation of the STAT3 pathway drives PD-L1 expression in natural killer/T-cell lymphoma. *Blood* **2018**, *132*, 1146–1158. [CrossRef] [PubMed]
46. Schimke, L.F.; Sawalle-Belohradsky, J.; Roesler, J.; Wollenberg, A.; Rack, A.; Borte, M.; Rieber, N.; Cremer, R.; Maaß, E.; Dopfer, R.; et al. Diagnostic approach to the hyper-IgE syndromes: Immunologic and clinical key findings to differentiate hyper-IgE syndromes from atopic dermatitis. *J. Allergy Clin. Immunol.* **2010**, *126*, 611–617. [CrossRef] [PubMed]
47. Couronné, L.; Scourzic, L.; Pilati, C.; Della Valle, V.; Duffourd, Y.; Solary, E.; Vainchenker, W.; Merlio, J.-P.; Beylot-Barry, M.; Damm, F.; et al. STAT3 mutations identified in human hematologic neoplasms induce myeloid malignancies in a mouse bone marrow transplantation model. *Haematol.* **2013**, *98*, 1748–1752. [CrossRef]
48. Kristensen, T.; Larsen, M.; Rewes, A.; Frederiksen, H.; Thomassen, M.; Møller, M.B. Clinical Relevance of Sensitive and Quantitative STAT3 Mutation Analysis Using Next-Generation Sequencing in T-Cell Large Granular Lymphocytic Leukemia. *J. Mol. Diagn.* **2014**, *16*, 382–392. [CrossRef]
49. Renner, E.D.; Rylaarsdam, S.; Añover-Sombke, S.; Rack, A.L.; Reichenbach, J.; Carey, J.C.; Zhu, Q.; Jansson, A.F.; Barboza, J.; Schimke, L.F.; et al. Novel signal transducer and activator of transcription 3 (STAT3) mutations, reduced T(H)17 cell numbers, and variably defective STAT3 phosphorylation in hyper-IgE syndrome. *J. Allergy Clin. Immunol.* **2008**, *122*, 181–187. [CrossRef]
50. Odio, C.D.; Milligan, K.L.; Mc Gowan, K.; Spergel, A.K.R.; Bishop, R.; Boris, L.; Urban, A.; Welch, P.; Heller, T.; Kleiner, D.; et al. Endemic mycoses in patients with STAT3-mutated hyper-IgE (Job) syndrome. *J. Allergy Clin. Immunol.* **2015**, *136*, 1411–1413. [CrossRef]
51. Kumánovics, A.; Wittwer, C.T.; Pryor, R.J.; Augustine, N.H.; Leppert, M.F.; Carey, J.C.; Ochs, H.D.; Wedgwood, R.J.; Faville, R.J.; Quie, P.G.; et al. Rapid Molecular Analysis of the STAT3 Gene in Job Syndrome of Hyper-IgE and Recurrent Infectious Diseases. *J. Mol. Diagn.* **2010**, *12*, 213–219. [CrossRef] [PubMed]
52. Ives, M.L.; Ma, C.S.; Palendira, U.; Chan, A.; Bustamante, J.; Boisson-Dupuis, S.; Arkwright, P.D.; Engelhard, D.; Averbuch, D.; Magdorf, K.; et al. Signal transducer and activator of transcription 3 (STAT3) mutations underlying autosomal dominant hyper-IgE syndrome impair human CD8 + T-cell memory formation and function. *J. Allergy Clin. Immunol.* **2013**, *132*, 400–411. [CrossRef] [PubMed]
53. Mogensen, T.H.; Jakobsen, M.A.; Larsen, C.S. Identification of a novel STAT3 mutation in a patient with hyper-IgE syndrome. *Scand. J. Infect. Dis.* **2013**, *45*, 235–238. [CrossRef] [PubMed]
54. Bellon, M.; Lu, L.; Nicot, C. Constitutive activation of Pim1 kinase is a therapeutic target for adult T-cell leukemia. *Blood* **2016**, *127*, 2439–2450. [CrossRef]

55. Giacomelli, M.; Tamassia, N.; Moratto, D.; Bertolini, P.; Bertulli, C.; Plebani, A.; Cassatella, M.; Ricci, G.; Bazzoni, F.; Badolato, R. SH2-domain mutations in STAT3 in hyper-IgE syndrome patients result in impairment of IL-10 function. *Eur. J. Immunol.* **2011**, *41*, 3075–3084. [CrossRef]
56. Jiao, H.; Tóth, B.; Erdős, M.; Fransson, I.; Rakoczi, E.; Balogh, I.; Magyarics, Z.; Dérfalvi, B.; Csorba, G.; Szaflarska, A.; et al. Novel and recurrent STAT3 mutations in hyper-IgE syndrome patients from different ethnic groups. *Mol. Immunol.* **2008**, *46*, 202–206. [CrossRef]
57. Shi, M.; He, R.; Feldman, A.L.; Viswanatha, D.S.; Jevremovic, D.; Chen, D.; Morice, W.G. STAT3 mutation and its clinical and histopathologic correlation in T-cell large granular lymphocytic leukemia. *Hum. Pathol.* **2018**, *73*, 74–81. [CrossRef]
58. Goncalves, M.R.; Junior, P.R. Association between STAT3 mutations and phenotypic features in Hyper-IgE Syndrome. *J. Allergy Clin. Immunol.* **2019**, *143*, AB111. [CrossRef]
59. Calderaro, J.; Nault, J.C.; Balabaud, C.; Couchy, G.; Saint-Paul, M.C.; Azoulay, D.; Mehdaoui, D.; Luciani, A.; Zafrani, E.S.; Bioulac-Sage, P.; et al. Inflammatory hepatocellular adenomas developed in the setting of chronic liver disease and cirrhosis. *Mod. Pathol.* **2016**, *29*, 43–50. [CrossRef]
60. Dufva, O.; Kankainen, M.; Kelkka, T.; Sekiguchi, N.; Awad, S.A.; Eldfors, S.; Yadav, B.; Kuusanmäki, H.; Malani, D.; Andersson, E.I.; et al. Aggressive natural killer-cell leukemia mutational landscape and drug profiling highlight JAK-STAT signaling as therapeutic target. *Nat. Commun.* **2018**, *9*, 1567. [CrossRef]
61. Kataoka, K.; Nagata, Y.; Kitanaka, A.; Shiraishi, Y.; Shimamura, T.; Yasunaga, J.-I.; Totoki, Y.; Chiba, K.; Sato-Otsubo, A.; Nagae, G.; et al. Integrated molecular analysis of adult T cell leukemia/lymphoma. *Nat. Genet.* **2015**, *47*, 1304–1315. [CrossRef] [PubMed]
62. Kiel, M.J.; Sahasrabuddhe, A.A.; Rolland, D.C.M.; Velusamy, T.; Chung, F.; Schaller, M.; Bailey, N.G.; Betz, B.L.; Miranda, R.N.; Porcu, P.; et al. Genomic analyses reveal recurrent mutations in epigenetic modifiers and the JAK–STAT pathway in Sézary syndrome. *Nat. Commun.* **2015**, *6*, 8470. [CrossRef] [PubMed]
63. Ishida, F.; Matsuda, K.; Sekiguchi, N.; Makishima, H.; Taira, C.; Momose, K.; Nishina, S.; Senoo, N.; Sakai, H.; Ito, T.; et al. STAT3 gene mutations and their association with pure red cell aplasia in large granular lymphocyte leukemia. *Cancer Sci.* **2014**, *105*, 342–346. [CrossRef] [PubMed]
64. Bergmann, A.K.; Fataccioli, V.; Castellano, G.; Martin-Garcia, N.; Pelletier, L.; Ammerpohl, O.; Bergmann, J.; Bhat, J.; Pau, E.C.; Martín-Subero, J.I.; et al. DNA methylation profiling of hepatosplenic t-cell lymphoma. *Haematologica* **2019**, *104*, e104–e107. [CrossRef] [PubMed]
65. Koskela, H.L.M.; Eldfors, S.; Ellonen, P.; van Adrichem, A.J.; Kuusanmäki, H.; Andersson, E.I.; Lagström, S.; Clemente, M.J.; Olson, T.; Jalkanen, S.E.; et al. Somatic STAT3 mutations in large granular lymphocytic leukemia. *N. Engl. J. Med.* **2012**, *366*, 1905–1913. [CrossRef] [PubMed]
66. Pilati, C.; Amessou, M.; Bihl, M.P.; Balabaud, C.; Van Nhieu, J.T.; Paradis, V.; Nault, J.C.; Izard, T.; Bioulac-Sage, P.; Couchy, G.; et al. Somatic mutations activating STAT3 in human inflammatory hepatocellular adenomas. *J. Exp. Med.* **2011**, *208*, 1359–1366. [CrossRef]
67. Jerez, A.; Clemente, M.J.; Makishima, H.; Koskela, H.; Leblanc, F.; Ng, K.P.; Olson, T.; Przychodzen, B.; Afable, M.; Gomez-Segui, I.; et al. STAT3 mutations unify the pathogenesis of chronic lymphoproliferative disorders of NK cells and T-cell large granular lymphocyte leukemia. *Blood* **2012**, *120*, 3048–3057. [CrossRef]
68. Ohgami, R.S.; Ma, L.; Merker, J.D.; Martinez, B.; Zehnder, J.L.; Arber, D.A. STAT3 mutations are frequent in CD30+ T-cell lymphomas and T-cell large granular lymphocytic leukemia. *Leukemia* **2013**, *27*, 2244–2247. [CrossRef]
69. Nicolae, A.; Xi, L.; Pittaluga, S.; Abdullaev, Z.; Pack, S.D.; Chen, J.; Waldmann, T.A.; Jaffe, E.S.; Raffeld, M. Frequent STAT5B mutations in $\gamma\delta$ hepatosplenic T-cell lymphomas. *Leuk.* **2014**, *28*, 2244–2248. [CrossRef]
70. Ma, C.S.; Chew, G.Y.; Simpson, N.; Priyadarshi, A.; Wong, M.; Grimbacher, B.; Fulcher, D.A.; Tangye, S.G.; Cook, M.C. Deficiency of Th17 cells in hyper IgE syndrome due to mutations in STAT3. *J. Exp. Med.* **2008**, *205*, 1551–1557. [CrossRef]
71. Flanagan, S.E.; Haapaniemi, E.; Russell, M.A.; Caswell, R.; Allen, H.L.; De Franco, E.; McDonald, T.J.; Rajala, H.; Ramelius, A.; Barton, J.; et al. Activating germline mutations in STAT3 cause early-onset multi-organ autoimmune disease. *Nat. Genet.* **2014**, *46*, 812–814. [CrossRef] [PubMed]
72. Fasan, A.; Kern, W.; Grossmann, V.; Haferlach, C.; Haferlach, T.; Schnittger, S. STAT3 mutations are highly specific for large granular lymphocytic leukemia. *Leukemia* **2013**, *27*, 1598–1600. [CrossRef] [PubMed]
73. Kim, M.S.; Lee, S.H.; Yoo, N.J.; Lee, S.H. STAT3 exon 21 mutation is rare in common human cancers. *Acta Oncol.* **2013**, *52*, 1221–1222. [CrossRef] [PubMed]

74. Liu, J.Y.; Li, Q.; Chen, T.T.; Guo, X.; Ge, J.; Yuan, L.X. Destructive pulmonary staphylococcal infection in a boy with hyper-IgE syndrome: A novel mutation in the signal transducer and activator of transcription 3 (STAT3) gene (p.Y657S). *Eur. J. Pediatr.* **2011**, *170*, 661–666. [CrossRef]
75. Milner, J.D.; Vogel, T.P.; Forbes, L.; Ma, C.A.; Stray-Pedersen, A.; Niemela, J.E.; Lyons, J.J.; Engelhardt, K.R.; Zhang, Y.; Topcagic, N.; et al. Early-onset lymphoproliferation and autoimmunity caused by germline STAT3 gain-of-function mutations. *Blood* **2015**, *125*, 591–599. [CrossRef]
76. Saikia, B.; Goel, S.; Suri, D.; Minz, R.W.; Rawat, A.; Singh, S. Novel Mutation in SH2 Domain of STAT3 (p.M660T) in Hyper-IgE Syndrome with Sterno-Clavicular and Paravertebral Abscesses. *Indian J. Pediatr.* **2017**, *203*, 244–495. [CrossRef]
77. Teramo, A.; Barila, G.; Calabretto, G.; Ercolin, C.; Lamy, T.; Moignet, A.; Roussel, M.; Pastoret, C.; Leoncin, M.; Gattazzo, C.; et al. STAT3 mutation impacts biological and clinical features of T-LGL leukemia. *Oncotarget* **2017**, *8*, 61876–61889. [CrossRef]
78. Crescenzo, R.; Abate, F.; Lasorsa, E.; Tabbo', F.; Gaudiano, M.; Chiesa, N.; Di Giacomo, F.; Spaccarotella, E.; Barbarossa, L.; Ercole, E.; et al. Convergent mutations and kinase fusions lead to oncogenic STAT3 activation in anaplastic large cell lymphoma. *Cancer Cell* **2015**, *27*, 516–532. [CrossRef]
79. Iwanaga, E.; Nakamura, M.; Nanri, T.; Kawakita, T.; Horikawa, K.; Mitsuya, H.; Asou, N. Acute promyelocytic leukemia harboring a STAT5B-RARA fusion gene and a G596V missense mutation in the STAT5B SH2 domain of the STAT5B-RARA. *Eur. J. Haematol.* **2009**, *83*, 499–501. [CrossRef]
80. Kiel, M.J.; Velusamy, T.; Rolland, D.; Sahasrabuddhe, A.A.; Chung, F.; Bailey, N.G.; Schrader, A.; Li, B.; Li, J.Z.; Ozel, A.B.; et al. Integrated genomic sequencing reveals mutational landscape of T-cell prolymphocytic leukemia. *Blood* **2014**, *124*, 1460–1472. [CrossRef]
81. Roberti, A.; Dobay, M.P.; Bisig, B.; Vallois, D.; Boéchat, C.; Lanitis, E.; Bouchindhomme, B.; Parrens, M.-C.; Bossard, C.; Quintanilla-Martinez, L.; et al. Type II enteropathy-associated T-cell lymphoma features a unique genomic profile with highly recurrent SETD2 alterations. *Nat. Commun.* **2016**, *7*, 12602–12613. [CrossRef] [PubMed]
82. Chia, D.J.; Subbian, E.; Buck, T.M.; Hwa, V.; Rosenfeld, R.G.; Skach, W.R.; Shinde, U.; Rotwein, P. Aberrant folding of a mutant Stat5b causes growth hormone insensitivity and proteasomal dysfunction. *J. Biol. Chem.* **2006**, *281*, 6552–6558. [CrossRef] [PubMed]
83. Schrader, A.; Crispatzu, G.; Oberbeck, S.; Mayer, P.; Pützer, S.; Von Jan, J.; Vasyutina, E.; Warner, K.; Weit, N.; Pflug, N.; et al. Actionable perturbations of damage responses by TCL1/ATM and epigenetic lesions form the basis of T-PLL. *Nat. Commun.* **2018**, *9*, 697. [CrossRef] [PubMed]
84. Rajala, H.L.M.; Eldfors, S.; Kuusanmäki, H.; Van Adrichem, A.J.; Olson, T.; Lagström, S.; Andersson, E.I.; Jerez, A.; Clemente, M.J.; Yan, Y.; et al. Discovery of somatic STAT5b mutations in large granular lymphocytic leukemia. *Blood* **2013**, *121*, 4541–4550. [CrossRef] [PubMed]
85. Babushok, D.V.; Perdigones, N.; Perin, J.C.; Olson, T.S.; Ye, W.; Roth, J.J.; Lind, C.; Cattier, C.; Li, Y.; Hartung, H.; et al. Emergence of clonal hematopoiesis in the majority of patients with acquired aplastic anemia. *Cancer Genet.* **2015**, *208*, 115–128. [CrossRef]
86. Lopez, C.; Bergmann, A.K.; Paul, U.; Penas, E.M.M.; Nagel, I.; Betts, M.; Johansson, P.; Ritgen, M.; Baumann, T.; Aymerich, M.; et al. Genes encoding members of the JAK-STAT pathway or epigenetic regulators are recurrently mutated in T-cell prolymphocytic leukaemia. *Br. J. Haematol.* **2016**, *173*, 265–273. [CrossRef]
87. Andersson, E.I.; Tanahashi, T.; Sekiguchi, N.; Gasparini, V.R.; Bortoluzzi, S.; Kawakami, T.; Matsuda, K.; Mitsui, T.; Eldfors, S.; Bortoluzzi, S.; et al. High incidence of activating STAT5B mutations in CD4-positive T-cell large granular lymphocyte leukemia. *Blood* **2016**, *128*, 2465–2468. [CrossRef]
88. Andersson, E.I.; Pützer, S.; Yadav, B.; Dufva, O.; Khan, S.; He, L.; Sellner, L.; Schrader, A.; Crispatzu, G.; Oleś, M.; et al. Discovery of novel drug sensitivities in T-PLL by high-throughput ex vivo drug testing and mutation profiling. *Leukemia* **2018**, *32*, 774–787. [CrossRef]
89. Bandapalli, O.R.; Schuessele, S.; Kunz, J.B.; Rausch, T.; Stütz, A.M.; Tal, N.; Geron, I.; Gershman, N.; Izraeli, S.; Eilers, J.; et al. The activating STAT5B N642H mutation is a common abnormality in pediatric T-cell acute lymphoblastic leukemia and confers a higher risk of relapse. *Haematol.* **2014**, *99*, e188–e192. [CrossRef]
90. Atak, Z.K.; Gianfelici, V.; Hulselmans, G.; De Keersmaecker, K.; Devasia, A.G.; Geerdens, E.; Mentens, N.;

Chiaretti, S.; Durinck, K.; Uyttebroeck, A.; et al. Comprehensive Analysis of Transcriptome Variation Uncovers Known and Novel Driver Events in T-Cell Acute Lymphoblastic Leukemia. *PLoS Genet.* **2013**, *9*, e1003997.

91. Nairismägi, M.-L.; Tan, J.; Lim, J.Q.; Nagarajan, S.; Ng, C.C.Y.; Rajasegaran, V.; Huang, D.; Lim, W.K.; Laurensia, Y.; Wijaya, G.C.; et al. JAK-STAT and G-protein-coupled receptor signaling pathways are frequently altered in epitheliotropic intestinal T-cell lymphoma. *Leuk.* **2016**, *30*, 1311–1319. [CrossRef] [PubMed]
92. Lavallée, V.-P.; Krošl, J.; Lemieux, S.; Boucher, G.; Gendron, P.; Pabst, C.; Boivin, I.; Marinier, A.; Guidos, C.J.; Meloche, S.; et al. Chemo-genomic interrogation of CEBPA mutated AML reveals recurrent CSF3R mutations and subgroup sensitivity to JAK inhibitors. *Blood* **2016**, *127*, 3054–3061. [CrossRef] [PubMed]
93. Luo, Q.; Shen, J.; Yang, Y.; Tang, H.; Shi, M.; Liu, J.; Liu, Z.; Shi, X.; Yi, Y. CSF3R T618I, ASXL1 G942 fs and STAT5B N642H trimutation co-contribute to a rare chronic neutrophilic leukaemia manifested by rapidly progressive leucocytosis, severe infections, persistent fever and deep venous thrombosis. *Br. J. Haematol.* **2018**, *180*, 892–894. [CrossRef] [PubMed]
94. Prasad, A.; Rabionet, R.; Espinet, B.; Zapata, L.; Puiggros, A.; Melero, C.; Puig, A.; Sarria-Trujillo, Y.; Ossowski, S.; García-Muret, M.P.; et al. Identification of Gene Mutations and Fusion Genes in Patients with Sézary Syndrome. *J. Investig. Dermatol.* **2016**, *136*, 1490–1499. [CrossRef]
95. Ma, X.; Wen, L.; Wu, L.; Wang, Q.; Yao, H.; Wang, Q.; Ma, L.; Chen, S. Rare occurrence of a STAT5B N642H mutation in adult T-cell acute lymphoblastic leukemia. *Cancer Genet.* **2015**, *208*, 52–53. [CrossRef]
96. Cross, N.C.P.; Hoade, Y.; Tapper, W.J.; Carreno-Tarragona, G.; Fanelli, T.; Jawhar, M.; Naumann, N.; Pieniak, I.; Lübke, J.; Ali, S.; et al. Recurrent activating STAT5B N642H mutation in myeloid neoplasms with eosinophilia. *Leukemia* **2019**, *33*, 415–425. [CrossRef]
97. Ma, C.A.; Xi, L.; Cauff, B.; DeZure, A.; Freeman, A.F.; Hambleton, S.; Kleiner, G.; Leahy, T.R.; O'Sullivan, M.; Makiya, M.; et al. Somatic STAT5b gain-of-function mutations in early onset nonclonal eosinophilia, urticaria, dermatitis, and diarrhea. *Blood* **2017**, *129*, 650–653. [CrossRef]
98. Baer, C.; Muehlbacher, V.; Kern, W.; Haferlach, C.; Haferlach, T. Molecular genetic characterization of myeloid/lymphoid neoplasms associated with eosinophilia and rearrangement of PDGFRA, PDGFRB, FGFR1 or PCM1-JAK2. *Haematol.* **2018**, *103*, e348–e350. [CrossRef]
99. Simpson, H.M.; Khan, R.Z.; Song, C.; Sharma, D.; Sadashivaiah, K.; Furusawa, A.; Liu, X.; Nagaraj, S.; Sengamalay, N.; Sadzewicz, L.; et al. Concurrent Mutations in ATM and Genes Associated with Common γ Chain Signaling in Peripheral T Cell Lymphoma. *PLoS ONE* **2015**, *10*, e0141906. [CrossRef]
100. Jiang, L.; Gu, Z.-H.; Yan, Z.-X.; Zhao, X.; Xie, Y.-Y.; Zhang, Z.-G.; Pan, C.-M.; Hu, Y.; Cai, C.-P.; Dong, Y.; et al. Exome sequencing identifies somatic mutations of DDX3X in natural killer/T-cell lymphoma. *Nat. Genet.* **2015**, *47*, 1061–1066. [CrossRef]
101. Kontro, M.; Kuusanmäki, H.; Eldfors, S.; Burmeister, T.; Andersson, E.I.; Bruserud, O.; Brümmendorf, T.H.; Edgren, H.; Gjertsen, B.T.; Itälä-Remes, M.; et al. Novel activating STAT5B mutations as putative drivers of T-cell acute lymphoblastic leukemia. *Leukemia* **2014**, *28*, 1738–1742. [CrossRef] [PubMed]
102. Menon, M.P.; Nicolae, A.; Meeker, H.; Raffeld, M.; Xi, L.; Jegalian, A.G.; Miller, D.C.; Pittaluga, S.; Jaffe, E.S. Primary CNS T-cell Lymphomas: A Clinical, Morphologic, Immunophenotypic, and Molecular Analysis. *Am. J. Surg. Pathol.* **2015**, *39*, 1719–1729. [CrossRef] [PubMed]
103. Varco-Merth, B.; Feigerlová, E.; Shinde, U.; Rosenfeld, R.G.; Hwa, V.; Rotwein, P. Severe growth deficiency is associated with STAT5b mutations that disrupt protein folding and activity. *Mol. Endocrinol.* **2013**, *27*, 150–161. [CrossRef] [PubMed]
104. Hwa, V. STAT5B deficiency: Impacts on human growth and immunity. *Growth Horm. IGF Res.* **2016**, *28*, 16–20. [CrossRef]
105. Cui, Y.; Riedlinger, G.; Miyoshi, K.; Tang, W.; Li, C.; Deng, C.-X.; Robinson, G.W.; Hennighausen, L. Inactivation of Stat5 in Mouse Mammary Epithelium during Pregnancy Reveals Distinct Functions in Cell Proliferation, Survival, and Differentiation. *Mol. Cell. Boil.* **2004**, *24*, 8037–8047. [CrossRef]
106. Hoelbl, A.; Kovacic, B.; Kerenyi, M.A.; Simma, O.; Warsch, W.; Cui, Y.; Beug, H.; Hennighausen, L.; Moriggl, R.; Sexl, V. Clarifying the role of Stat5 in lymphoid development and Abelson-induced transformation. *Blood* **2006**, *107*, 4898–4906. [CrossRef]

107. Klammt, J.; Neumann, D.; Gevers, E.F.; Andrew, S.F.; Schwartz, I.D.; Rockstroh, D.; Colombo, R.; Sanchez, M.A.; Vokurkova, D.; Kowalczyk, J.; et al. Dominant-negative STAT5B mutations cause growth hormone insensitivity with short stature and mild immune dysregulation. *Nat. Commun.* **2018**, *9*, 2105. [CrossRef]
108. Kanai, T.; Jenks, J.; Nadeau, K.C. The STAT5b Pathway Defect and Autoimmunity. *Front. Immunol.* **2012**, *3*, 3. [CrossRef]
109. Sallmyr, A.; Fan, J.; Datta, K.; Kim, K.-T.; Grosu, D.; Shapiro, P.; Small, D.; Rassool, F. Internal tandem duplication of FLT3 (FLT3/ITD) induces increased ROS production, DNA damage, and misrepair: Implications for poor prognosis in AML. *Blood* **2008**, *111*, 3173–3182. [CrossRef]
110. Warsch, W.; Kollmann, K.; Eckelhart, E.; Fajmann, S.; Cerny-Reiterer, S.; Hölbl, A.; Gleixner, K.V.; Dworzak, M.; Mayerhofer, M.; Hoermann, G.; et al. High STAT5 levels mediate imatinib resistance and indicate disease progression in chronic myeloid leukemia. *Blood* **2011**, *117*, 3409–3420. [CrossRef]
111. Ribeiro, D.; Melão, A.; Van Boxtel, R.; Santos, C.I.; Silva, A.; Silva, M.C.; Cardoso, B.A.; Coffer, P.J.; Barata, J.T. STAT5 is essential for IL-7–mediated viability, growth, and proliferation of T-cell acute lymphoblastic leukemia cells. *Blood Adv.* **2018**, *2*, 2199–2213. [CrossRef] [PubMed]
112. Wang, Z.; Bunting, K.D. STAT5 activation in B-cell acute lymphoblastic leukemia: Damned if you do, damned if you don't. *Cancer Cell Microenviron.* **2016**, *3*, 1186.
113. Chiorazzi, N. Cell proliferation and death: Forgotten features of chronic lymphocytic leukemia B cells. *Best Pr. Res. Clin. Haematol.* **2007**, *20*, 399–413. [CrossRef] [PubMed]
114. Rajala, H.L.M.; Mustjoki, S. STAT5b in LGL leukemia—A novel therapeutic target? *Oncotarget* **2013**, *4*, 808–809. [CrossRef]
115. Mitchell, T.J.; Whittaker, S.J.; John, S. Dysregulated expression of COOH-terminally truncated Stat5 and loss of IL2-inducible Stat5-dependent gene expression in Sezary Syndrome. *Cancer Res.* **2003**, *63*, 9048–9054.
116. Zhang, Q.; Wang, H.Y.; Liu, X.; A Wasik, M. STAT5A is epigenetically silenced by the tyrosine kinase NPM1-ALK and acts as a tumor suppressor by reciprocally inhibiting NPM1-ALK expression. *Nat. Med.* **2007**, *13*, 1341–1348. [CrossRef]
117. Kollmann, S.; Grundschober, E.; Maurer, B.; Warsch, W.; Grausenburger, R.; Edlinger, L.; Huuhtanen, J.; Lagger, S.; Hennighausen, L.; Valent, P.; et al. Twins with different personalities: STAT5B-but not STAT5A-has a key role in BCR/ABL-induced leukemia. *Leuk.* **2019**, *33*, 1583–1597. [CrossRef]
118. He, J.; Shi, J.; Xu, X.; Zhang, W.; Wang, Y.; Chen, X.; Du, Y.; Zhu, N.; Zhang, J.; Wang, Q.; et al. STAT3 mutations correlated with hyper-IgE syndrome lead to blockage of IL-6/STAT3 signalling pathway. *J. Biosci.* **2012**, *37*, 243–257. [CrossRef]
119. Pham, H.T.T.; Maurer, B.; Prchal-Murphy, M.; Grausenburger, R.; Grundschober, E.; Javaheri, T.; Nivarthi, H.; Boersma, A.; Kolbe, T.; Elabd, M.; et al. STAT5B N642H is a driver mutation for T cell neoplasia. *J. Clin. Investig.* **2018**, *128*, 387–401. [CrossRef]
120. De Araujo, E.D.; Manaswiyoungkul, P.; Israelian, J.; Park, J.; Yuen, K.; Farhangi, S.; Berger-Becvar, A.; Abu-Jazar, L.; Gunning, P.T. High-throughput thermofluor-based assays for inhibitor screening of STAT SH2 domains. *J. Pharm. Biomed. Anal.* **2017**, *143*, 159–167. [CrossRef]
121. Kofoed, E.M.; Hwa, V.; Woods, K.A.; Buckway, C.K.; Tsubaki, J.; Pratt, K.L.; Bezrodnik, L.; Tepper, A.; Little, B.; Jasper, H.; et al. Growth Hormone Insensitivity Associated with aSTAT5bMutation. *New Engl. J. Med.* **2003**, *349*, 1139–1147. [CrossRef] [PubMed]
122. Bocchini, C.E.; Nahmod, K.; Katsonis, P.; Kim, S.; Kasembeli, M.M.; Freeman, A.; Lichtarge, O.; Makedonas, G.; Tweardy, D.J. Protein stabilization improves STAT3 function in autosomal dominant hyper-IgE syndrome. *Blood* **2016**, *128*, 3061–3072. [CrossRef] [PubMed]
123. Brambilla, L.; Genini, D.; Laurini, E.; Merulla, J.; Perez, L.; Fermeglia, M.; Carbone, G.M.; Pricl, S.; Catapano, C.V. Hitting the right spot: Mechanism of action of OPB-31121, a novel and potent inhibitor of the Signal Transducer and Activator of Transcription 3 (STAT3). *Mol. Oncol.* **2015**, *9*, 1194–1206. [CrossRef] [PubMed]
124. Chandrasekaran, P.; Zimmerman, O.; Paulson, M.; Sampaio, E.P.; Freeman, A.F.; Sowerwine, K.J.; Hurt, D.; Alcántara-Montiel, J.C.; Hsu, A.P.; Holland, S.M. Distinct mutations at the same positions of STAT3 cause either loss or gain of function. *J. Allergy Clin. Immunol.* **2016**, *138*, 1222–1224. [CrossRef] [PubMed]

125. Avvisati, G.; Tallman, M.S. All-trans retinoic acid in acute promyelocytic leukaemia. *Best Pr. Res. Clin. Haematol.* **2003**, *16*, 419–432. [CrossRef]

126. Yao, L.; Wen, L.; Wang, N.; Liu, T.; Xu, Y.; Ruan, C.; Wu, D.; Chen, S. Identification of novel recurrent STAT3-RARA fusions in acute promyelocytic leukemia lacking t(15;17)(q22;q12)/PML-RARA. *Blood* **2018**, *131*, 935–939. [CrossRef] [PubMed]

3

Targeting STAT3 and STAT5 in Tumor-Associated Immune Cells to Improve Immunotherapy

Grégory Verdeil [1], Toby Lawrence [2,3], Anne-Marie Schmitt-Verhulst [2] and Nathalie Auphan-Anezin [2,*]

1 Laboratory Regulation of immune dysfunction in cancer, Department of Oncology, University of Lausanne, CH-1066 Epalinges, Switzerland; gregory.verdeil@unil.ch

2 Aix Marseille University, Centre National de la Recherche Scientifique (CNRS) UMR7280, Institut National de la Santé et de la Recherche Médicale (INSERM) U1104, Centre Immunologie Marseille-Luminy (CIML), Parc Scientifique de Luminy, Case 906, 13288 Marseille CEDEX 09, France; lawrence@ciml.univ-mrs.fr (T.L.); amsverhulst@gmail.com (A.-M.S.-V.)

3 Centre for Inflammation Biology and Cancer Immunology, School of Immunology & Microbial Sciences, Faculty of Life Sciences and Medicine, King's College London, London SE1 1UL, UK

* Correspondence: auphan@ciml.univ-mrs.fr

Abstract: Oncogene-induced STAT3-activation is central to tumor progression by promoting cancer cell expression of pro-angiogenic and immunosuppressive factors. STAT3 is also activated in infiltrating immune cells including tumor-associated macrophages (TAM) amplifying immune suppression. Consequently, STAT3 is considered as a target for cancer therapy. However, its interplay with other STAT-family members or transcription factors such as NF-κB has to be considered in light of their concerted regulation of immune-related genes. Here, we discuss new attempts at re-educating immune suppressive tumor-associated macrophages towards a CD8 T cell supporting profile, with an emphasis on the role of STAT transcription factors on TAM functional programs. Recent clinical trials using JAK/STAT inhibitors highlighted the negative effects of these molecules on the maintenance and function of effector/memory T cells. Concerted regulation of STAT3 and STAT5 activation in CD8 T effector and memory cells has been shown to impact their tumor-specific responses including intra-tumor accumulation, long-term survival, cytotoxic activity and resistance toward tumor-derived immune suppression. Interestingly, as an escape mechanism, melanoma cells were reported to impede STAT5 nuclear translocation in both CD8 T cells and NK cells. Ours and others results will be discussed in the perspective of new developments in engineered T cell-based adoptive therapies to treat cancer patients.

Keywords: inflammation; tumor-associated macrophages; adoptive T cell therapy; immune suppression; STAT transcription factors

---

1. Introduction

Inflammation is now considered as a hallmark of cancer [1] and the inflammatory context in many cancers is strongly linked to poor prognosis and resistance to therapy. Activating mutations in oncogenic RAS/BRAF/MEK pathways trigger a tumor-intrinsic inflammatory network with the concerted regulation of master transcription factors (TFs) including STAT3 [2], NF-κB and AP-1 [3,4] which in turn trigger the expression of cytokines, including IL-6, IL-1, IL-10, TNF and VEGF [5]. The presence of cytokines is a major regulator of immune cell differentiation/function and is a crucial factor to consider for immunotherapy protocols. Many of these cytokines signal through the stimulation of STAT TFs. In this review, we will comment on the role of STAT TFs (i) for the recruitment and function of tumor-associated macrophages (TAM) and (ii) for the regulation of T cell functions. As STAT

TFs are key players in the regulation of functions of these immune cells, their manipulation can have a beneficial or detrimental effect on the anti-tumor response depending on the targeted cell type.

2. Tumor-Induced Inflammation Drives Accumulation of Tumor-Infiltrating Myeloid Cells

Cytokine receptor-induced signaling sustains and amplifies the activation of STAT3, NF-κB and AP-1 in a positive amplification loop, fueling tumor-associated inflammation. As such, a core inflammation-related gene set regulated by STAT3, NF-κB and AP-1 has recently been proposed as an "inflammatory index" in breast cancer cell lines and patient samples [4]. Importantly, in correlation with this inflammatory index, this study reported a concerted regulation of (i) non-inflammatory genes related to angiogenesis, metastasis, and cell proliferation; (ii) tumor genome instability; and (iii) heterogeneity of the tumor microenvironment (TME), including the recruited immune cells. Remarkably, these co-regulated characteristics were found across several cancer types driven by distinct oncogenes [4].

Tumor-derived cytokines have been linked to the accumulation of immune-suppressive myeloid cells including both myeloid-derived suppressor cells (MDSCs; IMCs) and tumor-associated macrophages (TAM). In both human and mouse melanomas, IMCs have an important role in malignant progression and evasion from anti-tumor immunity that is linked to the suppression of T cell responses [6–9]. While increased TAM accumulation has been ascribed to a poor prognosis in established tumors [10], this notion should be refined given the extreme phenotypic and functional heterogeneity of these cells during tumor growth.

Cancer-related inflammation (i) promotes the recruitment of monocyte-derived cells into the tumor bed and (ii) acts systemically as shown by the dysregulated transcriptomic signature of circulating monocytes in breast cancer patients as compared to healthy controls [11]. Numerous therapeutic attempts (reviewed in [12]) to block cytokine-induced monocyte recruitment are under clinical trials using either blocking mAbs (anti-CCR2; anti-CSF1R) or small inhibitors for downstream cytokine receptor signaling (receptor tyrosine kinase inhibitor, Pexidartinib; CSF1R inhibitor, PLX3397).

Once recruited to the tumor, monocyte progenitors (CD11b$^+$ SiglecF$^-$ Ly-6G$^-$Ly6C$^+$ F4/80$^-$ CD169$^-$ MHC-II$^-$) undergo a multistep differentiation program [13,14], passing through an immature stage (Ly6C$^+$ F4/80$^-$ CD169^{int} MHC-II^{hi}) before reaching a mature state (Ly6C$^-$ F4/80$^+$ CD169^{hi} MHC-II$^{hi\ or\ low}$). Recently, the heterogeneity of TAM in several cancer types has been emphasized by single-cell RNA-sequencing paired with mass cytometry, including lung [15], kidney [16], breast and endometrial cancers [11], as well as in mouse sarcoma [17]. In the case of renal cell carcinoma, 17 TAM subsets have been characterized [16], most of them expressing CD169 while being discriminated by expression of CD163, CD204 and CD206. Of note, when compared to steady-state tissue-resident macrophages or monocytes, TAM exhibited peculiar gene expression profiles [11,16], highlighting a tumor-induced dysregulation.

There is compelling evidence for high levels of phenotypic plasticity in macrophages, exhibiting differential functional programs depending on their surrounding microenvironment. In response to microbial stimuli pro-inflammatory macrophages—often referred to as of "M1-type" - express cytokines supporting T cell activation. However, in malignancies, alternatively activated macrophages - referred as of "M2-type"-secrete cytokines that sustain tumor growth and exert immune suppressive functions. Therefore, differential signal transduction pathways downstream of cell surface sensors define gene expression programs underlying anti- or pro- tumor functions of macrophages [18,19]. As such, IFNγ stimulates STAT1/STAT2 and IRF1/8, which can further promote pro-inflammatory macrophages. While GM-CSF/STAT5 activates a pro-inflammatory signature in monocytes [20], it rather induces a unique reparative program in macrophages after sterile renal injury [21]. Tumor-induced inflammation involving the IL-6/gp130/STAT3 [22] and ERK5/STAT3 [23] axes was shown to drive a pro-tumor transcriptomic program. Additionally, we recently showed that ovarian cancer cells reprogram macrophages towards an IL-4/AKT/STAT6-mediated tumor-promoting phenotype through increased cholesterol efflux from the TAM membrane [24]. Moreover, IL-6 synergizes with IL-4 in the programming of human monocyte-derived macrophages through the concerted activation of STAT6 and STAT3 DNA-binding activities [25]. Given the spectrum of STAT3-regulated genes in TAM encoding pro-tumor and immune suppressive mediators (Table 1), STAT3-modulators are currently being developed to dampen the cancer supportive functions of TAM, as reported in this issue by Rébé and Ghiringhelli [26]. As such, the specific targeting of a highly immune suppressive TAM (CD11b+ CD163+) subset by liposome-encapsulated STAT3-inhibitors showed some success in reprogramming TAM towards a pro-inflammatory profile [27].

Table 1. STAT3–regulated genes in tumor-associated macrophages (TAM).

Target Genes	STAT3 Input	Cancer Type	TAM Phenotype
		Cytokines/Cytokine receptors	
Il10 *	positive	m-melanoma	CD11b+ [28]
		m-PDAC	CD68+, IL-10Ra+ [29]
Il23a *	positive	m-melanoma	CD11b+ CD11c− [30]
Il10ra, Il4ra	positive	m-PDAC	CD68+, IL-10Ra+ [29]
Tgfb1 *	positive	m-melanoma	CD11b+ CD11c− [30]
Il12a	negative	m-melanoma	CD11b+ [28]; CD11b+ CD11c− [30]
Ifng	negative	m-melanoma	CD11b+ [28]
		Chemokines/Chemokine Receptors	
Ccl5, Cxcl9-10-11	Negative	m-melanoma	CD11b+ [28]
Cxcl2, Cxcl12	positive	m-melanoma	BMDM+Tumor conditioned media [31] MDSC: CD11b+ GR1+ CD11c− [22]
		Scavenger receptors/Endocytosis	
Mrc1 (CD206)	positive	m-breast	CD11b+ Ly-6C^{lo} F4/80^{hi} CD24^{lo} MHC-II^{lo} [32]
		h-gastric	CD163+ CD209a+ [33]
CD163	positive	h-SCC	ERK5+ CD163+ [23]
		m-PDAC	CD68+, IL-10Ra+ [29]
Cd209a	positive	m-PDAC	CD68+, IL-10Ra+ [29]
		Immune suppression	
Arg1	positive	m-PDAC; h-PDAC	CD68+, IL-10Ra+ [29]; blood CD14+ [34]
Cox2	positive	m-melanoma	BMDM + Tumor conditioned media [31]
Ido1	positive	m-liver metastasis	liver-MDSC: CD11b+ Ly-6C$^{int/hi}$ Ly-6G^{+} [35]
		h- & m-glioma	h-CD68+; m-CD11b+ CD115+ [36]
Pdl1 (CD274)	positive	h-breast	CD163+ [37]
		m-liver metastasis	liver-MDSC: CD11b+ Ly-6C$^{int/hi}$ Ly-6G^{+} [35]
		Extra-cellular Matrix/Angiogenesis	
Mmp2	positive	m-melanoma	BMDM + Tumor conditioned media [31]
Vegf	positive	m-melanoma	CD11b+ [28]; MDSC: CD11b+ GR1+ CD11c- [22]
Cathepsin (B, L)	positive	m-PDAC	CD68+, IL-10Ra+ [29]
		Cell cycle/TFs	
Ccnd1	positive	m-melanoma	BMDM + Tumor conditioned media [31]
ATF6, sXBP1	positive	m-PDAC	CD68+, IL-10Ra+ [29]

* Immune suppressive cytokines.

3. Re-Educating TAM to Restore Anti-Tumor T Cell Functions.

Extensive studies are being conducted to reprogram pro-tumoral TAM towards an inflammatory T cell supporting profile (recently reviewed in [38]). Mature TAM exert both trophic functions—through the promotion of angiogenesis and tissue remodeling—and immune regulatory functions. Here we will focus on the immune aspects of TAM functions, even though these two activities might be closely inter-connected. Indeed, prolonged interactions between stromal TAM (mainly CD163^{+} CD206^{+}) and CD8 tumor-infiltrating lymphocytes (TILs) observed by dynamic imaging microscopy, are limiting CD8 T cell motility and their consecutive access to both human lung squamous cell carcinomas and mouse MMTV-PyMT tumors [39].

Recent parallel analyses of TAM and TILs from cancer patients have greatly expanded our knowledge on the reciprocal regulation of these cell lineages. Paired CyTOF-based analyses of CD8 TILs and TAM in human renal cell carcinomas [16] showed some correlation between exhausted CD8 TILs, CD4 regulatory T cells and a few peculiar TAM subpopulations (either CD169^{-} CD163^{-} CD68^{hi}

CD38^{hi} CD204^{+}; or CD169^{+} CD163^{+} CD68^{hi} CD38^{hi} CD204^{+} CD206^{+}). These molecular data had been further correlated with clinical features, with the result that patients with the former TIL/TAM subsets showed increased cancer progression.

We recently reported [13] that a subset of mature CD163^{+} TAM present in mouse melanomas, exhibit transcripts related to T cell immune suppression. Interestingly, a high proportion of CD163^{+} macrophages expressing phospho-STAT3 have been observed in human skin tumors [23]. Targeted-depletion of this minor CD163^{+} TAM subset enhanced melanoma-infiltration by CD8 T cells and promoted CD8 T cell-mediated tumor regression in mice [13]; this was also accompanied by the recruitment of fresh monocytes and immature macrophages with an immune stimulatory phenotype (Figure 1).

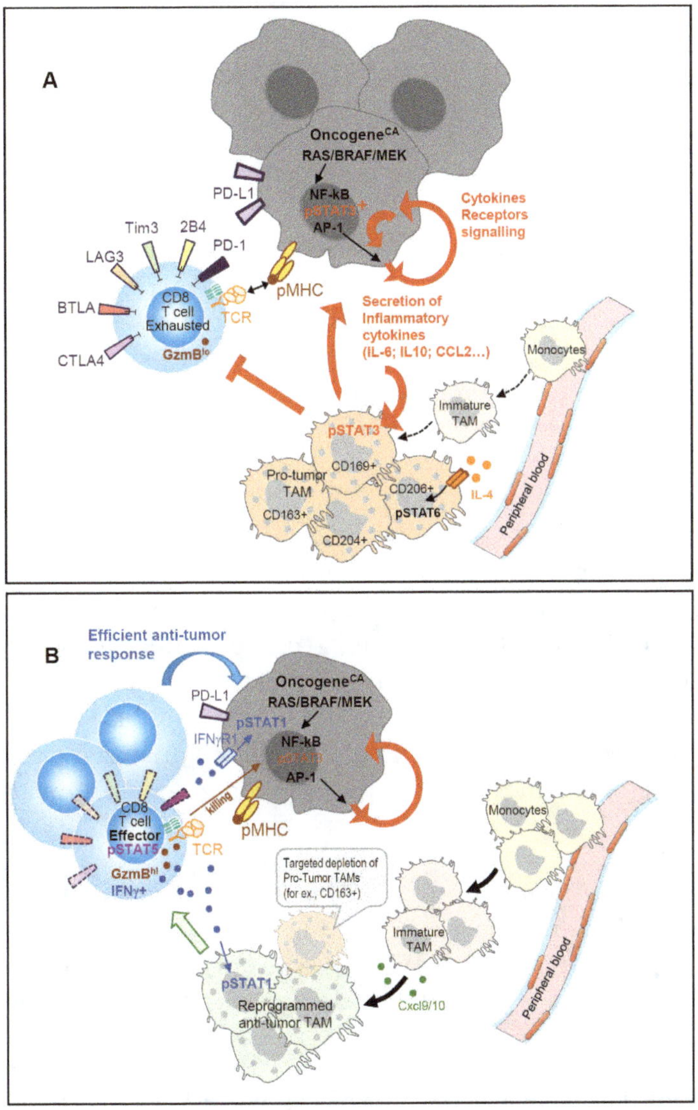

Figure 1. (**A**). Concerted regulation of tumor-induced inflammation promotes accumulation of immune-suppressive TAM. Oncogene activation in tumors induced secretion of inflammatory cytokines that activate STAT3 and promote the accumulation of immune-suppressive TAM; IL-4-derived signals through STAT6 sustain the pro-tumor TAM function that further sustains tumor growth in a positive feedback loop. (**B**). Targeted depletion of specific TAM subsets displaying strong T cell suppressive activity favors the recruitment of monocyte-derived immature TAM that secrete CXCL9/10 and display T cell activating capacities. Reinvigorated CD8 TILs with activated pSTAT5 secrete IFNγ that further maintains TAM anti-tumor functions and sensitizes tumors to T cell killing.

Cancer treatments have recently benefited from immune checkpoint therapies (ICT) targeting inhibitory signaling pathways in T lymphocytes (PD-1/PD-L1 and CTLA-4). Despite remarkable success in a subset of patients (objective responses ~20–30% for monotherapy and ~30–40% for combined therapy), primary resistance is observed in more than 50% of the patients and a subset of initial responders can later develop acquired resistance [40]. Analysis of pre-treatment tumor biopsy samples has revealed that patients with a pre-existing local CD8 T cell infiltrate (T cell inflamed) were more likely to show a clinical response to anti- PD-1/PD-L1 [41]. Furthermore, PD-L1-expression on dendritic cells and macrophages but not on cancer cells has been shown to shape the response to the PD-L1/PD-1 blockade [42,43].

Given the aforementioned reciprocal regulation of TAM and TILs, one should expect that ICT-based therapies could conjointly unleash tumor-specific T cells and reprogram TAM functions. Several groups exploring immune cells dynamics in vivo before and after ICT recently addressed this issue. In carcinoma-bearing mice, immune-PET monitoring showed that ICT induced an important infiltration of CD8 T cells within the tumor in responders as compared to non-responders; the responders displayed $CD11b^+$ TAM with a "M1-type" transcriptomic signature [44]. scRNA-seq and longitudinal CyTOF analyses also revealed ICT-induced dynamic changes in both TAM and TILs present in induced mouse sarcomas [17]. This study identified an ICT-induced decrease of both CD4 regulatory T cells and exhausted CD8 T cells. Meanwhile, conventional CD4 T cells and tumor-specific CD8 T cells displayed an activated profile as did recruited NK cells, with all these effector cells exhibiting an enhanced NF-κB and IFNγ-driven gene signatures. ICT consequently conferred a remarkable dynamic remodeling on intra-tumor monocytes and macrophages. Distinct TAM populations expressing IFNγ-induced iNOS, while down-regulating IL-4-responsive CD206 proteins, were enriched upon ICT Pathway analyses, which showed ICT-driven enrichment of IFNγ and NF-κB signaling as well as glucose metabolism. Concurrently, alternative "M2-type" TAM clusters with a $MerTK^{hi}$ $CD206^+$ $CCL2^+$ $CD274^+$ $IL4R\alpha^+$ phenotype were reduced by approximately one-third. Kinetic CyTOF analyses further highlighted an important crossroads between days 7 and 9—a time window where the TME drives the TAM behavior towards a pro-inflammatory/T cell supporting or an anti-inflammatory/immune suppressive program. The TME agent mediating monocyte/macrophage reprogramming was ascribed to be IFNγ secreted by ICT-unleashed tumor-specific T cells. Importantly, T cell produced IFNγ not only engages its receptor signaling on surrounding TAM but also on tumor cells themselves. As such, STAT1-activation was reported to sensitize hepatocarcinomas to T cell mediated killing [45] (see Figure 1). Therefore, the therapeutic use of STAT/JAK-modulators should be carefully evaluated for their specific targeting of STAT3 activity while preserving IFNγ-induced STAT1/2 signaling, which appears to be beneficial for anti-tumor immune responses.

In the large fraction of patients who are non-responsive to ICT other therapeutic approaches must be proposed to reinvigorate anti-tumor responses. Providing an infusion of autologous tumor-specific CD8 T cells manipulated to express an effector (IFNγ-proficient) program could be a way to fight cancer and induce TAM reprogramming. This will be addressed in the next section.

4. STAT5 versus STAT3 in Adaptive CD8 T Cell Responses to Cancer

Cytokines are major regulators of T cell differentiation/function and are crucial factors to consider for immunotherapy protocols. Many of these cytokines signal through the stimulation of STAT3 and/or STAT5. This makes these two TFs key players in the regulation of functions of T cells. Both STAT3 and STAT5 activation can have a beneficial or detrimental effect on the anti-tumor response depending on the T cell type targeted. In this part, we will focus on the T cell-intrinsic role of these TFs and on the possibility to manipulate them for improving CD8 T cell anti-tumor responses.

4.1. *STAT5 in the Adaptive T Cell Responses*

The STAT5 pathway is predominantly activated in T cells by members of the γc cytokine family (IL-2, -7, -9 and -15) (reviewed in [46]). These cytokines signal through receptors containing the γc (CD132) subunit and lead to the activation of the JAK3 tyrosine kinase. In addition, activation of JAK1 occurs through its interaction with the IL-2Rβ (CD122) (for IL-2 and IL-15), but also, with the IL-4Rα, IL-7Rα and IL-9Rα units. For IL-2, high-affinity binding to its receptor requires the association of an additional subunit (IL-2Rα or CD25) to the IL-2Rβ and the γc components. IL-15 signaling is further peculiar in that it requires the association "in-trans" of the IL-15Rα component with the IL-2Rβ and the γc components [47]. The specificity of signaling by these cytokines is thus partially explained by the recruited STAT proteins, but also by the differential expression of the relevant receptors. STAT5-activating cytokines have a general role in the maintenance and expansion of T cell subsets. IL-2 has a central role in the expansion phase of T cells following their primary antigenic stimulation [47,48]. The roles of IL-7 or IL-15 are rather associated with the maintenance of naïve or memory T cells [47,49,50].

In adaptive immunity, except for a population of CD4 T cells with a regulatory function (Treg), IL-2Rα (CD25) is not expressed at a significant level at the surface of naïve CD4 and CD8 T cells. Although the two other chains of the IL-2R are expressed at low basal levels on naïve T cells, IL-2 fails to activate these T cells, consistent with the report that only Tregs respond promptly to in vivo IL-2 exposure [51]. Thus, antigen stimulation of the TCR/CD3 complex is a pre-requisite for the secondary signaling by the IL-2R. TCR/CD3 initiated signals, which do not involve STAT activation, lead to transient expression of genes, including *il2ra*. IL-2R mediated signaling through STAT5 activation further increases CD25 expression at the cell surface and leads to the stabilization of a panel of genes initially induced by the TCR [52,53]. We and others reported that TCR-initiated signaling is influenced by the avidity of TCR-peptide/MHC interaction, which impacts strength and duration of TCR engagement [54–56]. Strong TCR/CD3 stimulation causes production of IL-2, leading to an autocrine effect on IL-2R signaling, which is not induced by low avidity Ags. In this latter case, exogenous IL-2 or expression of a constitutive-active STAT5 protein [52,53] can serve as a substitute for the lack of the IL-2/IL-2R amplification loop. Interestingly, a study evaluating the IL-2R/JAK-regulated phospho-proteome in CD8 CTL revealed a dominance of proteins that control mRNA stability and components of the protein translational machinery leading to an accumulation of cytokines and effector molecules, as well as proteins that support metabolic processes essential for cell "fitness" and important oxygen-sensing components [57]. Of note, active STAT5 does not substitute for all IL-2 induced signaling events that also involve MAP kinase- and phospho-inositol 3-kinase-dependent pathways [58]. Altogether, for CD8 T cells, depending on their state of activation and on the dose of cytokine provided, IL-2 may amplify effector function and proliferation and induce terminal differentiation or activation-induced cell death [47,48].

The synergistic action of TCR-induced TFs and STAT5 in CD8 T cells mirrors the cooperation between STAT5 and (i) TCR-induced GATA3 in CD4 Th-2 cells to control the accessibility of *Il4* gene locus [59]; (ii) Tbet in Th-1/Tc-1 for the regulation of the *Ifng* locus [60,61]; and (iii) BCL6 in B lymphocytes for the generation of memory B cells [62]. Additionally, STAT5 activation was shown to promote GM-CSF [63] and IL-9 [64], producing T cells and to be a prerequisite for Foxp3-expressing Tregs [65,66]. By contrast, STAT5 is a negative regulator of Th-17 [67] and T-Fh [68] by competing with STAT3 and BCL6, respectively. Altogether, STAT5 appears to control secondary decisions in adaptive immunity (see Table 2).

Table 2. Concerted gene regulation by STAT3 and STAT5 in helper and cytotoxic lymphocytes.

STAT3 and STAT5-Regulated Genes in T and NK cells				
Target Genes	**STAT3 Input**	**Cell Subsets**	**STAT5 Input**	**Cell Subsets**
		Cytokines/Cytokine receptors		
Il17	positive	hCD4 Th-17 [69]		
Il10	positive	mCD4 Th-2 [70]		
Il2ra (CD25)	positive	mCD4 Th-21 [71]	positive	mCD4 Th-1 [71], mCD8 [60], mNK [72]
Il7ra (CD127)			negative	mCD8 [60]
Il6st			negative	mCD8 [60]
Tgfb2r			negative	mCD8 [60]
		Homing		
CCR7			negative	mCD8 [60]
Sell (CD62L)			negative	mCD8 [60]
		TFs		
Prdm1 (Blimp)	positive	mCD4 Th-2 [70]		
Eomes			positive	mCD8 [60]
Tbx21 (Tbet)			positive	mCD8 [60]
		Cytotoxicity		
Gzmb			positive	mCD8 [60], mNK [73]
Prf1			positive	mCD8 [60], mNK [73]
Ifng			positive	mCD8 [60], mNK [73]
Fasl			positive	mCD8 [60]
		Cell cycle/Cell survival		
Myc	positive	hT lymphoma [74]	positive	mCD8 [60]
Pim1	positive	hT lymphoma [74]	positive	mCD8 [60,75]
Bcl2	positive	hT lymphoma [74]	positive	mCD8 [49,60]; NK [73]

Competitive gene regulation by STAT3 and STAT5 in T cells *			
Target Genes	**STAT3 Input**	**STAT5 Input**	**T Cell Subsets**
Il17	positive	competitor	mCD4 Th-17 [67]
Il9	competitor	positive	mCD4 Th-9 [64,76]
Bcl6	positive	competitor	mCD4 Tfh; mCD4 Th-1 [68,77]
Socs3	positive	positive	mCD4 Th-17/Treg balance [78]

* Mechanisms underlying competitive gene regulation by STAT3 and STAT5 are reviewed in [79].

Role of STAT5 in the Generation of Memory CD8 T Cells and Maintenance of Effector Functions

Several STAT5A mutants have been shown to confer cytokine-independent growth to Ba/F3 cells [72]. While a STAT5A S710F single-mutant displayed a strong constitutive activity sufficient to complement STAT5A^{null} bone marrow progenitors, a STAT5A double-mutant H298R/S710F was not able to complement STAT5A^{null} cells [80]. Further studies highlighted that the H298R mutation in the DNA-binding domain renders this protein inactive unless it can form heterodimers with endogenous wild-type STAT5 (see Figure 2). Therefore, the constitutive activity of STAT5 H298R/S710F is modest and limited by the bioavailability of wild-type STAT5 to pair with. By contrast, the single STAT5 S710F mutant exerts a strong constitutive activity in both CD8 T cells [81] and Ba/F3 cells [82].

Retroviral expression of STAT5A H298R/S710F (hereafter referred to as STAT5ca) in in vitro activated CD8 T cells led to the generation and maintenance of long-lived CD8 T effector cells upon their adoptive transfer [83]. Transcriptomic analyses of STAT5ca-expressing CD8 T cells highlighted a role for STAT5ca in the stabilization of a broad Tc-1 gene expression program initiated by TCR stimulation [60] (see Table 2, Figure 2). This observation is in agreement with the reported chromatin interactions of STAT5 in super-enhancers to activate IL-2 highly inducible genes [71].

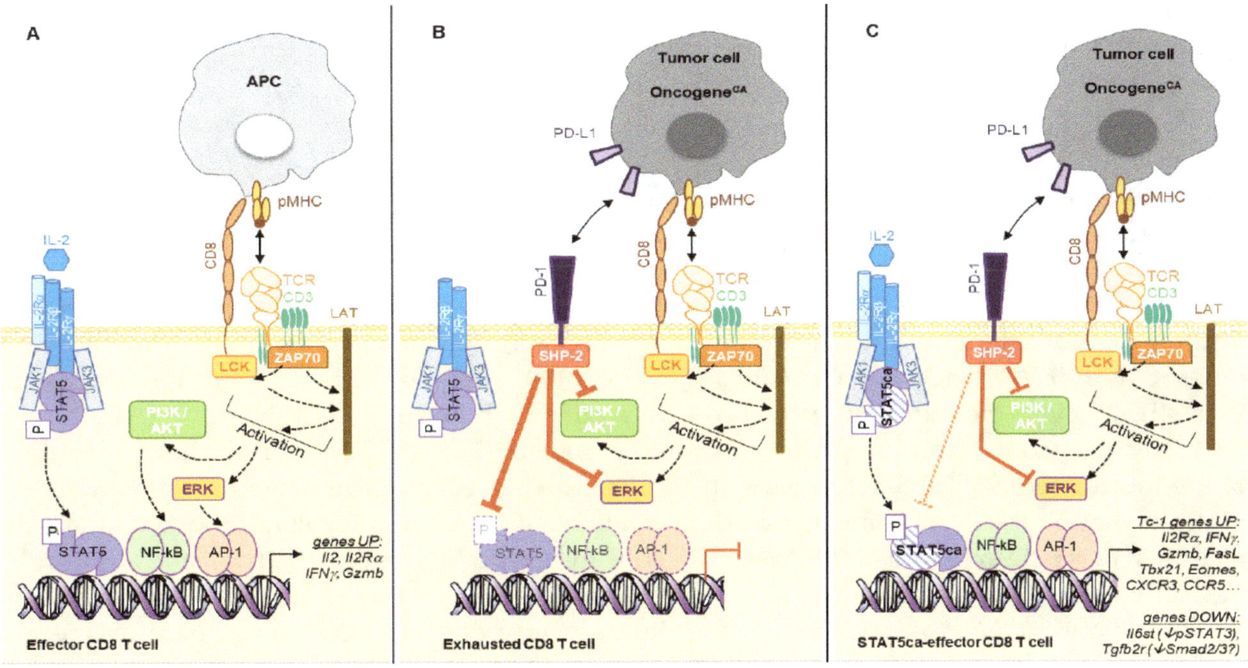

Figure 2. (**A**). Ag presented by APC (Ag-presenting cells) triggers a T cell activation cascade leading to gene transcription including *Il2* and *IL2Rα* genes. Binding of IL-2 to its receptor further amplifies the TCR-initiated gene transcription program. (**B**). Ag expressed on tumor cells mediates chronic TCR engagement on CD8 TILs leading to their "exhaustion", which is characterized by expression of multiple inhibitory receptors (as shown in Figure 1). For simplicity, we represent PD-1 only that recruits the phosphatase SHP-2 mediating inhibition of ERK and PI3K/AKT pathways as well as dephosphorylation of STAT5. (**C**). Expression of STAT5ca (H298R/S710F, here represented by dashed symbols as compared to the wild type (WT) protein) in CD8 T cells not only recapitulates the IL-2-mediated TCR-initiated gene transcription, but also stabilizes this functional program. This leads to a sustained Tc-1 program reminiscent of effector memory cells. Of note, while being PD-1^{hi} due to the chronic TCR engagement by their cognate Ag, STAT5ca-expressing T cells remain functional, as the S710F substitution reduces the SHP-2-mediated dephosphorylation. Additionally, STAT5ca represses the expression of *il6st* and *Tgfb2r* genes, rendering these cells insensitive to IL-6/STAT3 and TGFβ1/Smad signaling.

Of note, the in vivo maintenance of STAT5ca-expressing CD8 T cells remains under the control of γc-cytokines (IL-7, IL-15) and TCR tickling by self MHC class I [81]; these properties again point towards a moderate and controlled activity of this double-mutant. Accordingly, Kaech's group also reported that STAT5ca promoted memory CD8 T cells [49] that did not display any sign of transformation. However, Moriggl and colleagues recently demonstrated that high expression of S710F gain-of-function mutated STAT5A induced PTLC-nos (Peripheral T cell leukemia and lymphoma—not otherwise specified) cells when expressed during T cell development in transgenic mice [84].

Mice expressing a constitutively active STAT5Bca (H298R/S715F) transgene in the lymphoid lineage have been shown to present a selective expansion of memory-like CD8 T cells. Their analysis further suggested that moderate STAT5B activation underlies both IL-7/IL-15-dependent homeostatic proliferation of naive and memory CD8 T cells and IL-2-dependent development of CD4 CD25^{+} Tregs [85]. When expressed in the B cell lineage in mouse models, STAT5Bca (H298R/S715F) induces B cell acute lymphoblastic leukemia thanks to cooperative molecular events targeting JAK1 activity, tumor-suppressor genes, and pre-BCR signaling [86]. Indeed, mutated STAT5Bca was shown to antagonize preBCR-initiated TFs (NF-κB, IKAROS) for binding to B cell specific super enhancers [87]. Finally, mice which expressed a transgene, i.e., a human gain-of-function mutation of STAT5B (hSTAT5B N642H) identified in leukemic patients, developed lymphomas from multiple T cell subsets [88]. The recent crystal structure of hSTAT5B N642H highlighted important conformational changes in correlation to its resistance to dephosphorylation [89]. Overall, strong STAT5B hyperactivity appeared to trigger B or T lymphomas when express during lymphoid cell development and to directly influence disease aggressiveness and therapeutic resistance [87,89].

4.2. Role of STAT3 in T Cells

Several cytokines/cytokine receptors trigger STAT3 signaling in T cells, including IL-6-type cytokines (IL-6 and Oncostatin M), IL-10, IL-17, IL-21 and IL-27. Among the STAT3-activating cytokines, IL-21 is peculiar: While its receptor contains the γc (CD132) subunit, signals downstream of IL-21R converge on STAT3 and to a lesser extent on STAT1, rather than on STAT5 activation [46]. Intriguingly, IL-21 was shown to promote in vitro proliferation of CD8 T naïve and memory cells in synergy with STAT5-inducing cytokines IL-7/IL-15 [90]. Indeed, Leonard's group reported that IL-2 vs. IL-21 cytokine stimulation of pre-activated T cells induces STAT5 and STAT3 binding, respectively, to incompletely overlapping super enhancers [71]. Understanding the fine-tuning of cytokine-modulated STAT3/5 activities will require further effort as reviewed in [46]: This tight regulation relies on the T cell context, including cell lineage, differentiation state, and cytokine milieu, triggering synergistic/antagonistic STAT-mediated transcriptional regulation. Thus, the amplitude of STAT3 activation differs from one T cell subset to another in correlation with differential expression of the corresponding T cytokine receptor [91]. Interestingly, chronic TCR engagement was recently shown to enhance the sensitivity to IL-6/STAT3 signals [92], indicating again a cross-talk between TCR-induced and STAT TFs.

The function of STAT3 in various T cell subtypes is summarized in Table 2, but further details are described in this issue by both Rébé and Ghiringhelli [26] and Logotheti and Putzer [93].

The overall effect of STAT3 stimulation in T cells is generally correlated with a poor cytotoxic/increased regulatory response and as such, is associated with a defective anti-tumor immune response [94]. In the next part, we will focus on the role of STAT3 in the maintenance and formation of memory CD8 T cells.

4.2.1. Role of STAT3 in the Maintenance and Memory Formation of CD8 T Cells

Several studies have highlighted the role of IL-21 and STAT3 activation in T cell memory regulation. Using LCMV chronic infection in mice, Kaech's group showed that IL-10 and/or IL-21-induced STAT3 was required for the differentiation of memory CD8 T cells with a preserved replicative potential [95]. Indeed, in the absence of STAT3, memory precursor cells were replaced by T effector-like cells that failed to undergo homeostatic proliferation or to protect against secondary infection. Interestingly, STAT3 appeared to act both by induction of "pro-memory" TFs, such as Eomes and BCL6, and by dampening inflammation-driven TFs, including STAT4 and Tbet.

A similar role for STAT3 in human T cells [96] was reported in a cohort of patients suffering from autosomal-dominant hyper-IgE syndrome, which is caused by dominant-negative STAT3 mutations. These patients have increased numbers of naïve T cells but fewer central memory CD4$^+$ and CD8 memory T cells, leading to an increased susceptibility to EBV infections. This was associated with a defect of these naïve T cells to express the TFs important for memory formation.

Accordingly, IL-21 repressed the cytolytic effector program in tumor-specific CD8 T cells while preserving their replicative potential [97].

4.2.2. Role of STAT3 in the CD8 T Cell-Mediated Anti-Tumor Responses

STAT3-activating cytokines such as IL-6 and IL-10 are found in abundance within the tumor microenvironment. It was clearly shown that STAT3 inactivation in tumor-specific CD8 T cells increased their potential for tumor elimination after adoptive transfer [98,99]. Altogether, these studies suggest that a general inhibition of STAT3 in T cells would be a beneficial treatment for increasing tumor control. However, contradicting data exist in the literature [100]. In mice bearing transplanted tumors, a combination of anti-OX40 mAb and TGFβ/Smad inhibitors improved the CD8 T cell mediated tumor rejection. Use of OX40-Cre STAT3$^{fl/fl}$ mice further demonstrated that in absence of STAT3 in OX40-expressing T cells, the response to the treatment was lost [100]. These authors did not prove formally that the deletion of STAT3 in CD8 T effector cells only was mediating the same effect; but their data suggest that depending on the T cell subset or the immunotherapy used, inhibiting STAT3 could become detrimental and lead to poor survival of T cells and loss of the benefit of the treatment.

The reported discrepancies for the function of STAT3 in CD8 T cell mediated anti-tumor responses may rely on distinct roles of this TF depending on the T cell differentiation state (effector versus memory), the combined immunotherapy regimen and the STAT3-inducing cytokines in the TME. All these parameters may contribute to differential STAT3-activation thresholds triggering distinct T cell responses, a hypothesis that needs to be tested in refined analyses.

5. Adoptive CD8 T Cell Therapy and CAR-T Cell Generation for Cancer Immunotherapy

5.1. Increasing the Frequency of Tumor-Specific CD8 T Cells

As mentioned earlier in Section 3, beside tremendous achievements for patients with various types of cancers, immunotherapies aimed at blocking inhibiting receptors still failed for more than 50% of cancer patients. This could be the consequence of the paucity of tumor-specific CD8 T cells, an obstacle that could be circumvented by infusions of in vitro amplified tumor-specific T cells. Indeed, Adoptive Cell Transfer (ACT) of amplified TILs and Chimeric Antigenic Receptor (CAR) treatments are based on the use of the patient's T cells [101]. Historically, T cells used for ACT were obtained from tumor pieces/biopsies, amplified in vitro and transferred back into the patient when a sufficient number was reached (up to 10^{11} cells) [102]. The progress in gene engineering removed many hurdles to generate cancer specific T cells. CAR-T cells are gene-engineered products obtained from the expression in T cells of a construct encoding a domain of a single-chain variable antibody fragment recognizing a tumor antigen, fused to intracellular signaling motifs inducing T cell activation upon recognition of the target cells [103]. T cells from the blood are used for this therapy, allowing an increased potential to generate these cells on a large scale. CD19-directed CAR-T cells have shown impressive results in the treatment of patients with B-cell lymphoma [104]. However, evidence for the use of CAR-T cells against solid tumors is still sparse. The main limitation for application being the identification of Ags expressed exclusively on solid tumors and not on the non-transformed cell counterparts. Defining tumor-specific Ags for solid cancers is still a challenge [105,106]. Such an attempt was reported using mesothelin-specific CAR-T cells to treat patients bearing pancreatic ductal adenocarcinoma [107]. Of note, antibody-targeted chimeric T cells display receptors (i) of higher avidity for tumor-Ags than regular TCRs; (ii) which are not MHC restricted and thereby, are not impacted by tumor editing in the Ag processing/presentation pathway, (iii) interacting only with Ags expressed at the tumor cell surface.

Despite some clinical success using ACT or CAR-T cells, much effort is being made to improve T cell survival and resistance to immunosuppression in the frame of these therapies. Given the ability of IL-2 to expand CD8 T cells and to maintain their cytotoxic function, infusion of recombinant IL-2 in cancer patients was the first reported effective immunotherapy for human cancer [108]. However, IL-2 concomitantly acts on Tregs that suppress anti-tumor responses, and systemic IL-2 injections had severe adverse effects including vascular leak syndrome and pulmonary edema due to IL-2Rα expression on endothelial cells [109]. This has led to the development of (IL-2/anti-IL-2 mAb) complexes [110]: depending on the mAb the binding of the resulting complex is favored on IL-2Rβ/γc-expressing cells such as the memory CD8 T and NK cells, but prevented on IL-2Rα^+ Tregs and endothelial cells. Such approaches enhance the cytokine half-life in vivo and were shown to induce a massive (>100-fold) expansion of CD8 T cells in vivo [110,111] thereby boosting anti-tumor immune responses in mice and humans [112].

IL-21 is also considered to expand less differentiated CD8 T memory stem cells with both proliferative and multipotent potential [113] to be used in ACT.

The manipulation of cytokine-induced STAT-signaling in tumor-specific CD8 T lymphocytes may be another solution to potentiate adoptive T cell cancer therapies.

5.2. On CD8 T cell Intrinsic Modifications For adoptive T Cell Therapies

5.2.1. Promoting Effector Memory CD8 T Cells Through STAT5

Another hurdle for ACT is the persistence of the infused T cells, their capacity to home in tumor-invaded peripheral organs and to resist the local immune suppression. As such, CD19-directed CAR-T cells had limited capacities to control the growth of $CD19^+$ murine melanomas in relation with their scarcity in the tumor [114]. To infiltrate non hematologic solid tumors, T cells must acquire an effector phenotype: this includes the simultaneous loss of CD62L (L-selectin) and CCR7 expression, and acquisition of tissue-specific homing molecules such as adhesion molecules and chemokines/chemokine receptors [115]. Given the multiplicity of the molecular partners involved in T cell egress and migration, it is illusory to manipulate these targets, one by one or in combination. However, manipulating TFs known to be activated during T effector cell differentiation may have broader effects. We brought this proof of concept by expression of STAT5ca during the in vitro differentiation of CD8 T cells, which modified their in vivo migration upon ACT with increased infiltration of both non-lymphoid tissues in healthy mice and melanomas in tumor-bearing mice [60]. At the transcriptomic and protein levels, coincident down-regulation of CD62L and up-regulation of CCR2, CCR5 and CXCR3 was induced by STAT5ca as compared to standard CD8 T effector cells. Altogether, STAT5ca-CD8 T cells acquired a long-lived effector memory phenotype in correlation with a concerted STAT5-mediated regulation of *Tbx21* and *Eomes* genes (Table 2 and [60]). Coupled to their enhanced effector functions—Ag-driven cytotoxity and IFNγ production—these engineered STAT5ca-CD8 T cells mediated efficient melanoma rejection as compared with conventional CD8 T effector cells [83]. Importantly, this STAT5ca-induced reprogramming applies to both polyclonal and monoclonal (TCR transgenic) CD8 T cells, after primary or secondary stimulation [83]: these characteristics are of particular importance for translation to cancer patients' CD8 T cells. Finally, STAT5ca-expression in tumor-specific T cells had better therapeutic potential than the potentiation of standard CD8 T effector cells with combined infusions of IL-2 complexes, the effect of which disappeared at the end of treatment [83].

5.2.2. Promoting Central Memory CD8 T Cells Through STAT3

Recent studies have highlighted the importance of a memory-like CD8 T cell population to unleash an anti-tumor response by anti-PD-1 treatment [116,117]. In these studies, a small subset of CD8 TILs expressing PD-1 and the transcription factor TCF1 responded to anti-PD-1 immunotherapy by differentiating into highly cytotoxic TILs that mediated long-term tumor control. These studies highlight the importance of a long lasting, less differentiated population to mediate a more efficient control of the cancer.

This point is also valid for ACT, as transfer of expanded T cells that are too differentiated could lead to a failure of the treatment related to a lack of survival of the cells [118]. For that purpose, IL-21, a STAT3 stimulating cytokine, is efficient in driving the differentiation of central memory CAR or TCR engineered CD8 T cells in vitro [119]. Additionally, a recent study showed that CD19-directed CAR-T cells initially activated in vitro with optimal stimulation (anti-CD3/CD28) progressively acquired an "exhausted" phenotype upon transfer in tumor bearing mice. Thus, when retrieved from the tumor 12 days after their transfer, they presented a characteristic high surface expression of inhibitory receptors, diminished production of IFNγ and TNFα, and low cytolytic activity as well as the expression of the high-mobility group (HMG)-box TFs - TOX and TOX2. Expression of the latter TFs was recently described as resulting in commitment of CD8 T cells to an exhausted transcriptional and epigenetic developmental program distinct from that of functional CD8 T effector and T memory cells [120]. To understand further the factors associated with an efficient CAR response, Fraietta et al. [121] performed a transcriptomic profiling of CAR-T cells from complete-responding patients with chronic lymphocytic leukemia compared to non-responders. The gene signature was enriched in memory-related genes, including IL-6/STAT3 signatures, whereas T cells from non-responders upregulated programs involved in effector differentiation, glycolysis, exhaustion and apoptosis. Moreover, highly functional CAR-T cells from patients produced the STAT3-activating cytokine IL-6 and its concentration in serum was correlated with CAR-T cell expansion. These results showed STAT3 signaling is beneficial for an efficient CAR-T cell response [121]. This finding is further validated by the use of a new-generation CD19-CAR that encodes a truncated cytoplasmic domain from IL-2Rβ and a STAT3-binding tyrosine-X-X-glutamine motif. These CAR-T cells showed antigen-dependent activation of the JAK kinase and of the STAT3 and STAT5 TFs signaling pathways, which promoted their proliferation and prevented their terminal differentiation in vitro. The CAR-T cells demonstrated superior in vivo persistence and anti-tumor effects in models of hematologic malignancies as compared with CAR-T cells expressing a CD28 or 4-1BB co-stimulatory domain alone [114]. It should be noted that while a subtle increased STAT3 activation by these newly engineered IL-2Rβ-CAR-T cells was therapeutically beneficial, STAT3 gain-of-function mutants induced multi-organ autoimmunity and large granular lymphocytic leukemia [122].

In conclusion, these studies strengthen the interest of regulating STAT3/STAT5 activities in CD8 T cells to improve adoptive cell therapy: given their tightly balanced contribution to T cell memory fates, increased STAT3 or STAT5 activity is expected to improve the therapeutic success of hematological and non-hematological cancers, respectively. This hypothesis has to be validated in relevant preclinical mouse models.

5.2.3. On the STAT5 versus STAT3 Balance in T Cells

Several groups have provided data showing that the competitive binding of STAT3 and STAT5 dimers to DNA dictates the transcriptional regulation of certain target genes in T cells and thereby either trigger autoimmune disorders or promote tumor rejection (some examples are reported in Table 2). These data highlight the need for both in silico analyses [123] and appropriate cell/animal models to evaluate the outcome of competition between STAT TFs on T cell fates.

6. STAT5 and Resistance to Immunosuppression in the Tumor Microenvironment

Chronic stimulation of tumor-specific T cells promotes an exhausted phenotype, sharing strong [124] but not-completely overlapping similarities [125] with virus-induced exhausted CD8 T cells. Both the diversity and the high expression of inhibitory receptors by CD8 TILs (reviewed in [126]) can contribute to ICT resistance. However, combining blocking antibodies towards several inhibitory receptors to improve anti-tumor responses may further increase the adverse effects among which autoimmune attacks [127]. Therefore, manipulating CD8 T cells to resist local tumor-derived immune suppression may be of clinical benefit.

6.1. Immunosuppression by PD-1

PD-1 is related to the CD28 superfamily and is expressed on activated T cells, B cells, monocytes and macrophages. Engagement of PD-1 by its ligands (PD-L1 or PD-L2) induces inhibitory signals in T cells [128] through the induced phosphorylation of ITIM/ITSIM motives in its cytoplasmic domain, which leads to recruitment of the SHP-2/SHP-1 phosphatases. This dampens both TCR and CD28 signaling leading to abrogation of the PI3K/AKT and ERK pathways, as shown notably in primary CD4 T cells [129]. Interestingly, SHP-2 recruited by PD-1 was shown to counteract phospho-STAT5 signaling in human Tregs from HCV-infected patients' livers [130]. It was also demonstrated that PD-1 intrinsically regulates a subpopulation of high PD-1 expressing innate cells (ILC2) involved in helminth immunity (γc dependent proliferation) by inhibiting STAT5 phosphorylation through SHP-1/SHP-2 phosphatases [131]. Similarly, for T cells, the inhibitory effect of PD-1 is observed on populations expressing high levels of surface PD-1 such as exhausted T cells in contrast to acutely activated T cells [132]. However, in a melanoma model, in spite of upregulation of the PD-1/PD-L1 immunosuppressive pathway in the tumor microenvironment, STAT5ca-expressing CD8 T effector cells were found to be resistant to inhibition by PD-1/PD-L1 engagement as measured by their efficient IFNγ production, in contrast to their control counterpart [132]. Thus, the previously reported increased resistance to dephosphorylation of STAT5ca [72] may also contribute to its resistance to the phosphatases recruited to checkpoint inhibitors (Figure 2) [133,134].

6.2. Other Immune Suppressive Pathways

The diversity of immune suppressive mechanisms associated with inflammatory melanoma have previously been reported [133], with several involving tumor-derived proteins.

TGFβ1, an immunosuppressive cytokine produced by a number of cancer cells, was shown to inhibit both Th-1/Tc-1 cytokine production and Tc-1/NK cytolytic effector functions through the repression of *Ifng*, *Gzmb*, and *FasL* gene transcription [135,136]. Interestingly, STAT5ca-expressing T cells maintained efficient induction of both IFNγ and Gzmb in the presence of TGFβ1 [132]. The insensitivity to TGFβ1 may be linked to the STAT5ca-mediated negative regulation of *Tgfbr2* expression as well as its positive effects on *Ifng* and *Gzmb* gene transcription [60]; thus, STAT5ca-gene regulation counterbalances the transcriptional repression exerted by TGFβ1-induced Smad2/3. Indeed, two STAT5-activating cytokines, IL-2 [136] and IL-15 [137], have been shown to counteract TGFβ1-mediated immune suppression.

Of note, while TGFβ1 and IL-6 contribute to *Maf* up-regulation in exhausted CD8 T cells [125], STAT5ca-expressing T cells displayed reduced levels of *Il6st*, *Tgfbr2*, and *Maf* transcripts [60] and maintained a functional antitumor program.

Another tumor-secreted protein, the Dickkopf-related protein 2 (DKK2), was shown to be overexpressed in human colorectal cancers and melanomas, and to promote tumor progression by suppressing the activation of both CD8 T and NK cells [138]. Mechanistically, tumor cells secrete DKK2 that binds its receptor LRP5 inducing interactions between the intracellular domain of LRP5 and STAT5; while STAT5-phosphorylation was not precluded, STAT5 nuclear localization was impeded in cytotoxic cells. Conversely, DKK2 blockade enhanced cytotoxic immune cell activation.

Altogether, maintenance of active STAT5 signaling in cytotoxic cells appears to correlate with efficient anti-tumor immunity [73,83].

7. Conclusions

The frequency of tumor-specific CD8 T cells can now be increased in cancer patients through sophisticated personalized medical approaches including in vitro derived and expanded TILs or engineered CAR-T cells. Nevertheless the ability of adoptively transferred T cells to survive in cancer-invaded hosts and to efficiently penetrate into the tumor are dampened by the solid tumor landscape including cancer cells, tumor stroma and immune suppressive myeloid cells. Therefore, enhancing tumor T cell infiltration is one way to improve cancer immunotherapy. This could imply (i) manipulation of the T cells themselves through their transduction with chemokine receptors promoting non-hematopoietic tissue colonization [139,140] or manipulation of TFs that regulate expression of these homing receptors [60]; (ii) depletion of specific TAM subsets that exert trophic and/or immune suppressive functions either by ablation [13] or inactivation using STAT3 inhibitors [27]. The enhanced killing of cancer cells together with the recruitment of fresh monocytes will favor the engagement of the host immune system thanks to the presentation of tumor-derived Ags by professional APCs such as dendritic cells and/or immature TAM. This would result in spreading of tumor-derived epitopes ensuring a polyclonal anti-tumor response that could ultimately prevent antigen escape. Importantly, this favorable loop was observed when using STAT5ca-expressing CD8 T cells in ACT as their efficient capacity to infiltrate and kill inflammatory melanomas is accompanied by a concomitant infiltration of host T cells [83]. Compared to systemic treatment, such as IL-2 infusions, the targeted manipulation of STAT5 activity in tumor-specific CD8 T lymphocytes circumvents the negative stimulation of Tregs, which are also recruited into tumor beds. We here propose to transiently express (i.e., through mRNA transfection for example) the STAT5A H298R/S710F mutant in human CD8 T cells specific for Ags expressed on solid malignancies to be used in ACT: Both their efficient infiltration into tumors and IFNγ production resistant to tumor-derived suppression should help to restore endogenous T cell responses and to reprogram TAM. Although the IFNγ/STAT1 signature induced by T cells has recently been reported as a good prognostic factor for ICT response [141], a close control of this cytokine-induced signaling must be maintained since excess IFNγ can induce death of anti-tumor CD8 T cells at a certain stage of their differentiation/activation [142–144].

Acknowledgments: The authors thank the CIML imaging, cytometry and animal facilities personnel for assistance. The authors also thank Lee Leserman for editing the manuscript.

References

1. Hanahan, D.; Weinberg, R.A. Hallmarks of cancer: The next generation. *Cell* **2011**, *144*, 646–674. [CrossRef] [PubMed]
2. Yu, H.; Pardoll, D.; Jove, R. STATs in cancer inflammation and immunity: A leading role for STAT3. *Nat. Rev. Cancer* **2009**, *9*, 798–809. [CrossRef] [PubMed]
3. Fleming, J.D.; Giresi, P.G.; Lindahl-Allen, M.; Krall, E.B.; Lieb, J.D.; Struhl, K. STAT3 acts through pre-existing nucleosome-depleted regions bound by FOS during an epigenetic switch linking inflammation to cancer. *Epigenetics Chromatin* **2015**, *8*, 7. [CrossRef] [PubMed]
4. Ji, Z.; He, L.; Regev, A.; Struhl, K. Inflammatory regulatory network mediated by the joint action of NF-kB, STAT3, and AP-1 factors is involved in many human cancers. *Proc Natl. Acad. Sci. USA* **2019**, *116*, 9453–9462. [CrossRef]
5. Taniguchi, K.; Karin, M. IL-6 and related cytokines as the critical lynchpins between inflammation and cancer. *Semin. Immunol.* **2014**, *26*, 54–74. [CrossRef]
6. Gabrilovich, D.I.; Ostrand-Rosenberg, S.; Bronte, V. Coordinated regulation of myeloid cells by tumours. *Nat. Rev. Immunol.* **2012**, *12*, 253–268. [CrossRef]
7. Riesenberg, S.; Groetchen, A.; Siddaway, R.; Bald, T.; Reinhardt, J.; Smorra, D.; Kohlmeyer, J.; Renn, M.; Phung, B.; Aymans, P.; et al. MITF and c-Jun antagonism interconnects melanoma dedifferentiation with pro-inflammatory cytokine responsiveness and myeloid cell recruitment. *Nat. Commun.* **2015**, *6*, 8755. [CrossRef]
8. Soudja, S.M.; Wehbe, M.; Mas, A.; Chasson, L.; De Tenbossche, C.P.; Huijbers, I.; Van den Eynde, B.; Schmitt-Verhulst, A.M. Tumor-initiated inflammation overrides protective adaptive immunity in an induced melanoma model in mice. *Cancer Res.* **2010**, *70*, 3515–3525. [CrossRef]
9. Wehbe, M.; Soudja, S.M.; Mas, A.; Chasson, L.; Guinamard, R.; Powis de Tenbossche, C.; Verdeil, G.; Van den Eynde, B.; Schmitt-Verhulst, A.M. Epithelial-Mesenchymal-Transition-like and TGFβ pathways associated with autochthonous inflammatory melanoma development in mice. *PLoS ONE* **2012**, *7*, e49419. [CrossRef]
10. Noy, R.; Pollard, J.W. Tumor-associated macrophages: From mechanisms to therapy. *Immunity* **2014**, *41*, 49–61. [CrossRef]
11. Cassetta, L.; Fragkogianni, S.; Sims, A.H.; Swierczak, A.; Forrester, L.M.; Zhang, H.; Soong, D.Y.H.; Cotechini, T.; Anur, P.; Lin, E.Y.; et al. Human Tumor-Associated Macrophage and Monocyte Transcriptional Landscapes Reveal Cancer-Specific Reprogramming, Biomarkers, and Therapeutic Targets. *Cancer Cell* **2019**, *35*, 588–602. [CrossRef]
12. Bercovici, N.; Guerin, M.V.; Trautmann, A.; Donnadieu, E. The Remarkable Plasticity of Macrophages: A Chance to Fight Cancer. *Front. Immunol.* **2019**, *10*, 1563. [CrossRef] [PubMed]
13. Etzerodt, A.; Tsalkitzi, K.; Maniecki, M.; Damsky, W.; Delfini, M.; Baudoin, E.; Moulin, M.; Bosenberg, M.; Graversen, J.H.; Auphan-Anezin, N.; et al. Specific targeting of CD163(+) TAMs mobilizes inflammatory monocytes and promotes T cell-mediated tumor regression. *J. Exp. Med.* **2019**, *216*, 2394–2411. [CrossRef]
14. Movahedi, K.; Laoui, D.; Gysemans, C.; Baeten, M.; Stange, G.; Van den Bossche, J.; Mack, M.; Pipeleers, D.; In't Veld, P.; De Baetselier, P.; et al. Different tumor microenvironments contain functionally distinct subsets of macrophages derived from Ly6C(high) monocytes. *Cancer Res.* **2010**, *70*, 5728–5739. [CrossRef]
15. Lavin, Y.; Kobayashi, S.; Leader, A.; Amir, E.D.; Elefant, N.; Bigenwald, C.; Remark, R.; Sweeney, R.; Becker, C.D.; Levine, J.H.; et al. Innate Immune Landscape in Early Lung Adenocarcinoma by Paired Single-Cell Analyses. *Cell* **2017**, *169*, 750–765. [CrossRef]

16. Chevrier, S.; Levine, J.H.; Zanotelli, V.R.T.; Silina, K.; Schulz, D.; Bacac, M.; Ries, C.H.; Ailles, L.; Jewett, M.A.S.; Moch, H.; et al. An Immune Atlas of Clear Cell Renal Cell Carcinoma. *Cell* **2017**, *169*, 736–749. [CrossRef]
17. Gubin, M.M.; Esaulova, E.; Ward, J.P.; Malkova, O.N.; Runci, D.; Wong, P.; Noguchi, T.; Arthur, C.D.; Meng, W.; Alspach, E.; et al. High-Dimensional Analysis Delineates Myeloid and Lymphoid Compartment Remodeling during Successful Immune-Checkpoint Cancer Therapy. *Cell* **2018**, *175*, 1014–1030. [CrossRef]
18. Lawrence, T.; Natoli, G. Transcriptional regulation of macrophage polarization: Enabling diversity with identity. *Nat. Rev. Immunol.* **2011**, *11*, 750–761. [CrossRef]
19. Martinez, F.O.; Gordon, S. The M1 and M2 paradigm of macrophage activation: Time for reassessment. *F1000Prime Rep.* **2014**, *6*, 13. [CrossRef]
20. Croxford, A.L.; Lanzinger, M.; Hartmann, F.J.; Schreiner, B.; Mair, F.; Pelczar, P.; Clausen, B.E.; Jung, S.; Greter, M.; Becher, B. The Cytokine GM-CSF Drives the Inflammatory Signature of CCR2+ Monocytes and Licenses Autoimmunity. *Immunity* **2015**, *43*, 502–514. [CrossRef]
21. Huen, S.C.; Huynh, L.; Marlier, A.; Lee, Y.; Moeckel, G.W.; Cantley, L.G. GM-CSF Promotes Macrophage Alternative Activation after Renal Ischemia/Reperfusion Injury. *J. Am. Soc. Nephrol.* **2015**, *26*, 1334–1345. [CrossRef]
22. Kujawski, M.; Kortylewski, M.; Lee, H.; Herrmann, A.; Kay, H.; Yu, H. Stat3 mediates myeloid cell-dependent tumor angiogenesis in mice. *J. Clin. Investig.* **2008**, *118*, 3367–3377. [CrossRef]
23. Giurisato, E.; Xu, Q.; Lonardi, S.; Telfer, B.; Russo, I.; Pearson, A.; Finegan, K.G.; Wang, W.; Wang, J.; Gray, N.S.; et al. Myeloid ERK5 deficiency suppresses tumor growth by blocking protumor macrophage polarization via STAT3 inhibition. *Proc. Natl. Acad. Sci. USA* **2018**, *115*, E2801–E2810. [CrossRef] [PubMed]
24. Goossens, P.; Rodriguez-Vita, J.; Etzerodt, A.; Masse, M.; Rastoin, O.; Gouirand, V.; Ulas, T.; Papantonopoulou, O.; Van Eck, M.; Auphan-Anezin, N.; et al. Membrane Cholesterol Efflux Drives Tumor-Associated Macrophage Reprogramming and Tumor Progression. *Cell Metab.* **2019**, *29*, 1376–1389. [CrossRef] [PubMed]
25. Gupta, S.; Jain, A.; Syed, S.N.; Snodgrass, R.G.; Pfluger-Muller, B.; Leisegang, M.S.; Weigert, A.; Brandes, R.P.; Ebersberger, I.; Brune, B.; et al. IL-6 augments IL-4-induced polarization of primary human macrophages through synergy of STAT3, STAT6 and BATF transcription factors. *Oncoimmunology* **2018**, *7*, e1494110. [CrossRef] [PubMed]
26. Rebe, C.; Ghiringhelli, F. STAT3, a Master Regulator of Anti-Tumor Immune Response. *Cancers* **2019**, *11*, 1280. [CrossRef]
27. Andersen, M.N.; Etzerodt, A.; Graversen, J.H.; Holthof, L.C.; Moestrup, S.K.; Hokland, M.; Moller, H.J. STAT3 inhibition specifically in human monocytes and macrophages by CD163-targeted corosolic acid-containing liposomes. *Cancer Immunol. Immunother.* **2019**, *68*, 489–502. [CrossRef] [PubMed]
28. Lee, H.; Deng, J.; Xin, H.; Liu, Y.; Pardoll, D.; Yu, H. A requirement of STAT3 DNA binding precludes Th-1 immunostimulatory gene expression by NF-kappaB in tumors. *Cancer Res.* **2011**, *71*, 3772–3780. [CrossRef] [PubMed]
29. Yan, D.; Wang, H.W.; Bowman, R.L.; Joyce, J.A. STAT3 and STAT6 Signaling Pathways Synergize to Promote Cathepsin Secretion from Macrophages via IRE1alpha Activation. *Cell Rep.* **2016**, *16*, 2914–2927. [CrossRef]
30. Kortylewski, M.; Xin, H.; Kujawski, M.; Lee, H.; Liu, Y.; Harris, T.; Drake, C.; Pardoll, D.; Yu, H. Regulation of the IL-23 and IL-12 balance by Stat3 signaling in the tumor microenvironment. *Cancer Cell* **2009**, *15*, 114–123. [CrossRef]
31. Deng, J.; Liu, Y.; Lee, H.; Herrmann, A.; Zhang, W.; Zhang, C.; Shen, S.; Priceman, S.J.; Kujawski, M.; Pal, S.K.; et al. S1PR1-STAT3 signaling is crucial for myeloid cell colonization at future metastatic sites. *Cancer Cell* **2012**, *21*, 642–654. [CrossRef] [PubMed]
32. Jones, L.M.; Broz, M.L.; Ranger, J.J.; Ozcelik, J.; Ahn, R.; Zuo, D.; Ursini-Siegel, J.; Hallett, M.T.; Krummel, M.; Muller, W.J. STAT3 Establishes an Immunosuppressive Microenvironment during the Early Stages of Breast Carcinogenesis to Promote Tumor Growth and Metastasis. *Cancer Res.* **2016**, *76*, 1416–1428. [CrossRef] [PubMed]
33. Cheng, Z.; Zhang, D.; Gong, B.; Wang, P.; Liu, F. CD163 as a novel target gene of STAT3 is a potential therapeutic target for gastric cancer. *Oncotarget* **2017**, *8*, 87244–87262. [CrossRef] [PubMed]
34. Trovato, R.; Fiore, A.; Sartori, S.; Cane, S.; Giugno, R.; Cascione, L.; Paiella, S.; Salvia, R.; De Sanctis, F.; Poffe, O.; et al. Immunosuppression by monocytic myeloid-derived suppressor cells in patients with pancreatic ductal carcinoma is orchestrated by STAT3. *J. Immunother. Cancer* **2019**, *7*, 255. [CrossRef] [PubMed]

35. Thorn, M.; Guha, P.; Cunetta, M.; Espat, N.J.; Miller, G.; Junghans, R.P.; Katz, S.C. Tumor-associated GM-CSF overexpression induces immunoinhibitory molecules via STAT3 in myeloid-suppressor cells infiltrating liver metastases. *Cancer Gene.* **2016**, *23*, 188–198. [CrossRef] [PubMed]
36. Lamano, J.B.; Lamano, J.B.; Li, Y.D.; DiDomenico, J.D.; Choy, W.; Veliceasa, D.; Oyon, D.E.; Fakurnejad, S.; Ampie, L.; Kesavabhotla, K.; et al. Glioblastoma-Derived IL6 Induces Immunosuppressive Peripheral Myeloid Cell PD-L1 and Promotes Tumor Growth. *Clin. Cancer Res.* **2019**, *25*, 3643–3657. [CrossRef]
37. Zerdes, I.; Wallerius, M.; Sifakis, E.G.; Wallmann, T.; Betts, S.; Bartish, M.; Tsesmetzis, N.; Tobin, N.P.; Coucoravas, C.; Bergh, J.; et al. STAT3 Activity Promotes Programmed-Death Ligand 1 Expression and Suppresses Immune Responses in Breast Cancer. *Cancers* **2019**, *11*, 1479. [CrossRef] [PubMed]
38. Kowal, J.; Kornete, M.; Joyce, J.A. Re-education of macrophages as a therapeutic strategy in cancer. *Immunotherapy* **2019**, *11*, 677–689. [CrossRef]
39. Peranzoni, E.; Lemoine, J.; Vimeux, L.; Feuillet, V.; Barrin, S.; Kantari-Mimoun, C.; Bercovici, N.; Guerin, M.; Biton, J.; Ouakrim, H.; et al. Macrophages impede CD8 T cells from reaching tumor cells and limit the efficacy of anti-PD-1 treatment. *Proc Natl. Acad. Sci. USA* **2018**, *115*, E4041–E4050. [CrossRef]
40. O'Donnell, J.S.; Long, G.V.; Scolyer, R.A.; Teng, M.W.; Smyth, M.J. Resistance to PD1/PDL1 checkpoint inhibition. *Cancer Treat. Rev.* **2017**, *52*, 71–81. [CrossRef]
41. Tumeh, P.C.; Harview, C.L.; Yearley, J.H.; Shintaku, I.P.; Taylor, E.J.; Robert, L.; Chmielowski, B.; Spasic, M.; Henry, G.; Ciobanu, V.; et al. PD-1 blockade induces responses by inhibiting adaptive immune resistance. *Nature* **2014**, *515*, 568–571. [CrossRef] [PubMed]
42. Lin, H.; Wei, S.; Hurt, E.M.; Green, M.D.; Zhao, L.; Vatan, L.; Szeliga, W.; Herbst, R.; Harms, P.W.; Fecher, L.A.; et al. Host expression of PD-L1 determines efficacy of PD-L1 pathway blockade-mediated tumor regression. *J. Clin. Investig.* **2018**, *128*, 805–815. [CrossRef] [PubMed]
43. Tang, H.; Liang, Y.; Anders, R.A.; Taube, J.M.; Qiu, X.; Mulgaonkar, A.; Liu, X.; Harrington, S.M.; Guo, J.; Xin, Y.; et al. PD-L1 on host cells is essential for PD-L1 blockade-mediated tumor regression. *J. Clin. Investig.* **2018**, *128*, 580–588. [CrossRef] [PubMed]
44. Rashidian, M.; LaFleur, M.W.; Verschoor, V.L.; Dongre, A.; Zhang, Y.; Nguyen, T.H.; Kolifrath, S.; Aref, A.R.; Lau, C.J.; Paweletz, C.P.; et al. Immuno-PET identifies the myeloid compartment as a key contributor to the outcome of the antitumor response under PD-1 blockade. *Proc. Natl. Acad. Sci. USA* **2019**, *116*, 16971–16980. [CrossRef]
45. Wei, Y.; Zhao, Q.; Gao, Z.; Lao, X.M.; Lin, W.M.; Chen, D.P.; Mu, M.; Huang, C.X.; Liu, Z.Y.; Li, B.; et al. The local immune landscape determines tumor PD-L1 heterogeneity and sensitivity to therapy. *J. Clin. Investig.* **2019**, *129*, 3347–3360. [CrossRef]
46. Leonard, W.J.; Lin, J.X.; O'Shea, J.J. The gammac Family of Cytokines: Basic Biology to Therapeutic Ramifications. *Immunity* **2019**, *50*, 832–850. [CrossRef]
47. Raeber, M.E.; Zurbuchen, Y.; Impellizzieri, D.; Boyman, O. The role of cytokines in T-cell memory in health and disease. *Immunol Rev.* **2018**, *283*, 176–193. [CrossRef]
48. Spolski, R.; Li, P.; Leonard, W.J. Biology and regulation of IL-2: From molecular mechanisms to human therapy. *Nat. Rev. Immunol.* **2018**, *18*, 648–659. [CrossRef]
49. Hand, T.W.; Cui, W.; Jung, Y.W.; Sefik, E.; Joshi, N.S.; Chandele, A.; Liu, Y.; Kaech, S.M. Differential effects of STAT5 and PI3K/AKT signaling on effector and memory CD8 T-cell survival. *Proc. Natl. Acad. Sci. USA* **2010**, *107*, 16601–16606. [CrossRef]
50. Tripathi, P.; Kurtulus, S.; Wojciechowski, S.; Sholl, A.; Hoebe, K.; Morris, S.C.; Finkelman, F.D.; Grimes, H.L.; Hildeman, D.A. STAT5 is critical to maintain effector CD8+ T cell responses. *J. Immunol.* **2010**, *185*, 2116–2124. [CrossRef]
51. O'Gorman, W.E.; Dooms, H.; Thorne, S.H.; Kuswanto, W.F.; Simonds, E.F.; Krutzik, P.O.; Nolan, G.P.; Abbas, A.K. The initial phase of an immune response functions to activate regulatory T cells. *J. Immunol.* **2009**, *183*, 332–339. [CrossRef]
52. Verdeil, G.; Chaix, J.; Schmitt-Verhulst, A.M.; Auphan-Anezin, N. Temporal cross-talk between TCR and STAT signals for CD8 T cell effector differentiation. *Eur. J. Immunol.* **2006**, *36*, 3090–3100. [CrossRef]
53. Verdeil, G.; Puthier, D.; Nguyen, C.; Schmitt-Verhulst, A.M.; Auphan-Anezin, N. STAT5-mediated signals sustain a TCR-initiated gene expression program toward differentiation of CD8 T cell effectors. *J. Immunol.* **2006**, *176*, 4834–4842. [CrossRef]

54. Altan-Bonnet, G.; Germain, R.N. Modeling T cell antigen discrimination based on feedback control of digital ERK responses. *PLoS Biol.* **2005**, *3*, e356. [CrossRef]
55. Auphan-Anezin, N.; Mazza, C.; Guimezanes, A.; Barrett-Wilt, G.A.; Montero-Julian, F.; Roussel, A.; Hunt, D.F.; Malissen, B.; Schmitt-Verhulst, A.M. Distinct orientation of the alloreactive monoclonal CD8 T cell activation program by three different peptide/MHC complexes. *Eur. J. Immunol.* **2006**, *36*, 1856–1866. [CrossRef]
56. Chau, L.A.; Bluestone, J.A.; Madrenas, J. Dissociation of intracellular signaling pathways in response to partial agonist ligands of the T cell receptor. *J. Exp. Med.* **1998**, *187*, 1699–1709. [CrossRef]
57. Rollings, C.M.; Sinclair, L.V.; Brady, H.J.M.; Cantrell, D.A.; Ross, S.H. Interleukin-2 shapes the cytotoxic T cell proteome and immune environment-sensing programs. *Sci. Signal* **2018**, *11*, eaap8112. [CrossRef]
58. Ross, S.H.; Rollings, C.; Anderson, K.E.; Hawkins, P.T.; Stephens, L.R.; Cantrell, D.A. Phosphoproteomic Analyses of Interleukin 2 Signaling Reveal Integrated JAK Kinase-Dependent and -Independent Networks in CD8(+) T Cells. *Immunity* **2016**, *45*, 685–700. [CrossRef]
59. Cote-Sierra, J.; Foucras, G.; Guo, L.; Chiodetti, L.; Young, H.A.; Hu-Li, J.; Zhu, J.; Paul, W.E. Interleukin 2 plays a central role in Th2 differentiation. *Proc. Natl. Acad. Sci. USA* **2004**, *101*, 3880–3885. [CrossRef]
60. Grange, M.; Verdeil, G.; Arnoux, F.; Griffon, A.; Spicuglia, S.; Maurizio, J.; Buferne, M.; Schmitt-Verhulst, A.M.; Auphan-Anezin, N. Active STAT5 regulates T-bet and eomesodermin expression in CD8 T cells and imprints a T-bet-dependent Tc1 program with repressed IL-6/TGF-beta1 signaling. *J. Immunol.* **2013**, *191*, 3712–3724. [CrossRef]
61. Shi, M.; Lin, T.H.; Appell, K.C.; Berg, L.J. Janus-kinase-3-dependent signals induce chromatin remodeling at the Ifng locus during T helper 1 cell differentiation. *Immunity* **2008**, *28*, 763–773. [CrossRef]
62. Scheeren, F.A.; Naspetti, M.; Diehl, S.; Schotte, R.; Nagasawa, M.; Wijnands, E.; Gimeno, R.; Vyth-Dreese, F.A.; Blom, B.; Spits, H. STAT5 regulates the self-renewal capacity and differentiation of human memory B cells and controls Bcl-6 expression. *Nat. Immunol.* **2005**, *6*, 303–313. [CrossRef]
63. Sheng, W.; Yang, F.; Zhou, Y.; Yang, H.; Low, P.Y.; Kemeny, D.M.; Tan, P.; Moh, A.; Kaplan, M.H.; Zhang, Y.; et al. STAT5 programs a distinct subset of GM-CSF-producing T helper cells that is essential for autoimmune neuroinflammation. *Cell Res.* **2014**, *24*, 1387–1402. [CrossRef]
64. Olson, M.R.; Verdan, F.F.; Hufford, M.M.; Dent, A.L.; Kaplan, M.H. STAT3 Impairs STAT5 Activation in the Development of IL-9-Secreting T Cells. *J. Immunol.* **2016**, *196*, 3297–3304. [CrossRef]
65. Burchill, M.A.; Yang, J.; Vogtenhuber, C.; Blazar, B.R.; Farrar, M.A. IL-2 receptor beta-dependent STAT5 activation is required for the development of Foxp3+ regulatory T cells. *J. Immunol.* **2007**, *178*, 280–290. [CrossRef]
66. Yao, Z.; Kanno, Y.; Kerenyi, M.; Stephens, G.; Durant, L.; Watford, W.T.; Laurence, A.; Robinson, G.W.; Shevach, E.M.; Moriggl, R.; et al. Nonredundant roles for Stat5a/b in directly regulating Foxp3. *Blood* **2007**, *109*, 4368–4375. [CrossRef]
67. Yang, X.P.; Ghoreschi, K.; Steward-Tharp, S.M.; Rodriguez-Canales, J.; Zhu, J.; Grainger, J.R.; Hirahara, K.; Sun, H.W.; Wei, L.; Vahedi, G.; et al. Opposing regulation of the locus encoding IL-17 through direct, reciprocal actions of STAT3 and STAT5. *Nat. Immunol.* **2011**, *12*, 247–254. [CrossRef]
68. Nurieva, R.I.; Podd, A.; Chen, Y.; Alekseev, A.M.; Yu, M.; Qi, X.; Huang, H.; Wen, R.; Wang, J.; Li, H.S.; et al. STAT5 protein negatively regulates T follicular helper (Tfh) cell generation and function. *J. Biol. Chem.* **2012**, *287*, 11234–11239. [CrossRef]
69. Tripathi, S.K.; Chen, Z.; Larjo, A.; Kanduri, K.; Nousiainen, K.; Aijo, T.; Ricano-Ponce, I.; Hrdlickova, B.; Tuomela, S.; Laajala, E.; et al. Genome-wide Analysis of STAT3-Mediated Transcription during Early Human Th17 Cell Differentiation. *Cell Rep.* **2017**, *19*, 1888–1901. [CrossRef]
70. Poholek, A.C.; Jankovic, D.; Villarino, A.V.; Petermann, F.; Hettinga, A.; Shouval, D.S.; Snapper, S.B.; Kaech, S.M.; Brooks, S.R.; Vahedi, G.; et al. IL-10 induces a STAT3-dependent autoregulatory loop in TH2 cells that promotes Blimp-1 restriction of cell expansion via antagonism of STAT5 target genes. *Sci. Immunol.* **2016**, *1*, eaaf8612.
71. Li, P.; Mitra, S.; Spolski, R.; Oh, J.; Liao, W.; Tang, Z.; Mo, F.; Li, X.; West, E.E.; Gromer, D.; et al. STAT5-mediated chromatin interactions in superenhancers activate IL-2 highly inducible genes: Functional dissection of the Il2ra gene locus. *Proc. Natl. Acad. Sci. USA* **2017**, *114*, 12111–12119. [CrossRef]
72. Onishi, M.; Nosaka, T.; Misawa, K.; Mui, A.L.; Gorman, D.; McMahon, M.; Miyajima, A.; Kitamura, T.

Identification and characterization of a constitutively active STAT5 mutant that promotes cell proliferation. *Mol. Cell. Biol.* **1998**, *18*, 3871–3879. [CrossRef]

73. Gotthardt, D.; Putz, E.M.; Grundschober, E.; Prchal-Murphy, M.; Straka, E.; Kudweis, P.; Heller, G.; Bago-Horvath, Z.; Witalisz-Siepracka, A.; Cumaraswamy, A.A.; et al. STAT5 Is a Key Regulator in NK Cells and Acts as a Molecular Switch from Tumor Surveillance to Tumor Promotion. *Cancer Discov.* **2016**, *6*, 414–429. [CrossRef]
74. Cayrol, F.; Praditsuktavorn, P.; Fernando, T.M.; Kwiatkowski, N.; Marullo, R.; Calvo-Vidal, M.N.; Phillip, J.; Pera, B.; Yang, S.N.; Takpradit, K.; et al. THZ1 targeting CDK7 suppresses STAT transcriptional activity and sensitizes T-cell lymphomas to BCL2 inhibitors. *Nat. Commun.* **2017**, *8*, 14290. [CrossRef]
75. Nivarthi, H.; Prchal-Murphy, M.; Swoboda, A.; Hager, M.; Schlederer, M.; Kenner, L.; Tuckermann, J.; Sexl, V.; Moriggl, R.; Ermakova, O. Stat5 gene dosage in T cells modulates CD8+ T-cell homeostasis and attenuates contact hypersensitivity response in mice. *Allergy* **2015**, *70*, 67–79. [CrossRef]
76. Liao, W.; Spolski, R.; Li, P.; Du, N.; West, E.E.; Ren, M.; Mitra, S.; Leonard, W.J. Opposing actions of IL-2 and IL-21 on Th9 differentiation correlate with their differential regulation of BCL6 expression. *Proc. Natl. Acad. Sci. USA* **2014**, *111*, 3508–3513. [CrossRef]
77. Oestreich, K.J.; Mohn, S.E.; Weinmann, A.S. Molecular mechanisms that control the expression and activity of Bcl-6 in TH1 cells to regulate flexibility with a TFH-like gene profile. *Nat. Immunol.* **2012**, *13*, 405–411. [CrossRef]
78. Son, H.J.; Lee, S.H.; Lee, S.Y.; Kim, E.K.; Yang, E.J.; Kim, J.K.; Seo, H.B.; Park, S.H.; Cho, M.L. Oncostatin M Suppresses Activation of IL-17/Th17 via SOCS3 Regulation in CD4+ T Cells. *J. Immunol.* **2017**, *198*, 1484–1491. [CrossRef]
79. Wingelhofer, B.; Neubauer, H.A.; Valent, P.; Han, X.; Constantinescu, S.N.; Gunning, P.T.; Muller, M.; Moriggl, R. Implications of STAT3 and STAT5 signaling on gene regulation and chromatin remodeling in hematopoietic cancer. *Leukemia* **2018**, *32*, 1713–1726. [CrossRef]
80. Moriggl, R.; Sexl, V.; Kenner, L.; Duntsch, C.; Stangl, K.; Gingras, S.; Hoffmeyer, A.; Bauer, A.; Piekorz, R.; Wang, D.; et al. Stat5 tetramer formation is associated with leukemogenesis. *Cancer Cell* **2005**, *7*, 87–99. [CrossRef]
81. Grange, M.; Giordano, M.; Mas, A.; Roncagalli, R.; Firaguay, G.; Nunes, J.A.; Ghysdael, J.; Schmitt-Verhulst, A.M.; Auphan-Anezin, N. Control of CD8 T cell proliferation and terminal differentiation by active STAT5 and CDKN2A/CDKN2B. *Immunology* **2015**, *145*, 543–557. [CrossRef]
82. Freund, P.; Kerenyi, M.A.; Hager, M.; Wagner, T.; Wingelhofer, B.; Pham, H.T.T.; Elabd, M.; Han, X.; Valent, P.; Gouilleux, F.; et al. O-GlcNAcylation of STAT5 controls tyrosine phosphorylation and oncogenic transcription in STAT5-dependent malignancies. *Leukemia* **2017**, *31*, 2132–2142. [CrossRef]
83. Grange, M.; Buferne, M.; Verdeil, G.; Leserman, L.; Schmitt-Verhulst, A.M.; Auphan-Anezin, N. Activated STAT5 promotes long-lived cytotoxic CD8+ T cells that induce regression of autochthonous melanoma. *Cancer Res.* **2012**, *72*, 76–87. [CrossRef]
84. Maurer, B.; Nivarthi, H.; Wingelhofer, B.; Pham, H.T.T.; Schlederer, M.; Suske, T.; Grausenburger, R.; Schiefer, A.I.; Prchal-Murphy, M.; Chen, D.; et al. High activation of STAT5A drives peripheral T-cell lymphoma and leukemia. *Haematologica* **2019**. [CrossRef]
85. Burchill, M.A.; Goetz, C.A.; Prlic, M.; O'Neil, J.J.; Harmon, I.R.; Bensinger, S.J.; Turka, L.A.; Brennan, P.; Jameson, S.C.; Farrar, M.A. Distinct effects of STAT5 activation on CD4+ and CD8+ T cell homeostasis: Development of CD4+CD25+ regulatory T cells versus CD8+ memory T cells. *J. Immunol.* **2003**, *171*, 5853–5864. [CrossRef]
86. Heltemes-Harris, L.M.; Larson, J.D.; Starr, T.K.; Hubbard, G.K.; Sarver, A.L.; Largaespada, D.A.; Farrar, M.A. Sleeping Beauty transposon screen identifies signaling modules that cooperate with STAT5 activation to induce B-cell acute lymphoblastic leukemia. *Oncogene* **2016**, *35*, 3454–3464. [CrossRef]
87. Katerndahl, C.D.S.; Heltemes-Harris, L.M.; Willette, M.J.L.; Henzler, C.M.; Frietze, S.; Yang, R.; Schjerven, H.; Silverstein, K.A.T.; Ramsey, L.B.; Hubbard, G.; et al. Antagonism of B cell enhancer networks by STAT5 drives leukemia and poor patient survival. *Nat. Immunol.* **2017**, *18*, 694–704. [CrossRef]
88. Pham, H.T.T.; Maurer, B.; Prchal-Murphy, M.; Grausenburger, R.; Grundschober, E.; Javaheri, T.; Nivarthi, H.; Boersma, A.; Kolbe, T.; Elabd, M.; et al. STAT5BN642H is a driver mutation for T cell neoplasia. *J. Clin. Investig.* **2018**, *128*, 387–401. [CrossRef]

89. De Araujo, E.D.; Erdogan, F.; Neubauer, H.A.; Meneksedag-Erol, D.; Manaswiyoungkul, P.; Eram, M.S.; Seo, H.S.; Qadree, A.K.; Israelian, J.; Orlova, A.; et al. Structural and functional consequences of the STAT5B(N642H) driver mutation. *Nat. Commun.* **2019**, *10*, 2517. [CrossRef]
90. Zeng, R.; Spolski, R.; Finkelstein, S.E.; Oh, S.; Kovanen, P.E.; Hinrichs, C.S.; Pise-Masison, C.A.; Radonovich, M.F.; Brady, J.N.; Restifo, N.P.; et al. Synergy of IL-21 and IL-15 in regulating CD8+ T cell expansion and function. *J. Exp. Med.* **2005**, *201*, 139–148. [CrossRef]
91. Jones, L.L.; Alli, R.; Li, B.; Geiger, T.L. Differential T Cell Cytokine Receptivity and Not Signal Quality Distinguishes IL-6 and IL-10 Signaling during Th17 Differentiation. *J. Immunol.* **2016**, *196*, 2973–2985. [CrossRef]
92. Ashouri, J.F.; Hsu, L.Y.; Yu, S.; Rychkov, D.; Chen, Y.; Cheng, D.A.; Sirota, M.; Hansen, E.; Lattanza, L.; Zikherman, J.; et al. Reporters of TCR signaling identify arthritogenic T cells in murine and human autoimmune arthritis. *Proc. Natl. Acad. Sci. USA* **2019**, *116*, 18517–18527. [CrossRef]
93. Logotheti, S.; Putzer, B.M. STAT3 and STAT5 Targeting for Simultaneous Management of Melanoma and Autoimmune Diseases. *Cancers* **2019**, *11*, 1448. [CrossRef]
94. Wang, Y.; Shen, Y.; Wang, S.; Shen, Q.; Zhou, X. The role of STAT3 in leading the crosstalk between human cancers and the immune system. *Cancer Lett.* **2018**, *415*, 117–128. [CrossRef]
95. Cui, W.; Liu, Y.; Weinstein, J.S.; Craft, J.; Kaech, S.M. An interleukin-21-interleukin-10-STAT3 pathway is critical for functional maturation of memory CD8+ T cells. *Immunity* **2011**, *35*, 792–805. [CrossRef]
96. Siegel, A.M.; Heimall, J.; Freeman, A.F.; Hsu, A.P.; Brittain, E.; Brenchley, J.M.; Douek, D.C.; Fahle, G.H.; Cohen, J.I.; Holland, S.M.; et al. A critical role for STAT3 transcription factor signaling in the development and maintenance of human T cell memory. *Immunity* **2011**, *35*, 806–818. [CrossRef]
97. Hinrichs, C.S.; Spolski, R.; Paulos, C.M.; Gattinoni, L.; Kerstann, K.W.; Palmer, D.C.; Klebanoff, C.A.; Rosenberg, S.A.; Leonard, W.J.; Restifo, N.P. IL-2 and IL-21 confer opposing differentiation programs to CD8+ T cells for adoptive immunotherapy. *Blood* **2008**, *111*, 5326–5333. [CrossRef]
98. Kujawski, M.; Zhang, C.; Herrmann, A.; Reckamp, K.; Scuto, A.; Jensen, M.; Deng, J.; Forman, S.; Figlin, R.; Yu, H. Targeting STAT3 in adoptively transferred T cells promotes their in vivo expansion and antitumor effects. *Cancer Res.* **2010**, *70*, 9599–9610. [CrossRef]
99. Yue, C.; Shen, S.; Deng, J.; Priceman, S.J.; Li, W.; Huang, A.; Yu, H. STAT3 in CD8+ T Cells Inhibits Their Tumor Accumulation by Downregulating CXCR3/CXCL10 Axis. *Cancer Immunol. Res.* **2015**, *3*, 864–870. [CrossRef]
100. Triplett, T.A.; Tucker, C.G.; Triplett, K.C.; Alderman, Z.; Sun, L.; Ling, L.E.; Akporiaye, E.T.; Weinberg, A.D. STAT3 Signaling Is Required for Optimal Regression of Large Established Tumors in Mice Treated with Anti-OX40 and TGFbeta Receptor Blockade. *Cancer Immunol. Res.* **2015**, *3*, 526–535. [CrossRef]
101. Rosenberg, S.A.; Restifo, N.P. Adoptive cell transfer as personalized immunotherapy for human cancer. *Science* **2015**, *348*, 62–68. [CrossRef]
102. Dudley, M.E.; Wunderlich, J.R.; Yang, J.C.; Sherry, R.M.; Topalian, S.L.; Restifo, N.P.; Royal, R.E.; Kammula, U.; White, D.E.; Mavroukakis, S.A.; et al. Adoptive cell transfer therapy following non-myeloablative but lymphodepleting chemotherapy for the treatment of patients with refractory metastatic melanoma. *J. Clin. Oncol.* **2005**, *23*, 2346–2357. [CrossRef]
103. Sadelain, M.; Riviere, I.; Riddell, S. Therapeutic T cell engineering. *Nature* **2017**, *545*, 423–431. [CrossRef]
104. Schuster, S.J.; Svoboda, J.; Chong, E.A.; Nasta, S.D.; Mato, A.R.; Anak, O.; Brogdon, J.L.; Pruteanu-Malinici, I.; Bhoj, V.; Landsburg, D.; et al. Chimeric Antigen Receptor T Cells in Refractory B-Cell Lymphomas. *N. Engl. J. Med.* **2017**, *377*, 2545–2554. [CrossRef]
105. Majzner, R.G.; Mackall, C.L. Clinical lessons learned from the first leg of the CAR T cell journey. *Nat. Med.* **2019**, *25*, 1341–1355. [CrossRef]
106. Yamamoto, T.N.; Kishton, R.J.; Restifo, N.P. Developing neoantigen-targeted T cell-based treatments for solid tumors. *Nat. Med.* **2019**, *25*, 1488–1499. [CrossRef]
107. Beatty, G.L.; O'Hara, M.H.; Lacey, S.F.; Torigian, D.A.; Nazimuddin, F.; Chen, F.; Kulikovskaya, I.M.; Soulen, M.C.; McGarvey, M.; Nelson, A.M.; et al. Activity of Mesothelin-Specific Chimeric Antigen Receptor T Cells Against Pancreatic Carcinoma Metastases in a Phase 1 Trial. *Gastroenterology* **2018**, *155*, 29–32. [CrossRef]

108. Rosenberg, S.A. IL-2: The first effective immunotherapy for human cancer. *J. Immunol.* **2014**, *192*, 5451–5458. [CrossRef]
109. Krieg, C.; Letourneau, S.; Pantaleo, G.; Boyman, O. Improved IL-2 immunotherapy by selective stimulation of IL-2 receptors on lymphocytes and endothelial cells. *Proc. Natl. Acad. Sci. USA* **2010**, *107*, 11906–11911. [CrossRef]
110. Boyman, O.; Kovar, M.; Rubinstein, M.P.; Surh, C.D.; Sprent, J. Selective stimulation of T cell subsets with antibody-cytokine immune complexes. *Science* **2006**, *311*, 1924–1927. [CrossRef]
111. Verdeil, G.; Marquardt, K.; Surh, C.D.; Sherman, L.A. Adjuvants targeting innate and adaptive immunity synergize to enhance tumor immunotherapy. *Proc. Natl. Acad. Sci. USA* **2008**, *105*, 16683–16688. [CrossRef]
112. Boyman, O.; Arenas-Ramirez, N. Development of a novel class of interleukin-2 immunotherapies for metastatic cancer. *Swiss Med. Wkly.* **2019**, *149*, w14697. [CrossRef]
113. Sabatino, M.; Hu, J.; Sommariva, M.; Gautam, S.; Fellowes, V.; Hocker, J.D.; Dougherty, S.; Qin, H.; Klebanoff, C.A.; Fry, T.J.; et al. Generation of clinical-grade CD19-specific CAR-modified CD8+ memory stem cells for the treatment of human B-cell malignancies. *Blood* **2016**, *128*, 519–528. [CrossRef]
114. Kagoya, Y.; Tanaka, S.; Guo, T.; Anczurowski, M.; Wang, C.H.; Saso, K.; Butler, M.O.; Minden, M.D.; Hirano, N. A novel chimeric antigen receptor containing a JAK-STAT signaling domain mediates superior antitumor effects. *Nat. Med.* **2018**, *24*, 352–359. [CrossRef]
115. Sackstein, R.; Schatton, T.; Barthel, S.R. T-lymphocyte homing: An underappreciated yet critical hurdle for successful cancer immunotherapy. *Lab. Investig.* **2017**, *97*, 669–697. [CrossRef]
116. Miller, B.C.; Sen, D.R.; Al Abosy, R.; Bi, K.; Virkud, Y.V.; LaFleur, M.W.; Yates, K.B.; Lako, A.; Felt, K.; Naik, G.S.; et al. Subsets of exhausted CD8(+) T cells differentially mediate tumor control and respond to checkpoint blockade. *Nat. Immunol.* **2019**, *20*, 326–336. [CrossRef]
117. Siddiqui, I.; Schaeuble, K.; Chennupati, V.; Fuertes Marraco, S.A.; Calderon-Copete, S.; Pais Ferreira, D.; Carmona, S.J.; Scarpellino, L.; Gfeller, D.; Pradervand, S.; et al. Intratumoral Tcf1(+)PD-1(+)CD8(+) T Cells with Stem-like Properties Promote Tumor Control in Response to Vaccination and Checkpoint Blockade Immunotherapy. *Immunity* **2019**, *50*, 195–211. [CrossRef]
118. Robbins, P.F.; Dudley, M.E.; Wunderlich, J.; El-Gamil, M.; Li, Y.F.; Zhou, J.; Huang, J.; Powell, D.J., Jr.; Rosenberg, S.A. Cutting edge: Persistence of transferred lymphocyte clonotypes correlates with cancer regression in patients receiving cell transfer therapy. *J. Immunol.* **2004**, *173*, 7125–7130. [CrossRef]
119. Yang, S.; Ji, Y.; Gattinoni, L.; Zhang, L.; Yu, Z.; Restifo, N.P.; Rosenberg, S.A.; Morgan, R.A. Modulating the differentiation status of ex vivo-cultured anti-tumor T cells using cytokine cocktails. *Cancer Immunol. Immunother.* **2013**, *62*, 727–736. [CrossRef]
120. Khan, O.; Giles, J.R.; McDonald, S.; Manne, S.; Ngiow, S.F.; Patel, K.P.; Werner, M.T.; Huang, A.C.; Alexander, K.A.; Wu, J.E.; et al. TOX transcriptionally and epigenetically programs CD8(+) T cell exhaustion. *Nature* **2019**, *571*, 211–218. [CrossRef]
121. Fraietta, J.A.; Lacey, S.F.; Orlando, E.J.; Pruteanu-Malinici, I.; Gohil, M.; Lundh, S.; Boesteanu, A.C.; Wang, Y.; O'Connor, R.S.; Hwang, W.T.; et al. Determinants of response and resistance to CD19 chimeric antigen receptor (CAR) T cell therapy of chronic lymphocytic leukemia. *Nat. Med.* **2018**, *24*, 563–571. [CrossRef]
122. Milner, J.D.; Vogel, T.P.; Forbes, L.; Ma, C.A.; Stray-Pedersen, A.; Niemela, J.E.; Lyons, J.J.; Engelhardt, K.R.; Zhang, Y.; Topcagic, N.; et al. Early-onset lymphoproliferation and autoimmunity caused by germline STAT3 gain-of-function mutations. *Blood* **2015**, *125*, 591–599. [CrossRef]
123. Sadreev, I.I.; Chen, M.Z.Q.; Umezawa, Y.; Biktashev, V.N.; Kemper, C.; Salakhieva, D.V.; Welsh, G.I.; Kotov, N.V. The competitive nature of signal transducer and activator of transcription complex formation drives phenotype switching of T cells. *Immunology* **2018**, *153*, 488–501. [CrossRef]
124. McLane, L.M.; Abdel-Hakeem, M.S.; Wherry, E.J. CD8 T Cell Exhaustion During Chronic Viral Infection and Cancer. *Annu. Rev. Immunol.* **2019**, *37*, 457–495. [CrossRef]
125. Giordano, M.; Henin, C.; Maurizio, J.; Imbratta, C.; Bourdely, P.; Buferne, M.; Baitsch, L.; Vanhille, L.; Sieweke, M.H.; Speiser, D.E.; et al. Molecular profiling of CD8 T cells in autochthonous melanoma identifies Maf as driver of exhaustion. *EMBO J.* **2015**, *34*, 2042–2058. [CrossRef]
126. Speiser, D.E.; Ho, P.C.; Verdeil, G. Regulatory circuits of T cell function in cancer. *Nat. Rev. Immunol.* **2016**, *16*, 599–611. [CrossRef]
127. Ladak, K.; Bass, A.R. Checkpoint inhibitor-associated autoimmunity. *Best Pract. Res. Clin. Rheumatol.* **2018**, *32*, 781–802. [CrossRef]

128. Keir, M.E.; Butte, M.J.; Freeman, G.J.; Sharpe, A.H. PD-1 and its ligands in tolerance and immunity. *Annu. Rev. Immunol.* **2008**, *26*, 677–704. [CrossRef]
129. Celis-Gutierrez, J.; Blattmann, P.; Zhai, Y.; Jarmuzynski, N.; Ruminski, K.; Gregoire, C.; Ounoughene, Y.; Fiore, F.; Aebersold, R.; Roncagalli, R.; et al. Quantitative Interactomics in Primary T Cells Provides a Rationale for Concomitant PD-1 and BTLA Coinhibitor Blockade in Cancer Immunotherapy. *Cell Rep.* **2019**, *27*, 3315–3330. [CrossRef]
130. Franceschini, D.; Paroli, M.; Francavilla, V.; Videtta, M.; Morrone, S.; Labbadia, G.; Cerino, A.; Mondelli, M.U.; Barnaba, V. PD-L1 negatively regulates CD4+CD25+Foxp3+ Tregs by limiting STAT-5 phosphorylation in patients chronically infected with HCV. *J. Clin. Investig.* **2009**, *119*, 551–564. [CrossRef]
131. Taylor, D.K.; Walsh, P.T.; LaRosa, D.F.; Zhang, J.; Burchill, M.A.; Farrar, M.A.; Turka, L.A. Constitutive activation of STAT5 supersedes the requirement for cytokine and TCR engagement of CD4+ T cells in steady-state homeostasis. *J. Immunol.* **2006**, *177*, 2216–2223. [CrossRef] [PubMed]
132. Buferne, M.; Chasson, L.; Grange, M.; Mas, A.; Arnoux, F.; Bertuzzi, M.; Naquet, P.; Leserman, L.; Schmitt-Verhulst, A.M.; Auphan-Anezin, N. IFNgamma producing CD8+ T cells modified to resist major immune checkpoints induce regression of MHC class I-deficient melanomas. *Oncoimmunology* **2015**, *4*, e974959. [CrossRef] [PubMed]
133. Auphan-Anezin, N.; Verdeil, G.; Grange, M.; Soudja, S.M.; Wehbe, M.; Buferne, M.; Mas, A.; Schmitt-Verhulst, A.M. Immunosuppression in inflammatory melanoma: Can it be resisted by adoptively transferred T cells? *Pigment Cell Melanoma Res.* **2013**, *26*, 167–175. [CrossRef] [PubMed]
134. Verdeil, G.; Fuertes Marraco, S.A.; Murray, T.; Speiser, D.E. From T cell "exhaustion" to anti-cancer immunity. *Biochim. Biophys. Acta* **2016**, *1865*, 49–57. [CrossRef] [PubMed]
135. Sun, C.; Fu, B.; Gao, Y.; Liao, X.; Sun, R.; Tian, Z.; Wei, H. TGF-beta1 down-regulation of NKG2D/DAP10 and 2B4/SAP expression on human NK cells contributes to HBV persistence. *PLoS Pathog.* **2012**, *8*, e1002594. [CrossRef]
136. Thomas, D.A.; Massague, J. TGF-beta directly targets cytotoxic T cell functions during tumor evasion of immune surveillance. *Cancer Cell* **2005**, *8*, 369–380. [CrossRef]
137. Benahmed, M.; Meresse, B.; Arnulf, B.; Barbe, U.; Mention, J.J.; Verkarre, V.; Allez, M.; Cellier, C.; Hermine, O.; Cerf-Bensussan, N. Inhibition of TGF-beta signaling by IL-15: A new role for IL-15 in the loss of immune homeostasis in celiac disease. *Gastroenterology* **2007**, *132*, 994–1008. [CrossRef]
138. Xiao, Q.; Wu, J.; Wang, W.J.; Chen, S.; Zheng, Y.; Yu, X.; Meeth, K.; Sahraei, M.; Bothwell, A.L.M.; Chen, L.; et al. DKK2 imparts tumor immunity evasion through beta-catenin-independent suppression of cytotoxic immune-cell activation. *Nat Med.* **2018**, *24*, 262–270. [CrossRef]
139. Mardiana, S.; Lai, J.; House, I.G.; Beavis, P.A.; Darcy, P.K. Switching on the green light for chimeric antigen receptor T-cell therapy. *Clin. Transl. Immunol.* **2019**, *8*, e1046. [CrossRef]
140. Zhang, J.; Endres, S.; Kobold, S. Enhancing tumor T cell infiltration to enable cancer immunotherapy. *Immunotherapy* **2019**, *11*, 201–213. [CrossRef]
141. Ayers, M.; Lunceford, J.; Nebozhyn, M.; Murphy, E.; Loboda, A.; Kaufman, D.R.; Albright, A.; Cheng, J.D.; Kang, S.P.; Shankaran, V.; et al. IFN-gamma-related mRNA profile predicts clinical response to PD-1 blockade. *J. Clin. Investig.* **2017**, *127*, 2930–2940. [CrossRef] [PubMed]
142. Horton, B.L.; Williams, J.B.; Cabanov, A.; Spranger, S.; Gajewski, T.F. Intratumoral CD8(+) T-cell Apoptosis Is a Major Component of T-cell Dysfunction and Impedes Antitumor Immunity. *Cancer Immunol. Res.* **2018**, *6*, 14–24. [CrossRef] [PubMed]
143. Pai, C.S.; Huang, J.T.; Lu, X.; Simons, D.M.; Park, C.; Chang, A.; Tamaki, W.; Liu, E.; Roybal, K.T.; Seagal, J.; et al. Clonal Deletion of Tumor-Specific T Cells by Interferon-gamma Confers Therapeutic Resistance to Combination Immune Checkpoint Blockade. *Immunity* **2019**, *50*, 477–492. [CrossRef] [PubMed]
144. Zhu, J.; Powis de Tenbossche, C.G.; Cane, S.; Colau, D.; van Baren, N.; Lurquin, C.; Schmitt-Verhulst, A.M.; Liljestrom, P.; Uyttenhove, C.; Van den Eynde, B.J. Resistance to cancer immunotherapy mediated by apoptosis of tumor-infiltrating lymphocytes. *Nat. Commun.* **2017**, *8*, 1404. [CrossRef]

4

STAT3 and STAT5 Targeting for Simultaneous Management of Melanoma and Autoimmune Diseases

Stella Logotheti [1] **and Brigitte M. Pützer** [1,2,*]

[1] Institute of Experimental Gene Therapy and Cancer Research, Rostock University Medical Center, 18057 Rostock, Germany; Styliani.Logotheti@med.uni-rostock.de

[2] Department Life, Light & Matter, University of Rostock, 18059 Rostock, Germany

* Correspondence: brigitte.puetzer@med.uni-rostock.de

Abstract: Melanoma is a skin cancer which can become metastatic, drug-refractory, and lethal if managed late or inappropriately. An increasing number of melanoma patients exhibits autoimmune diseases, either as pre-existing conditions or as sequelae of immune-based anti-melanoma therapies, which complicate patient management and raise the need for more personalized treatments. STAT3 and/or STAT5 cascades are commonly activated during melanoma progression and mediate the metastatic effects of key oncogenic factors. Deactivation of these cascades enhances antitumor-immune responses, is efficient against metastatic melanoma in the preclinical setting and emerges as a promising targeting strategy, especially for patients resistant to immunotherapies. In the light of the recent realization that cancer and autoimmune diseases share common mechanisms of immune dysregulation, we suggest that the systemic delivery of STAT3 or STAT5 inhibitors could simultaneously target both, melanoma and associated autoimmune diseases, thereby decreasing the overall disease burden and improving quality of life of this patient subpopulation. Herein, we review the recent advances of STAT3 and STAT5 targeting in melanoma, explore which autoimmune diseases are causatively linked to STAT3 and/or STAT5 signaling, and propose that these patients may particularly benefit from treatment with STAT3/STAT5 inhibitors.

Keywords: melanoma; autoimmune disease; inflammation; STAT3; STAT5; immunotherapy; tumor–immune cell interactions

1. Introduction

Within the last decade, the cancer field has witnessed a rapid paradigm shift from traditional chemotherapy to immunotherapy. A major advantage of immunotherapeutics is that, instead of directly targeting and killing the tumor as cytotoxic drugs do, they stimulate a person's own immune system to recognize and destroy cancer cells. In this respect, they ally with the immune cells not only to shrink the primary tumor but also to establish durable responses against circulating cancer cells that might lurk beyond the primary site. Cancer immunotherapy approaches include (a) checkpoint inhibitors, which act by releasing the brakes that prevent T-cells from killing cancer cells, (b) monoclonal antibodies, that are designed to attach to cancer cell-specific antigens, (c) cancer vaccines, boosting the immune system's response to tumors, or (d) cell-based therapies, such as chimeric antigen receptor (CAR) T-cell therapy, where T cells taken from a patient's tumor are expanded and/or genetically engineered ex vivo and then administered back to the patient, a process termed adoptive transfer [1]. The field of successful application of immunotherapy includes, but is not limited to, metastatic melanoma [2], a type of cancer that arises from melanocytes and represents the deadliest form of skin cancer, with increasing prevalence. Once it becomes metastatic, the prognosis is very unfavorable and, thus, early diagnosis is crucial for effective management [3].

Since 2011, several next-generation immune-based formulations, such as the checkpoint inhibitors ipilimumab, pembrolizumab, and nivolumab, received approval by the Food and Drug Administration (FDA) for the indication of metastatic melanoma [2] and led to significant clinical improvements, either as monotherapies or in combination regimens [4]. However, despite their remarkable success, only up to 20% to 30% of patients have benefited from these treatments, while the rest are either non-responders (primary resistance) or partial responders (acquired resistance). Unresponsiveness is attributed to factors such as CD8+ T cell density in the tumor microenvironment, monocyte frequency, tumor heterogeneity, and neoantigen load, as well as the composition of patient's gut microbiota [4].

Other challenges regarding immunotherapy include immune-related toxicities. In particular, 85% of melanoma patients under ipilimumab treatment have experienced immune-related adverse events of any grade, with over one-third discontinuing therapy or requiring additional systemic treatment to manage side effects [5]. Immunotherapy faces limitations in patients with both an overactive (autoimmune disease patients) or a suppressed (organ transplant recipients) immune system. On the one hand, melanoma patients with pre-existing autoimmune diseases who receive ipilimumab treatment present frequent disease flares and exacerbations, requiring additional immunosuppression or therapy discontinuation [6,7]. On the other hand, solid organ transplant recipients are at increased risk of developing metastatic melanoma, and when they do, they exhibit a higher probability for graft rejection upon immune checkpoint inhibitor treatment [8,9]. In general, a dysregulated immune system poses as the Sword of Damocles in the decision of clinicians to prescribe immunotherapy. In this regard, there is an increasing need to develop drugs for the treatment of melanoma that are not only safer for such patients but are also able to manage this cancer along with a co-existing immune-related disease.

Herein, we hypothesize that therapeutic management of various clinical disorders simultaneously can be achieved by targeting their major common pathways. As a representative case, we consider the Janus kinase/signal transducers and activators of transcription (JAK/STAT) pathway, which is activated in a wide range of autoimmune diseases (AD), as well as in many different cancer types. It mediates immune responses to several insults from resisting infection to maintaining immune tolerance, enforcing barrier functions, and guarding against cancer [10]. In this review, we summarize ADs that are associated with malignant melanoma, we explore how STAT3 and STAT5 signaling contributes to their pathogenesis, and we evaluate STAT3/STAT5 inhibition as a feasible strategy to target these diseases in order to achieve their simultaneous management with a single drug.

2. Associations among Melanoma, Inflammation and Autoimmune Diseases

A cancer patient can frequently experience disorders, such as inflammation and autoimmune diseases, that occur as frequent pre-existing, predisposing, or intercurrent conditions [11–13]. Intriguingly, these diseases seem to be etiologically interrelated with one another. On one side, cancer has been linked with chronic inflammation. Moreover, there are interconnections between autoimmune diseases and cancer, since certain autoimmune disorders predispose to neoplasias [14]. Patients suffering from dermatomyositis, inflammatory bowel disease, systemic lupus erythematosus, rheumatoid arthritis, psoriasis or Sjögren syndrome may have increased risks for malignancies, whereas the type(s) of cancer they tend to develop depend on the type of the autoimmune disease [15]. For example, rheumatoid arthritis patients are at a greater risk of developing clonal expansions of large granular lymphocytes [16]. Although an autoimmune disorder does not necessarily lead to cancer, it is, however, a phenotypic manifestation of a deregulated immune system, which is generally a favorable background for cancer development [17]. Vice versa, cancer immunotherapy triggers autoimmunity towards several anatomical sites and can lead to conditions that range from relatively minor, such as skin depigmentation, to severe colitis, pancreatitis, lung or liver toxicity [18]. Furthermore, a persistent inflammation can be a fertile ground for the development of an AD [19]. Overall, an inflammation can potentially progress to a neoplasia or an autoimmune disorder, and this process can be facilitated by deregulation of the innate immune system [11,14] (Figure 1).

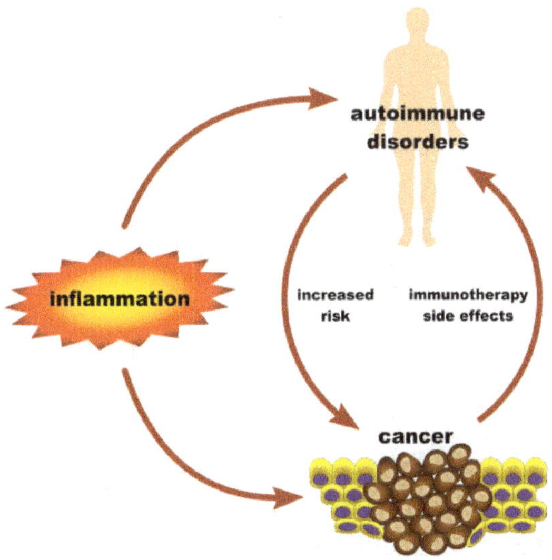

Figure 1. Associations between inflammation, cancer, and autoimmune disease. An inflammation can eventually lead to cancer or autoimmune disease. Some autoimmune disorders may predispose to malignancies. Cancer immunotherapy is associated to autoimmunity.

This interplay among ADs and cancer is evident in the case of melanoma patients. First of all, there is a long-standing inverse association between melanoma and vitiligo, a condition where the immune system produces autoantibodies against immunogenic, melanocytic-specific molecules (melanocytic-differentiation antigens, MDAs) that propel melanin production. These autoantibodies attack melanocytes, ultimately producing white skin patches. Thus, vitiligo patients show a lower melanoma risk because the antibodies against melanocytes confer natural cancer protection [20]. Vice versa, some melanoma patients develop a similar antibody-based condition, called melanoma-associated hypopigmentation or vitiligo-like depigmentation, which is usually considered as a predictor of better outcomes [21], although there are also reports demonstrating that hypopigmentation can be associated with disease progression [22–24]. Given that malignant melanoma co-evolves with immune cell phenotypes [25], this dynamic interaction between autoimmunity-based hypopigmentation and skin cancer could, in the long run, become a double-edged sword. Specifically, these tumors exhibit a high intratumoral heterogeneity and plasticity [25]. Therefore, over the course of the disease, tight immunosurveillance against MDA-expressing cells could serve as a microenvironmental cue that adds evolutionary pressure for immunoselection of low-MDA expressing cell variants that are poorly recognized by the autoantibodies. Such MDA-negative cells possess enhanced invasive capabilities. In this way, anti-MDA responses provoked by the melanoma tumor, can, in turn, promote clonal expansion of low-MDA-expressing cell variants with activated prometastatic programs that can migrate to distant sites, giving rise to secondary tumors [24].

Other autoimmune diseases are positively correlated with melanoma progression [2,26]. A retrospective meta-analysis assessed that the prevalence of pre-existing AD in melanoma patients increased by 1.7-fold within a decade. Prevalence rates were higher in metastatic melanoma patients compared to primary, non-metastatic skin cancer patients or the general population, suggesting that a pre-existing AD could possibly favor metastatic progression. The most common ADs among metastatic melanoma patients were myositis, peripheral neuropathy, type 1 diabetes mellitus, rheumatoid arthritis, psoriasis, autoimmune pancreatitis, autoimmune aplastic anemia, relapsing polychondritis, Hashimoto's encephalopathy, and inflammatory bowel disease. The authors suggested that disturbances in shared molecular or immune pathways could underlie increased susceptibility of AD patients to melanoma [2]. Another clinical study showed that only a small percentage of melanoma patients have a pre-existing AD, but in these patients, progression is faster and prognosis is worse.

This subpopulation has a significantly shorter median overall survival and disease-free survival after first metastasis versus cases with a primary tumor, while poorer prognosis was independent of the side effects of AD treatment. Those patients with an antibody-mediated AD had a worse prognosis in relation to those with a T cell-related AD. [27]. Together, these data unveil a potential link between malignant melanoma and immune dysregulation, implying that a pre-existing autoimmune disease could be a predisposing factor for melanoma development and progression. If that is indeed the case, further experimental investigations are needed.

The relationship between inflammation and cancer is well established [28] and inflammation contributes to melanoma initiation and progression [25]. Upregulation of key cancer-related inflammation genes, such as the transcription factors nuclear factor 'kappa-light-chain-enhancer' of activated B-cells (NF-κB) and STAT3, as well as several inflammatory cytokines and angiogenic factors, facilitate melanoma development. Indeed, inoculation of B16-F10 melanoma cells in chronic skin inflammation mouse models led to the formation of larger volume tumors in comparison with the non-inflamed controls, followed by increased periostin expression and M2 macrophage recruitment in the tumor microenvironment (TME) [29]. Similarly, in a mouse model of melanoma, repetitive UV exposure promoted metastasis via neutrophilic skin inflammation. In particular, UV irradiation-induced neutrophil recruitment and activation, which was initiated by the release of high mobility group box 1 (HMGB1) from UV-damaged epidermal keratinocytes. The UV-induced neutrophilic inflammatory response stimulated angiogenesis and increased the number of lung metastases through modulation of melanoma–endothelial cell interactions [30]. The association between inflammation and melanoma is also supported by the fact that anti-inflammatory drugs contribute to melanoma prevention or treatment. Population-based case-control studies showed that continuous use of low-dose non-steroid anti-inflammatory drugs (NSAIDs), such as diclofenac, ibuprofen, and naproxen, reduced the incidence of skin cancer, even though in a sex-dependent manner [31]. Other studies showed that combining celecoxib, a cyclooxygenase COX-2 selective NSAID, with chemotherapeutics can be an effective strategy for melanoma treatment [32].

3. A Basis for the Development of Multipotent Drugs against Melanoma, Inflammation, and Autoimmune Disorders

It is becoming increasingly evident that common molecular mechanisms underlie inflammatory-driven [12], as well as inflammatory/autoimmune-driven neoplasias [17]. The emerging similarities and interconnections among these diseases imply that despite their diverse clinical manifestations, outcome, and response to therapy, a limited number of mutual molecular events might drive their pathogenesis. In this regard, the mechanistic commonalities between cancer, inflammation, and ADs have created a basis for drug repurposing. For instance, anti-inflammatory drugs are used in combination with anticancer regimens [12,33]. Additionally, immunomodulatory drugs used for the treatment of ADs show efficacy against neoplastic diseases [34,35] and vice-versa, anticancer therapeutics can be applied to treat non-cancer immune-mediated diseases [36]. Recent network-based studies demonstrate that disorders with distinct clinical manifestations share a common genetic background [37]. Therefore, identifying shared signaling networks and cellular pathophenotypes at the core of these diseases is anticipated to further shape drug development in the future. We use the term 'multipotent drug' for any targeted inhibitor with the potential to act against two or more pathologies, even if these are different diseases, such as autoimmunity and cancer as an example. Moreover, given that they are mechanistically interrelated [11,12], we further postulate that the effectiveness of such a multipotent drug may depend on its interference with 'root' pathways that pose as common denominators in the pathology of these diseases. Hence, identification of these common traits is a prerequisite for the development of multipotent drugs, which could simultaneously manage cancer in conjunction with coexisting, pre-existing, or predisposing disorders (Figure 2).

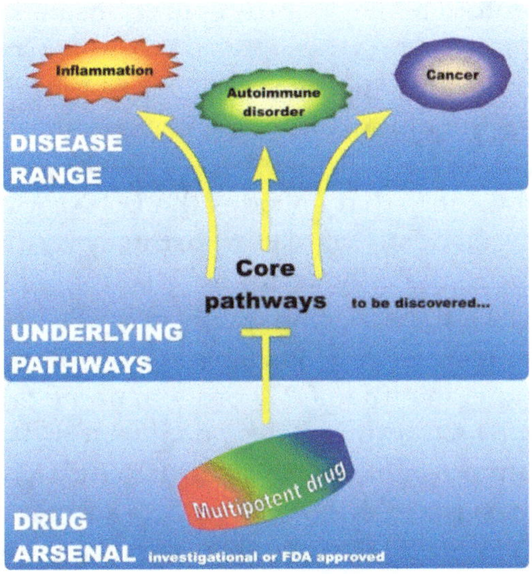

Figure 2. Proposed rationale for treating melanoma and associated inflammation or autoimmunity with multipotent drugs. Investigational or Food and Drug Administration (FDA)-approved drugs could exert anti-inflammatory, immunomodulatory, and anticancer effects. This, to an extent, might be due to their interference with signaling pathways commonly activated in inflammation, autoimmune disease, or cancer. These core pathways underlying all-three pathological conditions can be further characterized to facilitate simultaneous management of associated pathologies due to distinct diseases.

To this end, considering that deregulation of immunity is the main culprit in inflammation, autoimmune disease, and melanoma, we hypothesized that pathways mediating immune responses might be suitable therapeutic targets. Given that the JAK/STAT pathway is commonly activated in these diseases, we postulate that it is an emerging candidate 'core' pathway. Herein, we review the current knowledge of the effects of STAT3 and STAT5 signaling in melanoma, inflammation, and autoimmune disorders and estimate their value for concurrent management of these interconnected conditions.

4. STAT3 and STAT5 Signaling in Melanoma Initiation and Progression

STAT proteins, particularly STAT3 and, to a lesser extent, STAT5 govern fundamental oncogenic processes. STAT family members respond to cytokines, growth factors, and hormones, and transduce signals from the cell membrane to the nucleus to transactivate genes involved in cellular immunity, proliferation, apoptosis, and differentiation. The STAT family encompasses seven members, STAT1, STAT2, STAT3, STAT4, STAT5A, STAT5B, and STAT6, which show high homology in their functional domains. Their main difference lies in the C-terminal transactivation domain that varies among family members and modulates transcriptional activation of target genes. Under physiologic conditions, STAT signaling is stimulus-dependent and tightly regulated. The regulation of STAT activity via phosphorylation of a conserved C-terminal tyrosine residue has been previously described in detail [38,39]. Constitutive activation of STAT3 and STAT5 is involved in tumor formation and progression. However, not all STAT members are promoting cancer progression. STAT1, for instance, exerts proapoptotic and antiproliferative effects, and it seems that both, STAT3 and STAT5 can antagonize its function [40].

STAT3 is constitutively activated across many types of human cancers, including melanoma, as a consequence of aberrant autocrine or paracrine stimulation by cytokines and growth factors, such as interleukins (IL-6, IL-10, IL-12), interferons (IFNs), granulocyte-colony stimulating factor (G-CSF or CSF3), leptin, prolactin (PRL), growth hormone (HGH), epidermal growth factor (EGF), hepatocyte growth factor (HGF), basic fibroblast growth factor (FGF2), and virus proteins (e.g., v-Src, v-Fps, v-Sis). Permanent STAT3 activation can also result from receptors with intrinsic tyrosine kinase activities (such as erb-b2 receptor tyrosine kinase 2 (ERBB2), epidermal growth factor receptor (EGFR), and hepatocyte growth factor receptor HGFR), non-receptor tyrosine kinases (such as c-Src and c-abl), or G-protein coupled receptors [38,41]. An overactive STAT3 is associated with poor prognosis in melanoma patients and drives tumor initiation and malignant progression via induction of several cancer hallmarks, such as apoptosis inhibition, tumor angiogenesis, epithelial–mesenchymal transition (EMT), and stemness. In particular, upon c-Src activation, STAT3 promotes tumor cell survival and proliferation by transactivating *BCL2L1* (that encodes the Bcl-XL protein) and *MCL1*, two crucial anti-apoptotic genes that override cell death regulatory pathways. Additionally, STAT3 regulates the *MYC* gene, which mediates escape of melanoma tumor cells from both terminal differentiation and G0/G1 arrest. Beyond its function as a transcriptional activator, STAT3 can also suppress transcription of the well-established tumor suppressor *TP53* [38]. This suppression can provide an explanation on why melanomas that lack mutations in either *TP53* or its main negative regulator, such as *MDM2*, exhibit aggressive characteristics. STAT3 upregulates nodal factors of angiogenesis, mainly vascular endothelial growth factor (VEGF), hypoxia-inducible factor 1a (HIF-1α) and matrix metalloproteinase-2 (MMP-2) [38] and fosters brain metastasis in melanoma [42]. In addition, drivers of melanoma invasion and metastasis, such as ΔEx2/3p73 (named DNp73), a transactivation-deficient N-terminally truncated oncogenic isoform of the *TP73* gene, can trigger an IGF1R-AKT/STAT3 signaling cascade, which leads to the activation of EMT markers and acquisition of mesenchymal cell phenotypes [43,44]. Additionally, STAT3 is often mentioned in connection with ΔNp63 [45]. ΔNp63α indirectly drives STAT3 (Tyr705) phosphorylation in an autocrine loop by transactivating interleukin 6 (IL-6) and IL-8. Phosphorylated STAT3 stabilizes HIF-1α, resulting in an increased production of VEGF in ΔNp63α-overexpressing cells [44]. In melanoma, ΔEx2/3p73, but not ΔNp63α, mediates STAT3 (Tyr705) phosphorylation in an EPLIN/IGF-1R-dependent manner [43]. With respect to its ability to promote cancer through regulating cancer stem cell (CSC) activities [46], STAT3 upregulation mediates reprogramming of melanoma cells to melanoma stem cells by inducing expression of the Yamanaka factors, providing hints of STAT3 implication in cancer stemness [47]. Moreover, STAT3 increases chemoresistance of melanomas to selective inhibitors of BRAF, which are exploited in the treatment of unresectable or metastatic melanoma with a *BRAF-V600* gain-of-function mutation [48].

Similar to STAT3, STAT5 also exerts oncogenic functions. There are two distinct genes, *STAT5A* and *STAT5B*, that have arisen by gene duplication and encode protein products which share more than 90% peptide sequence similarity and differ primarily in the C-terminus-encoding region [49]. STAT5A is predominantly expressed in the mammary gland, while STAT5B is prevalent in muscle and liver. They respond to a number of factors, such as prolactin, Growth Hormone, erythropoietin, thrombopoietin, EGF, IL-2, IL-3, IL-6, IL-7, IL-9, and IL-15 [40]. STAT5 promotes malignant transformation in hematological malignancies, breast and prostate cancer, non-small cell lung carcinoma, and melanoma [50]. The initial correlation between STAT5 activation and aggressive characteristics of melanoma was first described in a Xiphophorus fish melanoma model [51]. Subsequently, Hassel and colleagues showed that constitutive activation of STAT5 correlated with the upregulation of its antiapoptotic target gene *BCL2L1*, an effect which was conserved in both, human melanoma cells and murine melanocytes [52]. In melanoma patients, STAT5B transcripts were significantly upregulated, whereas STAT5 was found phosphorylated in 62% of the metastatic cases versus normal human melanocytes and benign nevi. STAT5 activation is induced by the EGF/JAK1 axis in melanoma cell lines. Knockdown of *STAT5B* in these cells causes downregulation of BCL2, which triggers cell death and G1 arrest, thus underscoring that STAT5B acts as a survival factor in melanoma [50]. In addition to its antiapoptotic role in melanoma, STAT5 influences the sensitivity to anti-melanoma treatment, including interferon alpha (IFN-α) immunotherapy and BRAF inhibitors. For instance, in skin cancer patients under adjuvant IFN-α therapy, STAT5 expression emerged as an independent predictor of progression-free survival. Recurrence in patients with STAT5-expressing tumors was observed either during or after IFN-α therapy [53]. In accordance herewith, STAT5 has been shown to be overexpressed in IFNα-resistant melanoma cells [54]. Moreover, this transcription factor regulates the nicotinamide phosphoribosyltransferase (NAMPT), a key enzyme in the maintenance of cellular nicotinamide adenine dinucleotide (NAD+) levels, in response to activated B-Raf/extracellular signal-regulated kinases (BRAF/ERK) signaling. NAMPT induces melanoma cell proliferation accompanied by a phenotypic switch towards an invasive phenotype and resistance to BRAF inhibitors [55]. Consistently, a combination of the neuroleptic drug pimozide with indoleamine 2,3-dioxygenase sensitizes melanoma cells to apoptosis and inhibits cell migration via STAT5 suppression [56]. However, pimozide is not a direct STAT5 inhibitor, but rather targets upstream pathway activation for degradation.

5. STAT3 and STAT5 in the Crosstalk between Melanoma and Immune Cells

Melanomas display qualitative and quantitative changes in the density, composition, functional state, and organization of immune infiltrates, the so-called immune contexture, which render immune cells tolerant to tumors or exhaust their ability to attack tumor cells [57]. STAT3 influences the interplay between melanoma cells and components of the immune system, thus contributing to immune evasion. Tumor and immune cells expressing STAT3 develop sophisticated interactions to overall support an immunosuppressive tumor environment that propels metastatic progression. In detail, melanoma cells which overexpress STAT3 protein inhibit the expression of proinflammatory cytokines and chemokines, such as VEGF, IL-10, and IL-6. These, in turn, induce STAT3 activity in hematopoietic progenitor cells (HPCs) to promote the production of immature myeloid cells (IMCs) and plasmacytoid dendritic cells (pDCs). Through IL-10, IMCs block the maturation of dendritic cells into antigen-presenting cells. Thus, these immature dendritic cells are unable to stimulate the antitumor effects of CD8+ T cells and natural killer (NK) cells. In parallel, pDCs promote the accumulation of regulatory T cells (Treg) in the tumor microenvironment. IL-10 and TGF-β secreted by Treg cells further enhance the immunosuppressive microenvironment by restraining both, CD8+ effector T-cell function and DC maturation [38,58–60]. Direct STAT3 targeting in melanoma cell lines sufficed to modulate these crosstalks and enhanced antitumor activity through increasing interferon gamma (IFNγ) levels, mature dendritic cells, and CD8+ T cells. This resulted in reduced tumor growth and prolonged survival of tumor-bearing mice [61]. There is the first evidence that STAT3 activation in NK cells that trigger innate immune responses by the destruction of the tumor cells, can suppress their cytotoxicity against melanoma cells in vivo. The dual effect of STAT3 in melanoma, as well as tumor-attacking immune cells, is of great therapeutic interest since STAT3 inhibition not only blocks survival of cancer cells themselves but also boosts the cytotoxic behavior of infiltrating immune cells [62].

The effect of STAT5 on the melanoma–immune cell interplay is just beginning to be unveiled, mainly via studies in NK cells. The data demonstrate that STAT5 is indispensable for NK cell survival. Conditional knockdown of STAT5 in NK cells led to an almost entire loss of this cell population in transgenic mouse models. Subsequent intravenous injections of these mice with B16F10 melanoma cells increased tumor cell infiltration in the lungs when compared to the control groups [63]. In accordance with the results described above, Sathe et al. reported that an IL-15/JAK1/STAT5 pathway supports the generation of NK cells via transactivation of the antiapoptotic protein MCL1, and that *MCL1* conditional knockdown in NK cells in mice led to multiorgan metastases upon transplantation of melanoma tumors [64]. Other investigations revealed that forced expression of antiapoptotic *BCL2* rescues survival of STAT5-deficient NK cells [65]. Nevertheless, the presence of NK cells expressing high levels of BCL2, but lacking STAT5 was not sufficient to control tumor growth. As this study shows, lowering STAT5 levels in NK cells caused exacerbation of tumor growth in vivo, irrespective of the ability of NK cells to recognize and eradicate tumor cells [65]. They further demonstrated that upregulation of perforin, granzymes, and IFNγ by STAT5 is the key to the enhancement of NK cell cytotoxicity against melanoma [65]. In addition to NK cells, a STAT5-induced cytotoxic potential of immune cells towards skin cancer has also been reported for CD8+ T cells. In particular, genetic modification of CD8+ effector T cells with a constitutively active form of STAT5 gives them high efficiency for host colonization after adoptive transfer and transforms them into long-lived antigen-responsive cells. Upon transfer into melanoma-bearing hosts, these cells accumulate in the tumor site, become activated by tumor antigens, and express the cytolytic factor granzyme B, resulting in tumor regression [66]. It was recently shown that malignant melanoma cells induce inhibition of STAT5 signaling on cytotoxic NK and CD8+ T cells to achieve immune evasion and tumor progression. This effect is mediated by the melanoma-secreted dickkopf WNT signaling pathway inhibitor 2 (DKK2) [67].

In conclusion, STAT3 establishes a reciprocal relationship between melanoma cells and immune cells in favor of tumor immune evasion. STAT3-expressing cancer cells dysregulate immune cells, while at the same time, immune cells with high levels of STAT3 are unable to target melanoma cells. In contrast, STAT5 expression in tumor-attacking immune cells supports antitumor cytotoxicity (Figure 3). These sophisticated interactions between melanoma and immune cells via STAT proteins (and perhaps other factors) could provide a precocious basis towards interpreting the associations between melanoma and co-occurrent autoimmune conditions. Future studies are anticipated to shed more light on common mechanisms underlying melanoma and AD which could, at least in part, explain why these distinct pathologies of melanoma and autoimmunity appear, for example, in the same patients.

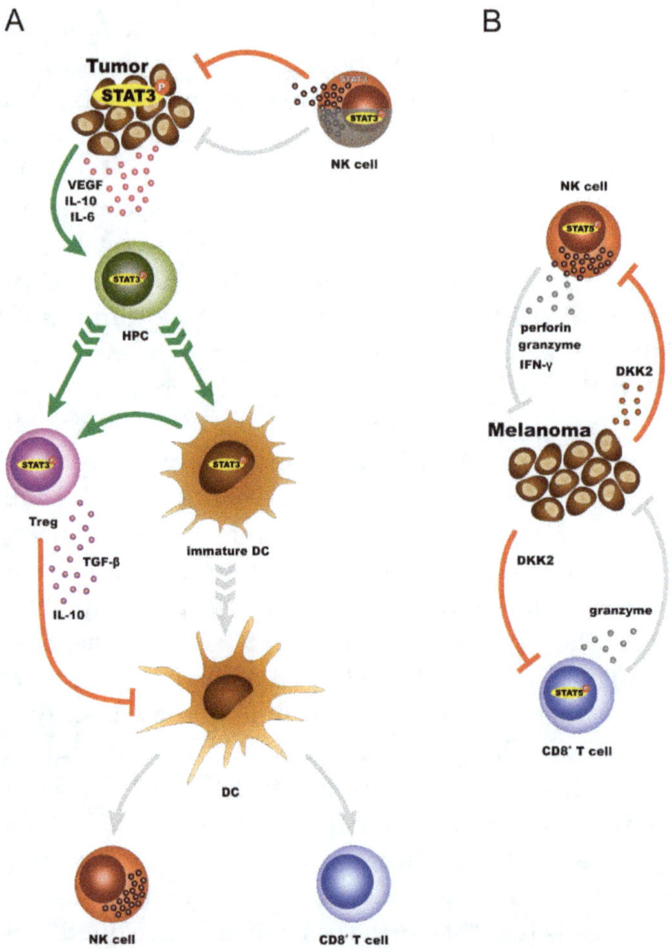

Figure 3. STAT3 and STAT5-mediated crosstalks between melanoma and immune cells create an immunosuppressive network that propels metastatic progression. (**A**) STAT3-expressing tumors secrete factors that upregulate STAT3 in hematopoietic progenitor cells (HPCs). This results in the accumulation of Tregs and immature dendritic cells in the tumor microenvironment, which further inhibit the maturation of these cells. Due to the lack of mature dendritic cells, the tumor-attacking CD8+ T cells and NK cells cannot be stimulated. NK cells with inactive STAT3 can repress tumors, while STAT3 activation in NK cells blocks their tumor-lysing properties. (**B**) STAT5-activated NK cells are effective against melanoma cells. This property is suppressed by secretion of DKK2 from melanoma cells (see main text for details).

6. STAT3 and STAT5 Pathways in Inflammation and Melanoma-Associated Autoimmune Diseases

During inflammation, lymphoid and myeloid cells are recruited to the site of the lesion. By secreting cytokines, immune cells and macrophages control the development of inflammation. Effective and timely management of an inflammation is crucial for maintaining the immune system homeostasis. Any factor that activates inflammation or triggers immune reactions could lead to an autoimmune disease, whenever immune regulation of the inflammatory response fails to manipulate the situation appropriately. Thus, the root cause of most autoimmune diseases is the failure of the immune response to orchestrate the dynamics or magnitude of an inflammatory response, limit it to a relevant body site, and terminate it at the proper time [19]. The balance between Th17 cells, a subset of proinflammatory T helper cells which are characterized by IL-17 production, and Tregs that maintain tolerance to self-antigens is a key determinant in the development of an AD, and the signals that induce Th17 differentiation from CD4+ T cells inhibit Treg differentiation [68]. STATs affect inflammatory disease since they control the development of hematopoietic cells that regulate inflammation and mediate the responses of target cells to inflammatory cytokines [69]. For instance, STAT members, such as STAT1 and STAT3, are highly interlinked with NF-κB [70,71]. Not only does STAT3 respond to NF-κB-induced IL-6, a critical mediator of the acute phase response in inflammation [72], but it also physically interacts with this transcription factor to co-regulate inflammatory gene targets [71]. However, as the damage response persists, chronic activation of STAT proteins leads to inflammatory, idiopathic, and autoimmune conditions [72]. In line with this, *STAT3* gain-of-function mutations can cause early-onset lymphoproliferation and autoimmunity [73] and have been associated with Th17 hyperactivation [74]. STAT5 signaling is also involved in autoimmunity. Patients with STAT5B deficiency have decreased numbers of Treg cells and exhibit immunological aberrations, whereas most of them suffer from severe eczema and AD [49]. Herein, we briefly summarize our current knowledge of how STAT3 and STAT5 are implicated in inflammatory and autoinflammatory conditions as well as in autoimmune diseases. The effect of STAT3 and STAT5 on autoimmune diseases with a demonstrated link to melanoma [2] is described in Section 6.1 to Section 6.8 and depicted in Table 1. STAT3/STAT5-related inflammatory and autoimmune diseases with a still understudied effect on melanoma incidence are also mentioned (Sections 6.9–6.12).

Table 1. Effects of STAT3/STAT5 in autoimmune diseases associated with melanoma (conditions are listed by decreasing prevalence rate in melanoma patients).

AD	STAT3 Input	STAT5 Input	STAT3 Inhibition	STAT5 Inhibition	Refs
Peripheral Neuropathy	activated JAK/STAT3 signaling pathway	n.d.	n.d.	n.d.	[75,76]
Type 1 Diabetes Mellitus	activated in T cells, premature differentiation of stem cells into cells of the pancreatic endocrine lineage	STAT5 phosphorylation in monocytes	therapeutic	n.d.	[77–79]
Rheumatoid Arthritis	activated in CD4+ T cells, increase of Th17/Treg ratio, induction of inflammatory and osteoclastogenic factors	decrease of Th17/Treg ratio	therapeutic	n.d.	[80–83]
Psoriasis	STAT3 activation in the skin	n.d.	therapeutic	n.d.	[84,85]
Autoimmune Pancreatitis	STAT3 loss-of-function mutation	n.d.	n.d.	n.d.	[86,87]

Table 1. *Cont.*

AD	STAT3 Input	STAT5 Input	STAT3 Inhibition	STAT5 Inhibition	Refs
Autoimmune Aplastic Anemia	STAT3 gain-of-function mutations in T cells	IL-2/STAT5B active in Tregs, STAT5B gain-of-function mutations in T cells	n.d.	n.d.	[88–90]
Hashimoto's Encephalopathy	n.d.	activation of neuroinflammation-promoting T helper cells	n.d.	n.d.	[91,92]
Inflammatory Bowel Disease	STAT3 activation in T-cells contributes to colitis, STAT3 activation in myeloid cells protects from colitis	proliferation of intestinal epithelial stem cells, regeneration of the crypt epithelium, regulation of Th17/Treg balance, protection of dendritic cells from apoptosis, mucosal wound healing, resistance to intestinal injury	therapeutic	n.d.	[72,93–97]

n.d.: not determined.

6.1. Peripheral Neuropathy

Peripheral neuropathy is an AD of paraneoplastic etiology, which may appear as melanoma comorbidity. It has been attributed to an immune response directed against antigens in the tumor that subsequently cross-react with the same or similar epitopes in the nervous system [75]. First evidence associates neuropathic pain with an activated JAK/STAT3 signaling pathway [76]. The exact role of STATs in this condition is yet to be determined.

6.2. Type 1 Diabetes Mellitus

Type 1 diabetes (T1D) is a chronic AD causing immune-mediated loss of pancreatic β cells. The key mediators of β cell destruction are the CD4+ and CD8+ T cells. Treg cells are also important for the maintenance of immune tolerance and prevention of autoimmunity. STAT3 is activated in T cells of T1D patients and favors their resistance to suppression [77]. It also influences diabetes by altering pancreatic cells development. This was shown in a study where an activating STAT3 mutation caused premature differentiation of stem cells into cells of the pancreatic endocrine lineage [78]. Similar to STAT3, STAT5 activation has been correlated with T1D, since persistent STAT5 phosphorylation characterizes monocytes of individuals with or at-risk for T1D and is suspected of altering the epigenetic regulation of inflammatory response genes [79].

6.3. Rheumatoid Arthritis

Rheumatoid arthritis (RA) is a chronic disorder manifested with continuous inflammation, swelling, destruction, and pain in multiple joints. Th17 cells are the pathogenic culprit in RA, while Treg cells suppress RA. STAT3 and STAT5 knockdown in RA demonstrated that STAT3 increases Th17 but decreases Treg proportions, whereas STAT5 has the opposite effects on these cell populations [80], providing insights that STAT5 counteracts STAT3 activity on the reciprocal balance of Th17 and Tregs in the context of RA. In addition, STAT3 induces factors that lead to inflammation and osteoclast genesis, while its conditional knockout in mice blocks joint inflammation and destruction and offers resistance to collagen-induced arthritis [81]. Consistently, STAT3 phosphorylation and subsequent upregulation of its downstream gene targets are discriminative for CD4+ T cells of RA patients [82]. It is possible that STAT5 counteracts STAT3 in the context of RA via exerting opposite effects in the Th17/Treg balance, which is crucial in the pathogenesis of this disease [83].

6.4. *Psoriasis*

Psoriasis is a chronic autoimmune disease characterized by patches of abnormal skin, which are typically red, dry, itchy, and scaly. Its most prevalent type is psoriasis vulgaris. It is considered a T cell-mediated AD modified by genetic susceptibility and environmental stimuli. Th17 lymphocytes, which differentiate from naïve T cells upon IL-6 induction, play a central role in its pathogenesis, and recent evidence suggests that inflammatory circuits are established among Th1 and Th17 cells and keratinocytes, promoting psoriasis. This leads to the hypothesis that STAT3 and STAT5, which regulate Th17, are possibly associated with psoriasis. Indeed, STAT3 activation has been observed in the skin of psoriatic patients [84]. Consistently, transgenic mice, in which keratinocytes express a constitutively active form of STAT3, develop psoriasis-like skin lesions. Topical administration of STAT3 inhibitor improved psoriatic lesions in both, these mice and in clinical patients [85]. The role of STAT5 in psoriasis needs to be assessed.

6.5. *Autoimmune Pancreatitis*

Autoimmune pancreatitis is a unique form of chronic pancreatitis initially reported in 1995. It exhibits characteristic histological features, frequent elevations of serum IgG4 antibodies, and a predictable response to steroid therapy. Potential long-term sequelae include pancreatic duct stones and malignancy [86]. A recent report describes a case of acute pancreatitis that presented in a patient with a loss-of-function STAT3 mutation [87]. The involvement of STATs in this newly-identified autoimmune condition remains to be elucidated.

6.6. *Autoimmune Aplastic Anemia*

Aplastic anemia (AA) is a non-malignant blood disorder, caused by immune destruction of hematopoietic and progenitor cells, which leads to a failure of bone marrow to sustain blood production. As a result, the patients develop pancytopenia, evidenced by low levels of all blood cell types. Clonal hematopoiesis with the formation of a genetically distinct subpopulation of blood cells has been suggested as a basis of this disease, where clonal cells have acquired the ability of increased proliferation and immune escape [88]. *STAT5B* [88] and *STAT3* [89] gain-of-function mutations have been found in T cells of AA patients, while an IL-2/STAT5B pathway characterized patients' Treg subpopulations [90]. Overall, these data link STATs with AA, although continued investigation into the mechanistic connections is necessary.

6.7. *Hashimoto's Encephalopathy*

Hashimoto's encephalopathy is a rare disease of autoimmune origin, characterized by high titers of antithyroid antibodies. It has been proposed that an abnormal function of the immune system causes neuronal inflammation, leading to impaired brain function. The condition co-exists with other ADs, such as T1D mellitus, systemic lupus erythematosus, and Sjögren syndrome [91]. Although the molecular mechanism of this rare disease remains elusive, a study showing that STAT5 programs a distinct subset of Granulocyte-macrophage colony-stimulating factor (GM-CSF)-producing T helper cells, which is essential for autoimmune neuroinflammation [92], could provide a potential link between STATs and this disorder. Future investigations could shed more light on possible associations of STATs with the etiopathology of encephalitis.

6.8. *Inflammatory Bowel Disease*

Inflammatory bowel disease (IBD) describes a group of chronic, relapsing, autoimmune diseases of complex etiology that become manifest at the small intestine and colon. It encompasses ulcerative colitis and Crohn's disease, which differ in the location of inflammation within the gastrointestinal tract. Several cytokines that activate STAT3 drive IBD pathogenesis. Data obtained from IBD patients showed that STAT3 is activated in their inflamed colons. Intriguingly, expression of STAT3 in different immune cell populations exerts opposing effects on IBD. In particular, phosphorylated protein in T-cells contributes to colitis, while its activation in myeloid cells (neutrophils and macrophages) and enterocytes is protective against colitis. In mouse models of IBD, several proinflammatory cytokines, such as IL-2, IL-6, IL-15, IL-21, IL-23, IL-17, and IL-18, have detrimental effects, whereas anti-inflammatory cytokines, including IFNα/β, IL-10, IL-11, and IL-22, are beneficial. STAT3 targeting with small molecule inhibitors ameliorates IBD in vivo and is under consideration as a new approach to IBD management, particularly in patients that are refractory to current therapies [72]. However, given the opposing functions of STAT3 on different immune cell types, targeting should be directed towards the specific cell population which promotes IBD, without jeopardizing those immune cells that protect from disease [93].

STAT5 has rather anti-inflammatory properties both in the intestinal epithelium and in adaptive immune cells and has been shown to oppose STAT3 functions in the context of IBD. A GH/STAT5 axis is protective against colitis in animal models. On one side, STAT5 is critical for the proliferation of intestinal epithelial stem cells and regeneration of the crypt epithelium. STAT5B-deficient mice are particularly susceptible to chemically induced colitis, a fact that was attributed to apoptosis of epithelial cells and damage of the mucosal barrier. In agreement, activated STAT5 promotes mucosal wound healing, increases intestinal epithelial stem cell proliferation, accelerates crypt regeneration, and confers resistance to intestinal injury [95,96]. Lack of active STAT5 predisposes to *Clostridium difficile* infection-induced colitis [97]. Otherwise, STAT5 regulates T cell differentiation, especially Treg cells. In addition, IL-2 signaling via STAT5 limits Th17 in favor of Treg development. This is opposed to STAT3 function, which induces Th17 differentiation and negatively controls Treg differentiation. The balance between Tregs and effector T cells is key in IBD suppression. Moreover, GM-CSF-induced STAT5 signaling protects dendritic cells from apoptosis, in contrast to the apoptotic effects of an IL-21/STAT3 axis in these cells [94].

6.9. *Asthma*

Asthma is a condition characterized by inflammation, which leads to hyperresponsiveness of the airways and remodeling of the airway wall. Airway inflammation and remodeling is accompanied by STAT3 activation and by increased levels of Th2- and Th17-type cytokines in the lung. STAT3 regulates immune cell recruitment, specifically Th2 cells, during allergic inflammation. Targeted STAT3 depletion in the airway epithelium prevents house dust mite-mediated allergic inflammation and airway hyperresponsiveness. Interestingly, other studies suggest that Th2 cells respond to STAT3 activation differentially, depending on their location in the lung [72]. In a similar manner, in animal models of asthma, the STAT5 pathway-regulates lymphocyte proliferation induced by ovalbumin [98], while a GM-CSF/STAT5 axis enhances survival of lung granulocytes [99]. Observations on a large cohort of hospitalized asthma patients revealed an increased cancer incidence, which, however, was highly cancer type-dependent. These patients presented an increased risk for stomach and colon cancer but decreased for endometrial cancer and melanoma [100]. Further studies which could also include the population of outpatient asthma patients are needed to investigate the potential link between asthma and several cancer types.

6.10. Cachexia and Polymyositis

Cachexia is an inflammation-driven metabolic syndrome, where impaired regulation of the balance between anabolism and catabolism results in the loss of adipose tissue and skeletal muscle, eventually leading to muscle atrophy. Mechanistic studies have shown that STAT3 phosphorylation in response to overexpression of its upstream cytokine IL-6 is associated with this condition [72]. In a similar manner, levels of phosphorylated STAT3 and cytokine IL-22 have been found elevated in muscle tissues of patients with polymyositis, an idiopathic inflammatory myopathy that causes muscle weakness [101]. Several known STAT3 inhibitors that directly target hyperphosphorylated STAT3 also reduced markers of cachexia in cell culture models and antagonized catabolic signaling in mice, supporting the concept that STAT3 is a valid target for cachexia treatment [72]. No study has correlated STAT5 and polymyositis thus far. An association between cachexia and melanoma has been suggested based on mice studies. In detail, B16F10 melanoma-bearing mice depicted skeletal muscle and epididymal fat mass reduction, muscle strength loss, and locomotor activity impairment, associated with elevated IL-6 levels in the plasma [102]. Further studies are needed to investigate if these effects are mediated by STATs.

6.11. Fibrosis

Tissue fibrosis is an inflammatory condition which is caused upon dysregulation of the tightly-controlled process of wound healing and is characterized by overproduction of the extracellular matrix (ECM) and excess matrix contraction. STAT3 drives wound healing following inflammation and contributes to fibrosis by inducing production of ECM or by transactivating profibrotic metalloproteases, such as MMP-9. The blockade of STAT3 phosphorylation with small molecule inhibitors could ameliorate the development of pulmonary fibrosis in mice exposed to bleomycin [72]. In contrast to the profibrotic function of STAT3, STAT5 seems to protect from fibrosis, perhaps through counteracting STAT3. In particular, loss of STAT5 causes liver fibrosis through STAT3 activation [103]. It was recently shown that the dorsal skin of mice contains multiple and diverse lineages of fibroblasts. One of those lineages is responsible for the fibrotic response to injury and cancer-stroma formation. Ablation of this specific lineage diminished connective tissue deposition in wounds and reduced melanoma growth in vivo [104]. This study provides an initial link between melanoma and fibrotic injury, although further investigation is required to confirm this finding in the cancer patient population and to unveil the underlying mechanisms.

6.12. Systemic Lupus Erythematosus

Systemic lupus erythematosus (SLE) is a chronic, systemic AD that distinguishes itself by autoreactive lymphocytes and proinflammatory cytokine production. It can often lead to renal injury and multiple organ damage due to the formation of autoantibodies against nuclear antigens, cell surface, and serum proteins [105]. Both STAT3 and STAT5 are implicated in SLE etiopathology and have been found activated in immune cells of SLE patients [106,107]. In T cells of SLE patients, STAT3 and STAT5 synergistically transactivate IL-10 through epigenetic remodeling [108]. In the development of SLE, dysregulation of the Th17/Treg balance may play an important role and could be responsible for an increased proinflammatory response, especially in the active form of the disease [109,110]. In this context, SLE has been recently associated with an active IL-17/STAT3 axis, accompanied by higher Th17 cell numbers [111]. STAT3 inhibitors in combination with immunosuppressive drugs, improve SLE via restoration of this balance [105], while agents inhibiting STAT3 phosphorylation have shown efficacy in the treatment of SLE [106]. STAT5 is also implicated in SLE, since activated STAT5 upregulates the antiapoptotic targets Bcl-2 and Ki-67 in CD4+ T cells, perhaps providing them with a survival and proliferative advantage over Treg cells [112]. A large patient population-based, retrospective study recently highlighted a statistically significant association between SLE and melanoma [113]. Dreyer et al. also described that SLE tends to be positively associated with melanoma, although the trend was not statistically significant [114]. However, another meta-analysis study reported a decreased risk of melanoma in SLE patients [115]. Further exploration of the association between malignant melanoma and SLE is anticipated to shed more light on this issue.

7. Perspectives, Challenges, and Limitations Towards Translating STAT3/STAT5 Targeting to Therapeutic Solutions for Patients with AD and Melanoma

Recent studies converge to the revolutionary idea of targeting a single nodal molecule to manage two inter-related pathological conditions simultaneously [116–118]. In line with this notion, we evaluated whether STAT targeting can be considered for the management of melanoma and its associated autoimmune comorbidities. An advantage of this approach is that there is an already established arsenal of STAT3 and STAT5 inhibitors, which are currently under investigation for the treatment of cancer or autoimmune diseases, as reviewed in detail by Loh and colleagues [40]. This arsenal is being further enriched by indirect epigenetic modifiers of STAT proteins [70,119,120]. STAT3 inhibitors have demonstrated their efficacy in animal tumor models [121] and are currently under ongoing clinical trials for melanoma treatment (ClinicalTrials.gov Identifiers: NCT01904123, NCT03195699). In a similar manner, these inhibitory molecules are also efficient in treating several autoimmune diseases in vivo [85,106] and are now tested in a clinical anti-T1D setting (ClinicalTrials.gov Identifier: NCT02641522), which has been reported as melanoma-associated comorbidity. Moreover, it has been reported that cancer patients who exhibit cachexia may benefit from STAT3 inactivation, as it preserves fat and tissue mass and rescues cachectic phenotypes, in addition to eliminating tumors [122]. Another approach for simultaneous disease management could be achieved through nutritherapeutic strategies. Several dietary compounds are potent inhibitors of STAT3 regulatory networks [123,124]. These nutriceuticals could have potential applications in patients with chronic ADs, in the sense that their long-term use as dietary supplements might not only mitigate AD symptoms, but also reduce the cancer risk. Hence, STAT3 inhibitors may hold therapeutic promise as multipurpose drugs for the treatment of melanoma in conjunction with associated ADs. Due to its roles in cancer and immunity, STAT5 is also a proposed therapeutic target [125]. Studies in AD animal models with transplanted melanoma tumors versus immunocompetent controls will not only provide proof-of-concept about the feasibility of using agents such as STAT inhibitors against different diseases but might also establish an experimental approach to facilitate insights into the complex interactions between melanoma and immune cells.

One challenge regarding the proposed approach remains, namely which melanoma–immune cell interactions would be suitable for modulation to achieve dual targeting of these diseases without reducing the beneficial effects of other immune cell populations. Following this direction, it is intriguing to hypothesize that a possible interplay among melanoma, Th17, and Treg cells could be manipulated towards this goal. In detail, it has been recognized that an unbalanced Th17/Treg response, on the one hand, mediates several melanoma-associated Ads, such as psoriasis, IBD, RA, and SLE, and on the other hand, contributes to carcinogenesis mainly via propelling chronic inflammation [126]. Interestingly, STAT3 and STAT5 emerge as fine-tuners of the Th17/Treg balance, since STAT3 is responsible for Treg cells and STAT5 mediates Th17 differentiation [126]. Given that Th17 [127] and Tregs [128] have been found dysregulated during melanoma progression, it is appealing to postulate that disturbance of the Th17/Treg homeostasis may favor melanoma cell proliferation in a STAT3/STAT5-dependent manner. Future studies could shed more light on this issue.

Targeting of the interplay between melanoma cells and NK cells poses as another challenge. While STAT3 inhibition reactivates NK cells against melanoma, STAT5 inhibition suppresses tumor cytotoxic activities of NK cells. A hypothetical explanation is that NK cells could be particularly sensitive to a still understudied equilibrium between STAT3 and STAT5. Such a scenario poses limitations to the straightforward inhibition of either STAT3 or STAT5 in NK cells and necessitates elucidating how the STAT3/STAT5 ratio is regulated and what is its contribution to the melanoma–NK cells interplay. In NK cells, STAT3 inhibition leads to STAT5 activation, and a delicate balance exists between STAT3-mediated suppression and STAT5-induced activation of NK-cell cytotoxicity [62]. It has been hypothesized that this inverse correlation between STAT3 and STAT5 could serve as a regulator of autoimmunity, given that both factors respond to the same cytokines. In particular, IL-15-induced STAT3 activation could counteract the IL-15-STAT5-mediated NK-cell cytotoxicity to prevent autoimmunity [62]. A detailed understanding of the mechanisms governing transactions between melanoma and immune cell populations could catalyze the development of anticancer strategies aiming at increasing the potential of killer cells while suppressing self-destruction.

Along with hopes, targeting of STAT factors has also raised skepticism, since its pleiotropic effects in non-tumor tissues are predicted to potentiate the risk of adverse events [129]. Indeed, STATs are points of convergence of several signal transduction pathways that affect diverse processes [130], and as such, their inhibition will have multiple effects, some of which may be manifested as side effects in nontumor tissues. However, this disadvantage can theoretically turn into an advantage in the event of multimorbid cancer patients, since in these patients systemic administration of inhibitors against pleiotropic molecules that are commonly activated in melanoma and associated comorbidities could, in the long run, simultaneously manage lesions. In this case, the side effect at a site outside the tumor could be proven beneficial if it actually counteracts a co-existing AD. Such directions could inspire next-generation therapeutics, especially in melanoma patients whose pre-existing conditions refrain them from getting benefit from current immunotherapy regimens.

8. Conclusions

Inflammation and autoimmune disorders emerge as comorbidities in melanoma, providing hints that deregulation in common processes may govern all-three diseases. Crosstalks are established among melanoma cells and several subpopulations of immune cells, reciprocally modifying their behavior. Molecular drivers of these crosstalks, such as STAT3 and STAT5 signaling pathways, could be targeted to manipulate interactions between melanoma cells and immune cells, to develop therapeutics that coordinately regulate skin cancer and inflammatory and/or autoimmune conditions. In this review, we (a) state that the high-risk patients with a non-competent immune system (i.e., those with a pre-existing AD or transplant organ recipients) constitute a special population which requires personalized management with novel therapeutics that are able to both kill tumor cells and suppress immune system responses, (b) evaluate if such an approach is feasible, based on the molecular commonalities between tumors, inflammation, and autoimmune disease, and (c) estimate STAT targeting as a representative example, although targeting of additional, probably still undiscovered molecules, may also exert a similar multipotent effect. Immunotherapeutics have taken center stage and emerge as the blockbusters of pharmacopoieia. Their favorable effects on cancer patients keep therapeutic hopes high. However, the use of cancer immunotherapy on patients with associated autoimmune disease could lead to life-threatening side effects. In contrast, drugs with an inherent ability to cause immune suppression which could theoretically counteract an overactive immune system might constitute a more suitable option in the context of personalized therapy. To this end, selected next-generation therapeutics, e.g., STAT inhibitors, may have the potential to shape the first line of treatment for these patient populations in the future.

Acknowledgments: The authors are especially grateful to Stephan Marquardt for support in image preparation.

References

1. Ventola, C.L. Cancer Immunotherapy, Part 1: Current Strategies and Agents. *Pharm. Ther.* **2017**, *42*, 375–383.
2. Ma, Q.; Shilkrut, M.; Zhao, Z.; Li, M.; Batty, N.; Barber, B. Autoimmune comorbidities in patients with metastatic melanoma: A retrospective analysis of us claims data. *BMC Cancer* **2018**, *18*, 145. [CrossRef] [PubMed]
3. Domingues, B.; Lopes, J.M.; Soares, P.; Pópulo, H. Melanoma treatment in review. *ImmunoTargets Ther.* **2018**, *7*, 35–49. [CrossRef] [PubMed]

4. Park, Y.J.; Kuen, D.S.; Chung, Y. Future prospects of immune checkpoint blockade in cancer: From response prediction to overcoming resistance. *Exp. Mol. Med.* **2018**, *50*, 109. [CrossRef] [PubMed]
5. Horvat, T.Z.; Adel, N.G.; Dang, T.O.; Momtaz, P.; Postow, M.A.; Callahan, M.K.; Carvajal, R.D.; Dickson, M.A.; D'Angelo, S.P.; Woo, K.M.; et al. Immune-Related Adverse Events, Need for Systemic Immunosuppression, and Effects on Survival and Time to Treatment Failure in Patients with Melanoma Treated with Ipilimumab at Memorial Sloan Kettering Cancer Center. *J. Clin. Oncol.* **2015**, *33*, 3193–3198. [CrossRef] [PubMed]
6. Johnson, D.B.; Sullivan, R.J.; Ott, P.A.; Carlino, M.S.; Khushalani, N.I.; Ye, F.; Guminski, A.; Puzanov, I.; Lawrence, D.P.; Buchbinder, E.I.; et al. Ipilimumab Therapy in Patients with Advanced Melanoma and Preexisting Autoimmune Disorders. *JAMA Oncol.* **2016**, *2*, 234–240. [CrossRef]
7. Menzies, A.M.; Johnson, D.B.; Ramanujam, S.; Atkinson, V.G.; Wong, A.N.M.; Park, J.J.; McQuade, J.L.; Shoushtari, A.N.; Tsai, K.K.; Eroglu, Z.; et al. Anti-PD-1 therapy in patients with advanced melanoma and preexisting autoimmune disorders or major toxicity with ipilimumab. *Ann. Oncol.* **2017**, *28*, 368–376. [CrossRef] [PubMed]
8. Tripathi, S.V.; Morris, C.R.; Alhamad, T.; Fields, R.C.; Linette, G.P.; Cornelius, L.A. Metastatic melanoma after solid organ transplantation: An interdisciplinary, institution-based review of management with systemic and targeted therapies. *J. Am. Acad. Dermatol.* **2018**, *78*, 184–185. [CrossRef]
9. Abdel-Wahab, N.; Safa, H.; Abudayyeh, A.; Johnson, D.H.; Trinh, V.A.; Zobniw, C.M.; Lin, H.; Wong, M.K.; Abdelrahim, M.; Gaber, A.O.; et al. Checkpoint inhibitor therapy for cancer in solid organ transplantation recipients: An institutional experience and a systematic review of the literature. *J. Immunother. Cancer* **2019**, *7*, 106. [CrossRef]
10. Villarino, A.V.; Kanno, Y.; Ferdinand, J.R.; O'Shea, J.J. Mechanisms of Jak/STAT signaling in immunity and disease. *J. Immunol.* **2015**, *194*, 21–27. [CrossRef]
11. Karin, M.; Lawrence, T.; Nizet, V. Innate immunity gone awry: Linking microbial infections to chronic inflammation and cancer. *Cell* **2006**, *124*, 823–835. [CrossRef] [PubMed]
12. Wogan, G.N.; Dedon, P.C.; Tannenbaum, S.R.; Fox, J.G. Infection, inflammation and colon carcinogenesis. *Oncotarget* **2012**, *3*, 737–738. [CrossRef] [PubMed]
13. Smith, A.W.; Reeve, B.B.; Bellizzi, K.M.; Harlan, L.C.; Klabunde, C.N.; Amsellem, M.; Bierman, A.S.; Hays, R.D. Cancer, comorbidities, and health-related quality of life of older adults. *Health Care Financ. Rev.* **2008**, *29*, 41–56. [PubMed]
14. Franks, A.L.; Slansky, J.E. Multiple associations between a broad spectrum of autoimmune diseases, chronic inflammatory diseases and cancer. *Anticancer Res.* **2012**, *32*, 1119–1136. [PubMed]
15. Beyaert, R.; Beaugerie, L.; Van Assche, G.; Brochez, L.; Renauld, J.C.; Viguier, M.; Cocquyt, V.; Jerusalem, G.; Machiels, J.P.; Prenen, H.; et al. Cancer risk in immune-mediated inflammatory diseases (IMID). *Mol. Cancer* **2013**, *12*, 98. [CrossRef] [PubMed]
16. Schwaneck, E.C.; Renner, R.; Junker, L.; Einsele, H.; Gadeholt, O.; Geissinger, E.; Kleinert, S.; Gernert, M.; Tony, H.P.; Schmalzing, M. Prevalence and Characteristics of Persistent Clonal T Cell Large Granular Lymphocyte Expansions in Rheumatoid Arthritis: A Comprehensive Analysis of 529 Patients. *Arthritis Rheumatol.* **2018**, *70*, 1914–1922. [CrossRef]
17. Pateras, I.S.; Havaki, S.; Nikitopoulou, X.; Vougas, K.; Townsend, P.A.; Panayiotidis, M.I.; Georgakilas, A.G.; Gorgoulis, V.G. The DNA damage response and immune signaling alliance: Is it good or bad? Nature decides when and where. *Pharmacol. Ther.* **2015**, *154*, 36–56. [CrossRef]
18. Amos, S.M.; Duong, C.P.; Westwood, J.A.; Ritchie, D.S.; Junghans, R.P.; Darcy, P.K.; Kershaw, M.H. Autoimmunity associated with immunotherapy of cancer. *Blood* **2011**, *118*, 499–509. [CrossRef]
19. Cohen, I.R. Activation of benign autoimmunity as both tumor and autoimmune disease immunotherapy: A comprehensive review. *J. Autoimmun.* **2014**, *54*, 112–117. [CrossRef]
20. Teulings, H.E.; Overkamp, M.; Ceylan, E.; Nieuweboer-Krobotova, L.; Bos, J.D.; Nijsten, T.; Wolkerstorfer, A.W.; Luiten, R.M.; van der Veen, J.P. Decreased risk of melanoma and nonmelanoma skin cancer in patients with vitiligo: A survey among 1307 patients and their partners. *Br. J. Dermatol.* **2013**, *168*, 162–171. [CrossRef]
21. Teulings, H.E.; Limpens, J.; Jansen, S.N.; Zwinderman, A.H.; Reitsma, J.B.; Spuls, P.I.; Luiten, R.M. Vitiligo-like depigmentation in patients with stage III-IV melanoma receiving immunotherapy and its association with survival: A systematic review and meta-analysis. *J. Clin. Oncol.* **2015**, *33*, 773–781. [CrossRef] [PubMed]
22. Cho, E.A.; Lee, M.A.; Kang, H.; Lee, S.D.; Kim, H.O.; Park, Y.M. Vitiligo-like Depigmentation Associated with Metastatic Melanoma of an Unknown Origin. *Ann. Dermatol.* **2009**, *21*, 178–181. [CrossRef]

23. Pinner, S.; Jordan, P.; Sharrock, K.; Bazley, L.; Collinson, L.; Marais, R.; Bonvin, E.; Goding, C.; Sahai, E. Intravital imaging reveals transient changes in pigment production and Brn2 expression during metastatic melanoma dissemination. *Cancer Res.* **2009**, *69*, 7969–7977. [CrossRef] [PubMed]
24. Fürst, K.; Steder, M.; Logotheti, S.; Angerilli, A.; Spitschak, A.; Marquardt, S.; Schumacher, T.; Engelmann, D.; Herchenröder, O.; Rupp, R.A.W.; et al. DNp73-induced degradation of tyrosinase links depigmentation with EMT-driven melanoma progression. *Cancer Lett.* **2019**, *442*, 299–309. [CrossRef] [PubMed]
25. Hölzel, M.; Tüting, T. Inflammation-Induced Plasticity in Melanoma Therapy and Metastasis. *Trends Immunol.* **2016**, *37*, 364–374. [CrossRef] [PubMed]
26. Wang, Y.; Deng, O.; Feng, Z.; Du, Z.; Xiong, X.; Lai, J.; Yang, X.; Xu, M.; Wang, H.; Taylor, D.; et al. RNF126 promotes homologous recombination via regulation of E2F1-mediated BRCA1 expression. *Oncogene* **2016**, *35*, 1363–1372. [CrossRef]
27. Bottoni, U.; Paolino, G.; Ambrifi, M.; Didona, D.; Albanesi, M.; Clerico, R.; Lido, P.; Brachini, A.; Corsetti, P.; Richetta, A.G.; et al. Association between autoimmune disease and cutaneous melanoma with regard to melanoma prognosis. *Clin. Exp. Dermatol.* **2015**, *40*, 254–259. [CrossRef]
28. Grivennikov, S.I.; Greten, F.R.; Karin, M. Immunity, inflammation, and cancer. *Cell* **2010**, *140*, 883–899. [CrossRef]
29. Ohno, F.; Nakahara, T.; Kido-Nakahara, M.; Ito, T.; Nunomura, S.; Izuhara, K.; Furue, M. Periostin Links Skin Inflammation to Melanoma Progression in Humans and Mice. *Int. J. Mol. Sci.* **2019**, *20*, 169. [CrossRef]
30. Bald, T.; Quast, T.; Landsberg, J.; Rogava, M.; Glodde, N.; Lopez-Ramos, D.; Kohlmeyer, J.; Riesenberg, S.; van den Boorn-Konijnenberg, D.; Hömig-Hölzel, C.; et al. Ultraviolet-radiation-induced inflammation promotes angiotropism and metastasis in melanoma. *Nature* **2014**, *507*, 109–113. [CrossRef]
31. Joosse, A.; Koomen, E.R.; Casparie, M.K.; Herings, R.M.; Guchelaar, H.J.; Nijsten, T. Non-steroidal anti-inflammatory drugs and melanoma risk: Large Dutch population-based case-control study. *J. Investig. Dermatol.* **2009**, *129*, 2620–2627. [CrossRef]
32. Gogas, H.; Polyzos, A.; Stavrinidis, I.; Frangia, K.; Tsoutsos, D.; Panagiotou, P.; Markopoulos, C.; Papadopoulos, O.; Pectasides, D.; Mantzourani, M.; et al. Temozolomide in combination with celecoxib in patients with advanced melanoma. A phase II study of the Hellenic Cooperative Oncology Group. *Ann. Oncol.* **2006**, *17*, 1835–1841. [CrossRef]
33. Logotheti, S.; Khoury, N.; Vlahopoulos, S.A.; Skourti, E.; Papaevangeliou, D.; Liloglou, T.; Gorgoulis, V.; Budunova, I.; Kyriakopoulos, A.M.; Zoumpourlis, V. N-bromotaurine surrogates for loss of antiproliferative response and enhances cisplatin efficacy in cancer cells with impaired glucocorticoid receptor. *Transl. Res.* **2016**, *173*, 58–73.e52. [CrossRef]
34. Ben-Ari, E.T. Dual purpose: Some cancer therapies used to treat autoimmune diseases. *J. Natl. Cancer Inst.* **2004**, *96*, 577–579. [CrossRef]
35. Chanan-Khan, A.A.; Swaika, A.; Paulus, A.; Kumar, S.K.; Mikhael, J.R.; Rajkumar, S.V.; Dispenzieri, A.; Lacy, M.Q. Pomalidomide: The new immunomodulatory agent for the treatment of multiple myeloma. *Blood Cancer J.* **2013**, *3*, e143. [CrossRef]
36. Lash, A.A. Anticancer drugs for noncancer diseases. *Medsurg Nurs.* **1996**, *5*, 177–180.
37. Kontou, P.I.; Pavlopoulou, A.; Dimou, N.L.; Pavlopoulos, G.A.; Bagos, P.G. Network analysis of genes and their association with diseases. *Gene* **2016**, *590*, 68–78. [CrossRef]
38. Kortylewski, M.; Jove, R.; Yu, H. Targeting STAT3 affects melanoma on multiple fronts. *Cancer Metastasis Rev.* **2005**, *24*, 315–327. [CrossRef]
39. Heppler, L.N.; Frank, D.A. Rare mutations provide unique insight into oncogenic potential of STAT transcription factors. *J. Clin. Investig.* **2018**, *128*, 113–115. [CrossRef]
40. Loh, C.Y.; Arya, A.; Naema, A.F.; Wong, W.F.; Sethi, G.; Looi, C.Y. Signal Transducer and Activator of Transcription (STATs) Proteins in Cancer and Inflammation: Functions and Therapeutic Implication. *Front. Oncol.* **2019**, *9*, 48. [CrossRef]
41. Lim, C.P.; Cao, X. Structure, function, and regulation of STAT proteins. *Mol. Biosyst.* **2006**, *2*, 536–550. [CrossRef]
42. Xie, T.X.; Huang, F.J.; Aldape, K.D.; Kang, S.H.; Liu, M.; Gershenwald, J.E.; Xie, K.; Sawaya, R.; Huang, S. Activation of stat3 in human melanoma promotes brain metastasis. *Cancer Res.* **2006**, *66*, 3188–3196. [CrossRef]

43. Steder, M.; Alla, V.; Meier, C.; Spitschak, A.; Pahnke, J.; Fürst, K.; Kowtharapu, B.S.; Engelmann, D.; Petigk, J.; Egberts, F.; et al. DNp73 exerts function in metastasis initiation by disconnecting the inhibitory role of EPLIN on IGF1R-AKT/STAT3 signaling. *Cancer Cell* **2013**, *24*, 512–527. [CrossRef]
44. Engelmann, D.; Pützer, B.M. Emerging from the shade of p53 mutants: N-terminally truncated variants of the p53 family in EMT signaling and cancer progression. *Sci. Signal.* **2014**, *7*, re9. [CrossRef]
45. Galoczova, M.; Coates, P.; Vojtesek, B. STAT3, stem cells, cancer stem cells and p63. *Cell. Mol. Biol. Lett.* **2018**, *23*, 12. [CrossRef]
46. Marquardt, S.; Solanki, M.; Spitschak, A.; Vera, J.; Pützer, B.M. Emerging functional markers for cancer stem cell-based therapies: Understanding signaling networks for targeting metastasis. *Semin. Cancer Biol.* **2018**, *53*, 90–109. [CrossRef]
47. Wang, Y.; Mou, Y.; Zhang, H.; Wang, X.; Li, R.; Cheng, Z.; Liu, X. Reprogramming Factors Remodel Melanoma Cell Phenotype by Changing Stat3 Expression. *Int. J. Med. Sci.* **2017**, *14*, 1402–1409. [CrossRef]
48. Liu, F.; Cao, J.; Wu, J.; Sullivan, K.; Shen, J.; Ryu, B.; Xu, Z.; Wei, W.; Cui, R. Stat3-targeted therapies overcome the acquired resistance to vemurafenib in melanomas. *J. Investig. Dermatol.* **2013**, *133*, 2041–2049. [CrossRef]
49. Kanai, T.; Jenks, J.; Nadeau, K.C. The STAT5b Pathway Defect and Autoimmunity. *Front. Immunol.* **2012**, *3*, 234. [CrossRef]
50. Mirmohammadsadegh, A.; Hassan, M.; Bardenheuer, W.; Marini, A.; Gustrau, A.; Nambiar, S.; Tannapfel, A.; Bojar, H.; Ruzicka, T.; Hengge, U.R. STAT5 phosphorylation in malignant melanoma is important for survival and is mediated through SRC and JAK1 kinases. *J. Investig. Dermatol.* **2006**, *126*, 2272–2280. [CrossRef]
51. Wellbrock, C.; Geissinger, E.; Gómez, A.; Fischer, P.; Friedrich, K.; Schartl, M. Signalling by the oncogenic receptor tyrosine kinase Xmrk leads to activation of STAT5 in Xiphophorus melanoma. *Oncogene* **1998**, *16*, 3047–3056. [CrossRef]
52. Hassel, J.C.; Winnemöller, D.; Schartl, M.; Wellbrock, C. STAT5 contributes to antiapoptosis in melanoma. *Melanoma Res.* **2008**, *18*, 378–385. [CrossRef]
53. Machiraju, D.; Moll, I.; Gebhardt, C.; Sucker, A.; Buder-Bakhaya, K.; Schadendorf, D.; Hassel, J.C. STAT5 expression correlates with recurrence and survival in melanoma patients treated with interferon-α. *Melanoma Res.* **2018**, *28*, 204–210. [CrossRef]
54. Wellbrock, C.; Weisser, C.; Hassel, J.C.; Fischer, P.; Becker, J.; Vetter, C.S.; Behrmann, I.; Kortylewski, M.; Heinrich, P.C.; Schartl, M. STAT5 contributes to interferon resistance of melanoma cells. *Curr. Biol.* **2005**, *15*, 1629–1639. [CrossRef]
55. Ohanna, M.; Cerezo, M.; Nottet, N.; Bille, K.; Didier, R.; Beranger, G.; Mograbi, B.; Rocchi, S.; Yvan-Charvet, L.; Ballotti, R.; et al. Pivotal role of NAMPT in the switch of melanoma cells toward an invasive and drug-resistant phenotype. *Genes Dev.* **2018**, *32*, 448–461. [CrossRef]
56. Jia, H.; Ren, W.; Feng, Y.; Wei, T.; Guo, M.; Guo, J.; Zhao, J.; Song, X.; Wang, M.; Zhao, T.; et al. The enhanced antitumour response of pimozide combined with the IDO inhibitor L-MT in melanoma. *Int. J. Oncol.* **2018**, *53*, 949–960. [CrossRef]
57. Fridman, W.H.; Zitvogel, L.; Sautès-Fridman, C.; Kroemer, G. The immune contexture in cancer prognosis and treatment. *Nat. Rev. Clin. Oncol.* **2017**. [CrossRef]
58. Lee, H.; Pal, S.K.; Reckamp, K.; Figlin, R.A.; Yu, H. STAT3: A target to enhance antitumor immune response. *Curr. Top. Microbiol. Immunol.* **2011**, *344*, 41–59. [CrossRef]
59. Wang, Y.; Shen, Y.; Wang, S.; Shen, Q.; Zhou, X. The role of STAT3 in leading the crosstalk between human cancers and the immune system. *Cancer Lett.* **2018**, *415*, 117–128. [CrossRef]
60. Yu, H.; Kortylewski, M.; Pardoll, D. Crosstalk between cancer and immune cells: Role of STAT3 in the tumour microenvironment. *Nat. Rev. Immunol.* **2007**, *7*, 41–51. [CrossRef]
61. Emeagi, P.U.; Maenhout, S.; Dang, N.; Heirman, C.; Thielemans, K.; Breckpot, K. Downregulation of Stat3 in melanoma: Reprogramming the immune microenvironment as an anticancer therapeutic strategy. *Gene Ther.* **2013**, *20*, 1085–1092. [CrossRef]
62. Gotthardt, D.; Sexl, V. STATs in NK-Cells: The Good, the Bad, and the Ugly. *Front. Immunol.* **2016**, *7*, 694. [CrossRef]
63. Eckelhart, E.; Warsch, W.; Zebedin, E.; Simma, O.; Stoiber, D.; Kolbe, T.; Rülicke, T.; Mueller, M.; Casanova, E.; Sexl, V. A novel Ncr1-Cre mouse reveals the essential role of STAT5 for NK-cell survival and development. *Blood* **2011**, *117*, 1565–1573. [CrossRef]

64. Sathe, P.; Delconte, R.B.; Souza-Fonseca-Guimaraes, F.; Seillet, C.; Chopin, M.; Vandenberg, C.J.; Rankin, L.C.; Mielke, L.A.; Vikstrom, I.; Kolesnik, T.B.; et al. Innate immunodeficiency following genetic ablation of Mcl1 in natural killer cells. *Nat. Commun.* **2014**, *5*, 4539. [CrossRef]
65. Gotthardt, D.; Putz, E.M.; Grundschober, E.; Prchal-Murphy, M.; Straka, E.; Kudweis, P.; Heller, G.; Bago-Horvath, Z.; Witalisz-Siepracka, A.; Cumaraswamy, A.A.; et al. STAT5 Is a Key Regulator in NK Cells and Acts as a Molecular Switch from Tumor Surveillance to Tumor Promotion. *Cancer Discov.* **2016**, *6*, 414–429. [CrossRef]
66. Grange, M.; Buferne, M.; Verdeil, G.; Leserman, L.; Schmitt-Verhulst, A.M.; Auphan-Anezin, N. Activated STAT5 promotes long-lived cytotoxic CD8+ T cells that induce regression of autochthonous melanoma. *Cancer Res.* **2012**, *72*, 76–87. [CrossRef]
67. Xiao, Q.; Wu, J.; Wang, W.J.; Chen, S.; Zheng, Y.; Yu, X.; Meeth, K.; Sahraei, M.; Bothwell, A.L.M.; Chen, L.; et al. DKK2 imparts tumor immunity evasion through β-catenin-independent suppression of cytotoxic immune-cell activation. *Nat. Med.* **2018**, *24*, 262–270. [CrossRef]
68. Lee, G.R. The Balance of Th17 versus Treg Cells in Autoimmunity. *Int. J. Mol. Sci.* **2018**, *19*, 730. [CrossRef]
69. Kaplan, M.H. STAT signaling in inflammation. *JAKSTAT* **2013**, *2*, e24198. [CrossRef]
70. Wieczorek, M.; Ginter, T.; Brand, P.; Heinzel, T.; Krämer, O.H. Acetylation modulates the STAT signaling code. *Cytokine Growth Factor Rev.* **2012**, *23*, 293–305. [CrossRef]
71. Yu, H.; Pardoll, D.; Jove, R. STATs in cancer inflammation and immunity: A leading role for STAT3. *Nat. Rev. Cancer* **2009**, *9*, 798–809. [CrossRef]
72. Kasembeli, M.M.; Bharadwaj, U.; Robinson, P.; Tweardy, D.J. Contribution of STAT3 to Inflammatory and Fibrotic Diseases and Prospects for its Targeting for Treatment. *Int. J. Mol. Sci.* **2018**, *19*, 2299. [CrossRef]
73. Milner, J.D.; Vogel, T.P.; Forbes, L.; Ma, C.A.; Stray-Pedersen, A.; Niemela, J.E.; Lyons, J.J.; Engelhardt, K.R.; Zhang, Y.; Topcagic, N.; et al. Early-onset lymphoproliferation and autoimmunity caused by germline STAT3 gain-of-function mutations. *Blood* **2015**, *125*, 591–599. [CrossRef]
74. Wienke, J.; Janssen, W.; Scholman, R.; Spits, H.; van Gijn, M.; Boes, M.; van Montfrans, J.; Moes, N.; de Roock, S. A novel human STAT3 mutation presents with autoimmunity involving Th17 hyperactivation. *Oncotarget* **2015**, *6*, 20037–20042. [CrossRef]
75. Kloos, L.; Sillevis Smitt, P.; Ang, C.W.; Kruit, W.; Stoter, G. Paraneoplastic ophthalmoplegia and subacute motor axonal neuropathy associated with anti-GQ1b antibodies in a patient with malignant melanoma. *J. Neurol. Neurosurg. Psychiatry* **2003**, *74*, 507–509. [CrossRef]
76. Tsuda, M.; Kohro, Y.; Yano, T.; Tsujikawa, T.; Kitano, J.; Tozaki-Saitoh, H.; Koyanagi, S.; Ohdo, S.; Ji, R.R.; Salter, M.W.; et al. JAK-STAT3 pathway regulates spinal astrocyte proliferation and neuropathic pain maintenance in rats. *Brain* **2011**, *134*, 1127–1139. [CrossRef]
77. Ihantola, E.L.; Viisanen, T.; Gazali, A.M.; Näntö-Salonen, K.; Juutilainen, A.; Moilanen, L.; Rintamäki, R.; Pihlajamäki, J.; Veijola, R.; Toppari, J.; et al. Effector T Cell Resistance to Suppression and STAT3 Signaling during the Development of Human Type 1 Diabetes. *J. Immunol.* **2018**, *201*, 1144–1153. [CrossRef]
78. Saarimäki-Vire, J.; Balboa, D.; Russell, M.A.; Saarikettu, J.; Kinnunen, M.; Keskitalo, S.; Malhi, A.; Valensisi, C.; Andrus, C.; Eurola, S.; et al. An Activating STAT3 Mutation Causes Neonatal Diabetes through Premature Induction of Pancreatic Differentiation. *Cell Rep.* **2017**, *19*, 281–294. [CrossRef]
79. Garrigan, E.; Belkin, N.S.; Alexander, J.J.; Han, Z.; Seydel, F.; Carter, J.; Atkinson, M.; Wasserfall, C.; Clare-Salzler, M.J.; Amick, M.A.; et al. Persistent STAT5 phosphorylation and epigenetic dysregulation of GM-CSF and PGS2/COX2 expression in Type 1 diabetic human monocytes. *PLoS ONE* **2013**, *8*, e76919. [CrossRef]
80. Ju, J.H.; Heo, Y.J.; Cho, M.L.; Jhun, J.Y.; Park, J.S.; Lee, S.Y.; Oh, H.J.; Moon, S.J.; Kwok, S.K.; Park, K.S.; et al. Modulation of STAT-3 in rheumatoid synovial T cells suppresses Th17 differentiation and increases the proportion of Treg cells. *Arthritis Rheum.* **2012**, *64*, 3543–3552. [CrossRef]
81. Oike, T.; Sato, Y.; Kobayashi, T.; Miyamoto, K.; Nakamura, S.; Kaneko, Y.; Kobayashi, S.; Harato, K.; Saya, H.; Matsumoto, M.; et al. Stat3 as a potential therapeutic target for rheumatoid arthritis. *Sci. Rep.* **2017**, *7*, 10965. [CrossRef]
82. Anderson, A.E.; Maney, N.J.; Nair, N.; Lendrem, D.W.; Skelton, A.J.; Diboll, J.; Brown, P.M.; Smith, G.R.; Carmody, R.J.; Barton, A.; et al. Expression of STAT3-regulated genes in circulating CD4+ T cells discriminates rheumatoid arthritis independently of clinical parameters in early arthritis. *Rheumatology* **2019**, *58*, 1250–1258. [CrossRef]

83. Lee, S.H.; Park, J.S.; Byun, J.K.; Jhun, J.; Jung, K.; Seo, H.B.; Moon, Y.M.; Kim, H.Y.; Park, S.H.; Cho, M.L. PTEN ameliorates autoimmune arthritis through down-regulating STAT3 activation with reciprocal balance of Th17 and Tregs. *Sci. Rep.* **2016**, *6*, 34617. [CrossRef]
84. Calautti, E.; Avalle, L.; Poli, V. Psoriasis: A STAT3-Centric View. *Int. J. Mol. Sci.* **2018**, *19*, 171. [CrossRef]
85. Miyoshi, K.; Takaishi, M.; Nakajima, K.; Ikeda, M.; Kanda, T.; Tarutani, M.; Iiyama, T.; Asao, N.; DiGiovanni, J.; Sano, S. Stat3 as a therapeutic target for the treatment of psoriasis: A clinical feasibility study with STA-21, a Stat3 inhibitor. *J. Investig. Dermatol.* **2011**, *131*, 108–117. [CrossRef]
86. Hart, P.A.; Kamisawa, T.; Brugge, W.R.; Chung, J.B.; Culver, E.L.; Czakó, L.; Frulloni, L.; Go, V.L.; Gress, T.M.; Kim, M.H.; et al. Long-term outcomes of autoimmune pancreatitis: A multicentre, international analysis. *Gut* **2013**, *62*, 1771–1776. [CrossRef]
87. Michaud, C.; Peppers, B.; Frith, J.; Tcheurekdjian, H.; Hostoffer, R. Idiopathic pancreatitis in a patient with a STAT3 mutation. *Allergy Rhinol.* **2016**, *7*, 42–44. [CrossRef]
88. Babushok, D.V.; Perdigones, N.; Perin, J.C.; Olson, T.S.; Ye, W.; Roth, J.J.; Lind, C.; Cattier, C.; Li, Y.; Hartung, H.; et al. Emergence of clonal hematopoiesis in the majority of patients with acquired aplastic anemia. *Cancer Genet.* **2015**, *208*, 115–128. [CrossRef]
89. Jerez, A.; Clemente, M.J.; Makishima, H.; Rajala, H.; Gómez-Seguí, I.; Olson, T.; McGraw, K.; Przychodzen, B.; Kulasekararaj, A.; Afable, M.; et al. STAT3 mutations indicate the presence of subclinical T-cell clones in a subset of aplastic anemia and myelodysplastic syndrome patients. *Blood* **2013**, *122*, 2453–2459. [CrossRef]
90. Kordasti, S.; Costantini, B.; Seidl, T.; Perez Abellan, P.; Martinez Llordella, M.; McLornan, D.; Diggins, K.E.; Kulasekararaj, A.; Benfatto, C.; Feng, X.; et al. Deep phenotyping of Tregs identifies an immune signature for idiopathic aplastic anemia and predicts response to treatment. *Blood* **2016**, *128*, 1193–1205. [CrossRef]
91. Mocellin, R.; Walterfang, M.; Velakoulis, D. Hashimoto's encephalopathy: Epidemiology, pathogenesis and management. *CNS Drugs* **2007**, *21*, 799–811. [CrossRef]
92. Sheng, W.; Yang, F.; Zhou, Y.; Yang, H.; Low, P.Y.; Kemeny, D.M.; Tan, P.; Moh, A.; Kaplan, M.H.; Zhang, Y.; et al. STAT5 programs a distinct subset of GM-CSF-producing T helper cells that is essential for autoimmune neuroinflammation. *Cell Res.* **2014**, *24*, 1387–1402. [CrossRef]
93. Sugimoto, K. Role of STAT3 in inflammatory bowel disease. *World J. Gastroenterol.* **2008**, *14*, 5110–5114. [CrossRef]
94. Zundler, S.; Neurath, M.F. Integrating Immunologic Signaling Networks: The JAK/STAT Pathway in Colitis and Colitis-Associated Cancer. *Vaccines* **2016**, *4*, 5. [CrossRef]
95. Gilbert, S.; Zhang, R.; Denson, L.; Moriggl, R.; Steinbrecher, K.; Shroyer, N.; Lin, J.; Han, X. Enterocyte STAT5 promotes mucosal wound healing via suppression of myosin light chain kinase-mediated loss of barrier function and inflammation. *EMBO Mol. Med.* **2012**, *4*, 109–124. [CrossRef]
96. Gilbert, S.; Nivarthi, H.; Mayhew, C.N.; Lo, Y.H.; Noah, T.K.; Vallance, J.; Rülicke, T.; Müller, M.; Jegga, A.G.; Tang, W.; et al. Activated STAT5 confers resistance to intestinal injury by increasing intestinal stem cell proliferation and regeneration. *Stem Cell Rep.* **2015**, *4*, 209–225. [CrossRef]
97. Liu, R.; Moriggl, R.; Zhang, D.; Li, H.; Karns, R.; Ruan, H.B.; Niu, H.; Mayhew, C.; Watson, C.; Bangar, H.; et al. Constitutive STAT5 activation regulates Paneth and Paneth-like cells to control. *Life Sci. Alliance* **2019**, *2*, e201900296. [CrossRef]
98. Li, G.; Liu, Z.; Ran, P.; Qiu, J.; Zhong, N. Activation of signal transducer and activator of transcription 5 (STAT5) in splenocyte proliferation of asthma mice induced by ovalbumin. *Cell Mol. Immunol.* **2004**, *1*, 471–474.
99. Turlej, R.K.; Fiévez, L.; Sandersen, C.F.; Dogné, S.; Kirschvink, N.; Lekeux, P.; Bureau, F. Enhanced survival of lung granulocytes in an animal model of asthma: Evidence for a role of GM-CSF activated STAT5 signalling pathway. *Thorax* **2001**, *56*, 696–702. [CrossRef]
100. Ji, J.; Shu, X.; Li, X.; Sundquist, K.; Sundquist, J.; Hemminki, K. Cancer risk in hospitalised asthma patients. *Br. J. Cancer* **2009**, *100*, 829–833. [CrossRef]
101. Ciccia, F.; Rizzo, A.; Alessandro, R.; Guggino, G.; Maugeri, R.; Saieva, L.; Cannizzaro, A.; Giardina, A.; De Leo, G.; Gerardo Iacopino, D.; et al. Activated IL-22 pathway occurs in the muscle tissues of patients with polymyositis or dermatomyositis and is correlated with disease activity. *Rheumatology* **2014**, *53*, 1307–1312. [CrossRef]

102. Voltarelli, F.A.; Frajacomo, F.T.; Padilha, C.S.; Testa, M.T.J.; Cella, P.S.; Ribeiro, D.F.; de Oliveira, D.X.; Veronez, L.C.; Bisson, G.S.; Moura, F.A.; et al. Syngeneic B16F10 Melanoma Causes Cachexia and Impaired Skeletal Muscle Strength and Locomotor Activity in Mice. *Front. Physiol.* **2017**, *8*, 715. [CrossRef]
103. Hosui, A.; Kimura, A.; Yamaji, D.; Zhu, B.M.; Na, R.; Hennighausen, L. Loss of STAT5 causes liver fibrosis and cancer development through increased TGF-{beta} and STAT3 activation. *J. Exp. Med.* **2009**, *206*, 819–831. [CrossRef]
104. Rinkevich, Y.; Walmsley, G.G.; Hu, M.S.; Maan, Z.N.; Newman, A.M.; Drukker, M.; Januszyk, M.; Krampitz, G.W.; Gurtner, G.C.; Lorenz, H.P.; et al. Skin fibrosis. Identification and isolation of a dermal lineage with intrinsic fibrogenic potential. *Science* **2015**, *348*, aaa2151. [CrossRef]
105. Park, J.S.; Kim, S.M.; Hwang, S.H.; Choi, S.Y.; Kwon, J.Y.; Kwok, S.K.; Cho, M.L.; Park, S.H. Combinatory treatment using tacrolimus and a STAT3 inhibitor regulate Treg cells and plasma cells. *Int. J. Immunopathol. Pharmacol.* **2018**, *32*, 2058738418778724. [CrossRef]
106. Slight-Webb, S.; Guthridge, J.M.; Chakravarty, E.F.; Chen, H.; Lu, R.; Macwana, S.; Bean, K.; Maecker, H.T.; Utz, P.J.; James, J.A. Mycophenolate mofetil reduces STAT3 phosphorylation in systemic lupus erythematosus patients. *JCI Insight* **2019**, *4*, 124575. [CrossRef]
107. Meshaal, S.; El Refai, R.; El Saie, A.; El Hawary, R. Signal transducer and activator of transcription 5 is implicated in disease activity in adult and juvenile onset systemic lupus erythematosus. *Clin. Rheumatol.* **2016**, *35*, 1515–1520. [CrossRef]
108. Hedrich, C.M.; Rauen, T.; Apostolidis, S.A.; Grammatikos, A.P.; Rodriguez Rodriguez, N.; Ioannidis, C.; Kyttaris, V.C.; Crispin, J.C.; Tsokos, G.C. Stat3 promotes IL-10 expression in lupus T cells through trans-activation and chromatin remodeling. *Proc. Natl. Acad. Sci. USA* **2014**, *111*, 13457–13462. [CrossRef]
109. Yang, J.; Yang, X.; Zou, H.; Chu, Y.; Li, M. Recovery of the immune balance between Th17 and regulatory T cells as a treatment for systemic lupus erythematosus. *Rheumatology* **2011**, *50*, 1366–1372. [CrossRef]
110. Talaat, R.M.; Mohamed, S.F.; Bassyouni, I.H.; Raouf, A.A. Th1/Th2/Th17/Treg cytokine imbalance in systemic lupus erythematosus (SLE) patients: Correlation with disease activity. *Cytokine* **2015**, *72*, 146–153. [CrossRef]
111. Chen, S.Y.; Liu, M.F.; Kuo, P.Y.; Wang, C.R. Upregulated expression of STAT3/IL-17 in patients with systemic lupus erythematosus. *Clin. Rheumatol.* **2019**, *38*, 1361–1366. [CrossRef]
112. Goropevšek, A.; Gorenjak, M.; Gradišnik, S.; Dai, K.; Holc, I.; Hojs, R.; Krajnc, I.; Pahor, A.; Avčin, T. STAT5 phosphorylation in CD4 T cells from patients with SLE is related to changes in their subsets and follow-up disease severity. *J. Leukoc. Biol.* **2017**, *101*, 1405–1418. [CrossRef]
113. Grushchak, S.; Mathieu, R.J.; Orrell, K.A.; Hagstrom, E.L.; Laumann, A.E.; West, D.P.; Nardone, B. Malignant melanoma association with systemic lupus erythematosus in a large midwestern U.S. patient population: A retrospective study. *Int. J. Dermatol.* **2018**, *57*, e34–e36. [CrossRef]
114. Dreyer, L.; Faurschou, M.; Mogensen, M.; Jacobsen, S. High incidence of potentially virus-induced malignancies in systemic lupus erythematosus: A long-term followup study in a Danish cohort. *Arthritis Rheum.* **2011**, *63*, 3032–3037. [CrossRef]
115. Cao, L.; Tong, H.; Xu, G.; Liu, P.; Meng, H.; Wang, J.; Zhao, X.; Tang, Y.; Jin, J. Systemic lupus erythematous and malignancy risk: A meta-analysis. *PLoS ONE* **2015**, *10*, e0122964. [CrossRef]
116. Colonna, M. TREM1 Blockade: Killing Two Birds with One Stone. *Trends Immunol.* **2019**, *40*, 781–783. [CrossRef]
117. Asteriou, E.; Gkoutzourelas, A.; Mavropoulos, A.; Katsiari, C.; Sakkas, L.I.; Bogdanos, D.P. Curcumin for the Management of Periodontitis and Early ACPA-Positive Rheumatoid Arthritis: Killing Two Birds with One Stone. *Nutrients* **2018**, *10*, 908. [CrossRef]
118. Cai, Z.; Zhang, J.; Li, H. Two Birds with One Stone: Regular Use of PDE5 Inhibitors for Treating Male Patients with Erectile Dysfunction and Cardiovascular Diseases. *Cardiovasc. Drugs Ther.* **2019**, *33*, 119–128. [CrossRef]
119. Pietschmann, K.; Bolck, H.A.; Buchwald, M.; Spielberg, S.; Polzer, H.; Spiekermann, K.; Bug, G.; Heinzel, T.; Böhmer, F.D.; Krämer, O.H. Breakdown of the FLT3-ITD/STAT5 axis and synergistic apoptosis induction by the histone deacetylase inhibitor panobinostat and FLT3-specific inhibitors. *Mol. Cancer Ther.* **2012**, *11*, 2373–2383. [CrossRef]
120. Kosan, C.; Ginter, T.; Heinzel, T.; Krämer, O.H. STAT5 acetylation: Mechanisms and consequences for immunological control and leukemogenesis. *JAKSTAT* **2013**, *2*, e26102. [CrossRef]

121. Lesinski, G.B. The potential for targeting the STAT3 pathway as a novel therapy for melanoma. *Future Oncol.* **2013**, *9*, 925–927. [CrossRef]
122. Piccirillo, R.; Giavazzi, R. Inactivating STAT3: Bad for tumor, good for muscle. *Cell Cycle* **2015**, *14*, 939–940. [CrossRef]
123. Trécul, A.; Morceau, F.; Dicato, M.; Diederich, M. Dietary compounds as potent inhibitors of the signal transducers and activators of transcription (STAT) 3 regulatory network. *Genes Nutr.* **2012**, *7*, 111–125. [CrossRef]
124. Li, T.; Fu, X.; Tse, A.K.; Guo, H.; Lee, K.W.; Liu, B.; Su, T.; Wang, X.; Yu, Z. Inhibiting STAT3 signaling is involved in the anti-melanoma effects of a herbal formula comprising Sophorae Flos and Lonicerae Japonicae Flos. *Sci. Rep.* **2017**, *7*, 3097. [CrossRef]
125. Rani, A.; Murphy, J.J. STAT5 in Cancer and Immunity. *J. Interferon Cytokine Res.* **2016**, *36*, 226–237. [CrossRef]
126. Knochelmann, H.M.; Dwyer, C.J.; Bailey, S.R.; Amaya, S.M.; Elston, D.M.; Mazza-McCrann, J.M.; Paulos, C.M. When worlds collide: Th17 and Treg cells in cancer and autoimmunity. *Cell. Mol. Immunol.* **2018**, *15*, 458–469. [CrossRef]
127. Chen, C.; Gao, F.H. Th17 Cells Paradoxical Roles in Melanoma and Potential Application in Immunotherapy. *Front. Immunol.* **2019**, *10*, 187. [CrossRef]
128. Jacobs, J.F.; Nierkens, S.; Figdor, C.G.; de Vries, I.J.; Adema, G.J. Regulatory T cells in melanoma: The final hurdle towards effective immunotherapy? *Lancet Oncol.* **2012**, *13*, e32–e42. [CrossRef]
129. Wong, A.L.A.; Hirpara, J.L.; Pervaiz, S.; Eu, J.Q.; Sethi, G.; Goh, B.C. Do STAT3 inhibitors have potential in the future for cancer therapy? *Expert Opin. Investig. Drugs* **2017**, *26*, 883–887. [CrossRef]
130. Harada, D.; Takigawa, N.; Kiura, K. The Role of STAT3 in Non-Small Cell Lung Cancer. *Cancers* **2014**, *6*, 708–722. [CrossRef]

5

STAT3 and STAT5 Activation in Solid Cancers

Sebastian Igelmann [1,2], Heidi A. Neubauer [3] and Gerardo Ferbeyre [1,2,*]

1 Department of Biochemistry and Molecular Medicine, Université de Montréal, C.P. 6128, Succ. Centre-Ville, Montréal, QC H3C 3J7, Canada; sebastian.igelmann@umontreal.ca
2 CRCHUM, 900 Saint-Denis St, Montréal, QC H2X 0A9, Canada
3 Institute of Animal Breeding and Genetics, University of Veterinary Medicine Vienna, Vienna 1210, Austria; Heidi.Neubauer@vetmeduni.ac.at
* Correspondence: g.ferbeyre@umontreal.ca

Abstract: The Signal Transducer and Activator of Transcription (STAT)3 and 5 proteins are activated by many cytokine receptors to regulate specific gene expression and mitochondrial functions. Their role in cancer is largely context-dependent as they can both act as oncogenes and tumor suppressors. We review here the role of STAT3/5 activation in solid cancers and summarize their association with survival in cancer patients. The molecular mechanisms that underpin the oncogenic activity of STAT3/5 signaling include the regulation of genes that control cell cycle and cell death. However, recent advances also highlight the critical role of STAT3/5 target genes mediating inflammation and stemness. In addition, STAT3 mitochondrial functions are required for transformation. On the other hand, several tumor suppressor pathways act on or are activated by STAT3/5 signaling, including tyrosine phosphatases, the sumo ligase Protein Inhibitor of Activated STAT3 (PIAS3), the E3 ubiquitin ligase TATA Element Modulatory Factor/Androgen Receptor-Coactivator of 160 kDa (TMF/ARA160), the miRNAs miR-124 and miR-1181, the Protein of alternative reading frame 19 (p19ARF)/p53 pathway and the Suppressor of Cytokine Signaling 1 and 3 (SOCS1/3) proteins. Cancer mutations and epigenetic alterations may alter the balance between pro-oncogenic and tumor suppressor activities associated with STAT3/5 signaling, explaining their context-dependent association with tumor progression both in human cancers and animal models.

Keywords: solid cancers; cell cycle; apoptosis; inflammation; mitochondria; stemness; tumor suppression

---

1. Introduction

Activation of Signal Transducer and Activator of Transcription (STAT) proteins has been linked to many human cancers. STATs were initially discovered as latent cytosolic transcription factors that are phosphorylated by the Janus Kinase (JAK) family upon stimulation of membrane-associated cytokine and growth factor receptors. Phosphorylation triggers STAT dimerization and translocation to the nucleus to bind specific promoters and regulate transcription [1]. Here, we review the role of STAT family members STAT3 and STAT5 in solid human malignancies, as well as the mechanisms that may explain their association with either worse or better prognosis.

2. STAT3 and STAT5 in Solid Cancers

The discovery of cancer genes has been propelled by genetic analyses and more recently by next generation DNA sequencing technologies. Combined, these studies have identified 127 significantly mutated cancer genes that cover diverse signaling pathways [2]. Mutations acting as drivers in cancer are positively selected during tumor growth and constitute solid proof of the involvement of a particular gene as a driver in the disease. Mutations in STAT3 and STAT5 have been reported in patients with solid cancers, but unlike hyperactivation of the JAK/STAT pathway, STAT3/5 mutations in cancer are relatively infrequent and occur mostly in hematological malignancies.

An overview of reported STAT3/5 mutations in solid cancers is illustrated in Figure 1, based on data collected from the Catalogue of Somatic Mutations in Cancer (COSMIC) database. Mutations in *STAT3* are more prevalent than mutations in *STAT5A* or *STAT5B* genes. Noticeably, gastrointestinal cancers have the highest rates of STAT3/5 mutations compared with other solid cancers (Figure 1). Missense mutations tend to cluster within the SH2 domain, where gain-of-function mutations were previously characterized [3,4], as well as within the DNA binding domain and to an extent the N-terminal domain (Figure 1A). Interestingly, the *STAT3* Tyrosine 640 into Phenylalanine (Y640F) hotspot gain-of-function mutation reported in various lymphoid malignancies has also been detected in patients with liver cancer (Figure 1A). Nonsense and frameshift mutations are less frequent and more disperse, likely representing loss-of-function events (Figure 1B). Notably, a hotspot frameshift mutation at position Q368 within the DNA binding domain of STAT5B has been reported in 24 patients with various types of carcinoma; this frameshift generates a stop codon shortly after the mutation and is therefore likely to be loss-of-function, although characterization of this mutation has not been performed.

As opposed to mutation rates, STAT3/5 activation is very frequent in human cancers, perhaps reflecting increased cytokine signaling or mutations in cytokine receptors or negative regulators. STAT3/5 activation can be detected using antibodies that measure total levels or activation marks in STAT3/5 proteins (e.g. tyrosine phosphorylation). A better assessment of STAT3/5 activation can be obtained by measuring downstream signaling targets (i.e., mRNA levels of STAT3 [5] and STAT5 [6] target genes). A recent metanalysis of 63 different studies concluded that STAT3 protein overexpression was significantly associated with a worse 3-year overall survival (OS) (OR = 2.06, 95% CI = 1.57 to 2.71, $p < 0.00001$) and 5-year OS (OR = 2.00, 95% CI = 1.53 to 2.63, $p < 0.00001$) in patients with solid tumors [7]. Elevated STAT3 expression was associated with poor prognosis in gastric cancer, lung cancer, gliomas, hepatic cancer, osteosarcoma, prostate cancer and pancreatic cancer. However, high STAT3 protein expression levels predicted a better prognosis for breast cancer [7]. This study mixed data of both STAT3 and phospho-STAT3 (p-STAT3) expression limiting its ability to associate pathway activation to prognosis. Here, we summarize the data linking activation of STAT3/5 to overall survival in several major human solid cancers identifying the biomarkers used in each study (Table 1). Taken together, the results clearly show that *STAT3* and *STAT5* are important cancer genes despite their relatively low mutation frequency.

STAT3 activation is clearly a factor linked to bad prognosis in patients with lung cancer, liver cancer, renal cell carcinoma (RCC) and gliomas. In other tumors, the association is not significant. In solid tumors, STAT3 activation is more frequent than STAT5 activation although no explanation for this difference was proposed. In prostate cancer, both STAT3 and STAT5 have been associated with castration-resistant disease and proposed as therapeutic targets [8,9]. In colon cancer, the association between p-STAT3 and survival varies according to the study, but a high p-STAT3/p-STAT5 ratio indicates bad prognosis [10]. Also in breast cancer, p-STAT5 levels are clearly associated with better prognosis [11]. In liver cancer, STAT5 has ambivalent functions that were recently reviewed by Moriggl and colleagues [12]. Understanding mechanistically how STAT3/5 promote transformation and tumor suppression is important for the eventual design of new treatments. Also, survival data is highly influenced by the response of patients to their treatment and may not always reflect all mechanistic links between STAT3/5 activity and tumor biology. Of note, the effect of any gene is conditioned by the genetic context of gene action. Some genes can clearly exert a tumor suppressor effect in the initial stages of carcinogenesis that is lost when cancer mutations or epigenetic changes inactivate key effectors of these tumor suppressor pathways [13]. Human studies are usually limited to late stage tumors because it is easier to collect samples at that point. Studies in model systems, including primary cells, organoids and mouse models are thus required for a full understanding of how cancer genes work specifically at early stages in tumorigenesis.

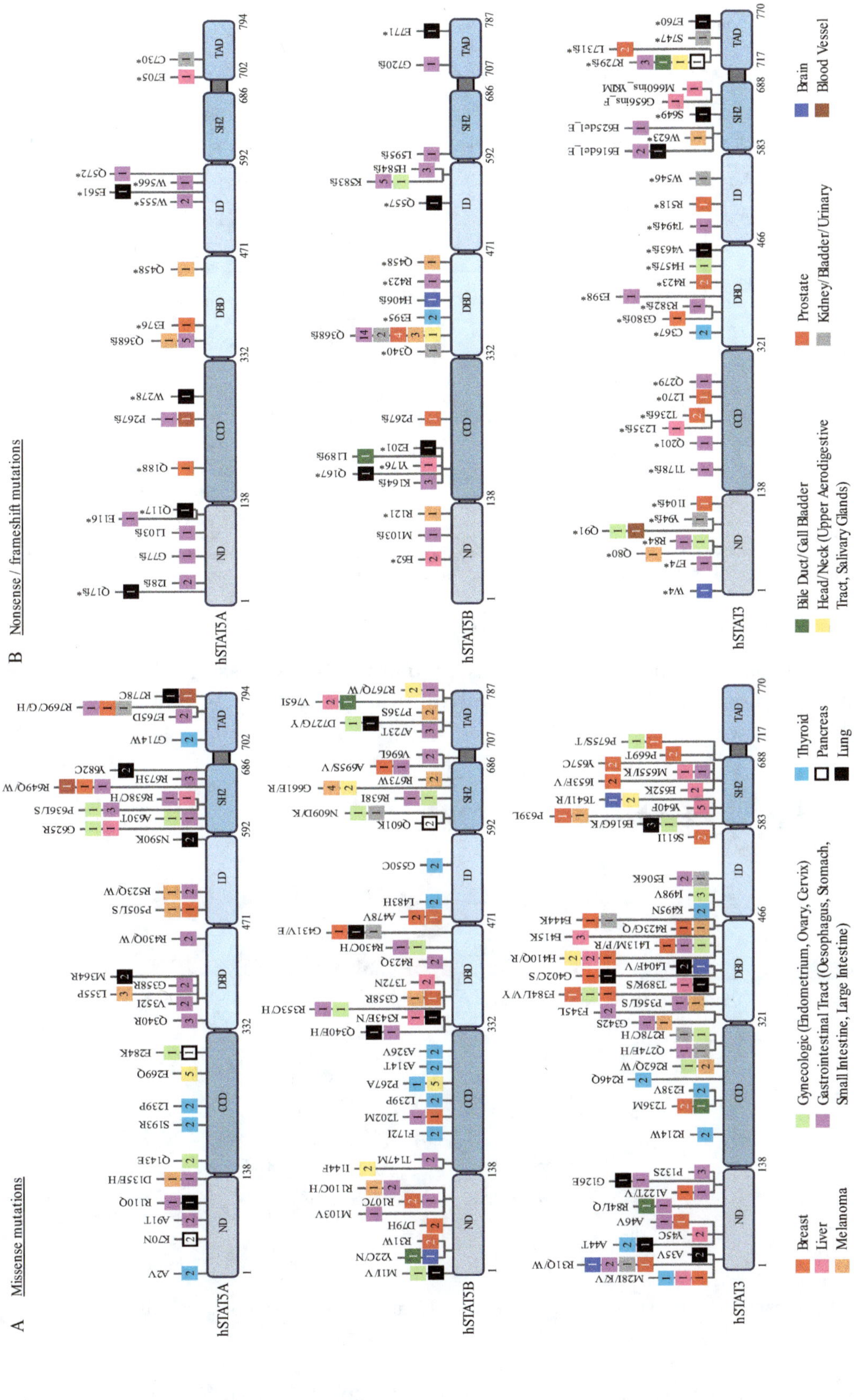

Figure 1. Map of somatic mutations detected in human Signal Transducer and Activator of Transcription (STAT)5A, STAT5B and STAT3 in patients with solid cancers. Individual missense mutations found in at least two patients (**A**), as well as all reported nonsense and frameshift mutations (**B**), are depicted. Numbers in each box represent the number of cases reported for each mutation. Data were mined from the Catalogue of Somatic Mutations In Cancer (COSMIC) database. ND, N-terminal domain; CCD, Coiled coil domain; DBD, DNA binding domain; LD, Linker domain; SH2, Src homology 2 domain; TAD, Transactivation domain.

Table 1. STAT3/5 activity and overall survival in major human solid tumors.

Tumor Type	Biomarker/Type of Study	Overall Survival	Ref
NSCLC	High p-STAT3/Meta-analysis of 9 studies	Log HR 0.67, 95% CI: 0.57–0.77, $p < 0.0001$	[14]
NSCLC	High p-STAT3/Cox regression multivariate analysis	HR 2.45, 95% CI: 1.084–5.556, $p = 0.031$	[15]
Lung cancer	High p-STAT3/Meta-analysis of 13 studies	HR 1.23, 95% CI: 1.04–1.46, $p = 0.02$	[16]
Pancreatic cancer	High p-STAT3/Log-rank test	No association $p > 0.05$	[17]
Liver cancer (HCC)	High p-STAT3/Meta-analysis of 8 studies	HR 1.69, 95% CI: 1.07–2.31, $p < 0.0001$ 3yr HR 1.67, 95% CI: 1.18–2.15, $p < 0.0001$ 5yr	[18]
Breast cancer	High p-STAT3/Meta-analysis of 12 studies	No association $p > 0.05$	[19]
Breast cancer (ER+)	High p-STAT3/Log-rank test	No association $p > 0.05$	[20]
GBM	High p-S727-STAT3/Cox regression multivariate analysis	HR 1.797, 95% CI: 1.028–3.142, $p = 0.040$	[21]
RCC	High p-S727-STAT3/Cox regression multivariate analysis	HR 3.32, 95% CI: 1.26–8.71, $p = 0.014$ 10yr	[22]
Colon cancer	High p-STAT3/p-STAT5 ratio/Cox regression multivariate analysis	HR 4.468, $p = 0.043$ 5yr	[10]
Colon cancer	High p-STAT3/Log-rank test	Worse overall survival, $p < 0.001$	[23]
Colon cancer	High p-STAT3/Cox regression multivariate analysis	HR 1.61, 95% CI: 1.11–2.34, $p = 0.015$	[24]
Breast cancer	Low p-STAT5/Cox regression multivariate analysis	HR 2.49, 95% CI: 1.23–5.05, $p = 0.012$ 5yr	[11]
Prostate cancer	High nuclear STAT5A/B/Cox regression multivariate analysis	HR 1.59, 95% CI: 1.04–2.44, $p = 0.034$	[9]

ER+, estrogen receptor-positive; HCC, hepatocellular carcinoma; GBM, glioblastoma multiforme; NSCLC, non-small-cell lung carcinoma; HR, hazard ratio; RCC, renal cell carcinoma.

3. Mechanisms of Transformation by STAT3/5 Proteins in Solid Cancers

STAT3 and STAT5 promote tumor progression by regulating the expression of cell cycle, survival and pro-inflammatory genes. In addition, they control mitochondrial functions, metabolism and stemness, as discussed below (Figure 2).

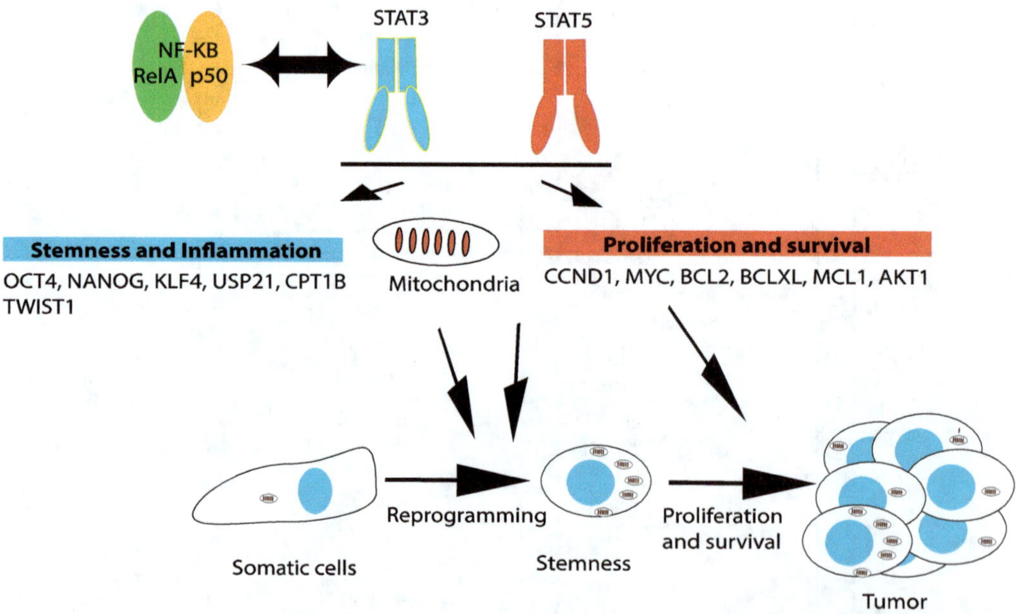

Figure 2. Mechanisms of tumorigenic activity of STAT3 and STAT5 signaling in solid tumors.

3.1. Cell Cycle and Apoptosis

As transcription factors, STAT3 and STAT5 regulate many genes required for cell cycle progression and cell survival. A major target of the transcriptional control of the mammalian cell cycle is cyclin

D. STAT3 regulates cyclin D expression in a complex with CD44 and the acetyltransferase p300. The latter acetylates STAT3 promoting its dimerization, nuclear translocation and binding to the cyclin D promoter [25]. Other cell cycle and survival genes regulated by STAT3 include *c-MYC (myc proto-oncogene)*, B-cell lymphoma 2 (*BCL2)*, *BCL2L1*/BCL-XL (B-cell lymphoma-extra large), *MCL1* (Myeloid Cell Leukemia Sequence 1) and *BIRC5*/survivin [26]. Recent studies combined ChIPSeq with whole transcriptome profiling in ABC DLBCL (activated B cell-like diffuse large B cell lymphoma) cell lines and revealed that STAT3 activates genes in the Phosphoinositide 3-Kinase (PI3K)/AKT/Mammalian Target of Rapamycin (mTOR) pathway, the Nuclear Factor Kappa-Light-Chain Enhancer of Activated B-Cells (NF-κB) pathway and the cell cycle regulation pathway, while repressing type I interferon signaling genes [27]. STAT5 also regulates the expression of cell cycle and cell survival genes [13] including *AKT1* [28], which encodes a pro-survival kinase.

3.2. *Inflammation and Innate Immunity*

Although the induction of cell proliferation and cell survival genes by STAT3/5 proteins contribute to their pro-cancer activity, in basal-like breast cancers the major genes associated with STAT3 activation control inflammation and the immune response [29]. Of note, inflammation is initially an adaptive response to pathological insults such as oncogenic stimuli, and it therefore exerts a tumor suppressive function. However, dysregulated inflammation in the long term provides a substrate for tumorigenesis [30]. STAT3 alone or in cooperation with NF-κB regulates the expression of many pro-inflammatory genes [31–33]. Starved tumor cells activate NF-κB and STAT3 via endoplasmic reticulum (ER) stress and secrete cytokines that stimulate tumor survival and clonogenic capacity [34]. The coactivation of these two transcription factors amplifies pro-inflammatory gene expression driving cancer-associated inflammation [35]. Of interest, the STAT3-NF-κB complex can repress the expression of DNA Damage Inducible Transcript 3 (DDIT3), an inhibitor of CCAAT Enhancer Binding Protein Beta (CEBPβ), another pro-inflammatory transcription factor [36].

Pharmacological agents that limit inflammation have been proposed for cancer prevention [37]. The use of metformin, a drug widely used to control diabetes, has been associated with a dramatic reduction in cancer incidence in many tissues [38]. Although the primary site of action of this drug is in mitochondria, a consequence of its effects is a potent reduction in the activation of NF-κB and STAT3, suggesting that the promising anticancer actions of metformin are related to its ability to curtail pro-inflammatory gene expression [39,40]. In contrast to STAT3, STAT5B inhibits NF-κB activity in the kidney fibroblast cell line COS by competing with coactivators of transcription [41], while it stimulates NF-κB in leukemia cells [42]. These results suggest the involvement of different regulatory mechanisms of STAT5 in hematopoietic cancers compared with solid cancers.

3.3. *Mitochondria*

In addition to their canonical roles in inflammation and immunity, STAT3 and STAT5 have been shown to localize to mitochondria. The mitochondrial localization of STAT3 is required for its ability to support malignant transformation in murine embryonic fibroblasts and breast cancer cells [43–46], and mito-STAT3 regulates mitochondrial metabolism and mitochondrial gene expression [45,47–51]. Several reports have suggested that STAT3 can be imported to mitochondria after phosphorylation on S727 [44,45] or upon acetylation [52,53]. Other studies have revealed that STAT3 mitochondrial translocation is mediated by interactions with Heat Shock Protein 22 (HSP22), Gene Associated with Retinoic and Interferon-Induced Mortality 19 (GRIM-19) or Translocase of Outer Mitochondrial Membrane 20 (TOM20) [54–56]. The mRNAs coding for some mitochondrial proteins are translated close to or in physical interaction with the import complex TOM [57,58]. The structural motifs mediating those interactions are located in the 3′ and 5′ UTRs of the mRNAs [59,60] and it will be interesting to investigate whether the mRNA of STAT3 also possesses RNA localization signals (zip codes) to localize in close proximity to mitochondria.

Whereas the role of mitochondrial STAT3 has been extensively studied, the role of STAT5 in mitochondria is less clear. The import of STAT5 to mitochondria is regulated by cytokines [43]. Once imported into the mitochondria, STAT5 binds the D-loop of mitochondrial DNA, although no increase in transcription of mitochondrial genes was observed [61]. Mito-STAT5 is also able to interact with the Pyruvate Dehydrogenase Complex (PDC) and was shown to regulate metabolism towards glycolysis, as observed in cells treated with cytokines [43,61]. In the same line, STAT3 was also shown to interact with the PDC in mitochondria [53].

3.4. Reprogramming and Stemness

The role of STAT3 in stem cell biology was initially recognized due to the requirement for the cytokine LIF to maintain pluripotency in cultures of mouse embryonic stem (ES) cells. STAT3 activation mediates the induction or repression of several genes in mouse ES cells including the pluripotency factors *Oct4, Klf4, Tfcp2l1* and polycomb proteins [62–64]. Many pluripotency factors, such as Homeobox Protein NANOG, are short-lived proteins. STAT3 controls protein stability by inducing the expression of the deubiquitinase Ubiquitin Specific Peptidase 21 (USP21), stabilizing NANOG in mouse ES cells. Induction of ES cell differentiation promotes the Extracellular Signal-Regulated Kinase (ERK)-dependent phosphorylation of USP21 and its dissociation from NANOG, leading to NANOG degradation [65]. STAT3 also plays a role in the reprogramming of somatic cells into induced pluripotent stem (IPS) cells [66] and it has been suggested that its effects depend on the demethylation of pluripotency factor promoters [67]. STAT3 also activates mitochondrial DNA transcription, promoting oxidative phosphorylation during maintenance and induction of pluripotency [68]. It is thus likely that the ability of STAT3 to stimulate stemness also plays a role in its oncogenic activity.

In many tumors, a subpopulation of cells possess a higher malignant capacity. These so-called tumor-initiating cells are suspected to regenerate the tumor after cancer chemotherapy and express many genes commonly expressed in ES cells [69]. It has been shown that STAT3 is required for the formation of tumor spheres and the viability of the cancer stem cell pool in many different tumors [39,40,70–83]. At least in breast cancer, a critical mechanism stimulated by STAT3 to regulate stemness involves genes in fatty acid oxidation [78,79] and the ability of STAT3 to adjust the levels of reactive oxygen species (ROS) produced in mitochondria [79]. In colorectal cancer cells, STAT3 forms a complex with the stem cell marker CD44 and the p300 acetyltransferase. Acetylation of STAT3 by this complex allows dimerization, nuclear translocation and binding to the promoters of genes required for stemness such as *c-MYC* and *TWIST1* [84].

The role of STAT5 in promoting cancer stemness does not affect many cell types and is mostly confined to hematopoietic cancers [85]. However, Nevalainen and colleagues reported that STAT5B induces stem cell properties in prostate cancer cells [86] in line with the increase in nuclear STAT5A/B observed in these tumors in correlation with bad prognosis [9]. Furthermore, transgenic mice with increased expression of prolactin in prostate epithelial cells displayed increases in the basal/stem cell compartment in association with activation of STAT5. This enrichment of stem cells was partially reversed by depletion of *Stat5a/b* [87]. The pro-stem cell oncogenic effect of STAT5 in the prostate contrasts with its effects in the mammary gland where STAT5 induces cell differentiation [88]. The ETS transcription factor Elf5 (E74-like factor 5) is a target of the prolactin-STAT5 axis and promotes mammary cell differentiation [89–91], supporting the tumor suppressive role of STAT5 in the mammary gland.

4. Tumor Suppressor Functions and Negative Regulation of STAT3/5 Signaling

The oncogenic activity of JAK/STAT signaling is controlled by several molecular barriers that limit the activation of this pathway. They include tyrosine phosphatases, E3 SUMO ligases of the Protein Inhibitor of Activated STAT3 (PIAS) family, E3 ubiquitin ligases and miRNAs. In addition, oncogenic STAT3/5 signaling can activate fail-safe tumor suppressors such as protein of alternative reading frame 19 (p19ARF), Suppressor of Cytokine Signaling 1 (SOCS1) and p53 that trigger apoptosis, ferroptosis and/or senescence in potentially malignant cells (Figure 3). Understanding these different responses to

STAT signaling in cancer is important to further distinguish tumors that would benefit from STAT3 or STAT5 inhibitors and those that would not.

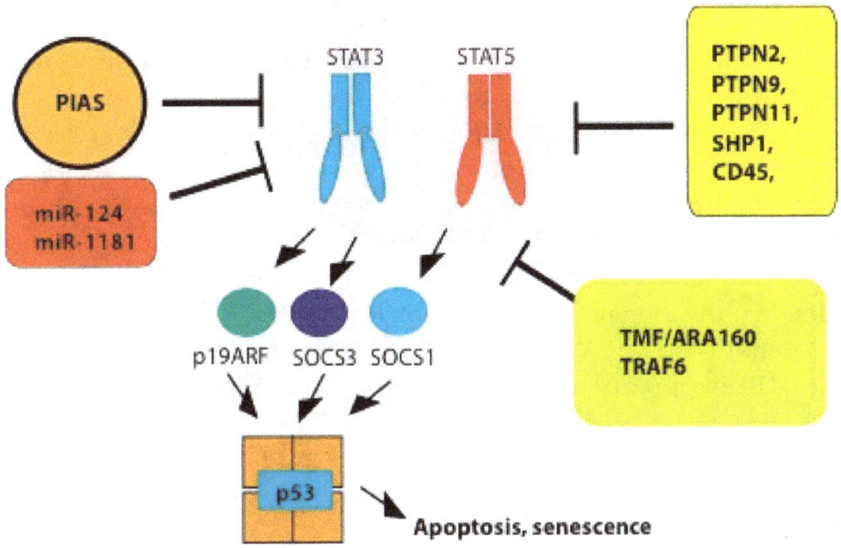

Figure 3. Tumor suppressor pathways acting on STAT3/5 activity (Protein Inhibitor of Activated STAT3 PIAS, miRNAs, E3 ligases, phosphatases) or activated by STAT3/5 transcriptional activity (Protein of alternative reading frame 19 (p19ARF) Suppressor of Cytokine Signaling 1 and 3 (SOCS1/3), p53). Abbreviations: (PTPN2 (Tyrosine-protein phosphatase non-receptor type 2), PTPN9/MEG2 (Tyrosine-protein phosphatase non-receptor type 9), PTPN11/SHP2 (Tyrosine-protein phosphatase non-receptor type 11), PTPN6/SHP1 (Tyrosine-protein phosphatase non-receptor type 6) and TNF receptor associated factor 6 (TRAF6)).

4.1. Tyrosine Phosphatases

Activation of STAT3 and STAT5 in tumors is often associated with tyrosine phosphorylation, a modification that can be reverted by several protein tyrosine phosphatases such as PTPN2 (Tyrosine-protein phosphatase non-receptor type 2), PTPN9/MEG2 (Tyrosine-protein phosphatase non-receptor type 9), PTPN11/SHP2 (Tyrosine-protein phosphatase non-receptor type 11) [92,93], CD45 [94] and PTPN6/SHP1 (Tyrosine-protein phosphatase non-receptor type 6) [95]. However, little is known about a possible role of these phosphatases in STAT3 activation in solid tumors. In liver cancers, SHP1 is downregulated in cells with mesenchymal features, and restoring its levels both reduced STAT3 phosphorylation and reversed the mesenchymal phenotype of liver cancer cells [95]. SHP1 and SHP2 also target STAT5 [96,97] but the significance of this regulation in solid tumors remains to be investigated.

4.2. PIAS

The Protein Inhibitor of Activated STAT3 (PIAS3) inhibits STAT3 transcriptional activity. In gliomas, PIAS3 expression is reduced [98]. Mechanistically, SMAD6 promotes PIAS3 degradation, promoting glioma cell growth and stem cell properties [76]. The PIAS proteins have SUMO E3 ligase activity acting on multiple proteins, and so their effects cannot be solely attributed to STAT3 inhibition [99]. Of interest, PIAS3 can bind NF-κB promoting its SUMOylation and inhibiting its activity [100,101], potentially targeting the expression of many pro-inflammatory genes required for tumor progression. Also, PIAS3 binds the N-terminus of p53 and prevents the interaction with its negative regulator MDM2, leading to p53 stabilization [102].

4.3. E3 Ligases

The Golgi resident and BC-box protein TATA Element Modulatory Factor/Androgen Receptor-Coactivator of 160 kDa (TMF/ARA160) was reported as an E3 ligase that catalyzes STAT3 ubiquitination leading to its proteasome-dependent degradation in myogenic C2C12 cells. The level of TMF/ARA160 was found to be significantly decreased in glioblastoma multiforme tumors, in benign meningioma and in malignant anaplastic meningioma, where STAT3 is known to play an oncogenic role [103]. TMF/ARA160 can also bind and ubiquitinate RELA/NF-κB leading to its proteasome-dependent degradation and a decrease in the expression of inflammatory genes [104]. Furthermore, the ubiquitin ligase TNF receptor associated factor 6 (TRAF6) binds and ubiquitinates STAT3 inhibiting the expression of STAT3 target genes [105]. During oncogene-induced senescence, STAT3 is degraded by the proteasome but the E3 ligase responsible has not been identified [106]. Recent results revealed that the long non-coding RNA (lncRNA) PVT1 (long non-coding RNA encoded by the human *PVT1* gene) binds STAT3 and protects it from ubiquitin-dependent degradation in gastric cancer [107]. PVT1 is upregulated in multiple cancers predicting poor prognosis for overall survival [108–110].

4.4. MiRNAs

The miRNA miR-124 regulates STAT3 signaling by targeting the mRNAs of interleukin-6 receptor (IL6R) [111] and STAT3 [112,113]. Suppression of this miRNA increases STAT3 phosphorylation and induces transformation in immortalized mouse hepatocytes. Of interest, systemic delivery of miR-124 prevented tumor growth in diethylnitrosamine (DEN)-treated mice, and miR-124 levels were found to be reduced in human hepatocellular carcinomas (HCC) [111]. In gliomas, miR-124 is poorly expressed but upregulation of its expression in glioma cancer stem cells inhibited the STAT3 pathway. In this model, STAT3 mediates immunosuppression, which was relieved upon systemic miR-124 delivery [114]. The circular RNA (circRNA) 100782 is upregulated in pancreatic cancer and its knockdown downregulates all miR-124 targets including IL6R and STAT3. This circRNA binds miR-124 suggesting that it may act as a miRNA sponge [115]. Furthermore, the miRNA miR-1181 also targets STAT3 and is downregulated in pancreatic cancer, predicting poorer overall survival. Overexpression of miR-1181 inhibited tumor formation and stem cell properties of pancreatic cancer cells [116].

4.5. The Suppressor of Cytokine Signaling SOCS

The members of the Suppressor of Cytokine Signaling (SOCS) family are major negative feedback regulators of JAK/STAT signaling and their expression is dysregulated in many human cancers [117–119]. These genes provide a barrier for cells with aberrant cytokine activation by inhibiting cytokine signaling [120]. In STAT3 driven cancers, SOCS3 seems to be the most important negative feedback regulator and mouse models of SOCS3 ablation show strong STAT3 activation [119,121–124]. On the other hand, in solid cancers where STAT5 plays a causal role such as liver and prostate cancer, in addition to SOCS3, SOCS1 is frequently inactivated and mouse models of SOCS1 ablation increase both liver and prostate tumorigenesis [125–132]. In addition to their role as JAK/STAT signaling barriers, SOCS1 and SOCS3 can bind p53 and activate tumor suppressor responses such as senescence and ferroptosis when their expression is induced by aberrant STAT5 signaling in primary cells [133–138]. In this way, SOCS1 and SOCS3 also act as fail-safe tumor suppressors in response to aberrant JAK/STAT signaling. So far, the SOCS1-p53-senescence axis has been demonstrated in primary fibroblasts and mammary epithelial cells [133,139–141]. This mechanism may explain the better prognosis of some solid cancers with high p-STAT5 [142–144] and the high frequency of SOCS1 inactivation in STAT5-driven cancers [125–132]. However, it is difficult to obtain evidence of a senescence tumor-suppression response by studying established tumors that have already circumvented this pathway. Senescence is particularly noticeable in premalignant lesions and benign tumors [40,106,145–150], and can be reactivated by cancer chemotherapy [151,152]. For this reason, evidence of STAT5-induced senescence in human cancers is not yet available and should be studied in samples from premalignant tumors or after chemotherapy.

The mechanisms that disable SOCS1 and SOCS3 in human cancers are often epigenetic, mediated either by miRNAs, promoter methylation or protein phosphorylation [127,128,130,131,137,153–162]. The SRC family of kinases (SFK) phosphorylate SOCS1 at Y80, interfering with p53-SOCS1 interactions. SFK inhibitors can reverse this effect and could be used to restore the SOCS1-p53 axis in tumors where these two proteins remain intact [162]. It is also possible to consider treatments that re-express SOCS1/3 in tumors. Indeed, in liver cancer *SOCS3* gene expression can be re-established by drugs that activate the Farnesoid X receptor (FXR) [163,164]. Gene therapy strategies are also under development to re-express SOCS1 or SOCS3 in tumors [165–167].

4.6. P19ARF-p53 Pathway

One of the first reports demonstrating that STAT3 can act as a tumor suppressor was shown in glioblastoma multiforme (GBM) [168] where a combination of low Phosphatase and tensin homolog (PTEN) expression and loss of STAT3 in astrocytes increased their tumorigenicity. This observation is in contrast to papers cited above on the requirement for STAT3 to maintain tumor stem cells in GBM [73,75,169]. This could be explained if STAT3 acts early in tumorigenesis as a tumor suppressor but gains oncogenic functions in the context of the cancer genome and epigenome. An interesting mechanism for the tumor suppressor role of STAT3 was recently described in the prostate where STAT3 induces the expression of p19ARF [170]. The latter is a tumor suppressor that activates p53 and inhibits ribosome biogenesis inducing cellular senescence and apoptosis [171–174]. Loss of STAT3 disrupts this STAT3-ARF-p53 axis and permits tumor progression [175]. STAT3 and other STATs can also induce p21 leading to cell cycle arrest or cellular senescence [176,177]. Further evidence for STAT3 as a tumor suppressor has been reported in lung [178], colon [179,180], thyroid [181], liver [182,183], skin [184], neck [185], nasopharynx, rectum [186], salivary gland [187] and breast cancers [188] but the mechanisms remain to be investigated.

5. Concluding Remarks

Context-dependent activities of STAT3 and STAT5 in solid human cancers justify detailed molecular studies that will clarify the specific molecular mechanisms of action of these two cancer genes. The cancer genome and transcriptome are shaped and selected to favor cancer cell survival and proliferation. Although restoring mutated genes is technologically difficult, reprograming the transcriptome to restore tumor suppression may be feasible. Drugs acting on STAT3/5 and their regulators may restore the control of cell proliferation in cancer cells.

Acknowledgments: We thank V. Bourdeau for comments.

References

1. Bromberg, J.; Darnell, J.E., Jr. The role of STATs in transcriptional control and their impact on cellular function. *Oncogene* **2000**, *19*, 2468–2473. [CrossRef] [PubMed]
2. Kandoth, C.; McLellan, M.D.; Vandin, F.; Ye, K.; Niu, B.; Lu, C.; Xie, M.; Zhang, Q.; McMichael, J.F.; Wyczalkowski, M.A.; et al. Mutational landscape and significance across 12 major cancer types. *Nature* **2013**, *502*, 333–339. [CrossRef] [PubMed]
3. de Araujo, E.D.; Erdogan, F.; Neubauer, H.A.; Meneksedag-Erol, D.; Manaswiyoungkul, P.; Eram, M.S.; Seo, H.S.; Qadree, A.K.; Israelian, J.; Orlova, A.; et al. Structural and functional consequences of the STAT5B(N642H) driver mutation. *Nat. Commun.* **2019**, *10*, 2517. [CrossRef] [PubMed]

4. Koskela, H.L.; Eldfors, S.; Ellonen, P.; van Adrichem, A.J.; Kuusanmaki, H.; Andersson, E.I.; Lagstrom, S.; Clemente, M.J.; Olson, T.; Jalkanen, S.E.; et al. Somatic STAT3 mutations in large granular lymphocytic leukemia. *N. Engl. J. Med.* **2012**, *366*, 1905–1913. [CrossRef] [PubMed]
5. Carpenter, R.L.; Lo, H.W. STAT3 Target Genes Relevant to Human Cancers. *Cancers (Basel)* **2014**, *6*, 897–925. [CrossRef]
6. Basham, B.; Sathe, M.; Grein, J.; McClanahan, T.; D'Andrea, A.; Lees, E.; Rascle, A. In vivo identification of novel STAT5 target genes. *Nucleic Acids Res.* **2008**, *36*, 3802–3818. [CrossRef]
7. Wu, P.; Wu, D.; Zhao, L.; Huang, L.; Shen, G.; Huang, J.; Chai, Y. Prognostic role of STAT3 in solid tumors: A systematic review and meta-analysis. *Oncotarget* **2016**, *7*, 19863–19883. [CrossRef]
8. Mohanty, S.K.; Yagiz, K.; Pradhan, D.; Luthringer, D.J.; Amin, M.B.; Alkan, S.; Cinar, B. STAT3 and STAT5A are potential therapeutic targets in castration-resistant prostate cancer. *Oncotarget* **2017**, *8*, 85997–86010. [CrossRef]
9. Mirtti, T.; Leiby, B.E.; Abdulghani, J.; Aaltonen, E.; Pavela, M.; Mamtani, A.; Alanen, K.; Egevad, L.; Granfors, T.; Josefsson, A.; et al. Nuclear Stat5a/b predicts early recurrence and prostate cancer-specific death in patients treated by radical prostatectomy. *Hum. Pathol.* **2013**, *44*, 310–319. [CrossRef]
10. Klupp, F.; Diers, J.; Kahlert, C.; Neumann, L.; Halama, N.; Franz, C.; Schmidt, T.; Lasitschka, F.; Warth, A.; Weitz, J.; et al. Expressional STAT3/STAT5 Ratio is an Independent Prognostic Marker in Colon Carcinoma. *Ann. Surg. Oncol.* **2015**, *22*, S1548–S1555. [CrossRef]
11. Peck, A.R.; Witkiewicz, A.K.; Liu, C.; Stringer, G.A.; Klimowicz, A.C.; Pequignot, E.; Freydin, B.; Tran, T.H.; Yang, N.; Rosenberg, A.L.; et al. Loss of nuclear localized and tyrosine phosphorylated Stat5 in breast cancer predicts poor clinical outcome and increased risk of antiestrogen therapy failure. *J. Clin. Oncol.* **2011**, *29*, 2448–2458. [CrossRef] [PubMed]
12. Kaltenecker, D.; Themanns, M.; Mueller, K.M.; Spirk, K.; Suske, T.; Merkel, O.; Kenner, L.; Luis, A.; Kozlov, A.; Haybaeck, J.; et al. Hepatic growth hormone-JAK2-STAT5 signalling: Metabolic function, non-alcoholic fatty liver disease and hepatocellular carcinoma progression. *Cytokine* **2018**. [CrossRef] [PubMed]
13. Ferbeyre, G.; Moriggl, R. The role of Stat5 transcription factors as tumor suppressors or oncogenes. *Biochim. Biophys. Acta* **2011**, *1815*, 104–114. [CrossRef] [PubMed]
14. Xu, Y.H.; Lu, S. A meta-analysis of STAT3 and phospho-STAT3 expression and survival of patients with non-small-cell lung cancer. *Eur. J. Surg. Oncol.* **2014**, *40*, 311–317. [CrossRef] [PubMed]
15. Sun, Z.G.; Zhang, M.; Yang, F.; Gao, W.; Wang, Z.; Zhu, L.M. Clinical and prognostic significance of signal transducer and activator of transcription 3 and mucin 1 in patients with non-small cell lung cancer following surgery. *Oncol. Lett.* **2018**, *15*, 4278–4288. [CrossRef] [PubMed]
16. Tong, M.; Wang, J.; Jiang, N.; Pan, H.; Li, D. Correlation between p-STAT3 overexpression and prognosis in lung cancer: A systematic review and meta-analysis. *PLoS ONE* **2017**, *12*, e0182282. [CrossRef] [PubMed]
17. Koperek, O.; Aumayr, K.; Schindl, M.; Werba, G.; Soleiman, A.; Schoppmann, S.; Sahora, K.; Birner, P. Phosphorylation of STAT3 correlates with HER2 status, but not with survival in pancreatic ductal adenocarcinoma. *APMIS* **2014**, *122*, 476–481. [CrossRef] [PubMed]
18. Liang, C.; Xu, Y.; Ge, H.; Li, G.; Wu, J. Clinicopathological significance and prognostic role of p-STAT3 in patients with hepatocellular carcinoma. *Onco-Targets Ther.* **2018**, *11*, 1203–1214. [CrossRef]
19. Liu, Y.; Huang, J.; Li, W.; Chen, Y.; Liu, X.; Wang, J. Meta-analysis of STAT3 and phospho-STAT3 expression and survival of patients with breast cancer. *Oncotarget* **2018**, *9*, 13060–13067. [CrossRef] [PubMed]
20. Sonnenblick, A.; Salgado, R.; Brohee, S.; Zahavi, T.; Peretz, T.; Van den Eynden, G.; Rouas, G.; Salmon, A.; Francis, P.A.; Di Leo, A.; et al. p-STAT3 in luminal breast cancer: Integrated RNA-protein pooled analysis and results from the BIG 2-98 phase III trial. *Int. J. Oncol.* **2018**, *52*, 424–432. [CrossRef]
21. Lin, G.S.; Chen, Y.P.; Lin, Z.X.; Wang, X.F.; Zheng, Z.Q.; Chen, L. STAT3 serine 727 phosphorylation influences clinical outcome in glioblastoma. *Int. J. Clin. Exp. Pathol.* **2014**, *7*, 3141–3149.
22. Vilardell, J.; Alcaraz, E.; Sarro, E.; Trilla, E.; Cuadros, T.; de Torres, I.; Plana, M.; Ramon, Y.C.S.; Pinna, L.A.; Ruzzene, M.; et al. Under-expression of CK2beta subunit in ccRCC represents a complementary biomarker of p-STAT3 Ser727 that correlates with patient survival. *Oncotarget* **2018**, *9*, 5736–5751. [CrossRef] [PubMed]
23. Kusaba, T.; Nakayama, T.; Yamazumi, K.; Yakata, Y.; Yoshizaki, A.; Inoue, K.; Nagayasu, T.; Sekine, I. Activation of STAT3 is a marker of poor prognosis in human colorectal cancer. *Oncol. Rep.* **2006**, *15*, 1445–1451. [CrossRef]

24. Morikawa, T.; Baba, Y.; Yamauchi, M.; Kuchiba, A.; Nosho, K.; Shima, K.; Tanaka, N.; Huttenhower, C.; Frank, D.A.; Fuchs, C.S.; et al. STAT3 expression, molecular features, inflammation patterns, and prognosis in a database of 724 colorectal cancers. *Clin. Cancer Res.* **2011**, *17*, 1452–1462. [CrossRef]
25. Lee, J.L.; Wang, M.J.; Chen, J.Y. Acetylation and activation of STAT3 mediated by nuclear translocation of CD44. *J. Cell Biol.* **2009**, *185*, 949–957. [CrossRef] [PubMed]
26. Banerjee, K.; Resat, H. Constitutive activation of STAT3 in breast cancer cells: A review. *Int. J. Cancer* **2016**, *138*, 2570–2578. [CrossRef] [PubMed]
27. Lu, L.; Zhu, F.; Zhang, M.; Li, Y.; Drennan, A.C.; Kimpara, S.; Rumball, I.; Selzer, C.; Cameron, H.; Kellicut, A.; et al. Gene regulation and suppression of type I interferon signaling by STAT3 in diffuse large B cell lymphoma. *Proc. Natl. Acad. Sci. USA* **2018**, *115*, E498–E505. [CrossRef] [PubMed]
28. Creamer, B.A.; Sakamoto, K.; Schmidt, J.W.; Triplett, A.A.; Moriggl, R.; Wagner, K.U. Stat5 promotes survival of mammary epithelial cells through transcriptional activation of a distinct promoter in Akt1. *Mol. Cell. Biol.* **2010**, *30*, 2957–2970. [CrossRef]
29. Tell, R.W.; Horvath, C.M. Bioinformatic analysis reveals a pattern of STAT3-associated gene expression specific to basal-like breast cancers in human tumors. *Proc. Natl. Acad. Sci. USA* **2014**, *111*, 12787–12792. [CrossRef]
30. Karki, R.; Kanneganti, T.D. Diverging inflammasome signals in tumorigenesis and potential targeting. *Nat. Rev. Cancer* **2019**, *19*, 197–214. [CrossRef]
31. Martincuks, A.; Andryka, K.; Kuster, A.; Schmitz-Van de Leur, H.; Komorowski, M.; Muller-Newen, G. Nuclear translocation of STAT3 and NF-kappaB are independent of each other but NF-kappaB supports expression and activation of STAT3. *Cell. Signal.* **2017**, *32*, 36–47. [CrossRef] [PubMed]
32. Goldstein, I.; Paakinaho, V.; Baek, S.; Sung, M.H.; Hager, G.L. Synergistic gene expression during the acute phase response is characterized by transcription factor assisted loading. *Nat. Commun.* **2017**, *8*, 1849. [CrossRef] [PubMed]
33. Grivennikov, S.I.; Karin, M. Dangerous liaisons: STAT3 and NF-kappaB collaboration and crosstalk in cancer. *Cytokine Growth Factor Rev.* **2010**, *21*, 11–19. [CrossRef] [PubMed]
34. Yoon, S.; Woo, S.U.; Kang, J.H.; Kim, K.; Shin, H.J.; Gwak, H.S.; Park, S.; Chwae, Y.J. NF-kappaB and STAT3 cooperatively induce IL6 in starved cancer cells. *Oncogene* **2012**, *31*, 3467–3481. [CrossRef] [PubMed]
35. Atsumi, T.; Singh, R.; Sabharwal, L.; Bando, H.; Meng, J.; Arima, Y.; Yamada, M.; Harada, M.; Jiang, J.J.; Kamimura, D.; et al. Inflammation amplifier, a new paradigm in cancer biology. *Cancer Res.* **2014**, *74*, 8–14. [CrossRef] [PubMed]
36. Canino, C.; Luo, Y.; Marcato, P.; Blandino, G.; Pass, H.I.; Cioce, M. A STAT3-NFkB/DDIT3/CEBPbeta axis modulates ALDH1A3 expression in chemoresistant cell subpopulations. *Oncotarget* **2015**, *6*, 12637–12653. [CrossRef] [PubMed]
37. Thi, H.T.H.; Hong, S. Inflammasome as a Therapeutic Target for Cancer Prevention and Treatment. *J. Cancer Prev.* **2017**, *22*, 62–73. [CrossRef] [PubMed]
38. Pollak, M.N. Investigating metformin for cancer prevention and treatment: The end of the beginning. *Cancer Discov.* **2012**, *2*, 778–790. [CrossRef]
39. Hirsch, H.A.; Iliopoulos, D.; Struhl, K. Metformin inhibits the inflammatory response associated with cellular transformation and cancer stem cell growth. *Proc. Natl. Acad. Sci. USA* **2013**, *110*, 972–977. [CrossRef]
40. Deschenes-Simard, X.; Parisotto, M.; Rowell, M.C.; Le Calve, B.; Igelmann, S.; Moineau-Vallee, K.; Saint-Germain, E.; Kalegari, P.; Bourdeau, V.; Kottakis, F.; et al. Circumventing senescence is associated with stem cell properties and metformin sensitivity. *Aging Cell* **2019**. [CrossRef]
41. Luo, G.; Yu-Lee, L. Stat5b inhibits NFkappaB-mediated signaling. *Mol. Endocrinol.* **2000**, *14*, 114–123. [CrossRef] [PubMed]
42. Kawashima, T.; Murata, K.; Akira, S.; Tonozuka, Y.; Minoshima, Y.; Feng, S.; Kumagai, H.; Tsuruga, H.; Ikeda, Y.; Asano, S.; et al. STAT5 induces macrophage differentiation of M1 leukemia cells through activation of IL-6 production mediated by NF-kappaB p65. *J. Immunol.* **2001**, *167*, 3652–3660. [CrossRef] [PubMed]
43. Chueh, F.Y.; Leong, K.F.; Yu, C.L. Mitochondrial translocation of signal transducer and activator of transcription 5 (STAT5) in leukemic T cells and cytokine-stimulated cells. *Biochem. Biophys. Res. Commun.* **2010**, *402*, 778–783. [CrossRef] [PubMed]
44. Gough, D.J.; Corlett, A.; Schlessinger, K.; Wegrzyn, J.; Larner, A.C.; Levy, D.E. Mitochondrial STAT3 supports Ras-dependent oncogenic transformation. *Science* **2009**, *324*, 1713–1716. [CrossRef] [PubMed]

45. Wegrzyn, J.; Potla, R.; Chwae, Y.J.; Sepuri, N.B.; Zhang, Q.; Koeck, T.; Derecka, M.; Szczepanek, K.; Szelag, M.; Gornicka, A.; et al. Function of mitochondrial Stat3 in cellular respiration. *Science* **2009**, *323*, 793–797. [CrossRef] [PubMed]
46. Zhang, Q.; Raje, V.; Yakovlev, V.A.; Yacoub, A.; Szczepanek, K.; Meier, J.; Derecka, M.; Chen, Q.; Hu, Y.; Sisler, J.; et al. Mitochondrial localized Stat3 promotes breast cancer growth via phosphorylation of serine 727. *J. Biol. Chem.* **2013**, *288*, 31280–31288. [CrossRef] [PubMed]
47. Macias, E.; Rao, D.; Carbajal, S.; Kiguchi, K.; DiGiovanni, J. Stat3 binds to mtDNA and regulates mitochondrial gene expression in keratinocytes. *J. Investig. Dermatol.* **2014**, *134*, 1971–1980. [CrossRef]
48. Rincon, M.; Pereira, F.V. A New Perspective: Mitochondrial Stat3 as a Regulator for Lymphocyte Function. *Int. J. Mol. Sci.* **2018**, *19*, 1656. [CrossRef]
49. Avalle, L.; Poli, V. Nucleus, Mitochondrion, or Reticulum? STAT3 a La Carte. *Int. J. Mol. Sci.* **2018**, *19*, 2820. [CrossRef]
50. Luo, D.; Fraga-Lauhirat, M.; Millings, J.; Ho, C.; Villarreal, E.M.; Fletchinger, T.C.; Bonfiglio, J.V.; Mata, L.; Nemesure, M.D.; Bartels, L.E.; et al. Phospho-valproic acid (MDC-1112) suppresses glioblastoma growth in preclinical models through the inhibition of STAT3 phosphorylation. *Carcinogenesis* **2019**. [CrossRef]
51. Sala, D.; Cunningham, T.J.; Stec, M.J.; Etxaniz, U.; Nicoletti, C.; Dall'Agnese, A.; Puri, P.L.; Duester, G.; Latella, L.; Sacco, A. The Stat3-Fam3a axis promotes muscle stem cell myogenic lineage progression by inducing mitochondrial respiration. *Nat. Commun.* **2019**, *10*, 1796. [CrossRef]
52. Bernier, M.; Paul, R.K.; Martin-Montalvo, A.; Scheibye-Knudsen, M.; Song, S.; He, H.J.; Armour, S.M.; Hubbard, B.P.; Bohr, V.A.; Wang, L.; et al. Negative regulation of STAT3 protein-mediated cellular respiration by SIRT1 protein. *J. Biol. Chem.* **2011**, *286*, 19270–19279. [CrossRef]
53. Xu, Y.S.; Liang, J.J.; Wang, Y.; Zhao, X.J.; Xu, L.; Xu, Y.Y.; Zou, Q.C.; Zhang, J.M.; Tu, C.E.; Cui, Y.G.; et al. STAT3 Undergoes Acetylation-dependent Mitochondrial Translocation to Regulate Pyruvate Metabolism. *Sci. Rep.* **2016**, *6*, 39517. [CrossRef]
54. Boengler, K.; Hilfiker-Kleiner, D.; Heusch, G.; Schulz, R. Inhibition of permeability transition pore opening by mitochondrial STAT3 and its role in myocardial ischemia/reperfusion. *Basic Res. Cardiol.* **2010**, *105*, 771–785. [CrossRef] [PubMed]
55. Tammineni, P.; Anugula, C.; Mohammed, F.; Anjaneyulu, M.; Larner, A.C.; Sepuri, N.B. The import of the transcription factor STAT3 into mitochondria depends on GRIM-19, a component of the electron transport chain. *J. Biol. Chem.* **2013**, *288*, 4723–4732. [CrossRef]
56. Qiu, H.; Lizano, P.; Laure, L.; Sui, X.; Rashed, E.; Park, J.Y.; Hong, C.; Gao, S.; Holle, E.; Morin, D.; et al. H11 kinase/heat shock protein 22 deletion impairs both nuclear and mitochondrial functions of STAT3 and accelerates the transition into heart failure on cardiac overload. *Circulation* **2011**, *124*, 406–415. [CrossRef] [PubMed]
57. Gadir, N.; Haim-Vilmovsky, L.; Kraut-Cohen, J.; Gerst, J.E. Localization of mRNAs coding for mitochondrial proteins in the yeast Saccharomyces cerevisiae. *RNA* **2011**, *17*, 1551–1565. [CrossRef]
58. Fox, T.D. Mitochondrial protein synthesis, import, and assembly. *Genetics* **2012**, *192*, 1203–1234. [CrossRef]
59. Zhang, Y.; Chen, Y.; Gucek, M.; Xu, H. The mitochondrial outer membrane protein MDI promotes local protein synthesis and mtDNA replication. *EMBO J.* **2016**, *35*, 1045–1057. [CrossRef]
60. Hansen, K.G.; Herrmann, J.M. Transport of Proteins into Mitochondria. *Protein J.* **2019**. [CrossRef]
61. Richard, A.J.; Hang, H.; Stephens, J.M. Pyruvate dehydrogenase complex (PDC) subunits moonlight as interaction partners of phosphorylated STAT5 in adipocytes and adipose tissue. *J. Biol. Chem.* **2017**, *292*, 19733–19742. [CrossRef] [PubMed]
62. Kidder, B.L.; Yang, J.; Palmer, S. Stat3 and c-Myc genome-wide promoter occupancy in embryonic stem cells. *PLoS ONE* **2008**, *3*, e3932. [CrossRef] [PubMed]
63. Hall, J.; Guo, G.; Wray, J.; Eyres, I.; Nichols, J.; Grotewold, L.; Morfopoulou, S.; Humphreys, P.; Mansfield, W.; Walker, R.; et al. Oct4 and LIF/Stat3 additively induce Kruppel factors to sustain embryonic stem cell self-renewal. *Cell Stem Cell* **2009**, *5*, 597–609. [CrossRef] [PubMed]
64. Ye, S.; Li, P.; Tong, C.; Ying, Q.L. Embryonic stem cell self-renewal pathways converge on the transcription factor Tfcp2l1. *EMBO J.* **2013**, *32*, 2548–2560. [CrossRef] [PubMed]
65. Jin, J.; Liu, J.; Chen, C.; Liu, Z.; Jiang, C.; Chu, H.; Pan, W.; Wang, X.; Zhang, L.; Li, B.; et al. The deubiquitinase USP21 maintains the stemness of mouse embryonic stem cells via stabilization of Nanog. *Nat. Commun.* **2016**, *7*, 13594. [CrossRef] [PubMed]

66. Yang, J.; van Oosten, A.L.; Theunissen, T.W.; Guo, G.; Silva, J.C.; Smith, A. Stat3 activation is limiting for reprogramming to ground state pluripotency. *Cell Stem Cell* **2010**, *7*, 319–328. [CrossRef]
67. Tang, Y.; Luo, Y.; Jiang, Z.; Ma, Y.; Lin, C.J.; Kim, C.; Carter, M.G.; Amano, T.; Park, J.; Kish, S.; et al. Jak/Stat3 signaling promotes somatic cell reprogramming by epigenetic regulation. *Stem Cells* **2012**, *30*, 2645–2656. [CrossRef]
68. Carbognin, E.; Betto, R.M.; Soriano, M.E.; Smith, A.G.; Martello, G. Stat3 promotes mitochondrial transcription and oxidative respiration during maintenance and induction of naive pluripotency. *EMBO J.* **2016**, *35*, 618–634. [CrossRef]
69. Ben-Porath, I.; Thomson, M.W.; Carey, V.J.; Ge, R.; Bell, G.W.; Regev, A.; Weinberg, R.A. An embryonic stem cell-like gene expression signature in poorly differentiated aggressive human tumors. *Nat. Genet.* **2008**, *40*, 499–507. [CrossRef]
70. Zhou, J.; Wulfkuhle, J.; Zhang, H.; Gu, P.; Yang, Y.; Deng, J.; Margolick, J.B.; Liotta, L.A.; Petricoin, E., 3rd; Zhang, Y. Activation of the PTEN/mTOR/STAT3 pathway in breast cancer stem-like cells is required for viability and maintenance. *Proc. Natl. Acad. Sci. USA* **2007**, *104*, 16158–16163. [CrossRef]
71. Marotta, L.L.; Almendro, V.; Marusyk, A.; Shipitsin, M.; Schemme, J.; Walker, S.R.; Bloushtain-Qimron, N.; Kim, J.J.; Choudhury, S.A.; Maruyama, R.; et al. The JAK2/STAT3 signaling pathway is required for growth of CD44(+)CD24(-) stem cell-like breast cancer cells in human tumors. *J. Clin. Investig.* **2011**, *121*, 2723–2735. [CrossRef] [PubMed]
72. Iliopoulos, D.; Hirsch, H.A.; Struhl, K. An epigenetic switch involving NF-kappaB, Lin28, Let-7 MicroRNA, and IL6 links inflammation to cell transformation. *Cell* **2009**, *139*, 693–706. [CrossRef] [PubMed]
73. Gong, A.H.; Wei, P.; Zhang, S.; Yao, J.; Yuan, Y.; Zhou, A.D.; Lang, F.F.; Heimberger, A.B.; Rao, G.; Huang, S. FoxM1 Drives a Feed-Forward STAT3-Activation Signaling Loop That Promotes the Self-Renewal and Tumorigenicity of Glioblastoma Stem-like Cells. *Cancer Res.* **2015**, *75*, 2337–2348. [CrossRef] [PubMed]
74. Peng, L.; Jiang, D. Resveratrol eliminates cancer stem cells of osteosarcoma by STAT3 pathway inhibition. *PLoS ONE* **2018**, *13*, e0205918. [CrossRef] [PubMed]
75. Man, J.; Yu, X.; Huang, H.; Zhou, W.; Xiang, C.; Huang, H.; Miele, L.; Liu, Z.; Bebek, G.; Bao, S.; et al. Hypoxic Induction of Vasorin Regulates Notch1 Turnover to Maintain Glioma Stem-like Cells. *Cell Stem Cell* **2018**, *22*, 104–118.e6. [CrossRef] [PubMed]
76. Jiao, J.; Zhang, R.; Li, Z.; Yin, Y.; Fang, X.; Ding, X.; Cai, Y.; Yang, S.; Mu, H.; Zong, D.; et al. Nuclear Smad6 promotes gliomagenesis by negatively regulating PIAS3-mediated STAT3 inhibition. *Nat. Commun.* **2018**, *9*, 2504. [CrossRef] [PubMed]
77. He, W.; Wu, J.; Shi, J.; Huo, Y.M.; Dai, W.; Geng, J.; Lu, P.; Yang, M.W.; Fang, Y.; Wang, W.; et al. IL22RA1/STAT3 Signaling Promotes Stemness and Tumorigenicity in Pancreatic Cancer. *Cancer Res.* **2018**, *78*, 3293–3305. [CrossRef]
78. Wang, T.; Fahrmann, J.F.; Lee, H.; Li, Y.J.; Tripathi, S.C.; Yue, C.; Zhang, C.; Lifshitz, V.; Song, J.; Yuan, Y.; et al. JAK/STAT3-Regulated Fatty Acid beta-Oxidation Is Critical for Breast Cancer Stem Cell Self-Renewal and Chemoresistance. *Cell Metab.* **2018**, *27*, 136–150. [CrossRef]
79. Kitajima, S.; Yoshida, A.; Kohno, S.; Li, F.; Suzuki, S.; Nagatani, N.; Nishimoto, Y.; Sasaki, N.; Muranaka, H.; Wan, Y.; et al. The RB-IL-6 axis controls self-renewal and endocrine therapy resistance by fine-tuning mitochondrial activity. *Oncogene* **2017**, *36*, 5145–5157. [CrossRef]
80. Chen, M.W.; Yang, S.T.; Chien, M.H.; Hua, K.T.; Wu, C.J.; Hsiao, S.M.; Lin, H.; Hsiao, M.; Su, J.L.; Wei, L.H. The STAT3-miRNA-92-Wnt Signaling Pathway Regulates Spheroid Formation and Malignant Progression in Ovarian Cancer. *Cancer Res.* **2017**, *77*, 1955–1967. [CrossRef]
81. Schroeder, A.; Herrmann, A.; Cherryholmes, G.; Kowolik, C.; Buettner, R.; Pal, S.; Yu, H.; Muller-Newen, G.; Jove, R. Loss of androgen receptor expression promotes a stem-like cell phenotype in prostate cancer through STAT3 signaling. *Cancer Res.* **2014**, *74*, 1227–1237. [CrossRef] [PubMed]
82. Tang, Y.; Kitisin, K.; Jogunoori, W.; Li, C.; Deng, C.X.; Mueller, S.C.; Ressom, H.W.; Rashid, A.; He, A.R.; Mendelson, J.S.; et al. Progenitor/stem cells give rise to liver cancer due to aberrant TGF-beta and IL-6 signaling. *Proc. Natl. Acad. Sci. USA* **2008**, *105*, 2445–2450. [CrossRef] [PubMed]
83. Thiagarajan, P.S.; Zheng, Q.; Bhagrath, M.; Mulkearns-Hubert, E.E.; Myers, M.G.; Lathia, J.D.; Reizes, O. STAT3 activation by leptin receptor is essential for TNBC stem cell maintenance. *Endocr. Relat. Cancer* **2017**, *24*, 415–426. [CrossRef] [PubMed]

84. Su, Y.J.; Lai, H.M.; Chang, Y.W.; Chen, G.Y.; Lee, J.L. Direct reprogramming of stem cell properties in colon cancer cells by CD44. *EMBO J.* **2011**, *30*, 3186–3199. [CrossRef] [PubMed]
85. Schepers, H.; van Gosliga, D.; Wierenga, A.T.; Eggen, B.J.; Schuringa, J.J.; Vellenga, E. STAT5 is required for long-term maintenance of normal and leukemic human stem/progenitor cells. *Blood* **2007**, *110*, 2880–2888. [CrossRef] [PubMed]
86. Talati, P.G.; Gu, L.; Ellsworth, E.M.; Girondo, M.A.; Trerotola, M.; Hoang, D.T.; Leiby, B.; Dagvadorj, A.; McCue, P.A.; Lallas, C.D.; et al. Jak2-Stat5a/b Signaling Induces Epithelial-to-Mesenchymal Transition and Stem-Like Cell Properties in Prostate Cancer. *Am. J. Pathol.* **2015**, *185*, 2505–2522. [CrossRef] [PubMed]
87. Boutillon, F.; Pigat, N.; Sala, L.S.; Reyes-Gomez, E.; Moriggl, R.; Guidotti, J.E.; Goffin, V. STAT5a/b Deficiency Delays, but does not Prevent, Prolactin-Driven Prostate Tumorigenesis in Mice. *Cancers (Basel)* **2019**, *11*, 929. [CrossRef] [PubMed]
88. Liu, X.; Robinson, G.W.; Wagner, K.U.; Garrett, L.; Wynshaw-Boris, A.; Hennighausen, L. Stat5a is mandatory for adult mammary gland development and lactogenesis. *Genes Dev.* **1997**, *11*, 179–186. [CrossRef] [PubMed]
89. Oakes, S.R.; Naylor, M.J.; Asselin-Labat, M.L.; Blazek, K.D.; Gardiner-Garden, M.; Hilton, H.N.; Kazlauskas, M.; Pritchard, M.A.; Chodosh, L.A.; Pfeffer, P.L.; et al. The ETS transcription factor Elf5 specifies mammary alveolar cell fate. *Genes Dev.* **2008**, *22*, 581–586. [CrossRef] [PubMed]
90. Metser, G.; Shin, H.Y.; Wang, C.; Yoo, K.H.; Oh, S.; Villarino, A.V.; O'Shea, J.J.; Kang, K.; Hennighausen, L. An autoregulatory enhancer controls mammary-specific STAT5 functions. *Nucleic Acids Res.* **2016**, *44*, 1052–1063. [CrossRef] [PubMed]
91. Stute, P.; Sielker, S.; Wood, C.E.; Register, T.C.; Lees, C.J.; Dewi, F.N.; Williams, J.K.; Wagner, J.D.; Stefenelli, U.; Cline, J.M. Life stage differences in mammary gland gene expression profile in non-human primates. *Breast Cancer Res. Treat.* **2012**, *133*, 617–634. [CrossRef] [PubMed]
92. Kim, M.; Morales, L.D.; Jang, I.S.; Cho, Y.Y.; Kim, D.J. Protein Tyrosine Phosphatases as Potential Regulators of STAT3 Signaling. *Int. J. Mol. Sci.* **2018**, *19*, 2708. [CrossRef] [PubMed]
93. Huang, Y.; Wang, J.; Cao, F.; Jiang, H.; Li, A.; Li, J.; Qiu, L.; Shen, H.; Chang, W.; Zhou, C.; et al. SHP2 associates with nuclear localization of STAT3: Significance in progression and prognosis of colorectal cancer. *Sci. Rep.* **2017**, *7*, 17597. [CrossRef] [PubMed]
94. Kumar, V.; Cheng, P.; Condamine, T.; Mony, S.; Languino, L.R.; McCaffrey, J.C.; Hockstein, N.; Guarino, M.; Masters, G.; Penman, E.; et al. CD45 Phosphatase Inhibits STAT3 Transcription Factor Activity in Myeloid Cells and Promotes Tumor-Associated Macrophage Differentiation. *Immunity* **2016**, *44*, 303–315. [CrossRef] [PubMed]
95. Fan, L.C.; Shiau, C.W.; Tai, W.T.; Hung, M.H.; Chu, P.Y.; Hsieh, F.S.; Lin, H.; Yu, H.C.; Chen, K.F. SHP-1 is a negative regulator of epithelial-mesenchymal transition in hepatocellular carcinoma. *Oncogene* **2015**, *34*, 5252–5263. [CrossRef] [PubMed]
96. Chen, Y.; Wen, R.; Yang, S.; Schuman, J.; Zhang, E.E.; Yi, T.; Feng, G.S.; Wang, D. Identification of Shp-2 as a Stat5A phosphatase. *J. Biol. Chem.* **2003**, *278*, 16520–16527. [CrossRef]
97. Xiao, W.; Ando, T.; Wang, H.Y.; Kawakami, Y.; Kawakami, T. Lyn- and PLC-beta3-dependent regulation of SHP-1 phosphorylation controls Stat5 activity and myelomonocytic leukemia-like disease. *Blood* **2010**, *116*, 6003–6013. [CrossRef]
98. Brantley, E.C.; Nabors, L.B.; Gillespie, G.Y.; Choi, Y.H.; Palmer, C.A.; Harrison, K.; Roarty, K.; Benveniste, E.N. Loss of protein inhibitors of activated STAT-3 expression in glioblastoma multiforme tumors: Implications for STAT-3 activation and gene expression. *Clin. Cancer Res.* **2008**, *14*, 4694–4704. [CrossRef] [PubMed]
99. Sundvall, M.; Korhonen, A.; Vaparanta, K.; Anckar, J.; Halkilahti, K.; Salah, Z.; Aqeilan, R.I.; Palvimo, J.J.; Sistonen, L.; Elenius, K. Protein inhibitor of activated STAT3 (PIAS3) protein promotes SUMOylation and nuclear sequestration of the intracellular domain of ErbB4 protein. *J. Biol. Chem.* **2012**, *287*, 23216–23226. [CrossRef]
100. Jang, H.D.; Yoon, K.; Shin, Y.J.; Kim, J.; Lee, S.Y. PIAS3 suppresses NF-kappaB-mediated transcription by interacting with the p65/RelA subunit. *J. Biol. Chem.* **2004**, *279*, 24873–24880. [CrossRef]
101. Liu, Y.; Bridges, R.; Wortham, A.; Kulesz-Martin, M. NF-kappaB repression by PIAS3 mediated RelA SUMOylation. *PLoS ONE* **2012**, *7*, e37636. [CrossRef]
102. Zhao, Z.; Wu, L.; Shi, H.; Wu, C. p53 Nterminal binding and stabilisation by PIAS3 inhibits MDM2induced p53 ubiquitination and regulates cell growth. *Mol. Med. Rep.* **2014**, *9*, 1903–1908. [CrossRef] [PubMed]

103. Perry, E.; Tsruya, R.; Levitsky, P.; Pomp, O.; Taller, M.; Weisberg, S.; Parris, W.; Kulkarni, S.; Malovani, H.; Pawson, T.; et al. TMF/ARA160 is a BC-box-containing protein that mediates the degradation of Stat3. *Oncogene* **2004**, *23*, 8908–8919. [CrossRef] [PubMed]
104. Abrham, G.; Volpe, M.; Shpungin, S.; Nir, U. TMF/ARA160 downregulates proangiogenic genes and attenuates the progression of PC3 xenografts. *Int. J. Cancer* **2009**, *125*, 43–53. [CrossRef] [PubMed]
105. Wei, J.; Yuan, Y.; Jin, C.; Chen, H.; Leng, L.; He, F.; Wang, J. The ubiquitin ligase TRAF6 negatively regulates the JAK-STAT signaling pathway by binding to STAT3 and mediating its ubiquitination. *PLoS ONE* **2012**, *7*, e49567. [CrossRef] [PubMed]
106. Deschenes-Simard, X.; Gaumont-Leclerc, M.F.; Bourdeau, V.; Lessard, F.; Moiseeva, O.; Forest, V.; Igelmann, S.; Mallette, F.A.; Saba-El-Leil, M.K.; Meloche, S.; et al. Tumor suppressor activity of the ERK/MAPK pathway by promoting selective protein degradation. *Genes Dev.* **2013**, *27*, 900–915. [CrossRef] [PubMed]
107. Zhao, J.; Du, P.; Cui, P.; Qin, Y.; Hu, C.; Wu, J.; Zhou, Z.; Zhang, W.; Qin, L.; Huang, G. LncRNA PVT1 promotes angiogenesis via activating the STAT3/VEGFA axis in gastric cancer. *Oncogene* **2018**. [CrossRef] [PubMed]
108. You, L.; Chang, D.; Du, H.Z.; Zhao, Y.P. Genome-wide screen identifies PVT1 as a regulator of Gemcitabine sensitivity in human pancreatic cancer cells. *Biochem. Biophys. Res. Commun.* **2011**, *407*, 1–6. [CrossRef] [PubMed]
109. Xie, Z.; Chen, X.; Li, J.; Guo, Y.; Li, H.; Pan, X.; Jiang, J.; Liu, H.; Wu, B. Salivary HOTAIR and PVT1 as novel biomarkers for early pancreatic cancer. *Oncotarget* **2016**, *7*, 25408–25419. [CrossRef]
110. Pan, X.; Li, B.; Fan, N.; Li, J.; Cai, F.; Zhao, G.; Zheng, G.; Gao, C. Long Noncoding RNA PVT1 as a Potent Predictor of Prognosis in Cancers: A Meta-Analysis. *Clin. Lab.* **2017**, *63*, 1657–1666. [CrossRef]
111. Hatziapostolou, M.; Polytarchou, C.; Aggelidou, E.; Drakaki, A.; Poultsides, G.A.; Jaeger, S.A.; Ogata, H.; Karin, M.; Struhl, K.; Hadzopoulou-Cladaras, M.; et al. An HNF4alpha-miRNA inflammatory feedback circuit regulates hepatocellular oncogenesis. *Cell* **2011**, *147*, 1233–1247. [CrossRef] [PubMed]
112. Cai, B.; Li, J.; Wang, J.; Luo, X.; Ai, J.; Liu, Y.; Wang, N.; Liang, H.; Zhang, M.; Chen, N.; et al. microRNA-124 regulates cardiomyocyte differentiation of bone marrow-derived mesenchymal stem cells via targeting STAT3 signaling. *Stem Cells* **2012**, *30*, 1746–1755. [CrossRef] [PubMed]
113. Zhang, J.; Lu, Y.; Yue, X.; Li, H.; Luo, X.; Wang, Y.; Wang, K.; Wan, J. MiR-124 suppresses growth of human colorectal cancer by inhibiting STAT3. *PLoS ONE* **2013**, *8*, e70300. [CrossRef] [PubMed]
114. Wei, J.; Wang, F.; Kong, L.Y.; Xu, S.; Doucette, T.; Ferguson, S.D.; Yang, Y.; McEnery, K.; Jethwa, K.; Gjyshi, O.; et al. miR-124 inhibits STAT3 signaling to enhance T cell-mediated immune clearance of glioma. *Cancer Res.* **2013**, *73*, 3913–3926. [CrossRef] [PubMed]
115. Chen, G.; Shi, Y.; Zhang, Y.; Sun, J. CircRNA_100782 regulates pancreatic carcinoma proliferation through the IL6-STAT3 pathway. *Onco-Targets Ther.* **2017**, *10*, 5783–5794. [CrossRef]
116. Jiang, J.; Li, Z.; Yu, C.; Chen, M.; Tian, S.; Sun, C. MiR-1181 inhibits stem cell-like phenotypes and suppresses SOX2 and STAT3 in human pancreatic cancer. *Cancer Lett.* **2015**, *356*, 962–970. [CrossRef] [PubMed]
117. Jiang, M.; Zhang, W.W.; Liu, P.; Yu, W.; Liu, T.; Yu, J. Dysregulation of SOCS-Mediated Negative Feedback of Cytokine Signaling in Carcinogenesis and Its Significance in Cancer Treatment. *Front. Immunol.* **2017**, *8*, 70. [CrossRef]
118. Ghafouri-Fard, S.; Oskooei, V.K.; Azari, I.; Taheri, M. Suppressor of cytokine signaling (SOCS) genes are downregulated in breast cancer. *World J. Surg. Oncol.* **2018**, *16*, 226. [CrossRef]
119. He, B.; You, L.; Uematsu, K.; Zang, K.; Xu, Z.; Lee, A.Y.; Costello, J.F.; McCormick, F.; Jablons, D.M. SOCS-3 is frequently silenced by hypermethylation and suppresses cell growth in human lung cancer. *Proc. Natl. Acad. Sci. USA* **2003**, *100*, 14133–14138. [CrossRef]
120. Inagaki-Ohara, K.; Kondo, T.; Ito, M.; Yoshimura, A. SOCS, inflammation, and cancer. *JAKSTAT* **2013**, *2*, e24053. [CrossRef]
121. Suzuki, A.; Hanada, T.; Mitsuyama, K.; Yoshida, T.; Kamizono, S.; Hoshino, T.; Kubo, M.; Yamashita, A.; Okabe, M.; Takeda, K.; et al. CIS3/SOCS3/SSI3 plays a negative regulatory role in STAT3 activation and intestinal inflammation. *J. Exp. Med.* **2001**, *193*, 471–481. [CrossRef] [PubMed]
122. Niwa, Y.; Kanda, H.; Shikauchi, Y.; Saiura, A.; Matsubara, K.; Kitagawa, T.; Yamamoto, J.; Kubo, T.; Yoshikawa, H. Methylation silencing of SOCS-3 promotes cell growth and migration by enhancing JAK/STAT and FAK signalings in human hepatocellular carcinoma. *Oncogene* **2005**, *24*, 6406–6417. [CrossRef] [PubMed]

123. Rigby, R.J.; Simmons, J.G.; Greenhalgh, C.J.; Alexander, W.S.; Lund, P.K. Suppressor of cytokine signaling 3 (SOCS3) limits damage-induced crypt hyper-proliferation and inflammation-associated tumorigenesis in the colon. *Oncogene* **2007**, *26*, 4833–4841. [CrossRef] [PubMed]
124. Lesina, M.; Kurkowski, M.U.; Ludes, K.; Rose-John, S.; Treiber, M.; Kloppel, G.; Yoshimura, A.; Reindl, W.; Sipos, B.; Akira, S.; et al. Stat3/Socs3 activation by IL-6 transsignaling promotes progression of pancreatic intraepithelial neoplasia and development of pancreatic cancer. *Cancer Cell* **2011**, *19*, 456–469. [CrossRef] [PubMed]
125. Gui, Y.; Yeganeh, M.; Ramanathan, S.; Leblanc, C.; Pomerleau, V.; Ferbeyre, G.; Saucier, C.; Ilangumaran, S. SOCS1 controls liver regeneration by regulating HGF signaling in hepatocytes. *J. Hepatol.* **2011**, *55*, 1300–1308. [CrossRef] [PubMed]
126. Yeganeh, M.; Gui, Y.; Kandhi, R.; Bobbala, D.; Tobelaim, W.S.; Saucier, C.; Yoshimura, A.; Ferbeyre, G.; Ramanathan, S.; Ilangumaran, S. Suppressor of cytokine signaling 1-dependent regulation of the expression and oncogenic functions of p21(CIP1/WAF1) in the liver. *Oncogene* **2016**, *35*, 4200–4211. [CrossRef] [PubMed]
127. Yoshikawa, H.; Matsubara, K.; Qian, G.S.; Jackson, P.; Groopman, J.D.; Manning, J.E.; Harris, C.C.; Herman, J.G. SOCS-1, a negative regulator of the JAK/STAT pathway, is silenced by methylation in human hepatocellular carcinoma and shows growth-suppression activity. *Nat. Genet.* **2001**, *28*, 29–35. [CrossRef] [PubMed]
128. Zhao, R.C.; Zhou, J.; He, J.Y.; Wei, Y.G.; Qin, Y.; Li, B. Aberrant promoter methylation of SOCS-1 gene may contribute to the pathogenesis of hepatocellular carcinoma: A meta-analysis. *J. BUON* **2016**, *21*, 142–151. [PubMed]
129. Suzuki, M.; Shigematsu, H.; Shivapurkar, N.; Reddy, J.; Miyajima, K.; Takahashi, T.; Gazdar, A.F.; Frenkel, E.P. Methylation of apoptosis related genes in the pathogenesis and prognosis of prostate cancer. *Cancer Lett.* **2006**, *242*, 222–230. [CrossRef]
130. Kobayashi, N.; Uemura, H.; Nagahama, K.; Okudela, K.; Furuya, M.; Ino, Y.; Ito, Y.; Hirano, H.; Inayama, Y.; Aoki, I.; et al. Identification of miR-30d as a novel prognostic maker of prostate cancer. *Oncotarget* **2012**, *3*, 1455–1471. [CrossRef]
131. Chevrier, M.; Bobbala, D.; Villalobos-Hernandez, A.; Khan, M.G.; Ramanathan, S.; Saucier, C.; Ferbeyre, G.; Geha, S.; Ilangumaran, S. Expression of SOCS1 and the downstream targets of its putative tumor suppressor functions in prostate cancer. *BMC Cancer* **2017**, *17*, 157. [CrossRef] [PubMed]
132. Villalobos-Hernandez, A.; Bobbala, D.; Kandhi, R.; Khan, M.G.; Mayhue, M.; Dubois, C.M.; Ferbeyre, G.; Saucier, C.; Ramanathan, S.; Ilangumaran, S. SOCS1 inhibits migration and invasion of prostate cancer cells, attenuates tumor growth and modulates the tumor stroma. *Prostate Cancer Prostatic Dis.* **2017**, *20*, 36–47. [CrossRef] [PubMed]
133. Calabrese, V.; Mallette, F.A.; Deschenes-Simard, X.; Ramanathan, S.; Gagnon, J.; Moores, A.; Ilangumaran, S.; Ferbeyre, G. SOCS1 links cytokine signaling to p53 and senescence. *Mol. Cell* **2009**, *36*, 754–767. [CrossRef] [PubMed]
134. Mallette, F.A.; Calabrese, V.; Ilangumaran, S.; Ferbeyre, G. SOCS1, a novel interaction partner of p53 controlling oncogene-induced senescence. *Aging* **2010**, *2*, 445–452. [CrossRef] [PubMed]
135. Saint-Germain, E.; Mignacca, L.; Vernier, M.; Bobbala, D.; Ilangumaran, S.; Ferbeyre, G. SOCS1 regulates senescence and ferroptosis by modulating the expression of p53 target genes. *Aging* **2017**, *9*, 2137–2162. [CrossRef] [PubMed]
136. Kong, X.; Feng, D.; Wang, H.; Hong, F.; Bertola, A.; Wang, F.S.; Gao, B. Interleukin-22 induces hepatic stellate cell senescence and restricts liver fibrosis in mice. *Hepatology* **2012**, *56*, 1150–1159. [CrossRef] [PubMed]
137. Bouamar, H.; Jiang, D.; Wang, L.; Lin, A.P.; Ortega, M.; Aguiar, R.C. MicroRNA 155 control of p53 activity is context dependent and mediated by Aicda and Socs1. *Mol. Cell. Biol.* **2015**, *35*, 1329–1340. [CrossRef] [PubMed]
138. Cui, X.; Shan, X.; Qian, J.; Ji, Q.; Wang, L.; Wang, X.; Li, M.; Ding, H.; Liu, Q.; Chen, L.; et al. The suppressor of cytokine signaling SOCS1 promotes apoptosis of intestinal epithelial cells via p53 signaling in Crohn's disease. *Exper. Mol. Pathol.* **2016**, *101*, 1–11. [CrossRef]
139. Mallette, F.A.; Gaumont-Leclerc, M.F.; Ferbeyre, G. The DNA damage signaling pathway is a critical mediator of oncogene-induced senescence. *Genes Dev.* **2007**, *21*, 43–48. [CrossRef]
140. Mallette, F.A.; Gaumont-Leclerc, M.F.; Huot, G.; Ferbeyre, G. Myc Down-regulation as a Mechanism to Activate the Rb Pathway in STAT5A-induced Senescence. *J. Biol. Chem.* **2007**, *282*, 34938–34944. [CrossRef]

141. Mallette, F.A.; Moiseeva, O.; Calabrese, V.; Mao, B.; Gaumont-Leclerc, M.F.; Ferbeyre, G. Transcriptome analysis and tumor suppressor requirements of STAT5-induced senescence. *Ann. N. Y. Acad. Sci.* **2010**, *1197*, 142–151. [CrossRef] [PubMed]
142. Barash, I. Stat5 in the mammary gland: Controlling normal development and cancer. *J. Cell. Physiol.* **2006**, *209*, 305–313. [CrossRef] [PubMed]
143. Nevalainen, M.T.; Xie, J.; Torhorst, J.; Bubendorf, L.; Haas, P.; Kononen, J.; Sauter, G.; Rui, H. Signal transducer and activator of transcription-5 activation and breast cancer prognosis. *J. Clin. Oncol.* **2004**, *22*, 2053–2060. [CrossRef]
144. Peck, A.R.; Witkiewicz, A.K.; Liu, C.; Klimowicz, A.C.; Stringer, G.A.; Pequignot, E.; Freydin, B.; Yang, N.; Ertel, A.; Tran, T.H.; et al. Low levels of Stat5a protein in breast cancer are associated with tumor progression and unfavorable clinical outcomes. *Breast Cancer Res.* **2012**, *14*, R130. [CrossRef] [PubMed]
145. Castro, P.; Giri, D.; Lamb, D.; Ittmann, M. Cellular senescence in the pathogenesis of benign prostatic hyperplasia. *Prostate* **2003**, *55*, 30–38. [CrossRef] [PubMed]
146. Gray-Schopfer, V.C.; Cheong, S.C.; Chong, H.; Chow, J.; Moss, T.; Abdel-Malek, Z.A.; Marais, R.; Wynford-Thomas, D.; Bennett, D.C. Cellular senescence in naevi and immortalisation in melanoma: A role for p16? *Br. J. Cancer* **2006**, *95*, 496–505. [CrossRef] [PubMed]
147. Maldonado, J.L.; Timmerman, L.; Fridlyand, J.; Bastian, B.C. Mechanisms of cell-cycle arrest in Spitz nevi with constitutive activation of the MAP-kinase pathway. *Am. J. Pathol.* **2004**, *164*, 1783–1787. [CrossRef]
148. Michaloglou, C.; Vredeveld, L.C.; Mooi, W.J.; Peeper, D.S. BRAF(E600) in benign and malignant human tumours. *Oncogene* **2008**, *27*, 877–895. [CrossRef]
149. Michaloglou, C.; Vredeveld, L.C.; Soengas, M.S.; Denoyelle, C.; Kuilman, T.; van der Horst, C.M.; Majoor, D.M.; Shay, J.W.; Mooi, W.J.; Peeper, D.S. BRAFE600-associated senescence-like cell cycle arrest of human naevi. *Nature* **2005**, *436*, 720–724. [CrossRef] [PubMed]
150. Vernier, M.; Bourdeau, V.; Gaumont-Leclerc, M.F.; Moiseeva, O.; Begin, V.; Saad, F.; Mes-Masson, A.M.; Ferbeyre, G. Regulation of E2Fs and senescence by PML nuclear bodies. *Genes Dev.* **2011**, *25*, 41–50. [CrossRef]
151. Dorr, J.R.; Yu, Y.; Milanovic, M.; Beuster, G.; Zasada, C.; Dabritz, J.H.; Lisec, J.; Lenze, D.; Gerhardt, A.; Schleicher, K.; et al. Synthetic lethal metabolic targeting of cellular senescence in cancer therapy. *Nature* **2013**, *501*, 421–425. [CrossRef] [PubMed]
152. Jing, H.; Kase, J.; Dorr, J.R.; Milanovic, M.; Lenze, D.; Grau, M.; Beuster, G.; Ji, S.; Reimann, M.; Lenz, P.; et al. Opposing roles of NF-kappaB in anti-cancer treatment outcome unveiled by cross-species investigations. *Genes Dev.* **2011**, *25*, 2137–2146. [CrossRef] [PubMed]
153. Zardo, G.; Tiirikainen, M.I.; Hong, C.; Misra, A.; Feuerstein, B.G.; Volik, S.; Collins, C.C.; Lamborn, K.R.; Bollen, A.; Pinkel, D.; et al. Integrated genomic and epigenomic analyses pinpoint biallelic gene inactivation in tumors. *Nat. Genet.* **2002**, *32*, 453–458. [CrossRef] [PubMed]
154. Liu, T.C.; Lin, S.F.; Chang, J.G.; Yang, M.Y.; Hung, S.Y.; Chang, C.S. Epigenetic alteration of the SOCS1 gene in chronic myeloid leukaemia. *Br. J. Haematol.* **2003**, *123*, 654–661. [CrossRef] [PubMed]
155. Chim, C.S.; Wong, K.Y.; Loong, F.; Srivastava, G. SOCS1 and SHP1 hypermethylation in mantle cell lymphoma and follicular lymphoma: Implications for epigenetic activation of the Jak/STAT pathway. *Leukemia* **2004**, *18*, 356–358. [CrossRef] [PubMed]
156. Ekmekci, C.G.; Gutierrez, M.I.; Siraj, A.K.; Ozbek, U.; Bhatia, K. Aberrant methylation of multiple tumor suppressor genes in acute myeloid leukemia. *Am. J. Hematol.* **2004**, *77*, 233–240. [CrossRef]
157. Sutherland, K.D.; Lindeman, G.J.; Choong, D.Y.; Wittlin, S.; Brentzell, L.; Phillips, W.; Campbell, I.G.; Visvader, J.E. Differential hypermethylation of SOCS genes in ovarian and breast carcinomas. *Oncogene* **2004**, *23*, 7726–7733. [CrossRef]
158. Hatirnaz, O.; Ure, U.; Ar, C.; Akyerli, C.; Soysal, T.; Ferhanoglu, B.; Ozcelik, T.; Ozbek, U. The SOCS-1 gene methylation in chronic myeloid leukemia patients. *Am. J. Hematol.* **2007**, *82*, 729–730. [CrossRef]
159. Jiang, S.; Zhang, H.W.; Lu, M.H.; He, X.H.; Li, Y.; Gu, H.; Liu, M.F.; Wang, E.D. MicroRNA-155 functions as an OncomiR in breast cancer by targeting the suppressor of cytokine signaling 1 gene. *Cancer Res.* **2010**, *70*, 3119–3127. [CrossRef]
160. Merkel, O.; Hamacher, F.; Griessl, R.; Grabner, L.; Schiefer, A.I.; Prutsch, N.; Baer, C.; Egger, G.; Schlederer, M.; Krenn, P.W.; et al. Oncogenic role of miR-155 in anaplastic large cell lymphoma lacking the t(2;5) translocation. *J. Pathol.* **2015**, *236*, 445–456. [CrossRef]

161. Zhao, X.D.; Zhang, W.; Liang, H.J.; Ji, W.Y. Overexpression of miR -155 promotes proliferation and invasion of human laryngeal squamous cell carcinoma via targeting SOCS1 and STAT3. *PLoS ONE* **2013**, *8*, e56395. [CrossRef]
162. Saint-Germain, E.; Mignacca, L.; Huot, G.; Acevedo, M.; Moineau-Vallee, K.; Calabrese, V.; Bourdeau, V.; Rowell, M.C.; Ilangumaran, S.; Lessard, F.; et al. Phosphorylation of SOCS1 inhibits the SOCS1-p53 tumor suppressor axis. *Cancer Res.* **2019**. [CrossRef] [PubMed]
163. Guo, F.; Xu, Z.; Zhang, Y.; Jiang, P.; Huang, G.; Chen, S.; Lyu, X.; Zheng, P.; Zhao, X.; Zeng, Y.; et al. FXR induces SOCS3 and suppresses hepatocellular carcinoma. *Oncotarget* **2015**, *6*, 34606–34616. [CrossRef]
164. Attia, Y.M.; Tawfiq, R.A.; Ali, A.A.; Elmazar, M.M. The FXR Agonist, Obeticholic Acid, Suppresses HCC Proliferation & Metastasis: Role of IL-6/STAT3 Signalling Pathway. *Sci. Rep.* **2017**, *7*, 12502. [CrossRef] [PubMed]
165. Sugase, T.; Takahashi, T.; Serada, S.; Fujimoto, M.; Hiramatsu, K.; Ohkawara, T.; Tanaka, K.; Miyazaki, Y.; Makino, T.; Kurokawa, Y.; et al. SOCS1 Gene Therapy Improves Radiosensitivity and Enhances Irradiation-Induced DNA Damage in Esophageal Squamous Cell Carcinoma. *Cancer Res.* **2017**, *77*, 6975–6986. [CrossRef] [PubMed]
166. Sugase, T.; Takahashi, T.; Serada, S.; Fujimoto, M.; Ohkawara, T.; Hiramatsu, K.; Nishida, T.; Hirota, S.; Saito, Y.; Tanaka, K.; et al. SOCS1 gene therapy has antitumor effects in imatinib-resistant gastrointestinal stromal tumor cells through FAK/PI3 K signaling. *Gastric Cancer* **2018**, *21*, 968–976. [CrossRef] [PubMed]
167. Yoneda, T.; Kunimura, N.; Kitagawa, K.; Fukui, Y.; Saito, H.; Narikiyo, K.; Ishiko, M.; Otsuki, N.; Nibu, K.I.; Fujisawa, M.; et al. Overexpression of SOCS3 mediated by adenovirus vector in mouse and human castration-resistant prostate cancer cells increases the sensitivity to NK cells in vitro and in vivo. *Cancer Gene Ther.* **2019**. [CrossRef] [PubMed]
168. de la Iglesia, N.; Konopka, G.; Puram, S.V.; Chan, J.A.; Bachoo, R.M.; You, M.J.; Levy, D.E.; Depinho, R.A.; Bonni, A. Identification of a PTEN-regulated STAT3 brain tumor suppressor pathway. *Genes Dev.* **2008**, *22*, 449–462. [CrossRef] [PubMed]
169. Sherry, M.M.; Reeves, A.; Wu, J.K.; Cochran, B.H. STAT3 is required for proliferation and maintenance of multipotency in glioblastoma stem cells. *Stem Cells* **2009**, *27*, 2383–2392. [CrossRef]
170. Pencik, J.; Schlederer, M.; Gruber, W.; Unger, C.; Walker, S.M.; Chalaris, A.; Marie, I.J.; Hassler, M.R.; Javaheri, T.; Aksoy, O.; et al. STAT3 regulated ARF expression suppresses prostate cancer metastasis. *Nat. Commun.* **2015**, *6*, 7736. [CrossRef]
171. Lessard, F.; Morin, F.; Ivanchuk, S.; Langlois, F.; Stefanovsky, V.; Rutka, J.; Moss, T. The ARF tumor suppressor controls ribosome biogenesis by regulating the RNA polymerase I transcription factor TTF-I. *Mol. Cell* **2010**, *38*, 539–550. [CrossRef] [PubMed]
172. Sherr, C.J. The INK4a/ARF network in tumour suppression. *Nat. Rev. Mol. Cell Biol.* **2001**, *2*, 731–737. [CrossRef] [PubMed]
173. Ko, A.; Han, S.Y.; Song, J. Regulatory Network of ARF in Cancer Development. *Mol. Cell* **2018**, *41*, 381–389. [CrossRef]
174. Ferbeyre, G.; de Stanchina, E.; Lin, A.W.; Querido, E.; McCurrach, M.E.; Hannon, G.J.; Lowe, S.W. Oncogenic ras and p53 cooperate to induce cellular senescence. *Mol. Cell. Biol.* **2002**, *22*, 3497–3508. [CrossRef] [PubMed]
175. Pencik, J.; Wiebringhaus, R.; Susani, M.; Culig, Z.; Kenner, L. IL-6/STAT3/ARF: The guardians of senescence, cancer progression and metastasis in prostate cancer. *Swiss Med. Wkly.* **2015**, *145*, w14215. [CrossRef] [PubMed]
176. Chin, Y.E.; Kitagawa, M.; Su, W.C.; You, Z.H.; Iwamoto, Y.; Fu, X.Y. Cell growth arrest and induction of cyclin-dependent kinase inhibitor p21 WAF1/CIP1 mediated by STAT1. *Science* **1996**, *272*, 719–722. [CrossRef] [PubMed]
177. Bellido, T.; O'Brien, C.A.; Roberson, P.K.; Manolagas, S.C. Transcriptional activation of the p21(WAF1,CIP1,SDI1) gene by interleukin-6 type cytokines. A prerequisite for their pro-differentiating and anti-apoptotic effects on human osteoblastic cells. *J. Biol. Chem.* **1998**, *273*, 21137–21144. [CrossRef] [PubMed]
178. Grabner, B.; Schramek, D.; Mueller, K.M.; Moll, H.P.; Svinka, J.; Hoffmann, T.; Bauer, E.; Blaas, L.; Hruschka, N.; Zboray, K.; et al. Disruption of STAT3 signalling promotes KRAS-induced lung tumorigenesis. *Nat. Commun.* **2015**, *6*, 6285. [CrossRef] [PubMed]

179. Musteanu, M.; Blaas, L.; Mair, M.; Schlederer, M.; Bilban, M.; Tauber, S.; Esterbauer, H.; Mueller, M.; Casanova, E.; Kenner, L.; et al. Stat3 is a negative regulator of intestinal tumor progression in Apc(Min) mice. *Gastroenterology* **2010**, *138*, 1003–1011. [CrossRef]

180. Lee, J.; Kim, J.C.; Lee, S.E.; Quinley, C.; Kim, H.; Herdman, S.; Corr, M.; Raz, E. Signal transducer and activator of transcription 3 (STAT3) protein suppresses adenoma-to-carcinoma transition in Apcmin/+ mice via regulation of Snail-1 (SNAI) protein stability. *J. Biol. Chem.* **2012**, *287*, 18182–18189. [CrossRef]

181. Couto, J.P.; Daly, L.; Almeida, A.; Knauf, J.A.; Fagin, J.A.; Sobrinho-Simoes, M.; Lima, J.; Maximo, V.; Soares, P.; Lyden, D.; et al. STAT3 negatively regulates thyroid tumorigenesis. *Proc. Natl. Acad. Sci. USA* **2012**, *109*, E2361–E2370. [CrossRef] [PubMed]

182. Wang, H.; Lafdil, F.; Wang, L.; Park, O.; Yin, S.; Niu, J.; Miller, A.M.; Sun, Z.; Gao, B. Hepatoprotective versus oncogenic functions of STAT3 in liver tumorigenesis. *Am. J. Pathol.* **2011**, *179*, 714–724. [CrossRef] [PubMed]

183. Schneller, D.; Machat, G.; Sousek, A.; Proell, V.; van Zijl, F.; Zulehner, G.; Huber, H.; Mair, M.; Muellner, M.K.; Nijman, S.M.; et al. p19(ARF)/p14(ARF) controls oncogenic functions of signal transducer and activator of transcription 3 in hepatocellular carcinoma. *Hepatology* **2011**, *54*, 164–172. [CrossRef] [PubMed]

184. Zhang, H.F.; Chen, Y.; Wu, C.; Wu, Z.Y.; Tweardy, D.J.; Alshareef, A.; Liao, L.D.; Xue, Y.J.; Wu, J.Y.; Chen, B.; et al. The Opposing Function of STAT3 as an Oncoprotein and Tumor Suppressor Is Dictated by the Expression Status of STAT3beta in Esophageal Squamous Cell Carcinoma. *Clin. Cancer Res.* **2016**, *22*, 691–703. [CrossRef] [PubMed]

185. Pectasides, E.; Egloff, A.M.; Sasaki, C.; Kountourakis, P.; Burtness, B.; Fountzilas, G.; Dafni, U.; Zaramboukas, T.; Rampias, T.; Rimm, D.; et al. Nuclear localization of signal transducer and activator of transcription 3 in head and neck squamous cell carcinoma is associated with a better prognosis. *Clin. Cancer Res.* **2010**, *16*, 2427–2434. [CrossRef]

186. Gordziel, C.; Bratsch, J.; Moriggl, R.; Knosel, T.; Friedrich, K. Both STAT1 and STAT3 are favourable prognostic determinants in colorectal carcinoma. *Br. J. Cancer* **2013**, *109*, 138–146. [CrossRef] [PubMed]

187. Ettl, T.; Stiegler, C.; Zeitler, K.; Agaimy, A.; Zenk, J.; Reichert, T.E.; Gosau, M.; Kuhnel, T.; Brockhoff, G.; Schwarz, S. EGFR, HER2, survivin, and loss of pSTAT3 characterize high-grade malignancy in salivary gland cancer with impact on prognosis. *Hum. Pathol.* **2012**, *43*, 921–931. [CrossRef] [PubMed]

188. Sato, T.; Neilson, L.M.; Peck, A.R.; Liu, C.; Tran, T.H.; Witkiewicz, A.; Hyslop, T.; Nevalainen, M.T.; Sauter, G.; Rui, H. Signal transducer and activator of transcription-3 and breast cancer prognosis. *Am. J. Cancer Res.* **2011**, *1*, 347–355. [PubMed]

6

JAK/STAT-Activating Genomic Alterations are a Hallmark of T-PLL

Linus Wahnschaffe [1,2,3,†], Till Braun [1,2,3,†], Sanna Timonen [4,5,6,†], Anil K. Giri [6], Alexandra Schrader [1,2,3], Prerana Wagle [2], Henrikki Almusa [6], Patricia Johansson [7], Dorine Bellanger [8,9], Cristina López [10,11], Claudia Haferlach [12], Marc-Henri Stern [8,9], Jan Dürig [7,13], Reiner Siebert [10,11], Satu Mustjoki [4,5], Tero Aittokallio [6,14] and Marco Herling [1,2,3,*]

1 Department I of Internal Medicine, Center for Integrated Oncology (CIO), Aachen-Bonn-Cologne-Duesseldorf, University of Cologne (UoC), 50937 Cologne, Germany; linus.wahnschaffe@uk-koeln.de (L.W.); till.braun@uk-koeln.de (T.B.); alexandra.schrader@uk-koeln.de (A.S.)
2 Excellence Cluster for Cellular Stress Response and Aging-Associated Diseases (CECAD), University of Cologne, 50937 Cologne, Germany; prerana.wagle@uk-koeln.de
3 Center for Molecular Medicine Cologne (CMMC), University of Cologne, 50937 Cologne, Germany
4 Hematology Research Unit Helsinki, Helsinki University Hospital Comprehensive Cancer Center, FI-00029 Helsinki, Finland; sanna.timonen@helsinki.fi (S.T.); satu.mustjoki@helsinki.fi (S.M.)
5 Translational Immunology Research program and Department of Clinical Chemistry and Hematology, University of Helsinki, FI-00014 Helsinki, Finland
6 Institute for Molecular Medicine Finland (FIMM), University of Helsinki, FI-00014 Helsinki, Finland; anil.kumar@helsinki.fi (A.K.G.); henrikki.almusa@helsinki.fi (H.A.); tero.aittokallio@helsinki.fi (T.A.)
7 Department of Hematology, University Hospital Essen, University of Duisburg-Essen, 45147 Essen, Germany; patricia.johansson@uk-essen.de (P.J.); jan.duerig@uk-essen.de (J.D.)
8 Institut Curie, Centre de Recherche, 75248 Paris, France; dorine.bellanger@curie.fr (D.B.); marc-henri.stern@curie.fr (M.-H.S.)
9 French National Institute of Health and Medical Research (INSERM) U830, 75248 Paris, France
10 Institute for Human Genetics, Christian-Albrechts-University Kiel & University Hospital Schleswig Holstein, 24105 Kiel, Germany; cristina.lopez@uni-ulm.de (C.L.); reiner.siebert@uni-ulm.de (R.S.)
11 Institute of Human Genetics, Ulm University, Ulm University Medical Center, D-89081 Ulm, Germany
12 MLL Munich Leukemia Laboratory, Max-Lebsche-Platz 31, 81377 Munich, Germany; claudia.haferlach@mll.com
13 German Cancer Consortium (DKTK), 69120 Heidelberg, Germany
14 Department of Mathematics and Statistics, University of Turku, FI-20014 Turku, Finland
* Correspondence: marco.herling@uk-koeln.de
† Equal contribution.

Abstract: T-cell prolymphocytic leukemia (T-PLL) is a rare and poor-prognostic mature T-cell leukemia. Recent studies detected genomic aberrations affecting *JAK* and *STAT* genes in T-PLL. Due to the limited number of primary patient samples available, genomic analyses of the JAK/STAT pathway have been performed in rather small cohorts. Therefore, we conducted—via a primary-data based pipeline—a meta-analysis that re-evaluated the genomic landscape of T-PLL. It included all available data sets with sequence information on *JAK* or *STAT* gene loci in 275 T-PLL. We eliminated overlapping cases and determined a cumulative rate of 62.1% of cases with mutated *JAK* or *STAT* genes. Most frequently, *JAK1* (6.3%), *JAK3* (36.4%), and *STAT5B* (18.8%) carried somatic single-nucleotide variants (SNVs), with missense mutations in the SH2 or pseudokinase domains as most prevalent. Importantly, these lesions were predominantly subclonal. We did not detect any strong association between mutations of a *JAK* or *STAT* gene with clinical characteristics. Irrespective of the presence of gain-of-function (GOF) SNVs, basal phosphorylation of STAT5B was elevated in all analyzed T-PLL. Fittingly, a significant proportion of genes encoding for potential negative regulators of

STAT5B showed genomic losses (in 71.4% of T-PLL in total, in 68.4% of T-PLL without any *JAK* or *STAT* mutations). They included *DUSP4, CD45, TCPTP, SHP1, SOCS1, SOCS3*, and *HDAC9*. Overall, considering such losses of negative regulators and the GOF mutations in *JAK* and *STAT* genes, a total of 89.8% of T-PLL revealed a genomic aberration potentially explaining enhanced STAT5B activity. In essence, we present a comprehensive meta-analysis on the highly prevalent genomic lesions that affect genes encoding JAK/STAT signaling components. This provides an overview of possible modes of activation of this pathway in a large cohort of T-PLL. In light of new advances in JAK/STAT inhibitor development, we also outline translational contexts for harnessing active JAK/STAT signaling, which has emerged as a 'secondary' hallmark of T-PLL.

Keywords: JAK; STAT; T-PLL; T-cell leukemia; meta-analysis; STAT5B signaling

---

1. Introduction

T-cell prolymphocytic leukemia (T-PLL) is an aggressive malignancy characterized by an expansion of mature T-lymphocytes [1]. Although with an incidence of <2.0/million/year in Western countries infrequently encountered, T-PLL is the most common mature T-cell leukemia [2]. Patients suffering from T-PLL typically present with exponentially rising white blood cell (WBC) counts accompanied by bone marrow (BM) infiltration and splenomegaly, and at lower frequencies by various other manifestations such as effusions or in skin [3]. Due to its chemotherapy-refractory behavior, T-PLL patients have a dismal prognosis with a median overall survival (OS) of <3 years [4–6]. Clinicians treating T-PLL face limited therapeutic options, mainly caused by a still incomplete mechanistic disease concept and, therefore, a rudimentary understanding of targetable vulnerabilities in T-PLL. The most potent single substance, the CD52-antibody alemtuzumab, leads to complete remissions in more than 80% of patients, however, nearly all eventually relapse (at median already within 12 months) [3,4,7].

Due to the limited number of primary patient samples available, genomic analyses studying the underlying disease mechanisms have been performed in rather small cohorts of T-PLL patients. In these studies, the most common molecular features revealed were rearrangements that involve chromosome 14 or X, resulting in juxtaposition of the *T-cell leukemia/lymphoma 1A (TCL1A)* or *Mature T-cell leukemia 1 (MTCP1)* proto-oncogenes to *TCRAD* gene enhancer elements [8]. The second most common lesions are genomic alterations of the tumor suppressor *ataxia telangiectasia mutated (ATM)*, found in >85% of cases [9]. In addition to these lesions, activating mutations targeting the Janus kinase (JAK)/signal transducer and activator of transcription (STAT) pathway components were identified in these series of genomic analyses [9–18].

The JAK/STAT pathway is a ubiquitous cytokine-mediated signaling cascade that regulates cell proliferation, differentiation, migration, and apoptosis [19]. After recruitment of JAKs (JAK1, JAK2, JAK3, TYK2) to cytokine receptors, they phosphorylate STAT proteins (STAT1, STAT2, STAT3, STAT4, STAT5A, STAT5B, STAT6), which then bind DNA and regulate target gene transcription [20]. Dysregulation of the JAK/STAT axis has been described as a key event in the pathogenesis of various hematologic malignancies [21]. Constitutively active JAK/STAT signaling induces T-cell tumors in mice [22,23]. Using different sequencing approaches, activating mutations of *JAK1, JAK3*, and *STAT5B* were identified as the most recurrent genomic aberrations affecting *JAK/STAT* genes in T-PLL [9–18]. However, prevalence of gene mutations, information on their allele frequencies, assessment of negative regulators of JAK/STAT signaling, and the phosphorylation status of the most recurrently affected JAK/STAT proteins vary considerably or are not reported in these studies [9–18].

Therapeutic approaches blocking JAK/STAT signaling have so far improved patient outcomes predominantly in autoimmune conditions and in graft-versus-host disease [24,25]. JAK inhibitors are currently tested for a number of new indications [26]. T-PLL cells have shown a notable in vitro sensitivity towards JAK inhibition, which was not directly linked to the *JAK/STAT* mutation status [15,16]. First reports present individual clinical activity of tofacitinib (pan JAK inhibitor) and ruxolitinib (JAK 1/2 inhibitor) in relapsed T-PLL [27,28].

Although many studies identified *JAK* and *STAT* genes to be commonly mutated in T-PLL, these analyses have been performed in rather small cohorts not providing a sufficient dataset to determine reliable mutation and variant allele frequencies (VAFs). In addition, the publication overlap of these studies was unresolved and a systematic assessment for other potential genomic causes (e.g., copy number alterations (CNAs)) has not been performed.

Here, we conducted a meta-analysis that was supplemented by new primary data, hence providing the largest cohort to date that evaluated the genomic aberrations affecting *JAK/STAT* signaling in T-PLL. In addition to summarizing information on the functional impact of the most recurrent lesions, we propose a model of potential mechanisms leading to constitutive JAK/STAT signaling in T-PLL cells.

2. Results

2.1. Characteristics and Overlaps of Included Studies

The meta-analysis considered all available publications that have analyzed variants of any *JAK* or *STAT* gene in cases of T-PLL, regardless of the sequencing approach used (Table S1). Redundantly sequenced cases were identified to eliminate overlaps between these 10 studies (Figure 1A). The most common sequencing approach was Sanger sequencing (Sanger seq., 7 studies), followed by targeted amplicon sequencing (TAS, 5 studies), whole exome sequencing (WES, 4 studies), and whole genome sequencing (WGS, 2 studies). *JAK3* (n = 272 T-PLL patients), *JAK1* (n = 246), and *STAT5B* (n = 209) were predominantly sequenced due to the bias by the targeted approaches. Germline controls were sequenced in 53 cases (19.3%). The number of analyzed patients varied from 3 to 71 patients across the 10 studies [9–18]. After subtracting all cases reported in more than one study, we identified 275 unique T-PLL cases as the core cohort.

Notably, data that were acquired by WGS, WES, and SNP array analysis were re-analyzed as primary data in cases, in which raw data were available (WES: 62.2%, n = 46/74 T-PLL patients; WGS: 50.0%, n = 4/8; SNP arrays: 100.0%, n = 71/71), while data gained through Sanger seq. or TAS were not re-evaluated. By re-analyzing the WES and SNP array data through a uniform pipeline, homogeneity of the resulting dataset was obtained. *JAK1, JAK2, JAK3, TYK2, STAT1, STAT2, STAT3, STAT4, STAT5A, STAT5B*, and *STAT6* are further referred to as 'any *JAK* or *STAT* gene'.

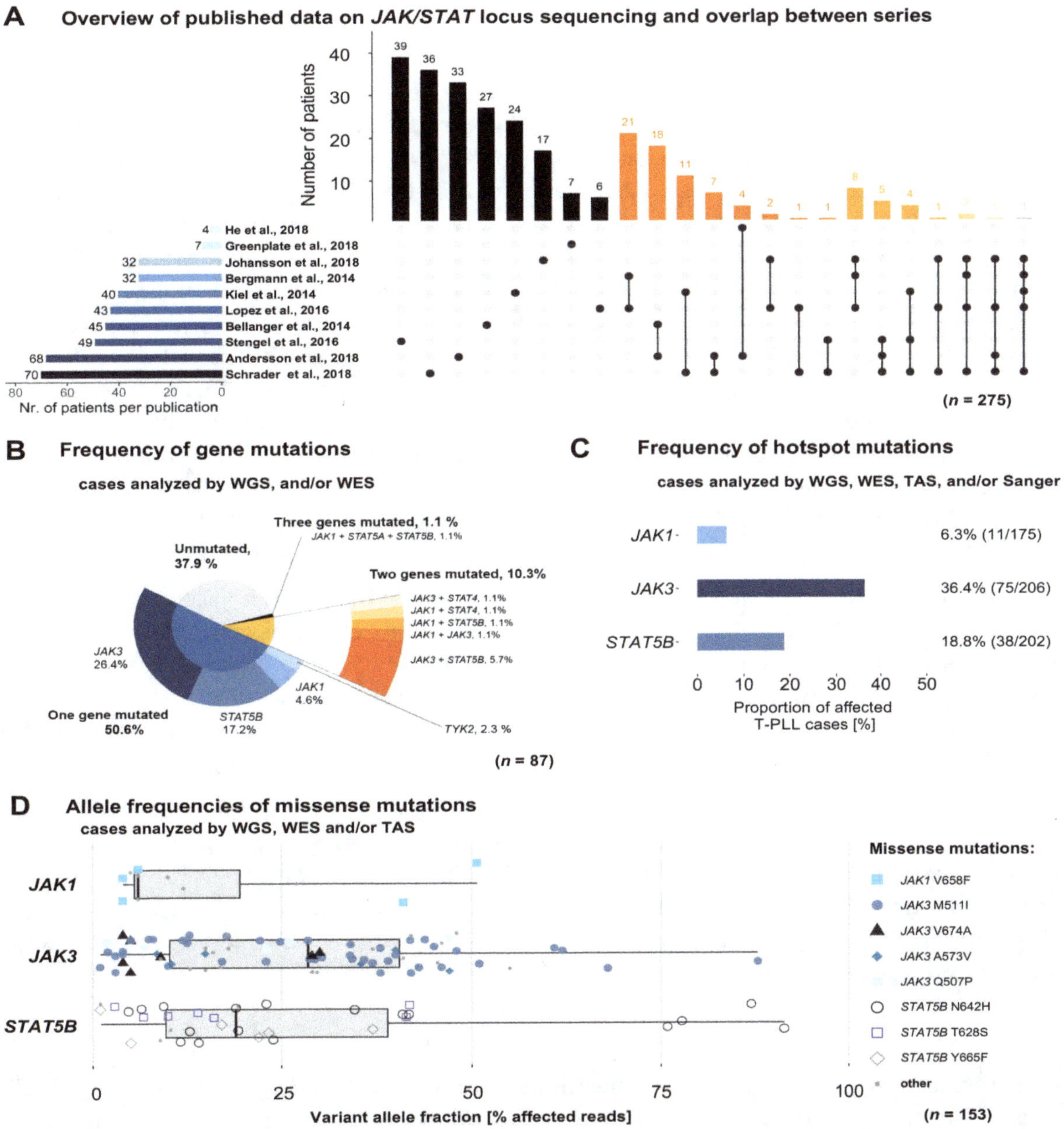

Figure 1. Meta-analyses of genomic profiling series in T-PLL underscore the high prevalence of mutations affecting *JAK* and *STAT* genes. (**A**) T-PLL patients (n = 275) sequenced for any *JAK* or *STAT* locus. Horizontal bar chart displays the total number of patients sequenced in each publication. Vertical bar chart indicates the size of intersections between sets of patients analyzed in one or more publications. Color-code of vertical bars indicates the number of studies reporting results of the same individual case (black: 1; dark-orange: 2; medium-orange: 3; light-orange: 4; light grey: 5). Dot connecting lines show the overlapping publications of each intersection. (**B**) Distribution of *JAK/STAT* mutations (n = 87 T-PLL analyzed by whole genome sequencing (WGS)/whole exome sequencing (WES)): in 62.1% of these cases (n = 54) at least one mutation in a gene of the *JAK/STAT* family was found to be mutated. (**C**) Relative frequencies of hotspot mutations of *JAK1*, *JAK3*, and *STAT5B* (as defined by the genomic region containing more than 90% of the respective mutations; n = 275 cases analyzed by WGS/WES/targeted amplicon sequencing (TAS)/Sanger sequencing). Every T-PLL case that was sequenced for the respective hotspot region of *JAK1* (Ex. 14–20), *JAK3* (Ex. 11–19), and/or *STAT5B* (Ex. 15–17), was included. (**D**) Box-whisker charted allele frequencies of missense mutations of *JAK1*, *JAK3*, and *STAT5B* (n = 153 T-PLL analyzed by WGS/WES and/or TAS) illustrate a high heterogeneity in variant allele fractions, with most lesions detected at lower frequencies (<50%).

2.2. Mutations in *JAK* and *STAT* Genes are Predominantly Found at Subclonal Levels

We included T-PLL cases with available data from WGS or WES in order to calculate the frequency of genomic variants in *JAK* and *STAT* genes. We identified a cumulative rate of 62.1% (n = 54/87, Figure 1B) cases with variants in any *JAK* or *STAT* gene. The vast majority of them were somatic single-nucleotide variants (SNVs) of missense type (96.0%, n = 72/75 of variants detected by WGS/WES). The remaining three lesions (4.0%, n = 3/75) were small in-frame deletions in *JAK1* or *JAK3*. In the following these SNVs and small in-frame deletions are referred to as 'mutations'. Somatic variants were called and known single nucleotide polymorphisms were filtered out in those tumor samples for which a matched germline sample was available. For T-PLL patients with a missing germline control (n = 38), we included only those variants which were detected in the WES with matched germline samples. *JAK3* (34.5%, n = 30/87), *STAT5B* (25.3%, n = 22/87), and *JAK1* (9.2%; n = 8/87) were the most recurrently mutated genes, while *TYK2* (2.3%, n = 2/87), *STAT4* (2.3%, n = 2/87), and *STAT5A* (1.1%, n = 1/87) were mutated at lower frequencies. Nine of 87 cases (10.3%) presented with mutations affecting two genes that encode for JAK or STAT proteins. Co-occuring ('double') *JAK1* and *JAK3* mutations were found in 1.1% of cases (n = 1/87), *JAK3* and *STAT4* in 1.1% (n = 1/87), and *JAK1* and *STAT4* mutations in 1.1% (n = 1/87); *JAK1* and *STAT5B* in 1.1% (n = 1/87), and *JAK3* and *STAT5B* in 5.8% (n = 5/87). Co-occuring *JAK1*, *STAT5A*, and *STAT5B* mutations ('triple') were detected in one case (1.1%).

Next, we calculated frequencies of missense mutations considering the hotspots of *JAK1* (Ex. 14–20), *JAK3* (Ex. 11–19), and *STAT5B* (Ex. 15–17). Hotspot regions were defined as genomic regions containing >90% of the respective mutations. By also including cases analyzed by TAS or Sanger seq. for the respective hotspot region, we arrived at a larger cohort for these analyses. Based on this, the hotspot of *JAK1* showed a relative mutation frequency of 6.3% (n = 11/175). For the hotspot of *JAK3* this was 36.4% (n = 75/206) and for the hotspot of *STAT5B* it was 18.8% (n = 38/202, Figure 1C).

As already described in smaller cohorts [9,16,18], most of these lesions presented as subclonal events with low VAFs (medians: *JAK1* 6.0%, *JAK3* 28.5%, *STAT5B* 19.0%, Figure 1D); however, we observed a high heterogeneity in VAFs. Notably, the N642H mutation of *STAT5B* was observed at a VAF of >50% in four cases and the M511I mutation of *JAK3* at VAFs >50% in five cases. Note that given the data provided in the reports, the percentage of treatment-naïve samples was 72.7%; sequential samples of individual T-PLL patients were not analyzed here.

2.3. Missense Mutations in *JAK1*, *JAK3*, and *STAT5B* Cluster Within the Conserved Pseudokinase and SH2 Domains

We further assessed the localization of the missense mutations of *JAK1*, *JAK3*, and *STAT5B* (Figure 2, upper protein schemes) as well as the frequencies of hotspot SNVs in these genes (lower inset). To assess the localization of the somatic SNVs of *JAK1*, *JAK3*, and *STAT5B*, we included all T-PLL cases which have been sequenced for the whole coding genome by WES or WGS. All T-PLL cases which have been sequenced for the respective lesion regardless of the sequencing approach were considered to determine the frequencies of hotspot mutations. The pseudokinase domain (JH2 domain) of *JAK1* was predominantly affected (62.5% of all *JAK1* mutations, n = 5/8) with V658F (3.7% of all analyzed cases, n = 9/246, regardless of the sequencing approach) as the most prominent lesion (Figure 2A). In *JAK3*, most somatic SNVs were found in the JH2-SH2-linker (69.7% of all *JAK3* missense mutations, n = 23/33 detected missense mutations), followed by the JH2 domain (27.3%, n = 9/33, Figure 2B). The M511I lesion was the most prevalent lesion in *JAK3* (27.2% of all analyzed cases, n = 74/272, regardless of the sequencing approach). Almost all missense mutations of *STAT5B* were found in the SH2 domain (96.2% of all *STAT5B* missense mutations, n = 25/26 detected missense mutations; Figure 2C). N642H (9.6% of all analyzed cases, n = 20/209, regardless of the sequencing approach), T628S (5.9%, n = 12/202), and Y665F (3.3%, n = 7/209) were the most recurrent mutations affecting *STAT5B*. Remarkably, we did not detect significant differences in the mutation frequencies with regard to the sequencing approach (see bars of the lower inset of Figure 2).

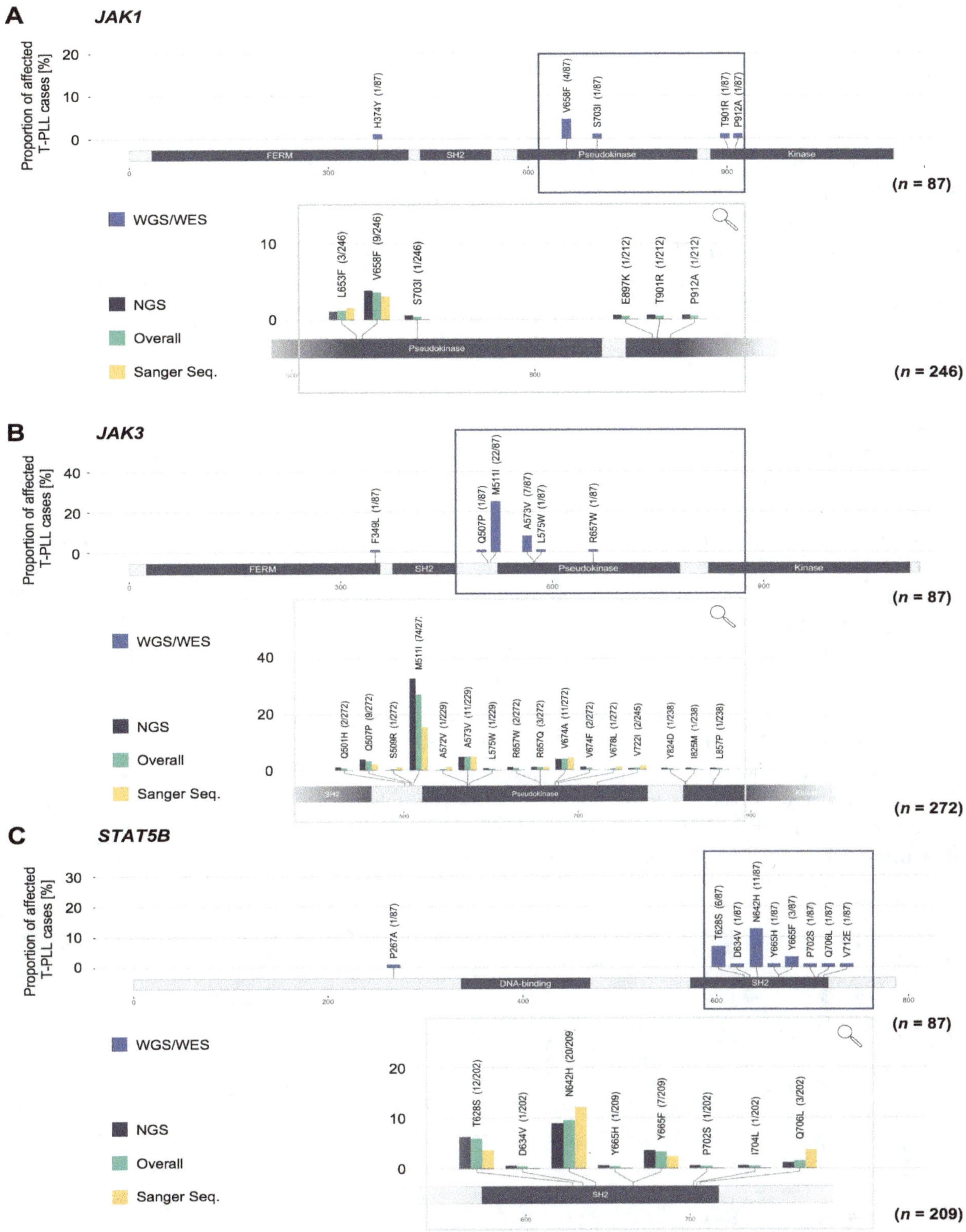

Figure 2. Missense mutations in *JAK1*/*JAK3*/*STAT5B* genes cluster within the conserved JH2 (pseudokinase) and SH2 domains. Upper protein scheme: gene-wide distribution of missense mutations of *JAK1* (**A**), *JAK3* (**B**), and *STAT5B* (**C**); $n = 87$ T-PLL analyzed by WES/WGS, representing the same cases as in Figure 1B. Lower inset for each sub-panel A–C: frequencies of hotspot mutations, stratified for applied sequencing methods ($n = 275$ cases analyzed with WES/WGS/TAS/Sanger seq). While *JAK1* and *JAK3* were predominately affected by lesions within the pseudokinase domains (JH2) and the SH2-JH2 linker regions, *STAT5B* missense mutations were presented mostly in the SH2 domain.

2.4. T-PLL Harboring any JAK or STAT Mutation Show Elevated TCL1A mRNA Level, but Present Comparable Clinical Outcomes

When analyzing associations of *JAK* and *STAT* mutations with immunophenotypic and cytogenetic data as well with the 18 most prevalent mutations found in T-PLL (as described by Schrader et al. [9]), we detected a decreased proportion of T-PLL cells with CD40L expression (p = 0.05, Fisher's exact test, Figure S1A) and an increased proportion of T-PLL cells harboring *NOTCH2* mutations (p = 0.03, Fisher's exact test, Figure S1B) in the *JAK3* mutated cohort (overview of tested associations is provided in Table S2). Notably, T-PLL with any *JAK* or *STAT* mutation showed elevated TCL1A mRNA levels as compared to patients without any *JAK* or *STAT* mutation (fold change (Fc) = 4.1, p = 0.01, Student's *t*-test, Figure 3A), further underlined by an increased proportion of cases harboring an inversion 14 (q11q32) in the *STAT5B* mutated cohort (p = 0.03, Fisher's exact test, Figure S1C). TCL1A mRNA levels were also elevated by just considering *JAK3* mutated cases (Fc = 6.5, p = 0.002, Student's *t*-test, Figure S1D) or *STAT5B* mutated cases (Fc = 3.6, p = 0.02, Student's *t*-test, Figure S1E) compared to T-PLL without either mutation, respectively. To assess the functional role of variants in *JAK* or *STAT* genes in T-PLL patients, we screened for significant associations between somatic *JAK/STAT* SNVs and clinical data, including outcome. For these analyses, we merged clinical information from nine studies [9–16,18]. As not all considered publications reported the same set of parameters, cohort sizes varied between the different analyses. When investigating an association of the *JAK/STAT* mutation status with overall survival, we did not observe differences in OS of T-PLL patients harboring any *JAK* or *STAT* mutation compared to patients without *JAK* or *STAT* mutation (p = 0.42, log rank test, Figure 3B). In contrast to studies of smaller cohorts [12,16], we could not observe a significantly shorter OS of *JAK3* mutated T-PLL patients (p = 0.26, log rank test, Figure S2A). Similarly, the *JAK3* M511 mutation was not associated with a shorter OS (p = 0.39, log rank test, Figure S2B). The OS of patients without any *JAK* or *STAT* mutations was comparable to those harboring a *STAT5B* (p = 0.55, log rank test, Figure S2C), *STAT5B* N642H (p = 0.60, log rank test, Figure S2D), or *JAK1* (p = 0.54, log rank test, Figure S2E) mutation. Interestingly, the *JAK1* L653F mutation status was associated with a significantly shorter OS (p = 0.003, log rank test, Figure S2F). In addition, cases with a *STAT5B* Y665F mutation also showed a shorter OS (p = 0.06, log rank test, Figure S2G). However, only two patients with a *JAK1* L653F mutation or five patients with a *STAT5B* Y665F mutation were included in the 'mutated' cohorts, so these results should be interpreted with caution. We did not detect any other association of clinical characteristics of T-PLL patients with the presence of *JAK* or *STAT* mutations (Table S3).

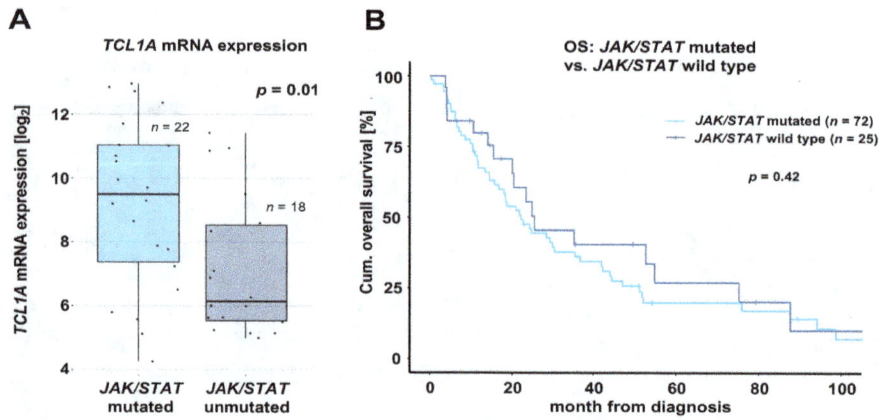

Figure 3. *JAK/STAT* mutation status shows association with elevated TCL1A mRNA expression, but not with patient outcomes. (**A**) TCL1A mRNA expression measured by array-based gene expression profiling (GEP) of *JAK/STAT* mutated cases compared to cases without any *JAK* or *STAT* mutation (fold change: 4.1; p = 0.01, Student's *t*-test). (**B**) Overall survival (OS) of *JAK/STAT* mutated cases (median OS: 21.0 months) compared to cases without any *JAK* or *STAT* mutation (median OS: 25.5 months, p = 0.42, log rank test). Significant associations between mutations affecting *JAK3* or *STAT5B* with immunophenotypic, mutational, and expression data are displayed in Figure S1. Associations of mutations affecting *JAK1*, *JAK3*, or *STAT5B* with OS are presented in Figure S2.

2.5. T-PLL Cells Show Basal STAT5B Phosphorylation, Regardless of Their JAK/STAT Mutation Status

Even though STAT5B was shown to be predominantly affected in T-PLL in previous series, its phosphorylation, and therefore activation state, was often not aligned with the genomic profiling data [9–11]. By analyzing primary samples of eight T-PLL cases, we observed noticeable basal STAT5B phosphorylation in every case (Figure 4A, no exposure to any culturing). We discovered no obvious association between STAT5B phosphorylation and the presence of any *JAK* or *STAT* mutation.

Samples without *JAK* or *STAT* mutation showed similar levels of high basal phospho-STAT5B to those that harbored such lesions, as already previously shown in a series of 6 T-PLL cases [9].

We further correlated the immunoblot data with alterations involving key regulators of STAT5B activity (either mutations or CNAs). For this, we pre-selected a set of 105 genes encoding for proteins known to regulate JAK/STAT signaling based on available literature (Table S4). We next identified of these 105 genes 7 which showed recurrent genomic lesions in the overall T-PLL cohort and which were reported to have a regulatory effect on STAT5B signaling in vitro or in vivo (Table S5). Overall, we identified recurrent mutations or genomic losses of seven negative regulators potentially leading to constitutive STAT5B activity (*DUSP4, CD45, TCPTP, SHP1, SOCS1, SOCS3,* and *HDAC9*) in 71.4% of analyzed T-PLL cases (n = 35/49 cases analyzed with WES/WGS and SNP array, Figure 4B). About 68.4% of T-PLL cases that did not reveal a mutation in any *JAK* or *STAT* gene showed such a CNA of a STAT5B signaling regulator. This resulted in a total of 89.8% of T-PLL cases that harbor a genomic lesion potentially explaining constitutive STAT5B signaling (either genomic losses of negative regulators, and/or mutations of *JAK* or *STAT* genes). Gene expression signatures (array-based) of cases that harbor a genomic loss or a mutation of a negative regulator of JAK/STAT signaling (and that lack a *JAK* or *STAT* mutation) were comparable to those of cases with a mutation in any *JAK* or *STAT* gene (principal component analysis in Figure S4A). Both cohorts showed similar activation (as per upregulated gene expression) of STAT5B target genes. All T-PLL with a mutation in a *JAK* or *STAT* gene and 90% of patients with a mutation or loss in a negative JAK/STAT regulator (and without any mutation in a *JAK* or *STAT* gene) showed overexpression of at least one STAT5 target gene. In contrast, the frequency of overexpressed STAT5 target genes was significantly lower in T-PLL without a genomic lesion potentially activating JAK/STAT signaling (60%, Figure S4B). In detail, *DUSP4, CD45, SOCS3, SHP1,* and *HDAC9* showed the highest prevalences of genomic losses with a higher frequency in T-PLL cases without any *JAK* or *STAT* mutation (Figure 4C). In addition, we identified genomic gains of *STAT2* (n = 1/49 T-PLL), *STAT3,* (n = 5/49 T-PLL), *STAT5A* (n = 5/49 T-PLL), and *STAT5B* (n = 5/49 T-PLL). These lesions were detected only in combination with mutations of a *JAK* or *STAT* gene or with genomic losses of a negative regulator of STAT5B signaling (Figure 4D).

Overall, we propose a model of constitutive JAK/STAT signaling induced by mutations of a predicted gain of function (GOF) in *JAK1, JAK3,* and *STAT5B* genes and by copy-number losses of negative regulators of STAT5B activity.

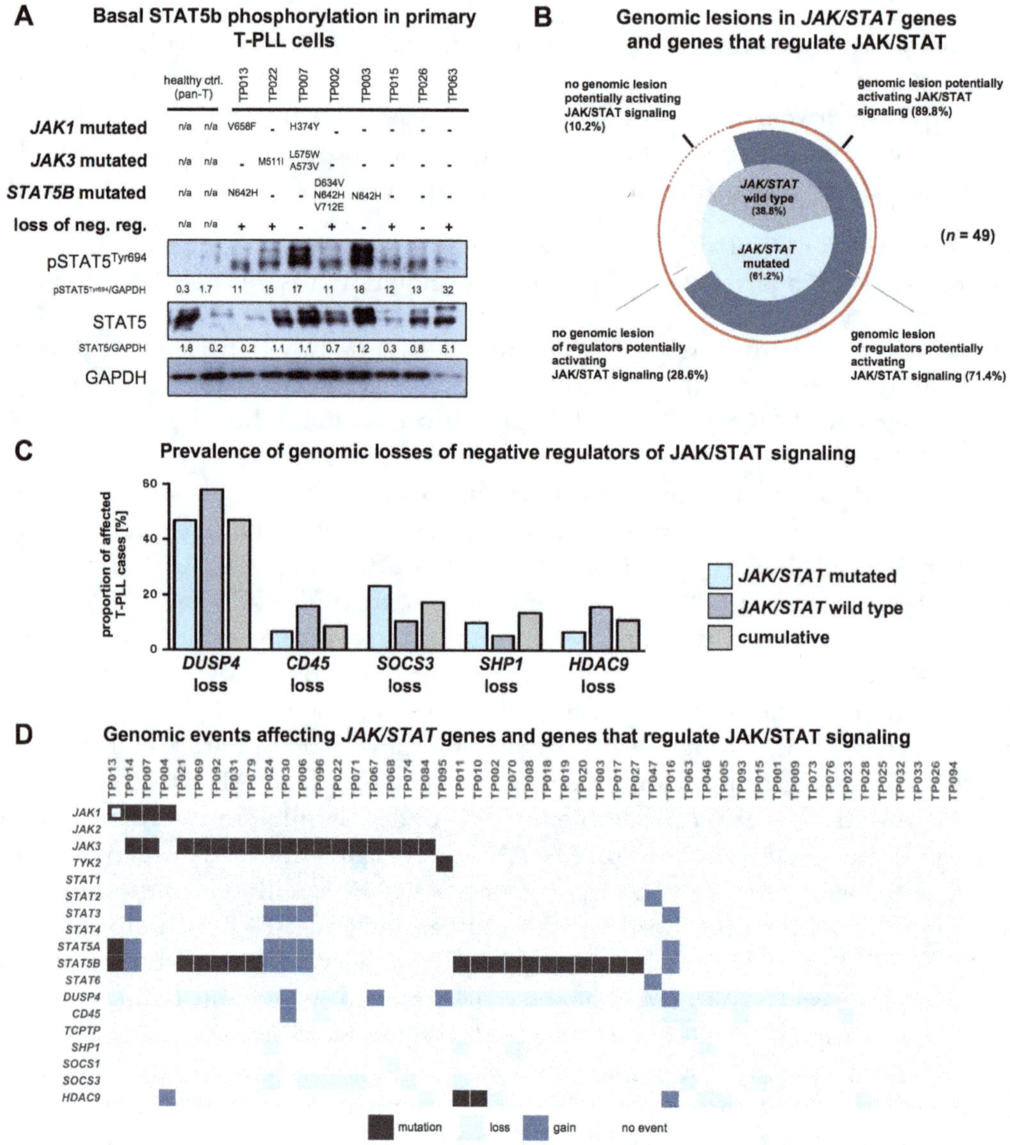

Figure 4. T-PLL cells show basal STAT5B phosphorylation, regardless of their *JAK/STAT* mutation status. (**A**) Elevated basal STAT5B phosphorylation levels of T-PLL cells. Controls: $CD3^{+}$ pan T-cells isolated from healthy individuals. 'Loss of neg. reg.': key regulators which negatively affect STAT5B activation (namely *DUSP4, CD45, TCPTP, SHP1, SOCS1, SOCS3,* and *HDAC*; see (D) for case-wise depiction) were considered based on available literature and based on data of their copy number alterations (CNA) in T-PLL. (**B**) Distribution of genomic lesions affecting any *JAK* or *STAT* gene and their regulators ($n = 49$ cases analyzed with WES/WGS and with SNP arrays). Inner pie chart: distribution of *JAK/STAT* mutations. Outer pie chart: Prevalence of genomic lesions of regulators activating JAK/STAT (either genomic losses of negative regulators or genomic gains of positive regulators). An overall proportion of 89.8% of T-PLL cases carried a genomic lesion potentially explaining constitutive STAT5B activation (mutation or CNA of JAK/STAT regulator). (**C**) Prevalence of the five most common genomic lesions affecting negative regulators of the JAK/STAT pathway ($n = 49$ cases analyzed with WES/WGS and SNP array): T-PLL cases without any mutation in a *JAK* or *STAT* gene showed a higher prevalence of genomic losses of *DUSP4, CD45,* and *HDAC9* as compared to *JAK/STAT* mutated cases. (**D**) Mapped genomic events involving *JAK* and *STAT* genes and their regulators ($n = 49$ cases analyzed with WES/WGS and SNP array). An overview of genomic lesions resulting in a suggested activation of the JAK/STAT pathway across all considered T-PLL cases is given in Figure S3.

3. Discussion

Here, we present a comprehensive meta-analysis of primary data from 275 T-PLL cases from 10 published studies that evaluated genomic lesions involving elements of JAK/STAT signaling. In this large cohort, we identified genomic aberrations potentially leading to constitutive JAK/STAT signaling in approximately 90% of cases, thus establishing this as a molecular hallmark of T-PLL. Our analysis provides an overview on the genomic causes of JAK/STAT signaling activation including *JAK/STAT* GOF mutations as well as CNAs of *JAK/STAT* genes or negative regulators of JAK/STAT signaling.

About 62% of T-PLL cases showed GOF mutations affecting any *JAK* or *STAT* gene, while previous publications reported a mutation frequency varying between 36% and 76% [10,18]. In accordance with these studies, we predominantly detected missense mutations in the SH2 or pseudokinase domains of *JAK1, JAK3,* and *STAT5B*, mostly occurring at a subclonal level. Mutations of genes encoding for components of the JAK/STAT pathway are frequently found in T-cell neoplasms (predominantly mutations of *JAK3, STAT3,* and *STAT5B*). Their reported incidences range from 10% (e.g., for Sézary syndrome [29]) to 70% (e.g., for intestinal T-cell lymphoma [30]). Compared to those, the cumulative mutation frequency of *JAK* and *STAT* genes in T-PLL documented in this meta-analysis is high [31].

Another important finding was the high basal phosphorylation of STAT5B in all analyzed T-PLL samples. In addition to a high proportion of T-PLL cases mutated in any *JAK* or *STAT* gene, we identified seven negative regulators to be commonly lost in T-PLL, potentially explaining cytokine-independent STAT5B activation. This affected 71.4% of all cases and 68.4% of those cases without a detectable *JAK/STAT* SNV. Of these negative regulators, *DUSP4, SOCS3,* and *CD45* were most frequently affected. While genomic losses of *DUSP4* and *SOCS3* were already reported in primary T-PLL [9,17,18], losses of *CD45* have not been described previously. Compared to $CD4^+$ T-cells isolated from healthy individuals, DUSP4 and CD45 mRNA was observed to be strongly downregulated in T-PLL cells [16]. Furthermore, the downregulation of CD45 transcripts was associated with an increased phosphorylation of STAT5, implicating a functional relevance of this negative regulator [17].

T-PLL cells usually show a complex karyotype and a high frequency of somatic CNAs [9,32]. In detail, the loci of the negative regulators *DUSP4* (chr.8p12) and of *SOCS3* (chr.17q25.3) are known to be highly affected by structural aberrations in T-PLL. Therefore, a secondary origin of the detected CNAs due to background imbalances has to be considered. T-PLL cases already harboring an activating mutation of a *JAK* or *STAT* gene or a genomic loss of a negative regulator showed in few cases (12.2%) also genomic gains of *JAK* or *STAT* genes, however, the functional impact of these genomic gains remains unclear.

Certainly, there is the possibility of other, yet-unknown regulators, which we did not include in our analysis. Furthermore, our analysis did not assess for epigenetic regulations or post-translational modifications of *JAK* and *STAT* genes or their regulators, as further causes of active JAK/STAT signaling. Moreover, constitutive T-cell-receptor or cytokine input of the malignant T-cell may represent other modes of (milieu-derived) JAK/STAT activation in T-PLL.

Another important result of the provided meta-analyses is the first description of elevated TCL1A in *JAK* and *STAT* mutated T-PLL. TCL1A overexpression is known to be associated with elevated levels of reactive oxygen species (ROS) [33]. In addition, an 8-oxoguanine DNA damage signature is characteristic for T-PLL, likely resulting from ROS-mediated DNA insults [9]. In this context, the initiating oncogene TCL1A is likely to contribute to the occurrence of new mutations, especially when the guardian of genome-integrity *ATM* is deleted or mutated, potentially explaining a higher prevalence of arising subclonal *JAK* and *STAT* mutations in T-PLL. Furthermore, a possible explanation for the association of reduced CD40L expression with the presence of *JAK3* mutations is a state of less T-cell receptor and cytokine dependent activation of T-PLL cells in the context of an acquired hyperactivating mutation of a signaling intermediate such as *JAK3*.

In line with our finding, that nearly every T-PLL case presents with a genomic aberration that potentially causes activated JAK/STAT signaling, we could not observe any differential association of the *JAK/STAT* mutation status with clinical characteristics, i.e., those indicating a more aggressive phenotype of T-PLL cells. Previous studies on small cohorts have shown a negative influence of the presence of *JAK3* mutations on OS [12,16]. However, as these studies used *JAK3* wild type T-PLL as a control group, they potentially included patients with mutations of other *JAK* or *STAT* genes, therefore not representing a proper control.

Although functional validations of the herein described genomic aberrations is outside the scope of this work, mechanistic analyses of many of the detected genomic aberrations and of their impact on tumorigenesis have been performed in various other entities. Such functional findings of mutations of *JAK1*, *JAK3*, and *STAT5B* are summarized in the following (an overview of literature is provided in Table S5).

JAK1, the third most frequently mutated *JAK* or *STAT* gene in this meta-analysis, showed a cumulative hotspot mutation rate of 6.3% in our analysis, in line with the mutation rates calculated in previous studies. V658F, the most prevalent lesion affecting *JAK1* in T-PLL, was initially described in the development of T-ALL [34]. The V658F lesion is homologous to the *JAK2* V617F mutation and was shown to lead to constitutive active JAK1 signaling in a cell line model [35]. Cells harboring the respective lesion presented enhanced basal JAK1, STAT5, and ERK phosphorylation and showed cytokine-independent growth [36]. S7031 and L653F, less frequently detected *JAK1* mutations, were also proven to act as GOF mutations [37,38]. While the S703I mutation was shown to mediate proliferative effects in vitro and in vivo, the L653F mutation is predicted to soften the negative regulation of JAK1 in a biophysical model. The *JAK1* V617F, S703I, and L653F mutations potentially mediate cytokine-independent phosphorylation of STAT5B in T-PLL.

JAK3 mutations were the most recurrent genomic aberration affecting *JAK/STAT* genes in this meta-analysis with a hotspot mutation rate of 36.4% (literature: 21% [12]–71% [17]). The oncogenic potential of the most frequent *JAK3* mutation M511I as well as the less frequently occurring mutations A573V and V674A was shown in various systems: M511I, A573V, as well as V674A mutant cell lines demonstrated high phosphorylation of STAT5 and ERK, leading to cytokine independent growth [39,40]. When transplanting mice with bone marrow progenitor cells harboring the M511I or A573V mutation in *JAK3*, they develop a T-ALL-like disease, characterized by an expansion of immature $CD8^+$ T-cells. In contrast, mice transplanted with V674A mutant bone marrow progenitor cells presented severe lymphadenopathy and splenomegaly without a significant increase of the WBC count [41]. The mentioned *JAK3* mutations were also described in T-ALL [42]. The Q507P mutation, the third most frequent genomic aberration affecting *JAK3* in T-PLL, was not discovered in other entities and has so far not been investigated for its functional relevance.

In this analysis, 18.8% of T-PLL cases were mutated within the hotspot region of *STAT5B*, while the mutation rate in the literature varied from 7% [16] to 36% [10]. The most frequently found N642H mutation is a well described GOF mutation: *STAT5B* N642H transduced cell lines showed prolonged phosphorylation and dimerization of STAT5B, resulting in an enhanced transcriptional activity [43,44]. The N642H mutation leads to a sustained stability to the anti-parallel dimer as shown by crystallization [45]. Transgenic mice harboring the *STAT5B* N642H lesion rapidly developed aggressive $CD8^+$ T-cell neoplasms [46]. The *STAT5B* Y665F mutation, which had a notable influence on OS of T-PLL patients in our analysis, revealed highly phosphorylated STAT5B, an enhanced transcriptional activity and increased proliferation in a cell culture model, comparable to the *STAT5B* N642H mutation. The above-mentioned genomic aberrations, which have also been described in the mutational landscape of T-LGL [47], may play an important role in the activation of JAK/STAT signaling in T-PLL. The functional role of the second most detected *STAT5B* aberration, the T628S mutation, is much less established. This genetic aberration is previously described in hepatosplenic T-cell lymphoma and associated with an increased phosphorylation of STAT5 in a cell line model [48]. Notably, the three commonly affected *JAK/STAT* genes (*JAK1, JAK3, STAT5B*) are crucial for IL-2 signaling, the cytokine secreted at highest levels in T-PLL [49]. Targeted approaches in appropriate models have to address the chronological role of such lesions as most of them were detected at subclonal levels.

Given that nearly every T-PLL case harbors a genomic aberration potentially activating JAK/STAT signaling, JAK and STAT proteins are clinically relevant targets for T-PLL therapy [50]. Interestingly, in a large panel of blood cancers, primary T-PLL patient cells showed high sensitivity towards JAK-targeting compounds. Moreover, JAK inhibitors were among the top 25 most effective drugs in an *ex vivo* drug screen of 39 T-PLL patient samples exposed to 301 different substances [15,16]. Previous case reports also showed the initial promising results of a combination therapy of the JAK inhibitors ruxolitinib (JAK 1/2 inhibitor) and tofacitinib (pan JAK inhibitor) [27,28]. However, previous studies have also argued that the *JAK/STAT* mutation status alone does not predict ex-vivo sensitivity towards JAK inhibitors [16]. This is in line with the observation of multiple, potentially distinct mechanisms, apart from missense mutations of *JAK/STAT* genes, that are required for activating this pathway. In general, predicting sensitivity of kinase inhibitors often requires larger panels of biomarkers, some of which may be outside of the target pathways or direct drivers of the disease. Therefore, therapeutic targeting of JAK/STAT signaling has to be expanded on various levels, including the development of novel STAT3/5 inhibitors and the extension of pre-clinical and clinical studies to large cohorts of T-PLL and other T-cell lymphomas, all with well-characterized tumor material (e.g., JAK/STAT activation state). Selective STAT5 inhibitors which bind to the SH2 domain of *STAT5* are currently under development [51].

4. Materials and Methods

4.1. Data Acquisition

Available literature was systematically screened for all genomic profiling studies that have information on the mutational status of any *JAK* or *STAT* gene in T-PLL, regardless of the sequencing technique. We identified a total of 10 publications meeting these criteria (Table S6). Raw data of these publications was obtained from different sources, either publicly available or kindly provided by the corresponding authors. Full descriptions of the composed data set and detailed information on the sources of data are provided in Table S6. Considered T-PLL patients had provided written informed consent and all the studies were originally approved by their institutional review boards.

4.2. Data Merging

Considering the rarity of T-PLL and the strong collaboration network in T-PLL research, we assumed a pronounced exchange of patient samples between different centers and studies. To determine all redundantly analyzed patients in our cohort, we requested basic patient information to allow us to precisely identify potential overlaps while still ensuring anonymity of all the patients (Figure 1A). In cases where genomic regions were sequenced by different methods, we included the information provided by the widest type of analysis, ranking WGS > WES > TAS > Sanger sequencing. In total, 275 distinct T-PLL patients were included in our analyses.

4.3. Raw Data Analysis

Data acquired through whole-exome sequencing and SNP-array analysis was re-analyzed for those cases in which raw data was available, while data obtained through Sanger sequencing or targeted amplicon sequencing was not re-analyzed. Studies where raw data was not available were included by applying the already analyzed data. Detailed information on the data sources are listed in Table S6 and on the applied tools with references in Table S7. The below subsections describe the various genomic analyses performed for the meta-analysis.

4.3.1. Whole-Exome Sequencing (WES)

The sequenced raw exome reads were trimmed of B blocks from the end using Trimmomatic (RWTH Aachen, Aachen, Germany). The trimmed data were aligned to the human reference genome (GRCh build 37) using Burrows Wheeler Aligner (bwa-0.7.12, Wellcome Trust Sanger Institute, Cambridge, UK). After alignment the potential PCR duplicates were removed using Picard (Broad Institute of Harvard and MIT, Cambridge, MA, USA), and BAM files were generated, sorted, and indexed using SAMtools (Wellcome Trust Sanger Institute, Cambridge, UK). Exomic regions were re-aligned and the base quality scores were re-calibrated according to the Genome Analysis Toolkit Best Practices recommendations (GATK 4.1.3.0). VarScan2.2.3 (The Genome Institute, St. Louis, MO, USA) was used to call somatic mutations with the following parameters: strand-filter 1, min-coverage-normal 8, min-coverage-tumor 6, somatic-*p*-value 0.01, min-var-freq 0.05. The putative somatic mutations were annotated for functional consequences using SnpEff 4.03 (Institute of Environmental Health Sciences, Detroit, MI, USA). Variants present in 1000 genome or dbSNP 2.0 Build were filtered out from the analysis.

In order to call somatic single-nucleotide variants in 38 patients without matched germline samples, MuTect v2 (Broad Institute of Harvard and MIT) was employed with default parameters. Because we were mostly interested in identifying sequence variants that were likely to contribute to T-PLL pathogenesis, we focused on those variations that were identified in our analysis of 22 patients with matched healthy control samples. Only these filtered mutations have been reported for the patients without matched germline samples.

4.3.2. Somatic Copy-Number Alterations (sCNAs)

Genotyping of Affymetrix GenomeWide SNP6 array (Thermo Fisher Scientific, Waltham, MA, USA) was performed using Genotype Console Software 4 (GTC4, Thermo Fisher Scientific) with the default parameters using Birdseed v2 algorithms (Broad Institute of Harvard and MIT). In order to infer copy number variations in the T-PLL genome, we used the pooled controls as a reference (non-tumor hematopoietic cell DNA as 'germline' from T-PLL patients, $n = 13$) created using the GTC pipeline. The Canary algorithm was used to call CN state using the default settings in GTC. We performed segmentation analysis on the basis of identified SNPs/CNVs using inbuilt algorithm. Copy number values and segmentation were visually assessed in the Integrative Genomics Viewer (Broad Institute, Cambridge, MA, USA). Since the segmentation algorithm only reports significantly altered segments/regions, we mapped identified genomic regions to genes based on version 75 of the Ensembl annotation using BiomaRt (version 2.38 and the GenomicRanges R package, version 1.34.0).

4.3.3. Gene Expression Profiling (GEP)

The processed normalized expression profiles generated with GenomeStudio were downloaded from GEO. Data were merged and adjusted for batch effects using linear regression. A differential expression analysis was performed using Student's *t*-test on expression values of patients and healthy controls (CD3+ pan T-cells from 10 healthy donors). The differentially expressed probes were mapped to the respective genes by Illumina provided annotation files. Principal component analysis of the whole gene expression set was performed with R.

4.4. Clinical Data and Statistical Analyses

All publications were screened for accompanying clinical data and authors were contacted for further information. In total, we obtained and merged clinical data from nine publications [9–16,18]. For patients who were reported in multiple studies, we included the most detailed clinical data set. To assess possible correlations between mutational status and clinical phenotypes, we performed a screening approach testing for a broad range of parameters (Table S3), where the patients were stratified by overall mutational status, mutational status of specific genes, and by specific mutations. As a control, we used clinical data from T-PLL patients, who were unmutated in all *JAK/STAT* genes analyzed with WES/WGS.

All statistical analyses were performed using R software and R packages (Table S7). Analysis of overall survival, as measured from day of diagnosis until day of event or censoring, was performed and graphed with R survival and R survminer packages. Log rank statistics were calculated to test for differences in survival distributions. Continuous clinical parameters were tested for normal distribution with Shapiro–Wilk test and further assessed for their associations to *JAK/STAT* mutational status with either Student's *t*-test or Wilcoxon rank sum test, depending on the normality test. Fisher's exact test was used for testing differences in categorical data in patients with *JAK/STAT* mutations compared to unmutated patients. A $p < 0.05$ was considered to be statistically significant.

4.5. Immunoblots

We performed Western blots of whole-cell lysates of primary T-PLL cells and CD3+ pan T-cell isolated from age matched healthy controls by magnetic-bead based cell enrichment. Positive selection of CD3+ pan T-cells of healthy controls was performed according to the manufactures instruction (Biolegend). Following antibodies from Cell Signaling Technology were used in a 1:1000 dilution according to the manufacturer's instruction: phospho-STAT5TYR694 (clone C11C5, catalogue #9359), STAT5 (polyclonal, #9363), and GAPDH (clone 14C10, #2118). As a secondary antibody we made use of HRP-coupled anti-rabbit (Dianova) in a 1:5000 dilution. Immunoblots were done using Western Bright ECL (Advansta, Menlo Park, CA, USA) and luminescence intensities were evaluated by densitometry (ImageJ software, National Institute of Health, Bethesda, MD, USA). Uncropped images of the immunoblots are displayed in Figure S5.

4.6. Data Accessibility

All genomic data analyzed in this study was gathered from published series. For detailed sources of raw data and/or information on *JAK/STAT* mutations, see Table S6.

5. Conclusions

Overall, this meta-analysis provides an overview of the lesional landscape of *JAK/STAT* associated genes in the largest cohort of T-PLL cases to date and summarizes the potential functional impact of the most common genomic aberrations. Nearly every T-PLL case in our cohort had a genetic aberration, which can be intuitively implicated in constitutively active JAK/STAT signaling. Besides GOF missense mutations in *JAK/STAT* genes, genomic losses of negative regulators of the JAK-STAT signaling axis are frequently found in T-PLL, linking the high basal phosphorylation of STAT5B to genomic causes. We propose a model for these distinct mechanisms implicated in constitutive STAT5B signaling in T-PLL (Figure 5). Our data provide a rational framework for strategies to inhibit JAK/STAT signaling in T-PLL, even in patients whose leukemia does not carry mutations in a *JAK* or *STAT* gene. Development of novel STAT inhibitors and their application, including with synergistic partners, in model systems and in T-PLL patients, represent future tasks.

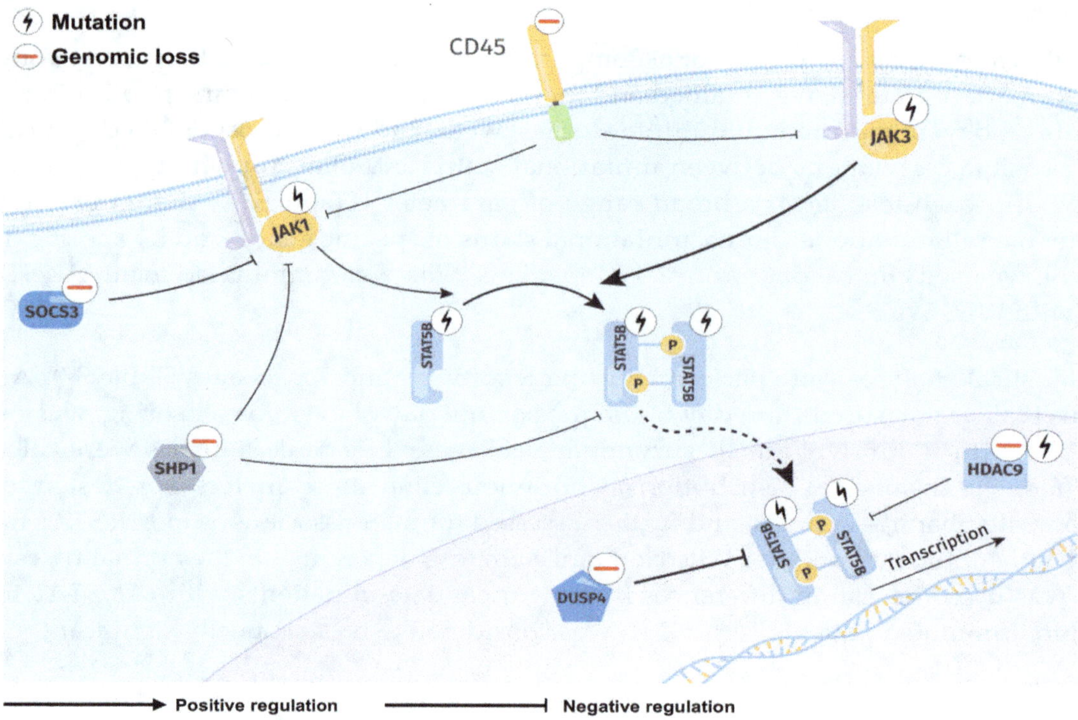

Figure 5. Proposed model of recurrent genomic lesions leading to an enhanced activation of STAT5B in T-PLL. Regulatory network summarizing detected genomic lesions (sCNAs, mutations) in *JAK/STAT* genes and their direct regulators. Mutations of *JAK* and *STAT* genes and genomic losses of negative STAT5B regulators being affected in more than 5% of T-PLL patients were included. Frequent missense mutations occur in the JH2 and SH2-JH2 linker of *JAK1* and *JAK3*, potentially leading to elevated phosphorylation and dimerization of STAT5B. Activation of JAK1 and JAK3 is potentially enhanced through genomic losses (*DUSP4, SOCS1, SOCS3, CD45, SHP1, HDAC9*, and *TCPTP*) and mutations (*HDAC9*) of negative regulators. STAT5B activation might be further increased through GOF mutations in its SH2 domain. Cytoplasmatic (*SHP1, TCPTP*) as well as nuclear (*DUSP4, HDAC9*) regulators are commonly affected by genomic losses in T-PLL, leading to intensified STAT5B signaling. Constitutive active STAT5B translocates into the nucleus and regulates transcription of many target genes relevant for T-cell development, differentiation, proliferation, migration, and apoptosis [52].

Supplementary Materials:
12/1833/s1, Figure S1: *JAK/STAT* mutation status shows association with the inversion 14 (q11q32) and elevated *TCL1A* mRNA expression; Figure S2: *JAK/STAT* mutation status shows no association with outcome in T-PLL patients; Figure S3: Overview of genomic lesions associated with an activation of the JAK/STAT pathway across all considered T-PLL cases; Figure S4: T-PLL cases harboring any *JAK* or *STAT* mutation show similar gene expression compared to T-PLL cases with a loss or mutation of a negative regulator potentially activating JAK/STAT signaling; Figure S5: Uncropped images of immunoblots; Table S1: Overview of considered publications; Table S2: Associations of *JAK* and *STAT* mutations with immunophenotypic, cytogenetic, and mutational data; Table S3: Screening of clinical parameters; Table S4: List of genes encoding for proteins which potentially regulate JAK/STAT signaling; Table S5: Overview of references; Table S6: Data sources; Table S7: Bioinformatic tools

Author Contributions: Conceptualization, L.W., T.B., A.S., and, M.H.; Formal analysis, L.W., S.T., A.K.G., H.A., and T.A.; Investigation, T.B.; Resources, D.B., P.J., C.L., C.H., M.-H.S., J.D., and R.S.; Data curation, L.W., S.T., and P.W.; Writing—original draft preparation, L.W., T.B., S.T., and A.K.G.; Writing—review and editing, A.S., R.S., S.M., T.A., and M.H.; Supervision, A.S., S.M., T.A., and M.H.; Project administration, L.W. and T.B.

Acknowledgments: The authors gratefully thank all the authors of the original publications for providing either the raw or already processed data for the meta-analyses. The authors thank Michael Gruen for his technical support with Figure 5 and all the patients with their families for their invaluable contributions.

References

1. Staber, P.B.; Herling, M.; Bellido, M.; Jacobsen, E.D.; Davids, M.S.; Kadia, T.M.; Shustov, A.; Tournilhac, O.; Bachy, E.; Zaja, F.; et al. Consensus criteria for diagnosis, staging, and treatment response assessment of T-cell prolymphocytic leukemia. *Blood* **2019**, *134*, 1132–1143. [CrossRef] [PubMed]
2. Herling, M.; Khoury, J.D.; Washington, L.T.; Duvic, M.; Keating, M.J.; Jones, D. A systematic approach to diagnosis of mature T-cell leukemias reveals heterogeneity among WHO categories. *Blood* **2004**, *104*, 328–335. [CrossRef] [PubMed]
3. Dearden, C. How i treat prolymphocytic leukemia. *Blood* **2012**, *120*, 538–551. [CrossRef] [PubMed]
4. Hopfinger, G.; Busch, R.; Pflug, N.; Weit, N.; Westermann, A.; Fink, A.M.; Cramer, P.; Reinart, N.; Winkler, D.; Fingerle-Rowson, G.; et al. Sequential chemoimmunotherapy of fludarabine, mitoxantrone, and cyclophosphamide induction followed by alemtuzumab consolidation is effective in T-cell prolymphocytic leukemia. *Cancer* **2013**, *119*, 2258–2267. [CrossRef] [PubMed]
5. Herling, M.; Patel, K.A.; Teitell, M.A.; Konopleva, M.; Ravandi, F.; Kobayashi, R.; Jones, D. High TCL1 expression and intact T-cell receptor signaling define a hyperproliferative subset of T-cell prolymphocytic leukemia. *Blood* **2008**, *111*, 328–337. [CrossRef] [PubMed]
6. Ravandi, F.; O'Brien, S.; Jones, D.; Lerner, S.; Faderl, S.; Ferrajoli, A.; Wierda, W.; Garcia-Manero, G.; Thomas, D.; Koller, C.; et al. T-cell prolymphocytic leukemia: A single-institution experience. *Clin. Lymhoma Myeloma* **2005**, *6*, 234–239. [CrossRef]
7. Dearden, C.E.; Khot, A.; Else, M.; Hamblin, M.; Grand, E.; Roy, A.; Hewamana, S.; Matutes, E.; Catovsky, D. Alemtuzumab therapy in T-cell prolymphocytic leukemia: Comparing efficacy in a series treated intravenously and a study piloting the subcutaneous route. *Blood* **2011**, *118*, 5799–5802. [CrossRef]
8. Hoh, F.; Yang, Y.-S.; Guignard, L.; Padilla, A.; Stern, M.-H.; Lhoste, J.-M.; van Tilbeurgh, H. Crystal structure of p14TCL1, an oncogene product involved in T-cell prolymphocytic leukemia, reveals a novel β-barrel topology. *Structure* **1998**, *6*, 147–155. [CrossRef]
9. Schrader, A.; Crispatzu, G.; Oberbeck, S.; Mayer, P.; Pützer, S.; von Jan, J.; Vasyutina, E.; Warner, K.; Weit, N.; Pflug, N.; et al. Actionable perturbations of damage responses by TCL1/ATM and epigenetic lesions form the basis of T-PLL. *Nat. Commun.* **2018**, *9*, 697. [CrossRef]
10. Kiel, M.J.; Velusamy, T.; Rolland, D.; Sahasrabuddhe, A.A.; Chung, F.; Bailey, N.G.; Schrader, A.; Li, B.; Li, J.Z.; Ozel, A.B.; et al. Integrated genomic sequencing reveals mutational landscape of T-cell prolymphocytic leukemia. *Blood* **2014**, *124*, 1460–1472. [CrossRef]
11. Bellanger, D.; Jacquemin, V.; Chopin, M.; Pierron, G.; Bernard, O.A.; Ghysdael, J.; Stern, M.-H. Recurrent *JAK1* and *JAK3* somatic mutations in T-cell prolymphocytic leukemia. *Leukemia* **2013**, *28*, 417. [CrossRef] [PubMed]
12. Stengel, A.; Kern, W.; Zenger, M.; Perglerová, K.; Schnittger, S.; Haferlach, T.; Haferlach, C. Genetic characterization of T-PLL reveals two major biologic subgroups and *JAK3* mutations as prognostic marker. *Genes Chromosom. Cancer* **2016**, *55*, 82–94. [CrossRef] [PubMed]
13. López, C.; Bergmann, A.K.; Paul, U.; Murga Penas, E.M.; Nagel, I.; Betts, M.J.; Johansson, P.; Ritgen, M.; Baumann, T.; Aymerich, M.; et al. Genes encoding members of the JAK-STAT pathway or epigenetic regulators are recurrently mutated in T-cell prolymphocytic leukaemia. *Br. J. Haematol.* **2016**, *173*, 265–273. [CrossRef] [PubMed]
14. He, L.; Tang, J.; Andersson, E.I.; Timonen, S.; Koschmieder, S.; Wennerberg, K.; Mustjoki, S.; Aittokallio, T. Patient-customized drug combination prediction and testing for T-cell prolymphocytic leukemia patients. *Cancer Res.* **2018**, *78*, 2407–2418. [CrossRef]
15. Dietrich, S.; Oleś, M.; Lu, J.; Sellner, L.; Anders, S.; Velten, B.; Wu, B.; Hüllein, J.; da Silva Liberio, M.; Walther, T.; et al. Drug-perturbation-based stratification of blood cancer. *J. Clin. Investig.* **2018**, *128*, 427–445. [CrossRef]
16. Andersson, E.I.; Pützer, S.; Yadav, B.; Dufva, O.; Khan, S.; He, L.; Sellner, L.; Schrader, A.; Crispatzu, G.; Oleś, M.; et al. Discovery of novel drug sensitivities in T-PLL by high-throughput ex vivo drug testing and mutation profiling. *Leukemia* **2017**, *32*, 774. [CrossRef]
17. Greenplate, A.; Wang, K.; Tripathi, R.M.; Palma, N.; Ali, S.M.; Stephens, P.J.; Miller, V.A.; Shyr, Y.; Guo, Y.; Reddy, N.M.; et al. Genomic profiling of T-Cell neoplasms reveals frequent *JAK1* and *JAK3* mutations with clonal evasion from targeted therapies. *JCO Precis. Oncol.* **2018**. [CrossRef]
18. Johansson, P.; Klein-Hitpass, L.; Choidas, A.; Habenberger, P.; Mahboubi, B.; Kim, B.; Bergmann, A.; Scholtysik, R.; Brauser, M.; Lollies, A.; et al. SAMHD1 is recurrently mutated in T-cell prolymphocytic leukemia. *Blood Cancer J.* **2018**, *8*, 11. [CrossRef]

19. Rawlings, J.S.; Rosler, K.M.; Harrison, D.A. The JAK/STAT signaling pathway. *J. Cell Sci.* **2004**, *117*, 1281–1283. [CrossRef]
20. Villarino, A.V.; Kanno, Y.; O'Shea, J.J. Mechanisms and consequences of Jak-STAT signaling in the immune system. *Nat. Immunol.* **2017**, *18*, 374–384. [CrossRef]
21. Furqan, M.; Mukhi, N.; Lee, B.; Liu, D. Dysregulation of JAK-STAT pathway in hematological malignancies and JAK inhibitors for clinical application. *Biomark. Res.* **2013**, *1*, 5. [CrossRef] [PubMed]
22. Heinrich, T.; Rengstl, B.; Muik, A.; Petkova, M.; Schmid, F.; Wistinghausen, R.; Warner, K.; Crispatzu, G.; Hansmann, M.-L.; Herling, M.; et al. Mature T-cell lymphomagenesis induced by retroviral insertional activation of Janus kinase 1. *Mol. Ther.* **2013**, *21*, 1160–1168. [CrossRef] [PubMed]
23. Maurer, B.; Nivarthi, H.; Wingelhofer, B.; Pham, H.T.T.; Schlederer, M.; Suske, T.; Grausenburger, R.; Schiefer, A.-I.; Prchal-Murphy, M.; Chen, D.; et al. High activation of STAT5A drives peripheral T-cell lymphoma and leukemia. *Haematologica* **2019**. [CrossRef] [PubMed]
24. Taylor, P.C. Clinical efficacy of launched JAK inhibitors in rheumatoid arthritis. *Rheumatology* **2019**, *58* (Suppl. 1), i17–i26. [CrossRef]
25. Mannina, D.; Kröger, N. Janus Kinase inhibition for graft-versus-host disease: Current status and future prospects. *Drugs* **2019**, *79*, 1499–1509. [CrossRef]
26. Schwartz, D.M.; Bonelli, M.; Gadina, M.; O'Shea, J.J. Type I/II cytokines, JAKs, and new strategies for treating autoimmune diseases. *Nat. Rev. Rheumatol.* **2016**, *12*, 25–36. [CrossRef]
27. Gomez-Arteaga, A.; Margolskee, E.; Wei, M.T.; van Besien, K.; Inghirami, G.; Horwitz, S. Combined use of tofacitinib (pan-JAK inhibitor) and ruxolitinib (a JAK1/2 inhibitor) for refractory T-cell prolymphocytic leukemia (T-PLL) with a JAK3 mutation. *Leuk. Lymphoma* **2019**, *60*, 1626–1631. [CrossRef]
28. Wei, M.; Koshy, N.; van Besien, K.; Inghirami, G.; Horwitz, S.M. Refractory T-cell prolymphocytic leukemia with JAK3 mutation: In Vitro and clinical synergy of Tofacitinib and Ruxolitinib. *Blood* **2015**, *126*, 5486. [CrossRef]
29. Kiel, M.J.; Sahasrabuddhe, A.A.; Rolland, D.C.M.; Velusamy, T.; Chung, F.; Schaller, M.; Bailey, N.G.; Betz, B.L.; Miranda, R.N.; Porcu, P.; et al. Genomic analyses reveal recurrent mutations in epigenetic modifiers and the JAK–STAT pathway in Sézary syndrome. *Nat. Commun.* **2015**, *6*, 8470. [CrossRef]
30. Nicolae, A.; Xi, L.; Pham, T.H.; Pham, T.-A.; Navarro, W.; Meeker, H.G.; Pittaluga, S.; Jaffe, E.S.; Raffeld, M. Mutations in the JAK/STAT and RAS signaling pathways are common in intestinal T-cell lymphomas. *Leuemia* **2016**, *30*, 2245. [CrossRef]
31. Lone, W.; Alkhiniji, A.; Manikkam Umakanthan, J.; Iqbal, J. Molecular Insights into pathogenesis of peripheral T cell lymphoma: A review. *Curr. Hematol. Malig. Rep.* **2018**, *13*, 318–328. [CrossRef] [PubMed]
32. Maljaei, S.H.; Brito-Babapulle, V.; Hiorns, L.R.; Catovsky, D. Abnormalities of chromosomes 8, 11, 14, and X in T-prolymphocytic leukemia studied by fluorescence in situ hybridization. *Cancer Genet. Cytogenet.* **1998**, *103*, 110–116. [CrossRef]
33. Prinz, C.; Vasyutina, E.; Lohmann, G.; Schrader, A.; Romanski, S.; Hirschhäuser, C.; Mayer, P.; Frias, C.; Herling, C.D.; Hallek, M.; et al. Organometallic nucleosides induce non-classical leukemic cell death that is mitochondrial-ROS dependent and facilitated by TCL1-oncogene burden. *Mol. Cancer* **2015**, *14*, 114. [CrossRef] [PubMed]
34. Jeong, E.G.; Kim, M.S.; Nam, H.K.; Min, C.K.; Lee, S.; Chung, Y.J.; Yoo, N.J.; Lee, S.H. Somatic mutations of *JAK1* and *JAK3* in acute leukemias and solid cancers. *Clin. Cancer Res.* **2008**, *14*, 3716–3721. [CrossRef] [PubMed]
35. Gordon, G.M.; Lambert, Q.T.; Daniel, K.G.; Reuther, G.W. Transforming JAK1 mutations exhibit differential signalling, FERM domain requirements and growth responses to interferon-γ. *Biochem. J.* **2010**, *432*, 255–265. [CrossRef]
36. Hornakova, T.; Staerk, J.; Royer, Y.; Flex, E.; Tartaglia, M.; Constantinescu, S.N.; Knoops, L.; Renauld, J.-C. Acute lymphoblastic leukemia-associated JAK1 mutants activate the Janus kinase/STAT pathway via interleukin-9 receptor alpha homodimers. *J. Biol. Chem.* **2009**, *284*, 6773–6781. [CrossRef] [PubMed]
37. Flex, E.; Petrangeli, V.; Stella, L.; Chiaretti, S.; Hornakova, T.; Knoops, L.; Ariola, C.; Fodale, V.; Clappier, E.; Paoloni, F.; et al. Somatically acquired *JAK1* mutations in adult acute lymphoblastic leukemia. *J. Exp. Med.* **2008**, *205*, 751–758. [CrossRef]
38. Yang, S.; Luo, C.; Gu, Q.; Xu, Q.; Wang, G.; Sun, H.; Qian, Z.; Tan, Y.; Qin, Y.; Shen, Y.; et al. Activating JAK1 mutation may predict the sensitivity of JAK-STAT inhibition in hepatocellular carcinoma. *Oncotarget* **2016**, *7*, 5461–5469. [CrossRef]

39. Degryse, S.; de Bock, C.E.; Demeyer, S.; Govaerts, I.; Bornschein, S.; Verbeke, D.; Jacobs, K.; Binos, S.; Skerrett-Byrne, D.A.; Murray, H.C.; et al. Mutant JAK3 phosphoproteomic profiling predicts synergism between JAK3 inhibitors and MEK/BCL2 inhibitors for the treatment of T-cell acute lymphoblastic leukemia. *Leukemia* **2018**, *32*, 788. [CrossRef]
40. Martinez, G.S.; Ross, J.A.; Kirken, R.A. Transforming mutations of Jak3 (A573V and M511I) show differential sensitivity to selective JAK3 inhibitors. *Clin. Cancer Drugs* **2016**, *3*, 131–137. [CrossRef]
41. Degryse, S.; de Bock, C.E.; Cox, L.; Demeyer, S.; Gielen, O.; Mentens, N.; Jacobs, K.; Geerdens, E.; Gianfelici, V.; Hulselmans, G.; et al. JAK3 mutants transform hematopoietic cells through JAK1 activation, causing T-cell acute lymphoblastic leukemia in a mouse model. *Blood* **2014**, *124*, 3092–3100. [CrossRef] [PubMed]
42. Vicente, C.; Schwab, C.; Broux, M.; Geerdens, E.; Degryse, S.; Demeyer, S.; Lahortiga, I.; Elliott, A.; Chilton, L.; Starza, R.L.; et al. Targeted sequencing identifies associations between IL7R-JAK mutations and epigenetic modulators in T-cell acute lymphoblastic leukemia. *Haematologica* **2015**, *100*, 1301–1310. [CrossRef] [PubMed]
43. Rajala, H.L.M.; Eldfors, S.; Kuusanmäki, H.; van Adrichem, A.J.; Olson, T.; Lagström, S.; Andersson, E.I.; Jerez, A.; Clemente, M.J.; Yan, Y.; et al. Discovery of somatic STAT5b mutations in large granular lymphocytic leukemia. *Blood* **2013**, *121*, 4541–4550. [CrossRef] [PubMed]
44. Küçük, C.; Jiang, B.; Hu, X.; Zhang, W.; Chan, J.K.C.; Xiao, W.; Lack, N.; Alkan, C.; Williams, J.C.; Avery, K.N.; et al. Activating mutations of STAT5B and STAT3 in lymphomas derived from $\gamma\delta$-T or NK cells. *Nat. Commun.* **2015**, *6*, 6025. [CrossRef]
45. de Araujo, E.D.; Erdogan, F.; Neubauer, H.A.; Meneksedag-Erol, D.; Manaswiyoungkul, P.; Eram, M.S.; Seo, H.S.; Qadree, A.K.; Israelian, J.; Orlova, A.; et al. Structural and functional consequences of the STAT5BN642H driver mutation. *Nat. Commun.* **2019**, *10*, 2517. [CrossRef]
46. Pham, H.T.T.; Maurer, B.; Prchal-Murphy, M.; Grausenburger, R.; Grundschober, E.; Javaheri, T.; Nivarthi, H.; Boersma, A.; Kolbe, T.; Elabd, M.; et al. STAT5BN642H is a driver mutation for T cell neoplasia. *J. Clin. Investig.* **2018**, *128*, 387–401. [CrossRef]
47. Andersson, E.I.; Tanahashi, T.; Sekiguchi, N.; Gasparini, V.R.; Bortoluzzi, S.; Kawakami, T.; Matsuda, K.; Mitsui, T.; Eldfors, S.; Bortoluzzi, S.; et al. High incidence of activating STAT5B mutations in CD4-positive T-cell large granular lymphocyte leukemia. *Blood* **2016**, *128*, 2465–2468. [CrossRef]
48. McKinney, M.; Moffitt, A.B.; Gaulard, P.; Travert, M.; de Leval, L.; Raffeld, A.N.M.; Jaffe, E.S.; Pittaluga, S.; Xi, L.; Heavican, T.; et al. The genetic basis of hepatosplenic T-cell lymphoma. *Cancer Discov.* **2017**, *7*, 369–379. [CrossRef]
49. O'Shea, J.J.; Schwartz, D.M.; Villarino, A.V.; Gadina, M.; McInnes, I.B.; Laurence, A. The JAK-STAT pathway: impact on human disease and therapeutic intervention. *Annu. Rev. Med.* **2015**, *66*, 311–328. [CrossRef]
50. Schrader, A.; Braun, T.; Herling, M. The dawn of a new era in treating T-PLL. *Oncotarget* **2019**, *10*, 626–628. [CrossRef]
51. Wingelhofer, B.; Maurer, B.; Heyes, E.C.; Cumaraswamy, A.A.; Berger-Becvar, A.; de Araujo, E.D.; Orlova, A.; Freund, P.; Ruge, F.; Park, J.; et al. Pharmacologic inhibition of STAT5 in acute myeloid leukemia. *Leukemia* **2018**, *32*, 1135–1146. [CrossRef] [PubMed]
52. Kanai, T.; Seki, S.; Jenks, J.A.; Kohli, A.; Kawli, T.; Martin, D.P.; Snyder, M.; Bacchetta, R.; Nadeau, K.C. Identification of STAT5A and STAT5B target genes in human T cells. *PLoS ONE* **2014**, *9*, e86790. [CrossRef] [PubMed]

7

A Novel Inhibitor of STAT5 Signaling Overcomes Chemotherapy Resistance in Myeloid Leukemia Cells

Marie Brachet-Botineau [1], Margaux Deynoux [1], Nicolas Vallet [1,2], Marion Polomski [3], Ludovic Juen [3], Olivier Hérault [1,4], Frédéric Mazurier [1], Marie-Claude Viaud-Massuard [3], Gildas Prié [3] and Fabrice Gouilleux [1,*]

1 LNOx, GICC, CNRS ERL 7001, University of Tours, 37000 Tours, France; marie.brachet@univ-tours.fr (M.B.-B.); margaux.deynoux@etu.univ-tours.fr (M.D.); nls.vallet@gmail.com (N.V.); olivier.herault@univ-tours.fr (O.H.); frederic.mazurier@inserm.fr (F.M.)

2 Service d'Hématologie et Thérapie Cellulaire, CHRU de Tours, 37000 Tours, France

3 IMT, GICC, EA 7501, University of Tours, 37000 Tours, France; marion.polomski@etu.univ-tours.fr (M.P.); ludovic.juen@mcsaf.fr (L.J.); marie-claude.viaud-massuard@univ-tours.fr (M.-C.V.-M.); gildas.prie@univ-tours.fr (G.P.)

4 Service d'Hematologie Biologique, CHRU de Tours, 37000 Tours, France

* Correspondence: fabrice.gouilleux@univ-tours.fr

Abstract: Signal transducers and activators of transcription 5A and 5B (STAT5A and STAT5B) are crucial downstream effectors of tyrosine kinase oncogenes (TKO) such as BCR-ABL in chronic myeloid leukemia (CML) and FLT3-ITD in acute myeloid leukemia (AML). Both proteins have been shown to promote the resistance of CML cells to tyrosine kinase inhibitors (TKI) such as imatinib mesylate (IM). We recently synthesized and discovered a new inhibitor (17f) with promising antileukemic activity. 17f selectively inhibits STAT5 signaling in CML and AML cells by interfering with the phosphorylation and transcriptional activity of these proteins. In this study, the effects of 17f were evaluated on CML and AML cell lines that respectively acquired resistance to IM and cytarabine (Ara-C), a conventional therapeutic agent used in AML treatment. We showed that 17f strongly inhibits the growth and survival of resistant CML and AML cells when associated with IM or Ara-C. We also obtained evidence that 17f inhibits STAT5B but not STAT5A protein expression in resistant CML and AML cells. Furthermore, we demonstrated that 17f also targets oncogenic STAT5B N642H mutant in transformed hematopoietic cells.

Keywords: pharmacological inhibitor; STAT5 signaling; chemotherapy resistance; myeloid leukemia

---

1. Introduction

STAT5A and STAT5B are two closely related signal transducers and activators of transcription family members. Both proteins are crucial downstream effectors of tyrosine kinase oncogenes (TKO) such as Fms-like receptor tyrosine kinase 3 with internal tandem duplications (Flt3-ITD), BCR-ABL and JAK2^{V617F} which cause AML, CML and other myeloproliferative diseases (MPD), respectively [1]. STAT5 proteins are recognized as major drivers in the development and/or maintenance of CML as well as in the proliferation and survival of AML cells [2–4]. The development of tyrosine kinase inhibitors (TKI) targeting BCR-ABL such as imatinib mesylate (IM) has revolutionized the treatment of CML. Despite this success story, IM is not totally curative and approximately 50% of patients remain therapy-free after IM discontinuation. The inability of IM to completely eradicate leukemic stem cells (LSC) is probably responsible for the relapse of CML patients [5]. Moreover, the occurrence of *BCR-ABL* mutations in progressive or relapsed disease promotes IM resistance of CML cells [6]. Therefore, there is a need for complementary therapeutic strategies to cure CML. STAT5 fulfils all the criteria of a major drug target in CML [7]. High STAT5 expression levels have been shown not only to enhance IM resistance in CML cells but also to trigger *BCR-ABL* mutations by inducing the production of reactive oxygen species (ROS) responsible for DNA damage [8,9]. Moreover, STAT5 was shown to play a key role in the maintenance of chemoresistant CML stem cells [10]. Thus, targeting STAT5 would also benefit relapsed CML patients who became resistant to TKI. Several approaches have been used to target STAT5 in leukemia. Among them, cell-based screening with small molecule libraries of already approved drugs allowed the identification of the psychotropic drug pimozide as a potential STAT5 inhibitor in CML cells [11]. Pimozide decreased the tyrosine phosphorylation of STAT5 and induced growth arrest and apoptosis in CML cells. In addition, pimozide was shown to target the deubiquitinating (DUB) enzyme, USP1, in leukemic cells indicating that the effects of pimozide on STAT5 activity might be indirect [12]. Indirubin derivatives were also reported to inhibit STAT5 phosphorylation in CML cells but the mechanism of inhibition is most likely suppression of upstream tyrosine kinases [13]. More recently, a number of small inhibitors that bind to the Src homology domain 2 (SH_2) required for STAT5 activation and dimer formation, have been described [14]. These compounds exhibit potent and selective binding activity for STAT5 by effectively disrupting phosphopeptide interactions. Some of these inhibitors bind STAT5 proteins in a nanomolar range and inhibit the tyrosine phosphorylation of STAT5 and CML/AML cell growth in a micromolar range [15–17]. A final approach is to target STAT5 activity through the activation of peroxisome proliferator-activated receptor gamma (PPARγ) [18]. Indeed, the existence of cross-talk between PPARγ and STAT5 has been discussed. For instance, antidiabetic drugs such as glitazones, which are PPARγ agonists, were shown to have antileukemic activity [19,20]. Activation of PPARγ by pioglitazone not only decreases the phosphorylation of STAT5 in CML cells but also reduces expression of *STAT5* genes in quiescent and resistant CML stem cells [10]. Importantly, the combined use of pioglitazone and IM triggers apoptosis of these leukemic cells suggesting that besides phosphorylation, inhibition of STAT5 expression is of prime importance for resistant CML stem cell eradication. Based on these different data, we sought to identify new STAT5 inhibitors in a library of PPARα/γ ligands that were synthetized in our laboratory [21,22]. The synthesis of derivatives of a "hit" compound identified in the library screening allowed the discovery of a new inhibitor of STAT5 signaling in CML and AML cells [23]. This molecule (17f) selectively inhibits the phosphorylation and transcriptional activity of STAT5 and induces apoptosis of CML and AML cells. Herein, we showed that 17f associated with IM or Ara-C resensitizes CML and AML cells, respectively, that acquired resistance to these drugs. We demonstrated that 17f treatment reduces STAT5B protein levels in resistant CML and AML cells, suggesting that 17f overcomes chemotherapy resistance though the downregulation of this protein. We also found that 17f suppresses expression of oncogenic $STAT5^{N642H}$ mutant in transformed Ba/F3 cells.

2. Results

2.1. *Effects of 17f Compound on Growth and Viability of IM-Sensitive and IM-Resistant BCR-ABL⁺ Cells*

Initial experiments were carried out to determine the effects of 17f alone (see structure in Figure S1) on K562 cells that are sensitive (K562S) or resistant (K562R) to IM treatment. These in vitro models are depicted in Figure 1A. Sensitive and resistant cells were treated with various concentrations of 17f (ranging from 1 to 10 μM). Growth and viability were determined by trypan blue exclusion (Figure 1B) and MTT (3-(4,5-dimethylthiazol-2-yl)-2,5-diphenyltetrazolium bromide) (Figure 1C) assays. Addition of 17f clearly blocked the growth of K562S cells while K562R cells remain insensitive to 17f treatment at the same concentration. The EC_{50} value was found to be two times higher in K562R cells than in K562S cells (14.5 ± 4.8 μM vs. 6.9 ± 1.7 μM). We also observed that treatment with 5 μM 17f did not affect the growth and viability of K562R cells and used this suboptimal concentration in most experiments to evaluate the combined effects of 17f and IM.

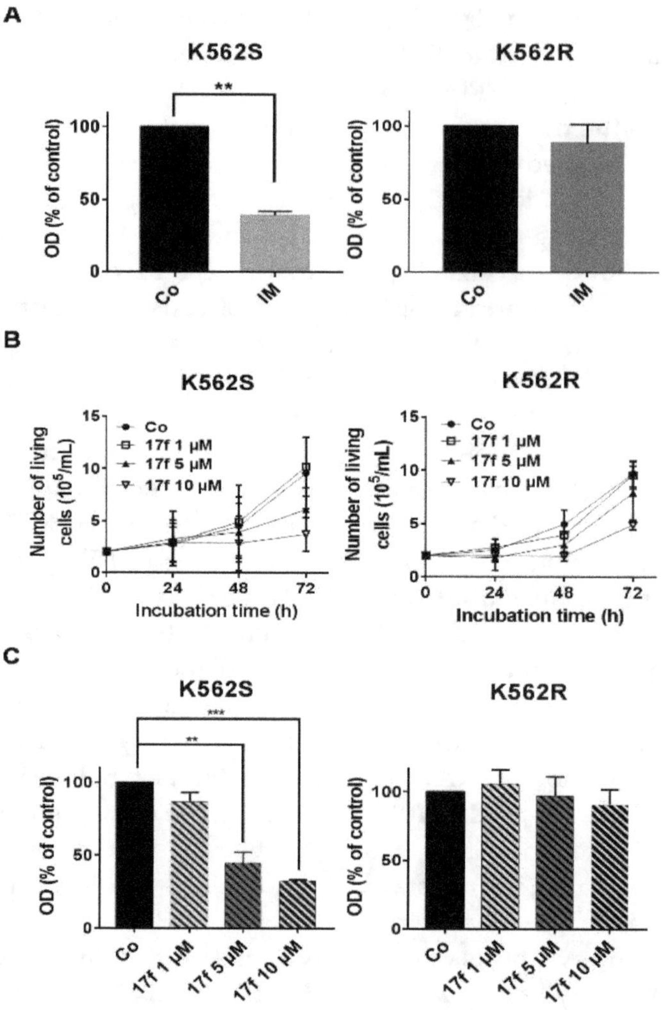

Figure 1. Effects of 17f molecule on K562S and K562R cell growth (**A**) Imatinib mesylate (IM)-sensitive K562 (K562S) and IM-resistant K562 cells (K562R) were treated with 1 μM IM or DMSO as control (Co) for 48 h. Cell viability was determined by MTT assays (data are presented as mean ± SD of three independent experiments ($n = 3$) in triplicates, *** $p < 0.001$; one sample t-test). (**B**) K562S and K562R cells were treated with 17f or DMSO as control (Co) for the indicated times. Growth kinetics were determined by trypan blue dye exclusion assays ($n = 3$ in triplicates, data are mean ± SD). (**C**) Cell viability was measured by MTT assays after treatment of K562S or K562R cells with increasing concentrations of 17f or DMSO as control (Co) during 48 h ($n = 3$ in triplicates, data are mean ± SD, ** $p < 0.01$, *** $p < 0.001$; one sample t-test).

2.2. *17f Induces Apoptosis and Cell Cycle Arrest in K562R Cells and Relieves the Resistance to IM*

We then addressed whether 17f in combination with IM might directly abrogate the resistance of K562R cells to IM. K562S and K562R cells were treated with 17f in the presence of IM and cell growth and viability were determined by MTT assays (Figure 2A). As expected, IM strongly inhibited the growth of K562S cells. This inhibition was further enhanced by 17f in a dose-dependent fashion. Interestingly, we found that the addition of 1 μM 17f in the presence of IM was already enough to significantly reduce the growth and viability of K562R cells. Treatment with 5 μM and 10 μM of 17f further increased this inhibitory effect. To analyze the growth-suppressive properties of 17f in K562R cells, we determined the impact of this small molecule on apoptosis and the cell cycle. 17f induced apoptosis and changes in cell cycle phase distribution in a concentration-dependent manner (Figure 2B,C). 17f significantly increased the number of cells in the G_0 phase indicating that treatment with this compound induced quiescence of K562R cells.

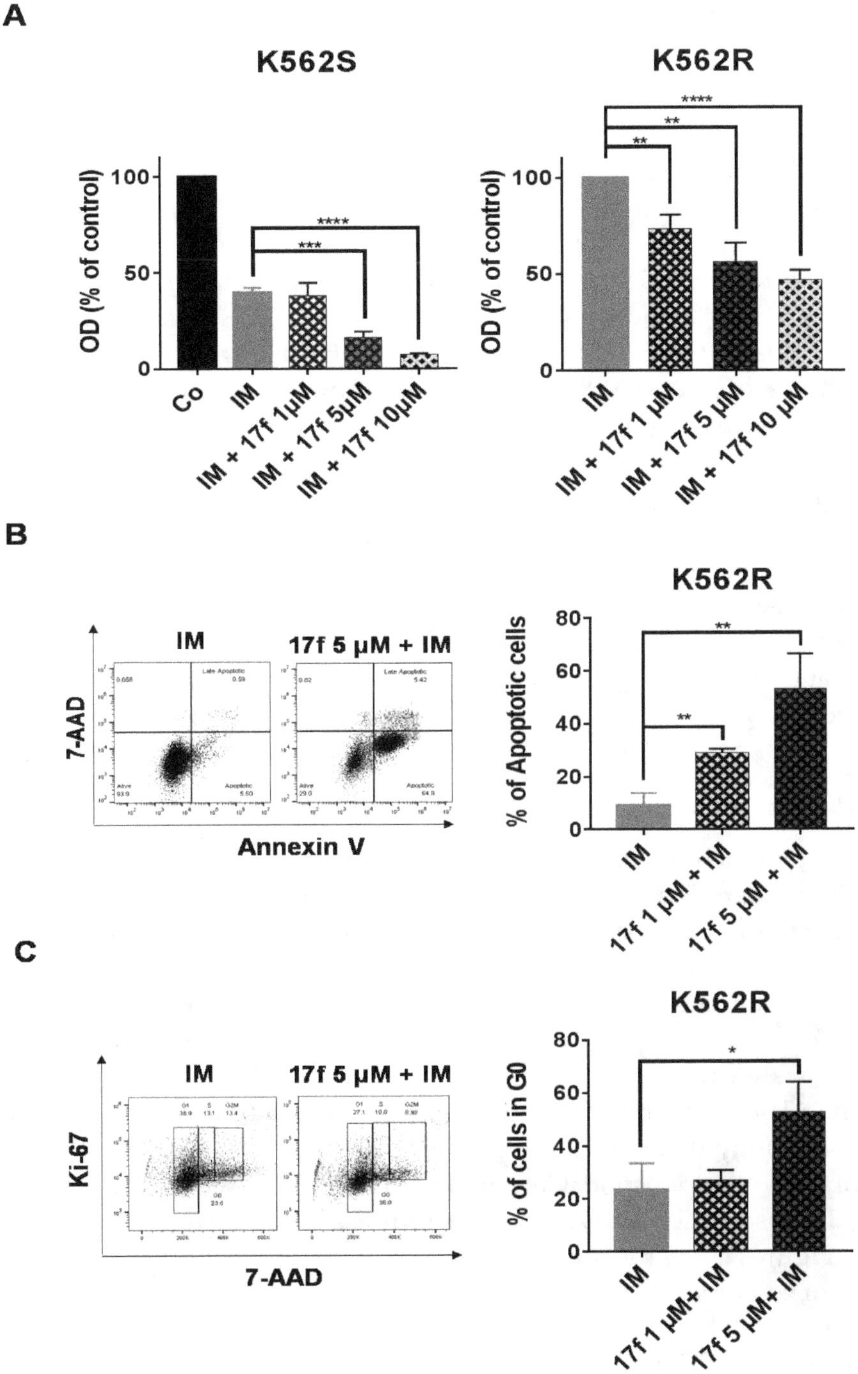

Figure 2. 17f overcomes the resistance of K562R cells to IM treatment. (**A**) K562S and K562R cells were treated with IM or not (Co) with or without 17f for 48 h. Cell viability was determined by MTT assays. (**B**) K562R cells cultured for 48 h with IM and 17f or IM vs. DMSO as control. Cells were stained with anti-annexin V coupled with FITC (fluorescein isothiocyanate) and with 7-amino-actinomycin D (7-AAD) to determine the percentages of apoptotic cells. One representative experiment is shown (left panel). (**C**) K562R cells treated for 48 h with IM and 17f or IM and DMSO as control were stained with 7-AAD and an Alexa Fluor 488-conjugated anti-Ki-67 antibody. Cell cycle phase distributions were then estimated by flow cytometry. The histogram presents the percentage of cells in the G_0 phase. One representative experiment is shown (left panel) ($n = 3$ in triplicates, data are mean ± SD, * $p < 0.05$, ** $p < 0.01$, *** $p < 0.001$, **** $p < 0.0001$).

2.3. 17f Inhibits STAT5-Dependent Transcriptional Activity in K562R Cells

We previously showed that 17f inhibits the transcriptional activity of STAT5 in CML cells. We then asked whether this small molecule also affects the activity of these proteins in IM-resistant K562R cells. We first determined the impact of this compound on the transcriptional activation of a reporter gene driven by a STAT5-specific promoter. K562S and K562R cells were transfected with a construct containing six tandem copies of the STAT5 response element in front of the minimal TK promoter fused to the luciferase reporter gene (6×(STAT5)-TK-luc). As control, cells were also transfected with a TK-luciferase vector without STAT5 response elements (TK-luc). Luciferase activity was determined 48 h post-transfection in K562S and K562R cells treated with DMSO as control, 17f (5 μM) and/or IM (1 μM). As expected, constitutive STAT5 activity induced by BCR-ABL increased luciferase activity in K562S cells transfected with the STAT5-dependent promoter construct compared to cells transfected with the control TK-luc vector (Figure 3A). This enhanced luciferase activity was strongly reduced after 17f or IM treatment. In sharp contrast, the luciferase activity remained elevated after treatment with IM in K562R cells transfected with the STAT5-dependent reporter construct, although this enzymatic activity was strongly decreased after the addition of 17f and IM. qRT-PCR experiments were then conducted to determine the effects of 17f on STAT5-dependent expression of target genes such as *PIM1* and *CISH* (Figure 3B). As expected, 17f or IM reduced expression of both genes in sensitive K562S cells while this effect was observed in resistant K562R cells after treatment with both compounds. Collectively, these data strongly suggest that 17f inhibits the transcriptional activity of STAT5 to bypass IM resistance in K562R cells.

2.4. 17f Inhibits STAT5B Protein Expression in IM-Resistant K562 Cells

We then determined the impact of 17f on BCR-ABL-induced tyrosine phosphorylation of STAT5 (P-$Y^{694/699}$-STAT5) by western blot and flow cytometry analysis (Figure 4A, Figures S2–S4). K562S and K562R cells were treated for 24 h instead of 48 h to analyze the early effects on STAT5 phosphorylation. IM strongly reduced P-Y-STAT5 levels in K562S, and the addition of 17f further enhanced this effect. P-Y-STAT5 levels were maintained in IM-treated K562R cells but were decreased after the addition of 17f. Interestingly, the level of STAT5 phosphorylation was strikingly enhanced in K562R cells after removal of IM and was weakly affected by the addition of 17f (Figure S5). To determine whether changes in P-Y-STAT5 levels reflect differences in protein abundance, immunoblots were performed with an anti-STAT5 antibody that recognizes STAT5A and STAT5B proteins (Figure 4B and Figure S2). As expected, IM inhibited the phosphorylation of STAT5 in sensitive and resistant cells. Interestingly, we observed that the association of 17f with IM reduces STAT5 expression in K562R cells but not in K562S cells (see Figure S3A,B for quantification). qRT-PCR experiments were then conducted to evaluate the impact of combination treatments on *STAT5A* and *STAT5B* gene expression in K562R cells. Results showed that *STAT5A/5B* mRNA levels were not affected by 17f when associated with IM (Figure 4B). In contrast, western blot analysis clearly evidenced that STAT5B protein expression was decreased after combination treatments suggesting that 17f sensitizes K562R cells to IM treatment by targeting STAT5B protein (Figure 4C).

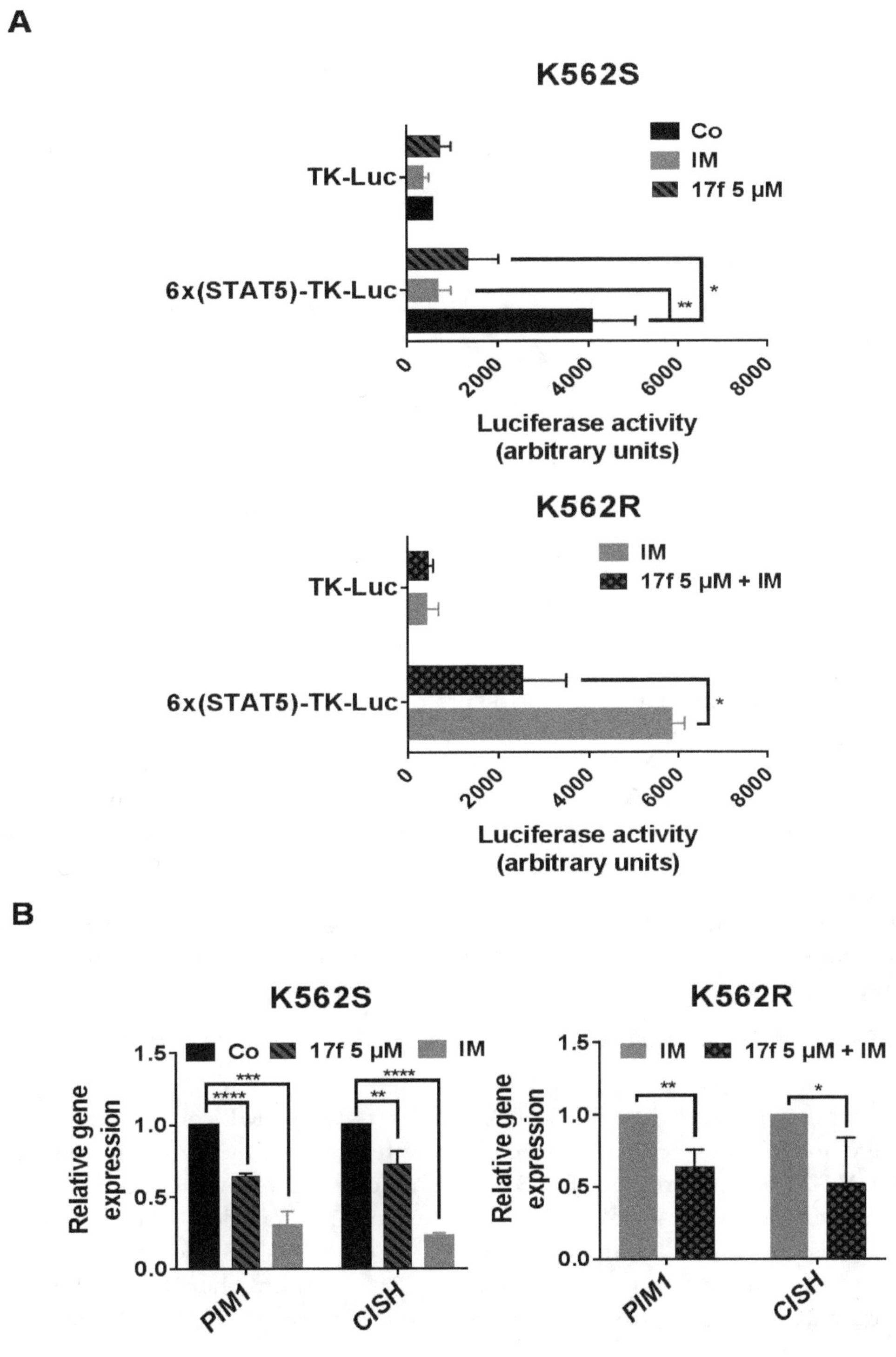

Figure 3. 17f associated with IM inhibit STAT5 activity in resistant K562R cells. (**A**) K562S or K562R cells transfected with a 6×(STAT5)-TK-luciferase reporter construct or a control TK-luciferase vector were treated or not (Co) with 17f (5 μM), IM (1 μM) or with the combination of 17f and IM for 48 h. Luciferase activities were then determined as described in Methods. Luciferase activity (arbitrary units) in the histogram represents the relative luminescence unit (rlu) values/mg of proteins (n = 3 in triplicates, data are mean ± SD, * $p < 0.05$, ** $p < 0.001$). (**B**) qRT-PCR analysis of *PIM1* and *CISH* expression in K562S and K562R treated or not (Co) with IM (1 μM),17f (5 μM) or with combined 17f and IM for 24 h. Results are presented as the fold change in *PIM1* and *CISH* gene expression in treated cells normalized to internal control genes (*GAPDH*, *ACTB* and *RPL13a*) and relative to control condition (normalized to 1) (n = 3 in triplicates, data are mean ± SD, * $p < 0.05$; one-sample t-test).

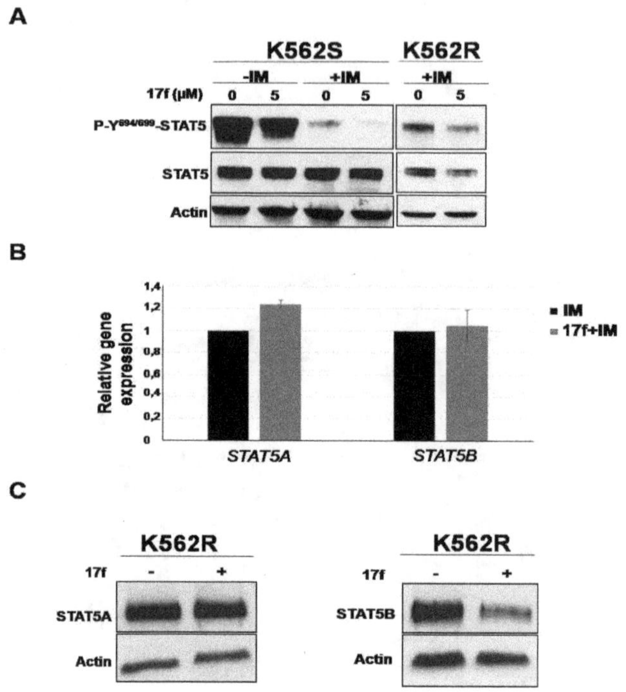

Figure 4. 17f associated with IM inhibits STAT5B protein expression in K562R cells (**A**) Protein extracts from K562S and K562R cells treated with 17f 5 μM or DMSO with or without IM for 24 h were analyzed by western blotting to detect P-$Y^{694/699}$-STAT5 and STAT5 protein expression (n = 2). Actin served as the loading control. (**B**) qRT-PCR analysis of *STAT5A* and *STAT5B* expression in K562R cultured with IM (1 μM) as control or treated with 17f (5μM) and IM for 24 h. Results are presented as the fold change in *STAT5A* and *STAT5B* gene expression in treated cells normalized to internal control genes (*GAPDH, ACTB* and *RPL13a*) and relative to control condition (normalized to 1) (n = 3 in triplicates, data are mean ± SD, * $p < 0.05$; one sample t-test). (**C**) Expression of STAT5A and STAT5B proteins in K562R cells treated or not with 17f (5 μM) was analyzed by western blot (n = 2). Actin served as the loading control.

2.5. *Effects of 17f on Growth and Viability of Ara-C-Sensitive and Ara-C-Resistant FLT3-ITD Expressing Leukemic Cells*

STAT5 is also phosphorylated by FLT3-ITD, a major TKO in AML cells. To exclude the possibility that 17f-mediated inhibition of STAT5 and cell growth is a peculiarity of IM-resistant BCR-ABL^+ cells, we used MV4-11 cells expressing FLT3-ITD that acquired resistance to Ara-C, a conventional therapeutic agent that affects DNA replication. Sensitive and resistant MV4-11 cell models are depicted in Figure 5A. We first evaluated the impact of 17f alone on MV4-11S and MV4-11R cell growth and showed that MV4-11R cells were more resistant to 17f treatment than MV4-11S cells (Figure 5B). Based on these data, IC_{50} values were found to be three-fold higher in MV4-11R than in MV11-4S cells (10.79 ± 3.2 vs. 3.55 ± 0.47).

2.6. *17f Sensitizes MV4-11R Cells to Ara-C Treatment*

We then analyzed the effects of 17f on MV4-11S and MV4-11R cell growth in the presence of Ara-C using trypan blue dye exclusion (Figure 6A) and MTT assays (Figure 6B). Addition of 17f significantly enhanced the growth inhibition and cytotoxic effect of Ara-C in MV4-11S cells. Importantly, 17f greatly reduced the growth of resistant MV4-11R cells cultured with Ara-C in a concentration-dependent fashion. This growth inhibition was already observed with 1 μM, a concentration that did not affect the growth of MV4-11R cells cultured in the absence of Ara-C. These data indicated that the addition of 17f overcomes the resistance of MV4-11R cells to Ara-C.

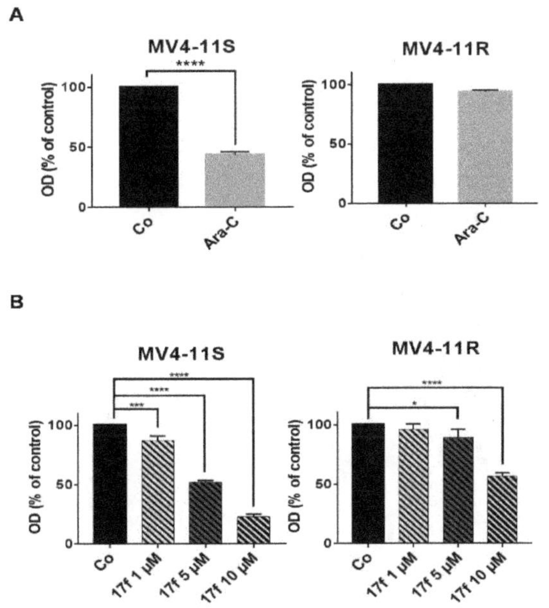

Figure 5. Effects of 17f on MV4-11S and MV4-11R cell growth (**A**) Ara-C-sensitive MV4-11 (MV4-11S) and Ara-C-resistant MV4-11 (MV4-11R) cells were treated with 1 µM Ara-C or DMSO as control (Co) for 48 h. Cell viability was then determined by MTT assays ($n = 3$ in triplicates, data are mean ± SD, **** $p < 0.0001$; one-sample t-test). (**B**) MV4-11S and MV4-11R cells were treated or not (Co) with increasing concentrations of 17f during 48 h. Cell viability was determined by MTT assays ($n = 3$ in triplicates, data are mean ± SD, ** $p < 0.01$, *** $p < 0.001$, **** $p < 0.0001$; one-sample t-test).

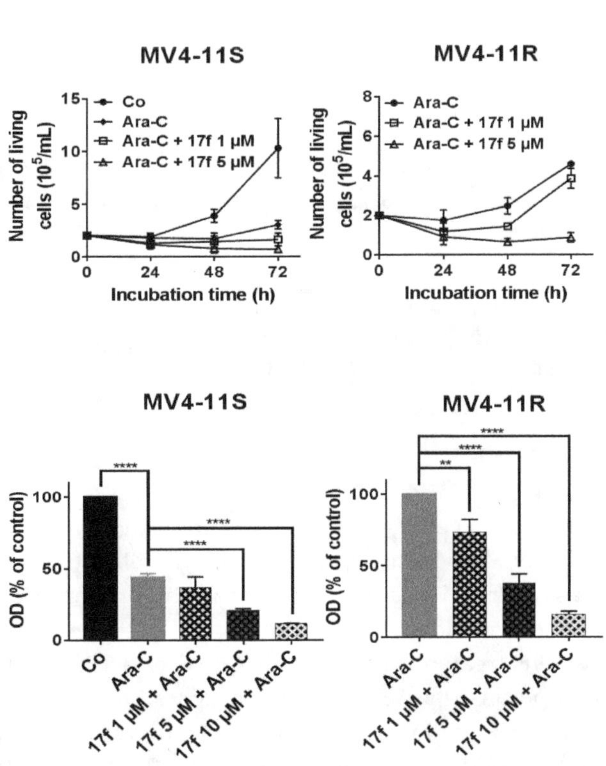

Figure 6. 17f relieves the resistance of MV4-11R cells to ARA-C treatment. (**A**) MV4-11S or MV4-11R cells were treated with Ara-C or not (Co) with or without 17f. Growth kinetics were determined by Trypan blue dye exclusion assays ($n = 3$ in triplicates, data are mean ± SD). (**B**) MV4-11S or MV4-11R cells were treated with Ara-C or not (Co) with or without 17f for 48 h. Cell viability was determined by MTT assays ($n = 3$ in triplicates, data are mean ± SD, * $p < 0.05$, ** $p < 0.01$, **** $p < 0.0001$; one-sample t-test).

2.7. 17f Triggers Apoptosis, Cell Cycle Arrest and Inhibition of STAT5B Expression in MV4-11R Cells

We then evaluated the effects of 17f on apoptosis and the cell cycle in MV4-11R cells. A significant increase in apoptotic cells was observed (Figure 7A) only after treatment with 5 μM 17f, while the addition of 1 μM was enough to enhance the number of cells in the G_0 phase of the cell cycle (Figure 7B). These results indicated that the growth-suppressive properties of 17f primarily affect the cell cycle in MV4-11R cells and apoptosis at higher concentrations. We then asked whether 17f interferes with STAT5 signaling in Ara-C-resistant AML cells and analyzed the impact of 17f on phosphorylation and expression of STAT5 in MV4-11R cells. In the absence of Ara-C, the level of STAT5 phosphorylation was slightly enhanced in MV4-11R cells (Figure S5C,D). The addition of 17f with or without Ara-C inhibited STAT5 expression in MV4-11R cells (Figure 7C and Figures S2B and S3C). Likewise, STAT5B expression was reduced after treatment with 17f alone or with Ara-C in resistant cells (Figure 7D).

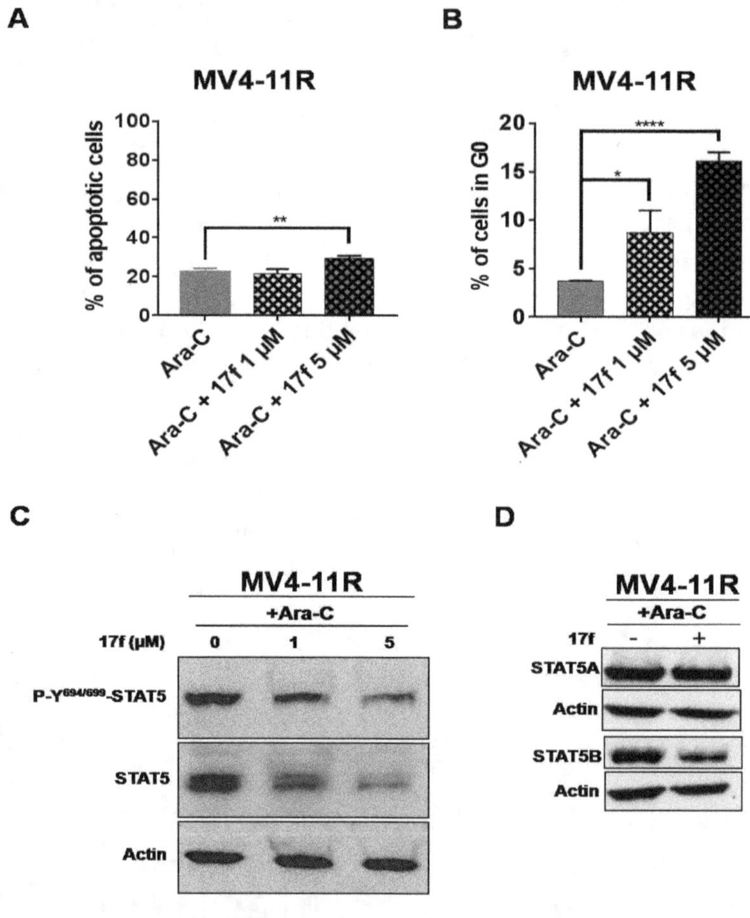

Figure 7. 17f promotes apoptosis, cell cycle arrest and inhibition of STAT5B protein expression in MV4-11R cells. (**A**) Flow cytometry histogram of MV4-11R cells cultured for 48 h with Ara-C and 17f or Ara-C and DMSO as control. Cells were stained with anti-annexin V coupled with FITC and with 7-AAD to determine the percentages of apoptotic cells ($n = 3$ in triplicates, data are mean ± SD, ** $p < 0.01$). (**B**) MV4-11R cells treated for 48 h with Ara-C and 17f or Ara-C and DMSO as control were stained with 7-AAD and an Alexa Fluor 488-conjugated anti-Ki67 antibody. Cell cycle phase distributions were then estimated by flow cytometry. The histogram presents the percentage of cells in the G_0 phase ($n = 3$ in triplicates, data are mean ± SD, * $p < 0.05$, *** $p < 0.001$). (**C**) Protein extracts from MV4-11R cells treated with Ara-C and 17f or Ara-C and DMSO for 24 h were analyzed by immunoblotting to detect P-$Y^{694/699}$-STAT5 and STAT5 protein expression ($n = 2$). Actin served as the loading control. (**D**) Expression of STAT5A and STAT5B proteins in MV4-11R cells treated or not with 17f (5 μM) was also analyzed by western blot ($n = 2$).

2.8. *17f Inhibits Expression of Oncogenic STAT5B^{N642H} Mutant*

Gain of function mutations of *STAT5B* have been described in hematopoietic malignancies. The recurrent hotspot mutation N642H has been identified in T cell leukemia and lymphomas and the STAT5B^{N642H} mutant was shown to induce T cell neoplasia in transgenic mice [24–27]. We therefore tested the ability of 17f to inhibit STAT5B^{N642H} expression and growth of hematopoietic cells transformed by this mutant. For this purpose, we used Ba/F3 cells expressing flag-tagged STAT5B^{N642H} or flag-tagged wild-type STAT5B (wtSTAT5B) as control [27]. We found that Ba/F3-STAT5B^{N642H} cells were more sensitive to 17f treatment than control Ba/F3-wtSTAT5B cells (Figure 8A). We then addressed whether STAT5^{N642H} expression was impacted by 17f and showed that 17f reduces expression of this mutant in Ba/F3 cells but does not affect wtSTAT5B or endogenous STAT5A expression after 24 h treatment (Figure 8B).

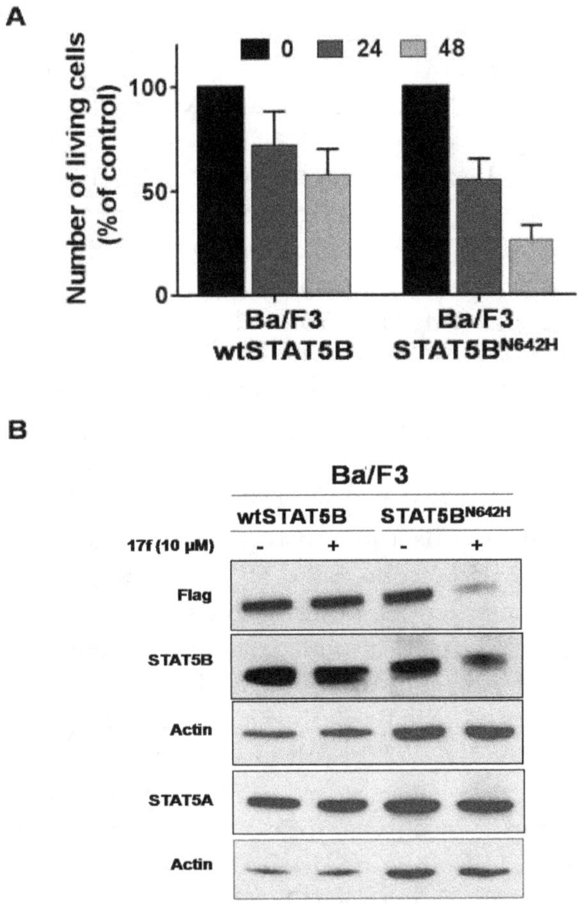

Figure 8. 17f inhibits STAT5B^{N642H} activity and expression in Ba/F3 cells. (**A**) Cells were treated or not with 17f (10 µM). Growth were then determined by Trypan blue dye exclusion assays at the indicated times (n = 5 in triplicates, data are mean ± SD). (**B**) Protein extracts from MV4-11R cells treated with 17f for 24 h were analyzed by immunoblotting to detect flag-tagged wtSTAT5B, STAT5B^{N642H} and endogenous STAT5A/STAT5B protein expression (n = 2). Actin served as the loading control.

3. Discussion

The development of pharmacological inhibitors targeting the JAK/STAT pathway has been the subject of intense investigation during the last decade. Among the STAT family members, STAT5 proteins are now recognized as important therapeutic targets in hematologic malignancies and also in certain solid tumors [28]. Distinct pharmacological compounds that directly or indirectly affect STAT5 activity and leukemia cell growth have been used or developed during these last years. We recently synthesized and discovered a new compound (17f) that inhibits STAT5 phosphorylation and transcriptional activity in various CML and AML cells, without detectable effects on other signal transduction molecules, such, as STAT3 and the protein kinases ERK1/2 and AKT [23]. We also demonstrated that 17f strongly reduces the growth of CML and AML cells with EC_{50} values below 10 μM close to EC_{50} values obtained with the STAT5 inhibitor pimozide (unpublished data) indicating that 17f as pimozide targets myeloid leukemia cells addicted to STAT5 signaling (see also Figure S1 for 17f and pimozide structures). In this study, we bring evidences that 17f also relieves the resistance of CML and AML cells to IM and Ara-C, respectively. Interestingly, we found that the concentrations of 17f required to restore the response to IM and Ara-C in resistant leukemic cells were much lower than EC_{50} values obtained for each resistant cell type. Indeed, inhibition of cell growth was already observed with 1 μM when combined with IM or Ara-C while EC_{50} values obtained for 17f compound alone were greater than 10 μM in these resistant cells. Depletion of IM or Ara-C in resistant cells might explain changes in the growth inhibitory effects of 17f. Indeed, we observed that the removal of IM strongly increases the phosphorylation of STAT5 in K562R cells. In these conditions, P-Y-STAT5 protein levels remain much higher in K562R cells after 17f treatment than in treated K562S cells, which are sensitive to lower concentrations of 17f. These data are in close agreement with a previously published study showing that high STAT5 levels mediate IM resistance in CML cells [8]. Although the removal of Ara-C results in a slight increase in STAT5 phosphorylation, the resistance of MV4-11R cells to this drug is not directly linked to overactivated STAT5. ERK1/2 and AKT kinases that also play a crucial role in cell survival, are involved in the resistance of MV4-11 cells to Ara-C [29]. It is then likely that Ara-C depletion may overexpress or overactivate these survival pathways in resistant MV4-11 cells. Whatever the resistance mechanism associated or not with STAT5 signaling, our data suggest that combination treatments with a STAT5 inhibitor might efficiently eliminate resistant CML and AML cells.

While 17f alone inhibited STAT5 phosphorylation in IM-depleted K562R cells, it decreased STAT5 expression in Ara-C-depleted MV4-11R cells. Importantly, combination treatments reduced expression of STAT5 in both resistant leukemic cells. The mechanisms involved in this downregulation remain unknown but are not associated with changes in *STAT5A* and *STAT5B* gene expression and specifically affect STAT5B protein. Importantly, we also demonstrated that 17f inhibits expression of $STAT5B^{N642H}$ protein expression in transformed Ba/F3 cells. $STAT5B^{N642H}$ is a driver mutation for T cell neoplasia and has been associated with aggressiveness, poor prognosis and an increased risk of relapse in T cell leukemia-lymphoma patients [24–27]. In addition to myeloid leukemia, 17f might be then employed to target lymphoproliferative disorders and lymphomas addicted to $STAT5B^{N642H}$ signaling.

It is likely that 17f inhibits STAT5B expression via the ubiquitin/proteasome-dependent degradation of this protein. Indeed, STAT5 proteins were previously shown to be ubiquitinated and several ubiquitination sites have been identified in STAT5A and STAT5B protein sequences [30,31]. Cbl, a well-known E3 ubiquitin ligase was found to interact with STAT5 and to induce its ubiquitination [30]. Moreover, cytokine-mediated STAT5 phosphorylation was enhanced in hematopoietic stem cells from *c-cbl* knockout mice [32]. 17f alone or associated with IM or Ara-C might then promote ubiquitination and proteasomal degradation of STAT5B protein in resistant leukemic cells as well as in $STAT5B^{N642H}$-expressing cells. In a similar vein, pimozide was shown to target USP1, a ubiquitin specific protease involved in the deubiquitination of transcription factors such as ID-1. Pimozide-mediated inhibition of USP-1 promotes ID1 degradation and inhibition of leukemic cell growth [12]. It is therefore conceivable that 17f activity is connected to *a* proteasome regulatory network that controls STAT5B protein degradation. Alternatively, the combination of 17f and IM or Ara-C might also target chaperone molecules such as the heat shock proteins HSP90 or HSP70 proteins which were previously shown to regulate expression and/or stability of STAT5 [33,34]. The dual inhibition of BCR-ABL and HSP90 was shown to abrogate the growth of IM-resistant CML cells [35]. Furthermore, a key role of STAT5 has been demonstrated in the synergistic effects of FLT3 and HSP90 inhibitors in FLT3-ITD-expressing leukemic cells [36]. Importantly, HSP90 inhibitors not only target STAT5 but also overcome the resistance of AML cells to FLT3 inhibitors [37]. HSP70 was also found to induce STAT5 expression and drug resistance in AML and CML cells and inhibition of STAT5 activity was sufficient to resensitize resistant leukemic cells to chemotherapy [34,38].

If the downregulation of STAT5A and STAT5B expression can occur via ubiquitin/proteasome-dependent protein degradation, the selective effect of 17f on STAT5B still remains unclear. Nevertheless, using a bacterial two-hybrid screening approach, we previously identified the tumor suppressor hTid1 as a specific binding partner of STAT5B [39]. hTid1 belongs to the DnaJ chaperone protein family, which contains the J domain, a highly conserved domain that binds to Hsp70. The DnaJ-Hsp70 complexes are involved in protein folding and protein degradation and hTid1 was shown to promote the ubiquitination and degradation of various cellular proteins including transcription factors [40]. We demonstrated that overexpression of hTid1 specifically suppresses STAT5B protein expression and the transforming potential of a constitutively active STAT5B variant (STAT5B1*6) in hematopoietic cells. 17f might then target specific effectors of STAT5B protein stability/degradation, a hypothesis that has yet to be experimentally tested.

Besides these potential mechanisms, the capacity of 17f to restore the sensitivity of resistant CML or AML cells to IM or Ara-C suggests that inhibitors targeting STAT5 expression would also benefit AML or CML patients who have developed resistance to chemotherapy. Accordingly, PPARγ agonists were shown to inhibit *STAT5A* and *STAT5B* gene expression and to synergize with IM to eradicate resistant CML stem cells [10]. Our findings suggest that targeting STAT5B protein is a promising therapeutic strategy to eradicate leukemic cells that acquired resistance to chemotherapeutic agents. This is also supported by previous works showing that STAT5B but not STAT5A plays a key role in BCR-ABL-induced leukemogenesis and in the sensitivity of CML cells to TKI treatment [41,42]. Recent studies indicated that STAT5 proteins also exert important non canonical functions in normal and cancer cells. For instance, unphosphorylated STAT5 (uSTAT5: non phosphorylated on Y694/699 residues) were shown to be transcriptionally active in self-renewing hematopoietic stem cells and to promote leukemia/lymphoma cell survival [43,44]. Selective inhibitors that only block tyrosine phosphorylation and dimer formation might then be insufficient to fully abrogate STAT5 activity and resistance to chemotherapy. Herein, we showed that that inhibition of STAT5B expression elicited by 17f might unlock drug resistance in CML and AML cells. Using these promising data as a lead, we carried out a rational search for new derivatives of 17f with enhanced antileukemic activity. Modeling work was initiated to identify a pharmacophore that could help to optimize the development of 17f derivatives working in the nanomolar range. These new compounds could represent promising drugs to overcome chemotherapy resistance in leukemia or lymphomas.

4. Materials and Methods

4.1. Cell Cultures and Reagents

IM-sensitive (K562S) and IM-resistant (K562R) BCR-ABL$^+$ cells and MV4-11 cells were obtained from American Type Culture Collection (ATCC) and Deutsche Sammlung von Mikroorganismens und Zellkulturen (DSMZ), respectively, and maintained according to the supplier's recommendations. K562R and Ara-C-resistant MV4-11 (MV4-11R) cells were obtained after cultures of K562S and sensitive MV4-11 (MV4-11S) cells with increasing concentrations of IM and Ara-C (until 1 μM). Ba/F3-STAT5B^{N642H} and Ba/F3-wtSTAT5B cells were previously described in [27]. All cell lines were cultured in RPMI 1640, with 10% fetal bovine serum, 2 mM glutamine, 100 U/mL penicillin and 100 μg/mL streptomycin at 37 °C, 5% CO_2. Resistant cells were cultured with 1 μM IM or Ara-C. IM was purchased from Selleckchem (Houston, TX, USA) and Ara-C from Sandoz France (Levallois-Perret, France). Ba/F3-wtSTAT5B were cultured with IL-3. The synthesis of the 17f compound was previously described in [23].

4.2. Cell Proliferation Assays

Cell viability and proliferation were studied using a MTT cell proliferation assay (Sigma-Aldrich, St Louis, MO, USA). Briefly, 2×10^4 leukemic cells were cultured in 100 μL of RPMI medium in 96-well plates and treated with drugs for 48 h. Cells were then incubated with 10 μL of MTT working solution (5 g/L of methylthiazolyldiphenyl-tetrazolium bromide) for 4 h. Cells were lysed overnight at 37 °C with 100 μL of SDS 10%, HCl 0.003%. Optical density (OD) at 570 nm was then measured using a spectrophotometer CLARIOstar® (BMG Labtech, Offenburg, Germany). Living cells were also enumerated using the trypan blue dye exclusion method.

4.3. Apoptosis and Cell Cycle Analysis

Cells were washed with PBS, then stained (10^6 cells) in buffer containing FITC-annexin V and 7-amino-actinomycin D (7-AAD) (Beckmann Coulter, Fullerton, CA, USA) for 15 min at 4 °C and analyzed by flow cytometry (Becton Dickinson Accuri™ C6 flow cytometer). For cell cycle analysis [45], cells were first incubated with fixing solution (PFA 2%, Hepes 1%, saponin 0.03%) for 15 min and then in PFS permeabilization solution (PBS 1×, SVF 10%, saponin 0.03%, Hepes 1%). Cells were next stained for 30 min at room temperature with anti-Ki67-Alexa Fluor 488 monoclonal antibody or the corresponding isotype as control (Becton-Dickinson, Franklin Lakes, NJ, USA) before analysis by flow cytometry (Becton Dickinson Accuri™ C6 flow cytometer). The FlowJo® software (V10.1, BD Biosciences, Franklin Lakes, NJ, USA) was used to analyze data.

4.4. Plasmids, Transfection and Luciferase Reporter Assays

The 6×(STAT5)-TK-luc containing six tandem copies of the STAT5 binding site linked to the minimal TK-luciferase reporter gene and control TK-luc plasmids have been described elsewhere [46]. For transient transfection assays, cells were electroporated (270 V, 950 μF) with the different constructs (50 μg). Transfected cells were expanded for 24 h in medium and then treated for 48 h. Cell extracts were then prepared in luciferase buffer according to the manufacturer's protocol (One Glo luciferase assay kit, Promega, Madison, WI, USA). Luciferase activities were measured in a luminometer CLARIOstar® (BMG Labtech, Offenburg, Germany).

4.5. Western Blot

Cells were suspended in Laemmli's 2× buffer (Bio-Rad, Hercules, CA, USA), separated on SDS/PAGE and blotted onto nitrocellulose membrane. Blots were incubated with the following antibodies (Abs): P-$Y^{694/699}$-STAT5, Actin (Cell Signaling Technology, Danvers, MA, USA), STAT5 (BD Transduction Laboratories, Franklin Lakes, NJ, USA), STAT5A and STAT5B (Zymed/ThermoFisher Scientific, Waltham, MA, USA). Membranes were developed with the ECL chemiluminescence detection system (GE Healthcare, Little Chalfont Buckinghamshire, UK) using specific peroxidase (HRP) conjugated to rabbit or mouse IgG antibodies (Cell Signaling Technology).

4.6. P-$Y^{694/699}$-STAT5 Flow Cytometry Analysis

Cells were washed in PBS and incubated with a fixing solution PFA 4% for 15 min at room temperature. The first permeabilization solution PBS/Triton X-100 0.2% was then added and incubated for 30 min at 37 °C. After being washed with PBS/BSA 0.5%, cells were suspended with the second permeabilization solution PBS/MeOH 50% and incubated for 10 min on ice. Cells were then stained with anti P-$Y^{694/699}$-STAT5 antibodies or the corresponding isotype as control (BD Biosciences, NJ, USA) for 30 min at room temperature before analysis by flow cytometry (FACS Canto II, BD Biosciences).

4.7. qRT-PCR Analysis

RNA samples were reverse-transcribed using the SuperScript®VILO cDNA synthesis kit (Invitrogen, Carlsbad, CA, USA) as recommended by the supplier. The resulting cDNAs were used for quantitative real-time PCR (qRT-PCR). PCR primers (*PIM1*: *for* 5′-TTTCGAGCATGACGAAGAGA-3′, *rev* 5′-GGGCCAAGCACCATCTAAT-3′; *CISH*: 5′- AGCCAAGACCTTCTCCTACCTT-3′, *rev* 5′-TGGCATCTTCTGCAGGTGT-3′; *STAT5A*: *for* 5′-TCCCTATAACATGTACCCACA-3′, *rev* 5′-ATGGTCTCATCCAGGTCGAA-3′; *STAT5B*: *for* 5′-TGAAGGCCACCATCATCAG-3′, *rev* 5′-TGTTCAAGATCTCGCCACTG-3′) were designed with the ProbeFinder software (Roche Applied Sciences, Basel, Switzerland) and used to amplify the RT-generated cDNAs. qRT-PCR analyses were performed on the Light Cycler 480 thermocycler II (Roche). *GAPDH* (glyceraldehyde-3-phosphate dehydrogenase), *ACTB* (actin beta) and *RPL13A* were used as reference genes for normalization of qRT-PCR experiments. Each reaction condition was performed in triplicate. Relative gene expression was analyzed using the $2^{-\Delta\Delta Ct}$ method [47].

5. Conclusions

In summary, this work shows for the first time that inhibition of STAT5B expression might be a promising targeting strategy to bypass the resistance of CML and AML cells to TKI or conventional chemotherapeutic agents. Investigations to elucidate the mechanisms involved in STAT5B downregulation induced by these combination therapies might help to design new inhibitors that specifically target cancer cells addicted to oncogenic STAT5B signaling.

Author Contributions: Conceptualization, M.B.-B., G.P. and F.G.; Formal analysis, M.B.-B. and F.G.; Funding acquisition, G.P. and F.G.; Investigation, M.B.-B., M.D., N.V., M.P. and L.J.; Methodology, M.B.-B., M.D., N.V., M.P. and L.J.; Project administration, G.P. and F.G.; Resources, G.P. and F.G.; Supervision, G.P.; Validation, M.B.-B., M.D., N.V., M.P., F.M., G.P. and F.G.; Visualization, F.G.; Writing—original draft, M.B.-B., G.P. and F.G.; Writing—review & editing, M.D., N.V., L.J., F.M., M.-C.V.-M. and O.H.

Acknowledgments: We would like to thank Emmanuel Pecnard, Farah Kouzi and Elodie Coste for technical assistance; Christina Maria Wagner and Heidi A. Neubauer for providing Ba/F3STAT5B^{N642H} and Ba/F3wtSTAT5B cells.

References

1. Bunting, K.D. STAT5 signaling in normal and pathologic hematopoiesis. *Front. Biosci.* **2007**, *12*, 2807–2820. [CrossRef] [PubMed]
2. Hoelbl, A.; Schuster, C.; Kovacic, B.; Zhu, B.; Wickre, M.; Hoelzl, M.A.; Fajmann, S.; Grebien, F.; Warsch, W.; Stengl, G.; et al. Stat5 is indispensable for the maintenance of Bcr/abl-positive leukemia. *Eur. Mol. Biol. Organ. Mol. Med.* **2010**, *2*, 98–110.
3. Ye, D.; Wolff, N.; Li, L.; Zhang, S.; Ilaria, R.L., Jr. STAT5 signaling is required for the efficient induction and maintenance of CML in mice. *Blood* **2006**, *107*, 4917–4925. [CrossRef] [PubMed]
4. Mizuki, M.; Fenski, R.; Halfter, H.; Matsumura, I.; Schmidt, R.; Müller, C.; Grüning, W.; Kratz-Albers, K.; Serve, S.; Steur, C.; et al. Flt3 mutations from patients with acute myeloid leukemia induce transformation of 32D cells mediated by the Ras and STAT5 pathways. *Blood* **2000**, *96*, 3907–3914. [CrossRef]
5. Chomel, J.C.; Bonnet, M.L.; Sorel, N.; Sloma, I.; Bennaceur-Griscelli, A.; Rea, D.; Legros, L.; Marfaing-Koka, A.; Bourhis, J.H.; Ame, S.; et al. Leukemic stem cell persistence in chronic myeloid leukemia patients in deep molecular response induced by tyrosine kinase inhibitors and the impact of therapy discontinuation. *Oncotarget* **2016**, *7*, 35293–35301. [CrossRef]
6. Gambacorti-Passerini, C.B.; Gunby, R.H.; Piazza, R.; Galietta, A.; Rostagno, R.; Scapozza, L. Molecular mechanisms of resistance to imatinib in Philadelphia-chromosome-positive leukaemias. *Lancet Oncol.* **2003**, *4*, 75–85. [CrossRef]
7. Cumaraswamy, A.A.; Todic, A.; Resetca, D.; Minden, M.D.; Gunning, P.T. Inhibitors of Stat5 protein signaling. *Med. Chem. Commun.* **2012**, *3*, 22–27. [CrossRef]
8. Warsch, W.; Kollmann, K.; Eckelhart, E.; Fajmann, S.; Cerny-Reiterer, S.; Hölbl, A.; Gleixner, K.V.; Dworzak, M.; Mayerhofer, M.; Hoermann, G.; et al. High STAT5 levels mediate imatinib resistance and indicate disease progression in chronic myeloid leukemia. *Blood* **2011**, *117*, 3409–3420. [CrossRef]

9. Warsch, W.; Grundschober, E.; Berger, A.; Gille, L.; Cerny-Reiterer, S.; Tigan, A.-S.; Hoelbl-Kovacic, A.; Valent, P.; Moriggl, R.; Sexl, V. STAT5 triggers BCR-ABL1 mutation by mediating ROS production in chronic myeloid leukemia. *Oncotarget* **2012**, *3*, 1669–1687. [CrossRef]
10. Prost, S.; Relouzat, F.; Spentchian, M.; Ouzegdouh, Y.; Saliba, J.; Massonnet, G.; Beressi, J.P.; Verhoeyen, E.; Raggueneau, V.; Maneglier, B.; et al. Erosion of the chronic myeloid leukemia stem cell pool by PPARγ agonists. *Nature* **2015**, *525*, 380–383. [CrossRef]
11. Nelson, E.A.; Walker, S.R.; Weisberg, E.; Bar-Natan, M.; Barrett, R.; Gashin, L.B.; Terrell, S.; Klitgaard, J.L.; Santo, L.; Addorio, M.R.; et al. The STAT5 inhibitor pimozide decreases survival of chronic myelogenous leukemia cells resistant to kinase inhibitors. *Blood* **2011**, *117*, 3421–3429. [CrossRef] [PubMed]
12. Mistry, H.; Hsieh, G.; Buhrlage, S.J.; Huang, M.; Park, E.; Cuny, G.D.; Galinsky, I.; Stone, R.M.; Gray, N.S.; D'Andrea, A.D.; et al. Small-molecule inhibitors of USP1 target ID1 degradation in leukemic cells. *Mol. Cancer Ther.* **2013**, *12*, 2651–2662. [CrossRef] [PubMed]
13. Nam, S.; Scuto, A.; Yang, F.; Chen, W.; Park, S.; Yoo, H.S.; Konig, H.; Bhatia, R.; Cheng, X.; Merz, K.H.; et al. Indirubin derivatives induce apoptosis of chronic myelogenous leukemia cells involving inhibition of Stat5 signaling. *Mol. Oncol.* **2012**, *6*, 276–283. [CrossRef] [PubMed]
14. Page, B.D.; Khoury, H.; Laister, R.C.; Fletcher, S.; Vellozo, M.; Manzoli, A.; Yue, P.; Turkson, J.; Minden, M.D.; Gunning, P.T. Small molecule STAT5-SH2 domain inhibitors exhibit potent antileukemia activity. *J. Med. Chem.* **2012**, *55*, 1047–1055. [CrossRef]
15. Cumaraswamy, A.A.; Lewis, A.M.; Geletu, M.; Todic, A.; Diaz, D.B.; Cheng, X.R.; Brown, C.E.; Laister, R.C.; Muench, D.; Kerman, K.; et al. Nanomolar-potency small molecule inhibitor of STAT5 protein. *Am. Chem. Soc. Med. Chem. Lett.* **2014**, *5*, 1202–1206. [CrossRef]
16. Elumalai, N.; Berg, A.; Rubner, S.; Blechschmidt, L.; Song, C.; Natarajan, K.; Matysik, J.; Berg, T. Rational development of Stafib-2: A selective, nanomolar inhibitor of the transcription factor STAT5b. *Sci. Rep.* **2017**, *7*, 819. [CrossRef]
17. Wingelhofer, B.; Maurer, B.; Heyes, E.C.; Cumaraswamy, A.A.; Berger-Becvar, A.; de Araujo, E.D.; Orlova, A.; Freund, P.; Ruge, F.; Park, J.; et al. Pharmacologic inhibition of STAT5 in acute myeloid leukemia. *Leukemia* **2018**, *32*, 1135–1146. [CrossRef]
18. Prost, S.; Le Dantec, M.; Augé, S.; Le Grand, R.; Derdouch, S.; Auregan, G.; Déglon, N.; Relouzat, F.; Aubertin, A.M.; Maillere, B.; et al. Human and simian immunodeficiency viruses deregulate early hematopoiesis through a Nef/PPARγ/STAT5 signaling pathway in macaques. *J. Clin. Investig.* **2008**, *118*, 1765–1775. [CrossRef]
19. Liu, H.; Zang, C.; Fenner, M.H.; Liu, D.; Possinger, K.; Koeffler, H.P.; Elstner, E. Growth inhibition and apoptosis in human Philadelphia chromosome-positive lymphoblastic leukemia cell lines by treatment with the dual PPARα/γ ligand TZD18. *Blood* **2006**, *107*, 3683–3692. [CrossRef]
20. Bertz, J.; Zang, C.; Liu, H.; Wächter, M.; Possinger, K.; Koeffler, H.P.; Elstner, E. Compound 48, a novel dual PPAR α/γ ligand, inhibits the growth of human CML cell lines and enhances the anticancer-effects of imatinib. *Leuk. Res.* **2009**, *33*, 686–692. [CrossRef]
21. Parmenon, C.; Guillard, J.; Caignard, D.-H.; Hennuyer, N.; Staels, B.; Audinot-Bouchez, V.; Boutin, J.A.; Dacquet, C.; Ktorza, A.; Viaud-Massuard, M.C. 4,4-Dimethyl-1,2,3,4-Tetrahydroquinoline-Based PPARα/γ agonists. Part I: Synthesis and pharmacological evaluation. *Bioorg. Med. Chem. Lett.* **2008**, *18*, 1617–1622. [CrossRef]
22. Parmenon, C.; Guillard, J.; Caignard, D.-H.; Hennuyer, N.; Staels, B.; Audinot-Bouchez, V.; Boutin, J.A.; Dacquet, C.; Ktorza, A.; Viaud-Massuard, M.C. 4,4-Dimethyl-1,2,3,4-Tetrahydroquinoline-Based PPARα/γ agonists. Part II: Synthesis and pharmacological evaluation of oxime and acidic head group structural variations. *Bioorg. Med. Chem. Lett.* **2009**, *19*, 2683–2687. [CrossRef]
23. Juen, L.; Brachet-Botineau, M.; Parmenon, C.; Bourgeais, J.; Hérault, O.; Gouilleux, F.; Viaud-Massuard, M.C.; Prié, G. New inhibitor targeting signal transducer and activator of transcription 5 (STAT5) signaling in myeloid leukemias. *J. Med. Chem.* **2017**, *60*, 6119–6136. [CrossRef]
24. Kontro, M.; Kuusanmäki, H.; Eldfors, S.; Burmeister, T.; Andersson, E.I.; Bruserud, O.; Brümmendorf, T.H.; Edgren, H.; Gjertsen, B.T.; Itälä-Remes, M.; et al. Novel activating STAT5B mutations as putative drivers of T-cell acute lymphoblastic leukemia. *Leukemia* **2014**, *28*, 1738–1742. [CrossRef]
25. Bandapalli, O.R.; Schuessele, S.; Kunz, J.B.; Rausch, T.; Stütz, A.M.; Tal, N.; Geron, I.; Gershman, N.; Izraeli, S.;

Eilers, J.; et al. The activating STAT5B N642H mutation is a common abnormality in pediatric T-cell acute lymphoblastic leukemia and confers a higher risk of relapse. *Haematologica* **2014**, *99*, 188–192. [CrossRef]

26. Nicolae, A.; Xi, L.; Pittaluga, S.; Abdullaev, Z.; Pack, S.D.; Chen, J.; Waldmann, T.A.; Jaffe, E.S.; Raffeld, M. Frequent STAT5B mutations in $\gamma\delta$ hepatosplenic T-cell lymphomas. *Leukemia* **2014**, *28*, 2244–2248. [CrossRef]
27. Pham, H.T.T.; Maurer, B.; Prchal-Murphy, M.; Grausenburger, R.; Grundschober, E.; Javaheri, T.; Nivarthi, H.; Boersma, A.; Kolbe, T.; Elabd, M.; et al. STAT5BN642H is a driver mutation for T cell neoplasia. *J. Clin. Investig.* **2018**, *128*, 387–401. [CrossRef]
28. Liao, Z.; Nevalainen, M.T. Targeting transcription factor Stat5a/b as a therapeutic strategy for prostate cancer. *Am. J. Transl. Res.* **2011**, *3*, 133–138.
29. Ko, Y.C.; Hu, C.Y.; Liu, Z.H.; Tien, H.F.; Ou, D.L.; Chien, H.F.; Lin, L.I. Cytarabine-Resistant FLT3-ITD Leukemia Cells are Associated with TP53 Mutation and Multiple Pathway Alterations—Possible Therapeutic Efficacy of Cabozantinib. *Int. J. Mol. Sci.* **2019**, *20*, 1230. [CrossRef]
30. Goh, E.L.; Zhu, T.; Leong, W.Y.; Lobie, P.E. c-Cbl is a negative regulator of GH-stimulated STAT5-mediated transcription. *Endocrinology* **2002**, *143*, 3590–3603. [CrossRef]
31. Chen, Y.; Dai, X.; Haas, A.L.; Wen, R.; Wang, D. Proteasome-dependent down-regulation of activated Stat5A in the nucleus. *Blood* **2006**, *108*, 566–574. [CrossRef]
32. Rathinam, C.; Thien, C.B.; Langdon, W.Y.; Gu, H.; Flavell, R.A. The E3 ubiquitin ligase c-Cbl restricts development and functions of hematopoietic stem cells. *Genes Dev.* **2008**, *22*, 992–997. [CrossRef]
33. Moulick, K.; Ahn, J.H.; Zong, H.; Rodina, A.; Cerchietti, L.; Gomes DaGama, E.M.; Caldas-Lopes, E.; Beebe, K.; Perna, F.; Hatzi, K.; et al. Affinity-based proteomics reveal cancer-specific networks coordinated by Hsp90. *Nat. Chem. Biol.* **2011**, *7*, 818–826. [CrossRef]
34. Guo, F.; Sigua, C.; Bali, P.; George, P.; Fiskus, W.; Scuto, A.; Annavarapu, S.; Mouttaki, A.; Sondarva, G.; Wei, S.; et al. Mechanistic role of heat shock protein 70 in Bcr-Abl-mediated resistance to apoptosis in human acute leukemia cells. *Blood* **2005**, *105*, 1246–1255. [CrossRef]
35. Wu, L.; Yu, J.; Chen, R.; Liu, Y.; Lou, L.; Wu, Y.; Huang, L.; Fan, Y.; Gao, P.; Huang, M.; et al. Dual inhibition of Bcr-Abl and Hsp90 by C086 potently inhibits the proliferation of imatinib-resistant CML cells. *Clin. Cancer Res.* **2015**, *21*, 833–843. [CrossRef]
36. Yao, Q.; Nishiuchi, R.; Kitamura, T.; Kersey, J.H. Human leukemias with mutated FLT3 kinase are synergistically sensitive to FLT3 and Hsp90 inhibitors: The key role of the STAT5 signal transduction pathway. *Leukemia* **2005**, *19*, 1605–1612. [CrossRef]
37. Katayama, K.; Noguchi, K.; Sugimoto, Y. Heat shock protein 90 inhibitors overcome the resistance to Fms-like tyrosine kinase 3 inhibitors in acute myeloid leukemia. *Oncotarget* **2018**, *9*, 34240–34258. [CrossRef]
38. Pocaly, M.; Lagarde, V.; Etienne, G.; Ribeil, J.A.; Claverol, S.; Bonneu, M.; Moreau-Gaudry, F.; Guyonnet-Duperat, V.; Hermine, O.; Melo, J.V.; et al. Overexpression of the heat-shock protein 70 is associated to imatinib resistance in chronic myeloid leukemia. *Leukemia* **2007**, *21*, 93–101. [CrossRef]
39. Dhennin-Duthille, I.; Nyga, R.; Yahiaoui, S.; Gouilleux-Gruart, V.; Régnier, A.; Lassoued, K.; Gouilleux, F. The tumor suppressor hTid1 inhibits STAT5b activity via functional interaction. *J. Biol. Chem.* **2011**, *286*, 5034–5042. [CrossRef]
40. Bae, M.K.; Jeong, J.W.; Kim, S.H.; Kim, S.Y.; Kang, H.J.; Kim, D.M.; Bae, S.K.; Yun, I.; Trentin, G.A.; Rozakis-Adcock, M.; et al. Tid-1 interacts with the von Hippel-Lindau protein and modulates angiogenesis by destabilization of HIF-1α. *Cancer Res.* **2005**, *65*, 2520–2525. [CrossRef]
41. Schaller-Schönitz, M.; Barzan, D.; Williamson, A.J.; Griffiths, J.R.; Dallmann, I.; Battmer, K.; Ganser, A.; Whetton, A.D.; Scherr, M.; Eder, M. BCR-ABL affects STAT5A and STAT5B differentially. *PLoS ONE* **2014**, *9*, e97243. [CrossRef]
42. Kollmann, S.; Grundschober, E.; Maurer, B.; Warsch, W.; Grausenburger, R.; Edlinger, L.; Huuhtanen, J.; Lagger, S.; Hennighausen, L.; Valent, P.; et al. Twins with different personalities: STAT5B-but not STAT5A-has a key role in BCR/ABL-induced leukemia. *Leukemia* **2019**, *33*, 1583–1597. [CrossRef]
43. Park, H.J.; Li, J.; Hannah, R.; Biddie, S.; Leal-Cervantes, A.I.; Kirschner, K.; Flores Santa Cruz, D.; Sexl, V.; Göttgens, B.; Green, A.R. Cytokine-induced megakaryocytic differentiation is regulated by genome-wide loss of a uSTAT transcriptional program. *Eur. Mol. Biol. Organ. J.* **2016**, *35*, 580–594. [CrossRef]
44. Nagy, Z.S.; Rui, H.; Stepkowski, S.M.; Karras, J.; Kirken, R.A. A preferential role for STAT5, not constitutively

active STAT3, in promoting survival of a human lymphoid tumor. *J. Immunol.* **2006**, *177*, 5032–5040. [CrossRef]

45. Vignon, C.; Debeissat, C.; Georget, M.-T.; Bouscary, D.; Gyan, E.; Rosset, P.; Herault, O. Flow cytometric quantification of all phases of the cell cycle and apoptosis in a two-color fluorescence plot. *PLoS ONE* **2013**, *7*, e68425. [CrossRef]
46. Moriggl, R.; Gouilleux-Gruart, V.; Jähne, R.; Berchtold, S.; Gartmann, C.; Liu, X.; Hennighausen, L.; Sotiropoulos, A.; Groner, B.; Gouilleux, F. Deletion of the carboxyl-terminal transactivation domain of MGF-Stat5 results in sustained DNA binding and a dominant negative phenotype. *Mol. Cell. Biol.* **1996**, *16*, 5691–5700. [CrossRef]
47. Livak, K.J.; Schmittgen, T.D. Analysis of relative gene expression data using real-time quantitative PCR and the $2^{-\Delta\Delta CT}$ method. *Methods* **2001**, *25*, 402–408. [CrossRef]

8

STAT3, a Master Regulator of Anti-Tumor Immune Response

Cédric Rébé * and François Ghiringhelli *

Platform of Transfer in Cancer Biology, Centre Georges François Leclerc, INSERM LNC UMR1231, University of Bourgogne Franche-Comté, F-21000 Dijon, France

* Correspondence: crebe@cgfl.fr (C.R.); fghiringhelli@cgfl.fr (F.G.)

Abstract: Immune cells in the tumor microenvironment regulate cancer growth. Thus cancer progression is dependent on the activation or repression of transcription programs involved in the proliferation/activation of lymphoid and myeloid cells. One of the main transcription factors involved in many of these pathways is the signal transducer and activator of transcription 3 (STAT3). In this review we will focus on the role of STAT3 and its regulation, e.g., by phosphorylation or acetylation in immune cells and how it might impact immune cell function and tumor progression. Moreover, we will review the ability of STAT3 to regulate checkpoint inhibitors.

Keywords: STAT3; cancer; $CD4^+$ T cells; $CD8^+$ T cells; myeloid cells; immune check point

---

1. Introduction

STAT3 is part of the Signal Transducer and Activator of Transcription (STAT) family which includes seven members encoded by distinct genes. STAT3 has evolutionary conserved amino acid sequences between *H. sapiens* and *S. harrisii* (99.09%) [1]. In resting cells, STAT3 remains in an inactive form in the cytoplasm. Once activated, mainly through phosphorylation, STAT3 translocates to the nucleus to play its transcription activity for specific target genes [2]. STAT3 phosphorylation on tyrosine (Y705) is mainly regulated by members of Janus-activated kinases (JAK), whereas its phosphorylation on serine (S727) is commonly regulated by mitogen-activated protein kinases, CDK5 and protein kinase C [3]. Finally, histone acetyltransferase-mediated reversible acetylation of STAT3 on a single lysine residue (K685) is a third mechanism of STAT3 activation through STAT3 dimer stabilization [4]. However, the phosphorylation on S727 is responsible for a mitochondrial relocalization of STAT3 where it exerts non-transcriptional roles. This mitochondrial localization enables STAT3 to increase cell respiration (through electron transport chain complex activation) and Ras transformation [5]. Non-nuclear STAT3 can also regulate glycolysis, thus enhancing lactate production leading to the protection of cells from apoptosis and senescence and can also regulate calcium homeostasis, energy production and apoptosis at the endoplasmic reticulum level [6].

Regulation of STAT protein activation is controlled by negative regulators, e.g., PIAS (protein inhibitor of activated STAT) and SOCS (suppressors of cytokine signaling) proteins as well as protein tyrosine phosphatases. PIAS are nuclear factors that negatively regulate STAT transcriptional activity through many mechanisms, especially by interacting and thus blocking the DNA binding activity [7]. SOCS proteins directly or indirectly interact with tyrosine kinase SH2 domains to prevent JAK from activating STAT3 [8]. Protein tyrosine phosphatases (such as CD45, SHP-1 and SHP-2) remove phosphates from activated STATs, which represent a third level of STAT modulation [9–11]. Lastly, STAT3 has also been shown to go through ubiquitination-dependent proteosomal degradation [12].

Moreover, because of their homologies, STATs can form homodimer and heterodimers. Specificity depends on the activator signal and leads to the transcription of different target genes. For example, STAT3 can heterodimerized with STAT1, under IL-6 treatment [13].

It is now well-established that STAT3 signaling is a major intrinsic pathway driving apoptosis, inflammation, cellular transformation, survival, proliferation, invasion, angiogenesis and metastasis in cancer [14–17]. Moreover, STAT3 in cancer cells affects stromal cells function, establishing crosstalk between cancer cells and its microenvironment. For example STAT3 can dampen STAT1-mediated upregulation of MHC class I, allowing immune escape [1]. The other way for STAT3 to drive tumor immune escape is to regulate the function of stromal cells and more particularly immune cells.

In general, all seven STAT family members have prominent roles in T-cell function or T-cell differentiation, survival or expansion. STAT4 is essential for Th1 and STAT6 is important for Th2 differentiation. Similarly, all STAT proteins have all seven prominent roles in myeloid cells and they all influence each other's expression and activity status on complex and not understood chromatin regulation. All that makes the interpretation of complex immune cell scenarios triggered by multiple action of cytokines, growth factors, hormones and chemokines a tricky business to correctly relate functions to this or that STAT family member. Importantly, T-cell expansion by common γ-chain cytokines and many T-cell effector functions such as CD8$^+$ T-cell, $\gamma\delta$ T-cell generations and cytokine release function and mounting a killing or efficient cytokine signaling response against foreign or mutated antigen is a STAT5-mediated affair together with proper recognition and signaling through the T-cell receptor (TCR), where again interplays are not carefully understood or worked out [18,19]. Furthermore, STAT5 is also essential to generate Treg cells, where both *Foxp3* and *Cd25* are direct STAT5 target genes [20]. STAT5 has also essential functions in erythropoiesis or macrophage or dendritic cell (DC) polarization, but due to space constrains and focus on fine-tuning and twisting immune responses in health or disease we will here illuminate STAT3 function in immune cells. We illuminate many important immune modulatory interplays of STAT3 signaling in distinct T-cell and myeloid cell compartments. We describe current knowledge on the impact of STAT3 activation in immune cells on the balance between immunosurveillance and immunoescape. We will describe how STAT3 affects both myeloid and lymphoid cells usually in a way to inhibit anti-tumor immune response and to promote tumor growth.

2. STAT3 and T-Cells

T lymphocytes or T-cells play a central role in host adaptive immune response to cancer [21]. Tumor-infiltrating CD4$^+$ and CD8$^+$ T-cells are associated with varying clinical outcomes and survival in many types of cancer such as colorectal, [22] breast [23] and lung cancers [24]. Cytokines can shape T-cells immune response and tune CD4$^+$ T-cells differentiation and CD8$^+$ T-cells activation [25]. Among T-cells, different subsets have been described (regulatory T-cells, cytotoxic T-cells, T helper cells) with distinct functions that could be regulated by STAT3 (Table 1).

2.1. Th1/Th2

CD4$^+$ T helper (Th) cells assist other hematopoietic cells in immune processes, including activation of cytotoxic T lymphocytes (CTLs), natural killer (NK) cells and macrophages. Th cells are activated when stimulated with a peptidic sequence of the antigen they specifically recognize. These peptides are presented to Th cells by antigen presenting cells (APCs), such as DCs through MHC class II molecules. Once activated, they rapidly proliferate and secrete cytokines that will inhibit or assist the active immune response [26].

Table 1. Impact of STAT3 in T-cell subsets.

Immune Cell Family	STAT3 Role in	STAT3 Modulators	Effects	Reference
CD4$^+$ T-cells	Th1	IL-27	↗ proliferation	[27]
	Th2	IL-21	IL-10 secretion	[28]
	Th17	KO STAT3	Inhibition of Differentiation	[29,30]
		IL-6, IL-21, IL-23	↗ RORγt and RORα → Differentiation (↗ IL-17)	[31–35]
		PPARγ ligand, Platelet factor 4	↗ SOCS3 → Inhibition of Differentiation	[36]
		SHP1	↘ pSTAT3 → Inhibition of Differentiation	[37]
		LOXL3	↘ STAT3 deacetylation → Differentiation	[38]
		Metformin, Resveratrol	SIRT1 activation → STAT3 acetylation → Th17 Differentiation	[39]
		IL-6 (+ TGF-β)	↗ STAT3 activation and ↘ Gfi-1 → ↗ CD39 and CD73 expression	[40]
		miR29a-3p, miR-21-5p	↘ STAT3 → Th17 Differentiation	[41]
	Treg	KO STAT3	↘ number of Treg	
		IL-2	↗ STAT3 + STAT5 → ↗ FOXP3 → ↗ inhibitory functions	[42–44]
		S1PR1	↗ STAT3 → Treg migration in the tumor	[45]
		IL-6, IL-27	↗ STAT3 → ↘ FOXP3 → ↘ Treg differentiation	[34,46]
		CDK5	↗ pSTAT3(S727) → ↗FOXP3	[47]
		GATA-3	↗ miR125a-5 → ↘ IL-6R + STAT3 → ↘ Treg conversion	[48]
		Wogonin	↘ pSTAT3(Y705) ↗ pSTAT3(S727) → ↘ Treg differentiation	[49]
		WP1066	↘ pSTAT3 → ↘ FOXP3$^+$ Treg	[50]
		compound9# (fluorinated β-amino-ketone)	↘ FOXP3$^+$ Treg	[51]
		anti- sense oligos + radiations	↘ FOXP3$^+$ Treg	[52]
	Tfh	KO STAT3 or STAT3 siRNA	↘ BCL6 ↗ GATA-3, IL-4 (Th2)	[53]
		STAT DNA Binding domain mutation	↘ STAT3 activity → ↘ IL-21	[54]
		TGF-β	↗ pSTAT3 → ↘ GATA-3, IL-4 (Th2)	[53,55]
		Intratumoral Tfh-like cells	→ ↗ IL-21, IFN-γ → ↗ M2b	[56]
	Th9	KO STAT3	↗ pSTAT5 → ↗ IL-9	[57]
		Murine IL-10	↗ pSTAT3 → ↘ IL-9	[58]
		Human IL-21	↗ pSTAT3 → ↘ T-BET → ↗ IL-9	[59]
CD8$^+$ T-cells		KO STAT3	↗ IFN-γ → ↗ CXCL10 production by myeloid cells	[60]
			↗ CXCR3 (CXCL10 receptor)	
			↗ CD8$^+$ proliferation and tumor invasion	[61]
		CD28 stimulation	↗ pSTAT3 → ↗ NKG2D	[62]

Expression levels of Th1 cell genes coding for Interferon-γ (IFNG), TAP1, Granzym B (GZMB) are significantly higher in colorectal tumors than in normal tissue. A high expression of Th1 cytotoxic genes was associated with significantly improved disease-free survival whereas a low expression of those genes lead to disease recurrence [63]. T-BET, the master transcriptional regulator for Th1 differentiation is induced by TCRs and IL-12 stimulation [64]. In contrast, GATA-3 is the master assessor for Th2 differentiation, after stimulation with IL-4 [65]. IL-27, a member of the IL-6/IL-12 family produced by macrophages and DCs, favors Th1 differentiation by up-regulating T-BET, down-regulating GATA-3 and suppressing proinflammatory cytokine production such as IL-2, IL-4, and IL-13 [27,66]. In this context, only the IL-27-dependent Th1 proliferation was mediated by STAT3 [27]. In contrast, in a different cytokine context, in patients harboring STAT3 dominant negative mutations or STAT1 or IL-21R loss of function mutations, it was shown that IL-21/IL-21R, STAT3 and STAT1 signaling are required for in vitro differentiation of IL-10-secreting cells, related to Th2 [28].

2.2. Th17

Th17 cells are $CD4^+$ T-cells induced by TCR triggering together with IL-6, transforming growth factor (TGF)-β, and IL-23, an IL-12 family member, stimulation [67]. Th17 cells have emerged as key drivers of a wide range of autoimmune disorders, including inflammatory bowel disease, psoriasis, and ankylosing spondylitis [68]. Th17 cell expansion was observed in human cancers such as ovarian, melanoma, breast or colon cancers [69]. In colorectal cancer, patients with low expression of Th17 genes seem to have a prolonged disease-free survival [63]. However, a positive role of Th17 was proposed in melanoma and ovarian cancer. Therefore, the role of Th17 cells in cancer immunity remains controversial [70].

Th17 are characterized by the expression of the transcription factors RORγt and RORα and the production of IL-17A [71]. In addition, STAT3 is also essential for Th17 cell differentiation, since STAT3 ablation in mice $CD4^+$ T-cells, abrogates Th17 differentiation [29,30]. Moreover, in patients harboring STAT3 dominant negative mutations, IL-21R loss of function mutations or STAT1 gain of function mutations, it was shown that IL-21/IL-21R/STAT3 signaling is required for in vitro production of IL-17A/F by Th17 cells whereas STAT1 overexpression inhibits it [28]. STAT3 can associate with Trim28 and RORγt to drive the transcription of target cytokines such as IL-17A/F [72]. Moreover, many in vitro studies have shown that STAT3 can be activated by several pro-inflammatory cytokines including IL-6, IL-21 and IL-23 leading to the regulation of RORγt and RORα expression, along with the development and the stabilization of Th17 cells [31–35]. We found that the n-3 fatty acid docosahexaenoic acid (DHA) was able to induce the expression of SOCS3 in a PPARγ-dependent manner. SOCS3 then inhibits pSTAT3 and Th17 differentiation [36]. Another regulator of STAT3 activation in Th17 is the tyrosine phosphatase SHP1, which dampens IL-6- and IL-21-driven Th17 development and limits colitis in mice [37]. Similarly, the Platelet Factor 4 (PF4) can also up-regulate SOCS3 expression leading to the inhibition of STAT3, Th17 differentiation and tumor growth [73].

The STAT3 acetylation profile is also involved in Th17 polarization. First, lysyl oxidase-like 3 (LOXL3) is able to deacetylate STAT3 and to inhibit its transcriptional activity. *Loxl3* deficiency leads to constitutive STAT3 K685 acetylation causing reduced Th17 differentiation associated with resistance to DSS-induced colitis in mice [38]. Second, we showed that metformin and resveratrol, two SIRT1 activators, entail STAT3 acetylation leading to Th17 differentiation impairment and limit tumor growth in mice. The capacity of metformin to promote acetylation of STAT3 and to decrease Th17 differentiation was also shown in patients [39].

We have shown that in vitro Th17 cells differentiated with IL-6 and TGF-β and in vivo tumor-infiltrating Th17 cells express CD39 and CD73 ectonucleotidases. This ectonucleotidase catalytic machinery entails the degradation of extracellular ATP into adenosine, an immunosuppressive molecule which suppresses effector T-cells. The expression of ectonucleotidases is dependent on IL-6-driven STAT3 activation and TGF-β-mediated downregulation of the zinc finger protein Growth Factor Independent-1 (Gfi-1), both required for the transcriptional regulation of ectonucleotidase expression during Th17 cell differentiation. CD39 expression at the surface of Th17 cells fosters tumor growth, suggesting that the immunosuppressive functions of Th17 cells in cancer are dictated by ectonucleotidase expression [40]. It has been reported that naive T-cells can be differentiated into Th17 cells with IL-1β, IL-6, IL-23 and without TGF-β. Unlike Th17 cells generated with TGF-β and IL-6, these Th17 cells were highly pathogenic in vivo [74] and didn't express ectonucleotidases [40]. These observations propose STAT3 and Gfi-1 as key determinants in the immunoregulatory function of Th17 cells, at least in part through the regulation of ectonucleotidase expression [40].

The mechanistic role of STAT3 in Th17 positive effects on anti-tumoral response is less documented. TAM-derived exosomes can deliver miR-29a-3p and miR-21-5p to $CD4^+$ T-cells leading to the inhibition of STAT3 and consequently to Th17 polarization in favor to Treg, which is beneficial for epithelial ovarian cancer progression [41].

2.3. Treg

Suppressor regulatory T-cells (Treg) maintain peripheral immune tolerance [75,76]. Co-stimulation of naive $CD4^+$ T-cells with TCR and TGF-β, triggers the generation of $CD4^+/CD25^+$ Treg cells. This leads to the expression of FOXP3, Tregs master transcription factor [77]. These T-cells accumulate in tumors and in cancer patients peripheral blood [78]. An increase in Treg frequency is generally considered as a marker of poor prognosis in cancer, probably because Treg mediate suppression of anti-tumor immunity [79–81].

The role of STAT3 in *Foxp3* expression regulation in Tregs appears to be context-dependent. In vitro, IL-2 induces the binding of STAT3 and STAT5 to a highly conserved STAT-binding site located within the first intron of the *Foxp3* gene, leading to FOXP3 expression up-regulation in purified $CD4^+CD25^+$ T-cells but not in $CD4^+CD25^-$ cells [42].

In tumor-infiltrating Tregs, both STAT3 and STAT5 bind to a STAT consensus site in the *Foxp3* promoter to enhance FOXP3 expression which seems to be important in maintaining Tregs inhibitory functions [42–44]. S1PR1 (Sphingosine-1 Phosphate Receptor 1) signaling has been shown to restrain Treg number and functions. An increase in S1PR1 in $CD4^+$ T-cells promotes STAT3 activation and JAK/STAT3-dependent Treg tumor migration, whereas STAT3 ablation in T-cells diminishes tumor-associated Treg accumulation and tumor growth [45]. Treatment of metastatic cancer or chronic myelogenous leukemia after allogeneic hematopoietic stem cell transplantation in patients with low-dose IL-2, leads to an increase of peripheral blood $CD4^+CD25^+$ cells and to FOXP3 expression in $CD3^+$ T-cells [42]. STAT3 and FOXP3 co-operatively control a subset of genes, responsible for Treg cell ability to suppress Th17 cell-mediated inflammation [82]. In contrast, IL-21 which activates STAT3 but not STAT5 has no effect on Treg viability, activation or function, suggesting that in this context IL-21-mediated STAT3 activation is not sufficient [83]. The regulation of *Foxp3* expression by STAT3 was strengthened by other studies. CDK5 increases *Foxp3* gene expression through phosphorylation of STAT3 at serine 727 [47]. GATA-3 controls the expression of miR-125a-5p, which in turn inhibits the expression of IL-6R and STAT3 and dampens Treg conversion [48]. In contrast, differentiation of naive T-cells into Tregs in vitro, is impaired when STAT3 is activated (by IL-6 or IL-27) [34,46]. In a different context, STAT3 binds to a silencer element within the *Foxp3* locus [84] and could also inhibit STAT5 interacting with the *Foxp3* promoter [85], to prevent FOXP3 expression.

One possible explanation for these ambivalent actions of STAT3 on Treg differentiation could be the phosphorylation site. Indeed, wogonin, a natural flavonoid from *Scutellaria baicalensis,* inhibits Treg induction by down-regulating ERK and STAT3-Y705 phosphorylation and promoting NF-κB and STAT3-S727 activation [49]. The modulation of STAT3 activity by molecular compounds could lead to inhibition of Tregs activity. Thus, WP1066 (an inhibitor of STAT3 signaling) enhances T-cell cytotoxicity against melanoma through inhibition of $FOXP3^+$ Tregs [50]. Compound9#, a fluorinated β-amino-ketone molecule, also inhibits Treg induction both in vitro and in vivo, via blockage of JAK2 signaling [51]. Finally, STAT3 inhibition with anti-sense oligonucleotides in association with radiation is a potent therapeutic target against Tregs [52]. All these studies suggest that STAT3 is required for immunosuppressive functions of Tregs.

2.4. T Follicular Helper Cells

Tfh differentiation is complex because it requires interaction with other cells such as B cells or DC. In mice, IL-6, IL-21 and IL-27 are essential for Tfh formation while in humans, Tfh generation relies on TGF-β, IL-12, IL-23. In both mammalian species of rodents or humans, Tfh cells express BCL6, ASCL2, IL-21, PD-1, and ICOS and produce IL-21 and CXCL13 [86,87]. While the role of Tfh is ambiguous in lymphoid tumors, many studies report that accumulation of Tfh in tertiary structures within the tumor is of good prognosis for breast, colon and non-small cell lung cancer patients [88,89]. Even if the protective effects of Tfh cells seem to be dependent on IL-21 and CXCL13-mediated recruitment of leucocytes, little is known about the accurate mechanism of Tfh anti-tumoral effects.

Generation of Tfh cells in patients with impaired STAT3 DNA-binding function is compromised due to the inability of IL-12 to induce IL-21 production without affecting its capacity to induce ICOS, BCL6 or CXCR5 expression [54]. When siRNA specific for STAT3 was used, TGF-β, IL-12, IL-23 failed to induce BCL6 expression in vitro [53]. However, the requirement of STAT3 seems to depend on the differentiation status of Tfh cells: It is required for Tfh generation but once these cells are generated it is no longer required [90]. In the same context, murine STAT3-deficient CD4$^+$ T-cells, Tfh cells expressed less or more BCL6 and IL-21 according to the immune environment [91,92]. Moreover, in conditions where STAT3 is necessary for Tfh differentiation, two studies showed that it cooperates with the IkZF transcription factors Aiolos and Ikaros. Moreover, the kinase activity of ROCK2 (Rho-associated coiled-coil kinase 2, an actin cytoskeleton assembly regulator) is required to induce STAT3 phosphorylation, nuclear relocalization and DNA binding to regulate *Bcl6* expression [93,94]. Finally, the importance of STAT3 in Tfh differentiation was strengthened by its capacity to block the expression of the Th2-associated genes *Gata3* and *Il4* [53,55].

A new protumorigenic IL-21$^+$ Tfh-like cell subset with a CXCR5$^-$PD-1$^-$ BTLA$^-$CD69^{hi} phenotype was identified in hepatocellular carcinoma (HCC). STAT1 and STAT3 activation are critical for these Tfh-like cell induction which operate via IL-21-IFN-γ pathways to induce plasma cells and create conditions for M2b macrophage polarization and tumor growth [56].

The importance of STAT3 in Tfh differentiation and its pro- or anti-tumoral role is not clear and could be dependent on differentiation stage, localization and environment.

2.5. Th9

Th9 cells have been characterized as a proinflammatory CD4 T-cell subset that can be generated through TGF-β and IL-4 stimulation. These cells are characterized by IL-9 secretion. Th9 harbor potent IL-9-dependent anti-cancer properties in most solid tumors and especially in melanoma while they can promote the development of many hematological human tumors, including Hodgkin's lymphoma and other B cell lymphoma. Th9 cells activate both innate and adaptive immune responses, thereby favoring anti-cancer immunity and tumor elimination [95].

In this CD4 T-cell subset, STAT3 was shown to dampen IL-9 production through STAT5 inhibition in Th9 cells [57]. In vitro, Th9 long term ability to secrete IL-9 is inhibited by pSTAT3 through an IL-10 receptor signaling [58]. In contrast, in humans Th9, pSTAT3 (mainly driven by IL-21 self-induction) inhibits pSTAT1-mediated T-BET induction, through SOCS3 induction. Since T-BET is an inhibitor of IL-9 transcription, this sustains IL-9 production. Patient-derived Th9 cells with dysfunctional STAT3, lose their capacity to produce IL-9, because of SOCS3 expression down-regulation, which leads to an increase pSTAT1 and T-BET expression. In the same study, the loss of function mutations observed in patients were recapitulated with deletion studies in mice, revealing that absence of STAT3 culminates into increased IL-9 production [59].

2.6. CD8$^+$

CD8$^+$ T lymphocytes are central players in cancer immune response, through their capacity to kill malignant cells. Upon recognition by the TCR of specific antigenic peptides presented on the surface of target cells by human leukocyte antigen class I (HLA-I)/beta-2-microglobulin (β2m) complexes, the CTL effector functions are activated. These functions are mediated either directly, through exocytosis of cytotoxic granules containing perforin and granzym into the target cells, resulting in cancer cell destruction, or indirectly, through secretion of cytokines, including IFN-γ and TNF [96].

The stimulation of the human and murine CD8$^+$ T-cells CD28, stabilizes the tyrosine kinase Lck activity and pSTAT3-mediated transcription of NKG2D. NKG2D expressing CD8$^+$ T-cells exert cytolytic activity against target tumor cells in vitro and significantly improve the antitumor therapeutic effects in vivo [62]. Even if IL-10 is considered as an immune suppressor it can also increase expansion and cytotoxic activity of CD8$^+$ cells. Tumor-resident CD8$^+$ T-cells express high levels of IL-10R, leading to high levels of activated pSTAT3 and pSTAT1 in response to IL-10 [97]. In contrast, circulating CD8$^+$ T-cells from peripheral blood of HCC patients present high amounts of pSTAT3 which is correlated with high amount of IL-4, IL-6 and IL-10 and low quantity of IFN-γ which may result in abnormal immune surveillance against tumor cells [98]. In murine CD8$^+$ T-cells, STAT3 has been shown to inhibit both IFN-γ-mediated CXCL10 production by myeloid cells and CD8$^+$ T-cells CXCR3 expression (the receptor of CXCL10), blocking the migration of these cells to the tumor site [60].

In an adoptive transfer therapeutic strategy in mice, ablating STAT3 in CD8$^+$ T-cells prior to transfer, allows efficient tumor infiltration and robust CD8$^+$ T-cell proliferation, resulting in increased tumor antigen-specific T-cell activity and tumor growth inhibition [61].

Altogether STAT3 seems to inhibit CD8$^+$ T-cell expansion and cytolytic activity except in some particular conditions.

3. STAT3 and Myeloid Cells

APCs dictate immune system response, since these cells have been shown to capture antigens in the periphery, migrate to the lymphoid organs, and present processed peptides to T-cells in a way that may lead either to priming or tolerance induction [99]. Among myeloid cells, different subsets have been described (Macrophages, DCs, Myeloid-Derived Suppressor Cells (MDSCs)) with distinct functions that could be regulated by STAT3 (Table 2).

Table 2. Impact of STAT3 in myeloid cells.

Immune Cell Family	STAT3 Role in	STAT3 Modulators	Effects	Reference
yeloid cells	Macrophages	KO STAT3	Inflammatory macrophages	[100]
			↗ CTL activation	[101]
			↗ TLR9 pathway (IFN-γ, TNF-α, IL-12)	[102]
			↗ IL-23 and ↘ IL-12	
		STAT3 oxerexpression	↗ CD163 (M2 marker)	[103]
		cancer cells (PAI-1, BMP6, IL-6)	↗ pSTAT3 → polarization of M1 into M2 (CD163)	[103–105]
		Tumor exosomes	↗ pSTAT3 → ↗ IL-6, IL-10, CCL2	[106]
		Corosolic acid, oleanic acid	↘ STAT3 activity → M1 polarization (↗ TNF-α, IFN-γ, IL-12, IL-2)	[107–109]
		ERK5	↗ pSTAT3 → pro-tumor macrophages	[110]
		M-CSF	↗ pSTAT3 → ↗ DC-SIGN	[111]
		KO SOCS3	↗ pSTAT3 → anti-tumor macrophages	[112]
		Tumor cells	↗ pSTAT3 → ↗ IL-10, VEGF, βFGF → angiogenesis	[113–115]
	Dendritic Cells	KO STAT3 or siRNA or shRNA	↗ DCs APC function and cytokine production (↗ IL-12, TNF-α and ↘ IL-10)	[102,116–121]
		Constitutive STAT3 activation	↘ MHC class II, ID-2	[117,122–124]
		Tumor-derived exosomes and IL-6	↘ PKCβII → DCs activation and differentiation	[125]
	MDSCs	KO STAT3 or siRNA or anti-sense oligonucleotides	↘ C/EBPβ	[126]
			↘ immunosuppressive functions	[117,127–130]
			→ MDSCs differentiation into DCs	
			↘ NOX2 → ↘ ROS → ↘ immunosuppression	[131,132]
		Tumor-derived exosomes (HSP70)	↗ pSTAT3 → ↗ immunosuppressive functions (with an IL-6 amplification loop)	[133]
		CCL2	↗ pSTAT3 → PMN-MDSCs-mediated T-cell suppression	
		IL-6	Early-stage MDSCs accumulation	
		G-CSF	↗ pSTAT3 → ↘ IRF8	[126,134]
		GM-CSF	↗ pSTAT3 → ↗ IDO → ↗ immunosuppression	[135]
		siRNA or STATTIC	↘ pSTAT3 → ↘ arginase-1 → ↘ immunosuppression	[136]
		JSI-124 (STAT3 inhibitor)	↘ pSTAT3 → ↘ IDO → ↘ immunosuppression	[137]
		CD45	↘ pSTAT3 → M-MDSCs differentiation into TAMs	[138]
		Embelin, PM01183, alisertib, STATTIC or BBI608	↘ pSTAT3	[139–142]
		Tumor cells	↗ pSTAT3 → ↗VEGF, βFGF → ↗ angiogenesis	[115]

3.1. Macrophages

Tumor-associated macrophages (TAMs) are subdivided into two subsets, M1 and M2 macrophages, based on their capacity to express or produce Nitric Oxide Synthase/IL-12/TNF-α or arginase-1/IL-10/TGF-β, respectively. M1 has potent microbicidal properties and promotes Th1 responses, whereas M2 supports Th2-associated effector functions [143,144]. M2 macrophages includes M2a, M2b or M2c subtypes. Tumor-derived signals, such as Macrophage-Colony Stimulating Factor (M-CSF/CSF-1), Monocyte Chemoattractant Protein-1 (MCP-1), or Chemokine (C-C motif) Ligand-2 (CCL2) entails the accumulation of M2 at the tumor site. M2 macrophages participate in tumor growth by releasing proangiogenic cytokines and growth factors, e.g. Epidermal Growth Factor (EGF), Vascular Endothelial Growth Factor (VEGF), Platelet-Derived Growth Factor (PDGF), Colony Stimulating Factor-1 (CSF-1), and basic Fibroblast Growth Factor (βFGF). They also generate arginase-1, IL-10 and TGF-β. These molecular messengers will inhibit the antitumor function of T-cells and NK cells. This will favor tumor tolerance and impairment of antitumor immunotherapies efficacy [145–147].

IL-6 inhibition of M-CSF-induced colony formation observed in animals was abolished in mice mutated for the gp130-STAT1/3 signaling, suggesting that the IL-6/STAT3 pathway could regulate macrophage homeostasis [148]. Moreover, breast cancer-derived exosomes are capable of inducing IL-6 secretion and a pro-tumoral phenotype (IL-6, IL-10, CCL2 production) in macrophages, partially via gp130/STAT3 signaling [106]. More particularly, STAT3 directly induces the expression of the M2 marker CD163, both in macrophages and tumor cells [103]. Prostate-cancer cells induce a change in macrophage phenotype from M1 into M2, through STAT3 activation [104]. This can be induced by Plasminogen Activating Inhibitor (PAI)-1 secreted by cancer cells [105].

The inhibition of STAT3 signaling in either macrophages or bone marrow-derived DCs is of great importance in cancer immunotherapy, because it allows these APCs to restore the responsiveness of tolerant T-cells from tumor-bearing mice. STAT3 signaling is a negative regulator in peritoneal elicited macrophages, as its targeted disruption gives a constitutively activated phenotype and an increased ability to produce inflammatory mediators in response to LPS. This may be the consequence of an increased STAT1 activity (leading to high production of inflammatory factors) or a lack of IL-10 production [100]. Moreover, macrophages derived from conditional STAT3 knockout mice are better than wild-type macrophages to prime cognate CTL responses and to cross-present tumor-derived antigen to CTLs in vitro. This leads to a more important proliferation of CTLs and an increased production of IFN-γ and TNF-α. Similarly, removing STAT3 in hematopoietic cells, leads to rapid activation of innate immunity by CpG (a TLR9 ligand), with enhanced activation of macrophages, neutrophils and NK cells and production of IFN-γ, TNF-α, IL-12 to eradicate B16 melanoma tumors [102]. Targeting STAT3 signaling therefore represents an attractive strategy to increase CTL responses in the tumor-bearing host [101]. Immunosuppressive activities of TAMs correlate with over-activated STAT3 signaling, whereas disruption of TAMs STAT3 activity can enhance rat immune response to breast cancer [149]. In glioblastoma patients, tumor-infiltrating macrophages were shown to be predominantly STAT3-positive M2 macrophages, which are associated with a poor prognosis [150]. The same team proposed that corosolic acid and oleanic acid can prevent tumor formation through their capacity to suppress macrophages M2 polarization and tumor cell proliferation by inhibiting STAT3 activation [107,108]. CD163-targeted corosolic acid-containing liposomes were also shown to reprogram M2 macrophages into M1 (increased expression of TNF-α, IFN-γ, IL-12, IL-2 and decreased expression of IL-10) [109]. Since ERK5 mediates Y705 phosphorylation of STAT3 in myeloid cells, blocking ERK5 might constitute a treatment strategy to reprogram macrophages toward an antitumor state by inhibiting STAT3-induced gene expression [110]. In intrahepatic cholangiocarcinoma (ICC), patients with high counts of $CD163^+$ M2 macrophages showed poor disease-free survival. Tumor cell supernatant from HuCCT1 ICC cell lines induces the production of IL-10 and VEGF-A by macrophages through activation of STAT3 and polarization towards the M2 phenotype [113]. Similarly, renal cell carcinoma-derived BMP (Bone Morphogenetic Protein)-6 mediates IL-10 expression in macrophages through Smad5 and STAT3, and M2 polarization [114]. These observations were confirmed by the fact that macrophages isolated from mouse tumors displayed activated STAT3 and induced angiogenesis in an in vitro tube formation assay via STAT3 induction of angiogenic factors, including VEGF and βFGF [115]. STAT3 signaling within the tumor microenvironment induces the production of IL-23, a procarcinogenic cytokine, via direct transcriptional activation of the IL-23/p19 gene in TAMs, while inhibiting the production of IL-12, a central anticarcinogenic cytokine, thereby shifting the balance of tumor immunity towards carcinogenesis [44]. The M-CSF-inducible DC-SIGN (Dendritic cell-specific ICAM-3-grabbing nonintegrin or CD209) expression along monocyte-to-macrophage differentiation is dependent on JNK and STAT3 activation. DC-SIGN contributes to the release of IL-10 that would maintain STAT3 activation in tumor cells, thus implying that DC-SIGN favors the maintenance of an activated STAT3 context in the tumor stroma. This will compromise the ability of TAMs and DCs to generate an effective antitumor response and to maintain an immunosuppressive environment [111]. This effect is potentiated by STAT3-activating cytokines IL-6 and IL-10 produced by STAT3-activated tumor cells. In the same way, IL-6-derived from gastric cancer cells induces normal macrophages differentiation to M2 macrophages with higher IL-10 and TGF-β expression, and lower IL-12 expression, via STAT3 phosphorylation. IL-6-induced M2 macrophages exert a pro-tumor function by promoting GC cell proliferation and migration [151].

However, an anti-tumoral role of STAT3 in macrophages has also been proposed, based on studies that investigated the importance of STAT3 in macrophages through an indirect manner, using SOCS3 conditional knockout mice in macrophages. Hyperactivation of STAT3 in myeloid cells simultaneously exerted anti-inflammatory as well as anti-tumor effects [112]. Thus, Lipoxin A4 induces STAT3 phosphorylation and mediates differentiation of monocytic-like cells into M2 subtypes with anti-tumorigenic activities [152]. The discrepancies between these studies could be explained by the fact that SOCS3 and lipoxin signaling should regulate other pathways such as NF-κB.

3.2. Dendritic Cells (DCs)

DCs are another differentiated stage of monocytes and are the key APCs of the immune system. DCs play a main role as immune sentinels in the initiation of T-cell response against microbial pathogens, tumors and inflammation [153,154].

The first evidence that STAT3 is important for DCs fate was made in mice lacking STAT3 expression in hematopoietic progenitors. These animals present a profound deficiency in DCs which are unresponsive to Flt3L stimulation [116]. However, the same mice bearing a tumor, present enhanced DC, T-cell, NK cell and neutrophil functions and a decreased tumor progression [117]. DCs derived from $LysM^{cre}/STAT3^{flox/flox}$ mice display higher cytokine production in response to TLR stimulation and activate more efficiently T-cells. Intratumoral administration of these DCs significantly inhibits MC38 tumor growth [119]. Moreover, ablating STAT3 in myeloid cells increases CpG-induced DCs maturation, T-cell activation, tumor antigen-specific T-cells generation and long-lasting antitumor immunity in B16 melanoma tumor model [102]. Similarly, CpG was used to administer STAT3 siRNA specifically to myeloid and B cells. Ablation of STAT3 in these cells increases DC engagement and adoptively transferred $CD8^+$ T-cells effector functions in vivo, with an upregulation of effector molecules such as perforin, granzym B, and IFN-γ [118]. Mice without STAT3 in myeloid compartment of tumor stroma, including DCs and macrophages, present reduced numbers of tumor-infiltrating $CD4^+CD25^+/FOXP3^+/LAG3^+$ Tregs, along with an increase in $CD8^+$ effector T-cells [117]. Constitutive STAT3 activation in tumor-residing DCs reduces expression of MHC class II and costimulatory molecules, impairs the antigen-presenting function of DC and contributes to the expansion of tumor-infiltrating $FOXP3^+$ T-cells and attenuates $CD4^+$ Th cell responses [117,122,123]. This can be partly explained by the fact that STAT3 inhibits the ID2 (inhibitor of differentiation 2) expression which promotes tumor immunity [124]. Finally, IL-6 is a suppressor of bone marrow-derived DC activation/maturation and a regulator of DC differentiation in vivo, through STAT3 phosphorylation. Then, DC differentiation/maturation is controlled by IL-6-gp130-STAT3, suggesting that this amplification loop may represent a target for controlling T-cell-mediated immune responses [155]. Similarly, mammary tumor-derived exosomes inhibit the differentiation of murine myeloid precursor cells into DCs in vitro. This was correlated with an increased IL-6 level and phosphorylated STAT3 and was blocked in bone marrow cells derived from IL-6 knockout mice. This suggests that tumor cells can dampen DCs differentiation through an autocrine activation of STAT3 by IL-6 [125].

In humans, tumor-derived factors suppress DC generation through STAT3-mediated PKCβII reduced expression [156]. STAT3-depleted DCs with adenoviral STAT3 short hairpin RNA (shRNA) or siRNA presented an altered cytokines production profile under TLR stimulation (such as more IL-12 and TNF-α and less IL-10), and induced tumor Ag-specific T-cells and IFN-γ-producing $\gamma\delta$ T lymphocytes more efficiently than control DCs [119–121]. The impact on IL-12 can be explained by a competition of STAT3 with CDK9 on a binding site on the IL-12p35 promoter [157]. The effects of STAT3 on IL-10 expression can be explained by the fact that HDAC6 forms a complex with STAT3, recruited to a specific DNA sequence element in the *Il10* gene promoter [158].

3.3. Myeloid-Derived Suppressor Cells (MDSCs)

MDSCs have been identified in humans and mice as a population of immature myeloid cells with the ability to suppress T-cell activation [159]. In tumor-bearing mice, these cells have been shown to markedly expand in lymphoid organs and blood [160]. In addition, an increased MDSCs frequency was detected in the blood of patients with different types of cancers [161,162]. In mice and humans, MDSCs from tumor bearers induce antigen-specific MHC class I restricted tolerance of $CD8^+$ T-cells and are one of the major suppressors of antitumor immunity [163]. In humans the phenotype of MDSCs is a matter of debate. However, two major subsets of MDSCs have been identified: monocytic MDSCs (M-MDSCs), similar to monocytes and polymorphonuclear MDSCs (PMN-MDSCs) sharing phenotypic and morphologic features with neutrophils [164].

STAT3 is probably one of the main transcription factors that regulate MDSCs functions. MDSCs from tumor-bearing mice present high levels of phosphorylated STAT3, compared with immature myeloid cells from naive mice [128]. Moreover, ablation of STAT3 expression through the use of conditional knockout mice or selective STAT3 inhibitors (JSI-124) markedly reduce the expansion of MDSCs, promote accumulation of DCs and increase T-cell responses in tumor-bearing mice [117,127,128]. In mice, when STAT3 was specifically deleted in myeloid cells, the ability of MDSCs to inhibit $CD4^+$ and $CD8^+$ T-cell-dependent apoptosis by cell-cell contact and to induce Treg polarization through TGF-β, IL-10 and NOX2 secretion was decreased [131]. When STAT3 was specifically turned off in myeloid cells expressing TLR9 from prostate cancer patients, using a CpG-STAT3 siRNA or CpG-STAT3 antisense oligonucleotides, it abrogated the immunosuppressive effects of patient-derived MDSCs on effector $CD8^+$ T-cells [129,130]. In contrast, deletion of SOCS3 in myeloid cells leads to an increased activation of the STAT3 and to differentiation into $Gr\text{-}1^+CD11b^+Ly6G^+$ MDSCs, enhancing tumor growth [165]. STAT3 can also be regulated in MDSCs by the epigenetic-associated protein, p66a, which may physically interact with STAT3 to suppress its activity through posttranslational modification [166]. We have shown that tumor-derived exosome (TDE)-associated HSP70 led to STAT3 activation in MDSCs. This activation depends on TLR2/MyD88 and autocrine production of IL-6. TDEs from human tumor cell lines activate human MDSCs suppressive functions but not their expansion in an HSP70/TLR2-dependent manner, showing that the mechanism described in mice is also relevant in cancer patients [133]. In tumor cell supernatants, tumor soluble factors induce activation of ERK, which results in MDSCs expansion, while TDEs trigger STAT3 activation without promoting MDSCs expansion [133]. How can these discrepancies be explained? It is well known that STAT3 signaling in myeloid cells, entails the expression of Bcl-xL, c-myc, cyclin D1 or survivin, which favors cell proliferation and inhibits cell apoptosis and differentiation to mature cell types [15,167].

STAT3 controls the G-CSF-and G-MCSF responsive induction of C/EPBβ (CCAAT-enhancer-binding protein β) expression and the interferon regulatory factor 8 (IRF8) downregulation in myeloid cells [126,134]. The transcription factor C/EBPβ was reported to play a crucial role in controlling the differentiation of myeloid precursors to functional MDSCs [126] whereas IRF8 attenuated MDSC accumulation, phenotype and function [134]. These data suggest also a link between CSF and STAT3 pathway in the regulation of MDSC biology.

Finally, recent studies highlighted the importance of signaling pathways downstream STAT3 in MDSCs differentiation. MDSCs isolated from mouse tumors present activated STAT3. STAT3 favors the production of angiogenic factors, including VEGF and βFGF to induce angiogenesis in an in vitro tube formation assay [115]. STAT3 as well as STAT5 control the cytokine-induced expression of the cytoplasmic NADPH oxidase NOX2 [168], being e.g., crucial for DNA damage response in AML cells, leading together with mitochondrial ROS production, which is a predominant STAT3 affair to the production of ROS, responsible for MDSCs-induced immune suppression in murine colon, lung, mammary carcinoma, thymoma, sarcoma models and in patients with head and neck cancers [132]. STAT3 also favors immunosuppressive functions of MDSCs by inducing the expression and the activity of IDO (Indoleamine 2,3-dioxygenase 1) in breast [137] and liver [135] cancers or arginase-1 in head and neck squamous cell carcinoma [136]. STAT3-inducible up-regulation of the myeloid-related protein S100A9 enhances MDSCs production in cancer. Mice lacking this protein mount potent antitumor immune responses and reject implanted tumors, an effect reversed by administration of wild-type MDSCs [169].

However, STAT3 activity can be endogenously controlled in intra-tumoral MDSCs. Thus, tumor hypoxia led to CD45 protein tyrosine phosphatases activation, resulting in STAT3 activity downregulation and in M-MDSC differentiation into tumor-promoting TAMs [138].

Moreover, many inhibitors were proposed such as the XIAP inhibitor embelin [139], PM01183 a novel synthetic agent derived from trabectedin [140], alisertib (MLN8237), a small-molecule inhibitor of Auror-A kinase [141], STATTIC or BBI608 [142] to inhibit STAT3 in MDSCs with a potential clinical application to favor anti-tumor response.

4. STAT3 and Check Points Inhibitors

The emergence of immune 'checkpoint inhibitors', blocking negative regulators of T-cell immunity opened new clinical applications of cancer immunotherapies. The more widely studied are cytotoxic T lymphocyte antigen 4 (CTLA-4) and programmed death receptor 1 (PD-1). CTLA-4 is mainly expressed on T helper and Treg cells and binds to its ligands B7–1 (CD80) and B7–2 (CD86) on APCs [170]. PD-1 expression is induced both on activated $CD8^+$ T-cells, Tfh and Treg present in tumor microenvironment, and on activated B cells and NK cells. PD-1 has two ligands: PD-L1 (B7-H1) and PD-L2 (B7-DC). PD-1 signaling contributes to T-cell exhaustion [170]. Other checkpoints can also be implicated in tumor immune escape such as Lymphocyte activation gene 3 protein (LAG-3) and T-cell immunoglobulin and mucin domain-containing 3 (TIM-3), IDO1, B- and T-lymphocyte attenuator (BTLA), V-domain immunoglobulin suppressor of T-cell activation (VISTA) and the A2A adenosine receptor (A2A-R) [170,171].

STAT3 can bind the promoter of murine *Pdcd1* gene coding for PD-1 in T-cells [172]. STAT3 has been demonstrated to bind to the *Pdcd1l1* promoter (coding for PD-L1) to regulate its transcriptional expression in cancer cells. It requires either mutated oncogene chimeric nucleophosmin/anaplastic lymphoma kinase (ALK) in T-cell lymphoma [173], Latent membrane protein-1 (LMP1) of Epstein–Barr virus in nasopharyngeal carcinoma [174], HDAC6 in osteosarcoma [175], NF-κB in melanoma [176] or HIF-1α in pulmonary adenocarcinoma [177]. In contrast, a study shows that STAT3 is necessary for docetaxel-mediated inhibition of PD-1 expression [178].

In CRC patients, FGFR2 expression is correlated to PD-L1 expression. FGFR2 stimulation leads to STAT3 activation, PD-L1 expression and colon cancer cell death [179]. The EGFR signaling pathway can also regulate PD-L1 expression through the IL-6/JAK/STAT3 pathway in non-small cell lung cancer (NSCLC) cells [180,181]. The expression of PD-L1 is associated with a poor prognosis and inhibition of PD-L1 expression (e.g., through STAT3 or its partner inhibition) is associated to a decrease in cell proliferation and/or an increase in tumor cell death in most of these studies. However, the effects on T-cell anti-tumor response were not tested here.

PD-L1/L2 can be expressed in non-tumoral cells. In liver MDSCs, GM-CSF is responsible for STAT3 activation which in turn induces PD-L1 and IDO1 expression [135]. GBM cells secrete IL-6 which in turn activates STAT3 in infiltrated myeloid cells leading to STAT3 activation and PD-L1 expression. An anti-IL-6 therapy decreases PD-L1 expression and tumor size in a $CD8^+$ T-cell-dependent manner [182]. In HCC, a similar regulation was observed. In this setting, the HCC-associated fibroblasts produce IL-6 which in turn increases PD-L1 expression in neutrophils [183]. Similarly, in prostate carcinoma, DC generated in the presence of stromal myofibroblasts factors expressed significantly elevated levels of PD-L1 in a STAT3 and IL-6-dependent manner [184]. In chronic lymphocytic leukemia (CLL), STAT3 is required to PD-L1 expression and IL-10 production which in turn seems to be responsible for PD-1 expression in $CD4^+$ and $CD8^+$ T-cells [185]. In adult T-cell lymphoma, IL-27B production by Lymphoma cells and IL-27p28 production by macrophages lead to STAT3 activation and PD-L1/L2 expression in macrophages [186]. TGF-β is another cytokine secreted by inflammatory or tumor cells that can increase PD-L1 expression in DC in a STAT3-dependent manner [187]. The use of IFN-α in clinical oncology for many types of cancers is reconsidered, as IFN-α induces the expression of PD-L1 molecule, in the majority of the specific immune cell populations, particularly in DCs [188]. However, it should be noted that interferons are highly liver toxic and they act on all cell types in the body, where many unwanted side effects from neurotoxic problems to fever symptoms were reported in therapy, making their window of opportunity in fragile patients delicate.

Little is known about the ability of STAT3 to regulate other checkpoints. One study shows that STAT3/IRF1 are required for PD-L2 expression in melanoma cells [189]. In a non-cancerous context, it has been shown that CTLA-4 as well as PD-1, LAG-3 and TIM-3 expression is induced in HIV-infected DCs in a STAT3-dependent manner [190].

In contrast, the immunosuppressive effect of these checkpoints can be dependent on STAT3 activation in target-cells. For example, IDO1 may promote EMT (Epithelial-Mesenchymal Transition) by activation of the IL-6/STAT3/PD-L1 signaling pathway [191]. $TIM\text{-}3^+$ endothelial cells modulate T-cell response to lymphoma surrogate antigens by suppressing activation of $CD4^+$ T lymphocytes through the activation of the IL-6-STAT3 pathway, inhibiting Th1 polarization and providing protective immunity [192]. Finally, CTLA-4 critically shapes the characteristics of IL-17 producing $CD8^+$ cells (Tc17 a pro-tumoral population) in a STAT3 activation-dependent manner and inhibition of CTLA-4-induced STAT3 activity reverses Tc17 signature to Tc1-like cells with enhanced cytotoxic potential [193].

5. Conclusions

STAT3 regulates genes involved in biological functions of cancer and immune cells, rendering this pathway an interesting therapeutic target. STAT3 could be inhibited directly by peptides or natural compounds or indirectly by blocking upstream signaling pathways such as IL-6 and JAK2 pathways (For review see [194,195]). However, the complexity of STAT3 biology and its broad effects may render its clinical development complex. This review underlines the ambivalent effects of STAT3 on the antitumoral immune response, with both positive or negative effects, depending on the context or cell types involved. Additional translational studies on patients treated with STAT3 inhibitors are awaited to understand their effects on the complexity of tumor biology.

Acknowledgments: We thank Isabel Gregoire for carefully reading the manuscript.

References

1. Kosack, L.; Wingelhofer, B.; Popa, A.; Orlova, A.; Agerer, B.; Vilagos, B.; Majek, P.; Parapatics, K.; Lercher, A.; Ringler, A.; et al. The ERBB-STAT3 Axis Drives Tasmanian Devil Facial Tumor Disease. *Cancer Cell* **2019**, *35*, 125–139. [CrossRef] [PubMed]

2. Yoshimura, A.; Naka, T.; Kubo, M. SOCS proteins, cytokine signalling and immune regulation. *Nat. Rev. Immunol.* **2007**, *7*, 454–465. [CrossRef] [PubMed]
3. Hirano, T.; Ishihara, K.; Hibi, M. Roles of STAT3 in mediating the cell growth, differentiation and survival signals relayed through the IL-6 family of cytokine receptors. *Oncogene* **2000**, *19*, 2548–2556. [CrossRef] [PubMed]
4. Yuan, Z.L.; Guan, Y.J.; Chatterjee, D.; Chin, Y.E. Stat3 dimerization regulated by reversible acetylation of a single lysine residue. *Science* **2005**, *307*, 269–273. [CrossRef] [PubMed]
5. Meier, J.A.; Larner, A.C. Toward a new STATe: The role of STATs in mitochondrial function. *Semin. Immunol.* **2014**, *26*, 20–28. [CrossRef]
6. Avalle, L.; Poli, V. Nucleus, Mitochondrion, or Reticulum? STAT3 a La Carte. *Int. J. Mol. Sci* **2018**, *19*, 2820. [CrossRef] [PubMed]
7. Shuai, K.; Liu, B. Regulation of gene-activation pathways by PIAS proteins in the immune system. *Nat. Rev. Immunol.* **2005**, *5*, 593–605. [CrossRef]
8. Alexander, W.S.; Hilton, D.J. The role of suppressors of cytokine signaling (SOCS) proteins in regulation of the immune response. *Annu Rev. Immunol.* **2004**, *22*, 503–529. [CrossRef]
9. Migone, T.S.; Cacalano, N.A.; Taylor, N.; Yi, T.; Waldmann, T.A.; Johnston, J.A. Recruitment of SH2-containing protein tyrosine phosphatase SHP-1 to the interleukin 2 receptor; loss of SHP-1 expression in human T-lymphotropic virus type I-transformed T cells. *Proc. Natl. Acad. Sci. USA* **1998**, *95*, 3845–3850. [CrossRef]
10. Schaper, F.; Gendo, C.; Eck, M.; Schmitz, J.; Grimm, C.; Anhuf, D.; Kerr, I.M.; Heinrich, P.C. Activation of the protein tyrosine phosphatase SHP2 via the interleukin-6 signal transducing receptor protein gp130 requires tyrosine kinase Jak1 and limits acute-phase protein expression. *Biochem. J.* **1998**, *335*, 557–565. [CrossRef]
11. Irie-Sasaki, J.; Sasaki, T.; Matsumoto, W.; Opavsky, A.; Cheng, M.; Welstead, G.; Griffiths, E.; Krawczyk, C.; Richardson, C.D.; Aitken, K.; et al. CD45 is a JAK phosphatase and negatively regulates cytokine receptor signalling. *Nature* **2001**, *409*, 349–354. [CrossRef] [PubMed]
12. Daino, H.; Matsumura, I.; Takada, K.; Odajima, J.; Tanaka, H.; Ueda, S.; Shibayama, H.; Ikeda, H.; Hibi, M.; Machii, T.; et al. Induction of apoptosis by extracellular ubiquitin in human hematopoietic cells: Possible involvement of STAT3 degradation by proteasome pathway in interleukin 6-dependent hematopoietic cells. *Blood* **2000**, *95*, 2577–2585. [PubMed]
13. Delgoffe, G.M.; Vignali, D.A. STAT heterodimers in immunity: A mixed message or a unique signal? *JAKSTAT* **2013**, *2*, e23060. [CrossRef] [PubMed]
14. Bromberg, J.; Darnell, J.E., Jr. The role of STATs in transcriptional control and their impact on cellular function. *Oncogene* **2000**, *19*, 2468–2473. [CrossRef] [PubMed]
15. Yu, H.; Pardoll, D.; Jove, R. STATs in cancer inflammation and immunity: A leading role for STAT3. *Nat. Rev. Cancer* **2009**, *9*, 798–809. [CrossRef] [PubMed]
16. Rebe, C.; Vegran, F.; Berger, H.; Ghiringhelli, F. STAT3 activation: A key factor in tumor immunoescape. *JAKSTAT* **2013**, *2*, e23010.
17. Zhang, H.F.; Lai, R. STAT3 in Cancer-Friend or Foe? *Cancers* **2014**, *6*, 1408–1440. [CrossRef] [PubMed]
18. Burchill, M.A.; Goetz, C.A.; Prlic, M.; O'Neil, J.J.; Harmon, I.R.; Bensinger, S.J.; Turka, L.A.; Brennan, P.; Jameson, S.C.; Farrar, M.A. Distinct effects of STAT5 activation on CD4+ and CD8+ T cell homeostasis: Development of CD4+CD25+ regulatory T cells versus CD8+ memory T cells. *J. Immunol.* **2003**, *171*, 5853–5864. [CrossRef]
19. Agnello, D.; Lankford, C.S.; Bream, J.; Morinobu, A.; Gadina, M.; O'Shea, J.J.; Frucht, D.M. Cytokines and transcription factors that regulate T helper cell differentiation: New players and new insights. *J. Clin. Immunol.* **2003**, *23*, 147–161. [CrossRef]
20. Yao, Z.; Kanno, Y.; Kerenyi, M.; Stephens, G.; Durant, L.; Watford, W.T.; Laurence, A.; Robinson, G.W.; Shevach, E.M.; Moriggl, R.; et al. Nonredundant roles for Stat5a/b in directly regulating Foxp3. *Blood* **2007**, *109*, 4368–4375. [CrossRef]
21. Shiku, H. Importance of CD4+ helper T-cells in antitumor immunity. *Int. J. Hematol* **2003**, *77*, 435–438. [CrossRef] [PubMed]
22. Galon, J.; Costes, A.; Sanchez-Cabo, F.; Kirilovsky, A.; Mlecnik, B.; Lagorce-Pages, C.; Tosolini, M.; Camus, M.; Berger, A.; Wind, P.; et al. Type, density, and location of immune cells within human colorectal tumors predict clinical outcome. *Science* **2006**, *313*, 1960–1964. [CrossRef] [PubMed]

23. Marrogi, A.J.; Munshi, A.; Merogi, A.J.; Ohadike, Y.; El-Habashi, A.; Marrogi, O.L.; Freeman, S.M. Study of tumor infiltrating lymphocytes and transforming growth factor-beta as prognostic factors in breast carcinoma. *Int. J. Cancer* **1997**, *74*, 492–501. [CrossRef]
24. Hiraoka, K.; Miyamoto, M.; Cho, Y.; Suzuoki, M.; Oshikiri, T.; Nakakubo, Y.; Itoh, T.; Ohbuchi, T.; Kondo, S.; Katoh, H. Concurrent infiltration by CD8+ T cells and CD4+ T cells is a favourable prognostic factor in non-small-cell lung carcinoma. *Br. J. Cancer* **2006**, *94*, 275–280. [CrossRef] [PubMed]
25. Tuting, T.; Storkus, W.J.; Lotze, M.T. Gene-based strategies for the immunotherapy of cancer. *J. Mol. Med.* **1997**, *75*, 478–491. [CrossRef]
26. Knutson, K.L.; Disis, M.L. Tumor antigen-specific T helper cells in cancer immunity and immunotherapy. *Cancer Immunol. Immunother.* **2005**, *54*, 721–728. [CrossRef]
27. Owaki, T.; Asakawa, M.; Morishima, N.; Mizoguchi, I.; Fukai, F.; Takeda, K.; Mizuguchi, J.; Yoshimoto, T. STAT3 is indispensable to IL-27-mediated cell proliferation but not to IL-27-induced Th1 differentiation and suppression of proinflammatory cytokine production. *J. Immunol.* **2008**, *180*, 2903–2911. [CrossRef]
28. Ma, C.S.; Wong, N.; Rao, G.; Nguyen, A.; Avery, D.T.; Payne, K.; Torpy, J.; O'Young, P.; Deenick, E.; Bustamante, J.; et al. Unique and shared signaling pathways cooperate to regulate the differentiation of human CD4+ T cells into distinct effector subsets. *J. Exp. Med.* **2016**, *213*, 1589–1608. [CrossRef]
29. Harris, T.J.; Grosso, J.F.; Yen, H.R.; Xin, H.; Kortylewski, M.; Albesiano, E.; Hipkiss, E.L.; Getnet, D.; Goldberg, M.V.; Maris, C.H.; et al. Cutting edge: An in vivo requirement for STAT3 signaling in TH17 development and TH17-dependent autoimmunity. *J. Immunol.* **2007**, *179*, 4313–4317. [CrossRef]
30. Zhang, Y.; Ma, C.A.; Lawrence, M.G.; Break, T.J.; O'Connell, M.P.; Lyons, J.J.; Lopez, D.B.; Barber, J.S.; Zhao, Y.; Barber, D.L.; et al. PD-L1 up-regulation restrains Th17 cell differentiation in STAT3 loss- and STAT1 gain-of-function patients. *J. Exp. Med.* **2017**, *214*, 2523–2533. [CrossRef]
31. Nishihara, M.; Ogura, H.; Ueda, N.; Tsuruoka, M.; Kitabayashi, C.; Tsuji, F.; Aono, H.; Ishihara, K.; Huseby, E.; Betz, U.A.; et al. IL-6-gp130-STAT3 in T cells directs the development of IL-17+ Th with a minimum effect on that of Treg in the steady state. *Int. Immunol.* **2007**, *19*, 695–702. [CrossRef] [PubMed]
32. Zhou, L.; Ivanov, I.I.; Spolski, R.; Min, R.; Shenderov, K.; Egawa, T.; Levy, D.E.; Leonard, W.J.; Littman, D.R. IL-6 programs T(H)-17 cell differentiation by promoting sequential engagement of the IL-21 and IL-23 pathways. *Nat. Immunol.* **2007**, *8*, 967–974. [CrossRef] [PubMed]
33. Yang, X.O.; Panopoulos, A.D.; Nurieva, R.; Chang, S.H.; Wang, D.; Watowich, S.S.; Dong, C. STAT3 regulates cytokine-mediated generation of inflammatory helper T cells. *J. Biol Chem* **2007**, *282*, 9358–9363. [CrossRef] [PubMed]
34. Laurence, A.; Tato, C.M.; Davidson, T.S.; Kanno, Y.; Chen, Z.; Yao, Z.; Blank, R.B.; Meylan, F.; Siegel, R.; Hennighausen, L.; et al. Interleukin-2 signaling via STAT5 constrains T helper 17 cell generation. *Immunity* **2007**, *26*, 371–381. [CrossRef] [PubMed]
35. Yang, X.O.; Pappu, B.P.; Nurieva, R.; Akimzhanov, A.; Kang, H.S.; Chung, Y.; Ma, L.; Shah, B.; Panopoulos, A.D.; Schluns, K.S.; et al. T helper 17 lineage differentiation is programmed by orphan nuclear receptors ROR alpha and ROR gamma. *Immunity* **2008**, *28*, 29–39. [CrossRef]
36. Berger, H.; Vegran, F.; Chikh, M.; Gilardi, F.; Ladoire, S.; Bugaut, H.; Mignot, G.; Chalmin, F.; Bruchard, M.; Derangere, V.; et al. SOCS3 transactivation by PPARgamma prevents IL-17-driven cancer growth. *Cancer Res.* **2013**, *73*, 3578–3590. [CrossRef] [PubMed]
37. Mauldin, I.S.; Tung, K.S.; Lorenz, U.M. The tyrosine phosphatase SHP-1 dampens murine Th17 development. *Blood* **2012**, *119*, 4419–4429. [CrossRef] [PubMed]
38. Ma, L.; Huang, C.; Wang, X.J.; Xin, D.E.; Wang, L.S.; Zou, Q.C.; Zhang, Y.S.; Tan, M.D.; Wang, Y.M.; Zhao, T.C.; et al. Lysyl Oxidase 3 Is a Dual-Specificity Enzyme Involved in STAT3 Deacetylation and Deacetylimination Modulation. *Mol. Cell* **2017**, *65*, 296–309. [CrossRef] [PubMed]
39. Limagne, E.; Thibaudin, M.; Euvrard, R.; Berger, H.; Chalons, P.; Vegan, F.; Humblin, E.; Boidot, R.; Rebe, C.; Derangere, V.; et al. Sirtuin-1 Activation Controls Tumor Growth by Impeding Th17 Differentiation via STAT3 Deacetylation. *Cell Rep.* **2017**, *19*, 746–759. [CrossRef]
40. Chalmin, F.; Mignot, G.; Bruchard, M.; Chevriaux, A.; Vegran, F.; Hichami, A.; Ladoire, S.; Derangere, V.; Vincent, J.; Masson, D.; et al. Stat3 and Gfi-1 transcription factors control Th17 cell immunosuppressive activity via the regulation of ectonucleotidase expression. *Immunity* **2012**, *36*, 362–373. [CrossRef]

41. Zhou, J.; Li, X.; Wu, X.; Zhang, T.; Zhu, Q.; Wang, X.; Wang, H.; Wang, K.; Lin, Y.; Wang, X. Exosomes Released from Tumor-Associated Macrophages Transfer miRNAs That Induce a Treg/Th17 Cell Imbalance in Epithelial Ovarian Cancer. *Cancer Immunol. Res.* **2018**, *6*, 1578–1592. [CrossRef] [PubMed]
42. Zorn, E.; Nelson, E.A.; Mohseni, M.; Porcheray, F.; Kim, H.; Litsa, D.; Bellucci, R.; Raderschall, E.; Canning, C.; Soiffer, R.J.; et al. IL-2 regulates FOXP3 expression in human CD4+CD25+ regulatory T cells through a STAT-dependent mechanism and induces the expansion of these cells in vivo. *Blood* **2006**, *108*, 1571–1579. [CrossRef] [PubMed]
43. Wan, Y.Y.; Flavell, R.A. Regulatory T-cell functions are subverted and converted owing to attenuated Foxp3 expression. *Nature* **2007**, *445*, 766–770. [CrossRef] [PubMed]
44. Kortylewski, M.; Xin, H.; Kujawski, M.; Lee, H.; Liu, Y.; Harris, T.; Drake, C.; Pardoll, D.; Yu, H. Regulation of the IL-23 and IL-12 balance by Stat3 signaling in the tumor microenvironment. *Cancer Cell* **2009**, *15*, 114–123. [CrossRef] [PubMed]
45. Priceman, S.J.; Shen, S.; Wang, L.; Deng, J.; Yue, C.; Kujawski, M.; Yu, H. S1PR1 is crucial for accumulation of regulatory T cells in tumors via STAT3. *Cell Rep.* **2014**, *6*, 992–999. [CrossRef] [PubMed]
46. Huber, M.; Steinwald, V.; Guralnik, A.; Brustle, A.; Kleemann, P.; Rosenplanter, C.; Decker, T.; Lohoff, M. IL-27 inhibits the development of regulatory T cells via STAT3. *Int. Immunol.* **2008**, *20*, 223–234. [CrossRef] [PubMed]
47. Lam, E.; Choi, S.H.; Pareek, T.K.; Kim, B.G.; Letterio, J.J. Cyclin-dependent kinase 5 represses Foxp3 gene expression and Treg development through specific phosphorylation of Stat3 at Serine 727. *Mol. Immunol.* **2015**, *67*, 317–324. [CrossRef] [PubMed]
48. Li, D.; Kong, C.; Tsun, A.; Chen, C.; Song, H.; Shi, G.; Pan, W.; Dai, D.; Shen, N.; Li, B. MiR-125a-5p Decreases the Sensitivity of Treg cells Toward IL-6-Mediated Conversion by Inhibiting IL-6R and STAT3 Expression. *Sci Rep.* **2015**, *5*, 14615. [CrossRef] [PubMed]
49. Xiao, W.; Yin, M.; Wu, K.; Lu, G.; Deng, B.; Zhang, Y.; Qian, L.; Jia, X.; Ding, Y.; Gong, W. High-dose wogonin exacerbates DSS-induced colitis by up-regulating effector T cell function and inhibiting Treg cell. *J. Cell Mol. Med.* **2017**, *21*, 286–298. [CrossRef] [PubMed]
50. Kong, L.Y.; Wei, J.; Sharma, A.K.; Barr, J.; Abou-Ghazal, M.K.; Fokt, I.; Weinberg, J.; Rao, G.; Grimm, E.; Priebe, W.; et al. A novel phosphorylated STAT3 inhibitor enhances T cell cytotoxicity against melanoma through inhibition of regulatory T cells. *Cancer Immunol. Immunother.* **2009**, *58*, 1023–1032. [CrossRef] [PubMed]
51. He, W.; Zhu, Y.; Mu, R.; Xu, J.; Zhang, X.; Wang, C.; Li, Q.; Huang, Z.; Zhang, J.; Pan, Y.; et al. A Jak2-selective inhibitor potently reverses the immune suppression by modulating the tumor microenvironment for cancer immunotherapy. *Biochem. Pharmacol.* **2017**, *145*, 132–146. [CrossRef] [PubMed]
52. Oweida, A.J.; Darragh, L.; Phan, A.; Binder, D.; Bhatia, S.; Mueller, A.; Van Court, B.; Milner, D.; Raben, D.; Woessner, R.; et al. The role of regulatory T cells in the response to radiation therapy in head and neck cancer. *J. Natl. Cancer Inst.* **2019**. [CrossRef] [PubMed]
53. Schmitt, N.; Liu, Y.; Bentebibel, S.E.; Munagala, I.; Bourdery, L.; Venuprasad, K.; Banchereau, J.; Ueno, H. The cytokine TGF-beta co-opts signaling via STAT3-STAT4 to promote the differentiation of human TFH cells. *Nat. Immunol.* **2014**, *15*, 856–865. [CrossRef] [PubMed]
54. Ma, C.S.; Avery, D.T.; Chan, A.; Batten, M.; Bustamante, J.; Boisson-Dupuis, S.; Arkwright, P.D.; Kreins, A.Y.; Averbuch, D.; Engelhard, D.; et al. Functional STAT3 deficiency compromises the generation of human T follicular helper cells. *Blood* **2012**, *119*, 3997–4008. [CrossRef] [PubMed]
55. Hercor, M.; Anciaux, M.; Denanglaire, S.; Debuisson, D.; Leo, O.; Andris, F. Antigen-presenting cell-derived IL-6 restricts the expression of GATA3 and IL-4 by follicular helper T cells. *J. Leukoc. Biol.* **2017**, *101*, 5–14. [CrossRef] [PubMed]
56. Chen, M.M.; Xiao, X.; Lao, X.M.; Wei, Y.; Liu, R.X.; Zeng, Q.H.; Wang, J.C.; Ouyang, F.Z.; Chen, D.P.; Chan, K.W.; et al. Polarization of Tissue-Resident TFH-Like Cells in Human Hepatoma Bridges Innate Monocyte Inflammation and M2b Macrophage Polarization. *Cancer Discov.* **2016**, *6*, 1182–1195. [CrossRef]
57. Olson, M.R.; Verdan, F.F.; Hufford, M.M.; Dent, A.L.; Kaplan, M.H. STAT3 Impairs STAT5 Activation in the Development of IL-9-Secreting T Cells. *J. Immunol.* **2016**, *196*, 3297–3304. [CrossRef]
58. Ulrich, B.J.; Verdan, F.F.; McKenzie, A.N.; Kaplan, M.H.; Olson, M.R. STAT3 Activation Impairs the Stability of Th9 Cells. *J. Immunol.* **2017**, *198*, 2302–2309. [CrossRef]

59. Zhang, Y.; Siegel, A.M.; Sun, G.; Dimaggio, T.; Freeman, A.F.; Milner, J.D. Human TH9 differentiation is dependent on signal transducer and activator of transcription (STAT) 3 to restrain STAT1-mediated inhibition. *J. Allergy Clin. Immunol.* **2019**, *143*, 1108–1118. [CrossRef]
60. Yue, C.; Shen, S.; Deng, J.; Priceman, S.J.; Li, W.; Huang, A.; Yu, H. STAT3 in CD8+ T Cells Inhibits Their Tumor Accumulation by Downregulating CXCR3/CXCL10 Axis. *Cancer Immunol. Res.* **2015**, *3*, 864–870. [CrossRef]
61. Kujawski, M.; Zhang, C.; Herrmann, A.; Reckamp, K.; Scuto, A.; Jensen, M.; Deng, J.; Forman, S.; Figlin, R.; Yu, H. Targeting STAT3 in adoptively transferred T cells promotes their in vivo expansion and antitumor effects. *Cancer Res.* **2010**, *70*, 9599–9610. [CrossRef] [PubMed]
62. Hu, J.; Batth, I.S.; Xia, X.; Li, S. Regulation of NKG2D(+)CD8(+) T-cell-mediated antitumor immune surveillance: Identification of a novel CD28 activation-mediated, STAT3 phosphorylation-dependent mechanism. *OncoImmunology* **2016**, *5*, e1252012. [CrossRef] [PubMed]
63. Tosolini, M.; Kirilovsky, A.; Mlecnik, B.; Fredriksen, T.; Mauger, S.; Bindea, G.; Berger, A.; Bruneval, P.; Fridman, W.H.; Pages, F.; et al. Clinical impact of different classes of infiltrating T cytotoxic and helper cells (Th1, th2, treg, th17) in patients with colorectal cancer. *Cancer Res.* **2011**, *71*, 1263–1271. [CrossRef] [PubMed]
64. Szabo, S.J.; Kim, S.T.; Costa, G.L.; Zhang, X.; Fathman, C.G.; Glimcher, L.H. A novel transcription factor, T-bet, directs Th1 lineage commitment. *Cell* **2000**, *100*, 655–669. [CrossRef]
65. Zheng, W.; Flavell, R.A. The transcription factor GATA-3 is necessary and sufficient for Th2 cytokine gene expression in CD4 T cells. *Cell* **1997**, *89*, 587–596. [CrossRef]
66. Yoshimoto, T.; Yasuda, K.; Mizuguchi, J.; Nakanishi, K. IL-27 suppresses Th2 cell development and Th2 cytokines production from polarized Th2 cells: A novel therapeutic way for Th2-mediated allergic inflammation. *J. Immunol.* **2007**, *179*, 4415–4423. [CrossRef] [PubMed]
67. Chen, Z.; O'Shea, J.J. Th17 cells: A new fate for differentiating helper T cells. *Immunol. Res.* **2008**, *41*, 87–102. [CrossRef]
68. Van den Berg, W.B.; Miossec, P. IL-17 as a future therapeutic target for rheumatoid arthritis. *Nat. Rev. Rheumatol.* **2009**, *5*, 549–553. [CrossRef]
69. Su, X.; Ye, J.; Hsueh, E.C.; Zhang, Y.; Hoft, D.F.; Peng, G. Tumor microenvironments direct the recruitment and expansion of human Th17 cells. *J. Immunol.* **2010**, *184*, 1630–1641. [CrossRef]
70. Hemdan, N.Y. Anti-cancer versus cancer-promoting effects of the interleukin-17-producing T helper cells. *Immunol. Lett* **2013**, *149*, 123–133. [CrossRef]
71. Ivanov, I.I.; McKenzie, B.S.; Zhou, L.; Tadokoro, C.E.; Lepelley, A.; Lafaille, J.J.; Cua, D.J.; Littman, D.R. The orphan nuclear receptor RORgammat directs the differentiation program of proinflammatory IL-17+ T helper cells. *Cell* **2006**, *126*, 1121–1133. [CrossRef] [PubMed]
72. Jiang, Y.; Liu, Y.; Lu, H.; Sun, S.C.; Jin, W.; Wang, X.; Dong, C. Epigenetic activation during T helper 17 cell differentiation is mediated by Tripartite motif containing 28. *Nat. Commun.* **2018**, *9*, 1424. [CrossRef]
73. Fang, S.; Liu, B.; Sun, Q.; Zhao, J.; Qi, H.; Li, Q. Platelet factor 4 inhibits IL-17/Stat3 pathway via upregulation of SOCS3 expression in melanoma. *Inflammation* **2014**, *37*, 1744–1750. [CrossRef] [PubMed]
74. Ghoreschi, K.; Laurence, A.; Yang, X.P.; Tato, C.M.; McGeachy, M.J.; Konkel, J.E.; Ramos, H.L.; Wei, L.; Davidson, T.S.; Bouladoux, N.; et al. Generation of pathogenic T(H)17 cells in the absence of TGF-beta signalling. *Nature* **2010**, *467*, 967–971. [CrossRef] [PubMed]
75. Sakaguchi, S. Regulatory T cells: Key controllers of Immunol.ogic self-tolerance. *Cell* **2000**, *101*, 455–458. [CrossRef]
76. Shevach, E.M. CD4+ CD25+ suppressor T cells: More questions than answers. *Nat. Rev. Immunol.* **2002**, *2*, 389–400. [CrossRef] [PubMed]
77. Chen, W.; Jin, W.; Hardegen, N.; Lei, K.J.; Li, L.; Marinos, N.; McGrady, G.; Wahl, S.M. Conversion of peripheral CD4+CD25- naive T cells to CD4+CD25+ regulatory T cells by TGF-beta induction of transcription factor Foxp3. *J. Exp. Med.* **2003**, *198*, 1875–1886. [CrossRef] [PubMed]
78. Nishikawa, H.; Sakaguchi, S. Regulatory T cells in tumor immunity. *Int. J. Cancer* **2010**, *127*, 759–767. [CrossRef] [PubMed]
79. Curiel, T.J.; Coukos, G.; Zou, L.; Alvarez, X.; Cheng, P.; Mottram, P.; Evdemon-Hogan, M.; Conejo-Garcia, J.R.; Zhang, L.; Burow, M.; et al. Specific recruitment of regulatory T cells in ovarian carcinoma fosters immune privilege and predicts reduced survival. *Nat. Med.* **2004**, *10*, 942–949. [CrossRef]

80. Bates, G.J.; Fox, S.B.; Han, C.; Leek, R.D.; Garcia, J.F.; Harris, A.L.; Banham, A.H. Quantification of regulatory T cells enables the identification of high-risk breast cancer patients and those at risk of late relapse. *J. Clin. Oncol.* **2006**, *24*, 5373–5380. [CrossRef]
81. Perrone, G.; Ruffini, P.A.; Catalano, V.; Spino, C.; Santini, D.; Muretto, P.; Spoto, C.; Zingaretti, C.; Sisti, V.; Alessandroni, P.; et al. Intratumoural FOXP3-positive regulatory T cells are associated with adverse prognosis in radically resected gastric cancer. *Eur. J. Cancer* **2008**, *44*, 1875–1882. [CrossRef] [PubMed]
82. Chaudhry, A.; Rudra, D.; Treuting, P.; Samstein, R.M.; Liang, Y.; Kas, A.; Rudensky, A.Y. CD4+ regulatory T cells control TH17 responses in a Stat3-dependent manner. *Science* **2009**, *326*, 986–991. [CrossRef] [PubMed]
83. Wuest, T.Y.; Willette-Brown, J.; Durum, S.K.; Hurwitz, A.A. The influence of IL-2 family cytokines on activation and function of naturally occurring regulatory T cells. *J. Leukoc. Biol.* **2008**, *84*, 973–980. [CrossRef] [PubMed]
84. Xu, L.; Kitani, A.; Stuelten, C.; McGrady, G.; Fuss, I.; Strober, W. Positive and negative transcriptional regulation of the Foxp3 gene is mediated by access and binding of the Smad3 protein to enhancer I. *Immunity* **2010**, *33*, 313–325. [CrossRef] [PubMed]
85. Laurence, A.; Amarnath, S.; Mariotti, J.; Kim, Y.C.; Foley, J.; Eckhaus, M.; O'Shea, J.J.; Fowler, D.H. STAT3 Transcription Factor Promotes Instability of nTreg Cells and Limits Generation of iTreg Cells during Acute Murine Graft-versus-Host Disease. *Immunity* **2012**, *37*, 209–222. [CrossRef] [PubMed]
86. Eivazi, S.; Bagheri, S.; Hashemzadeh, M.S.; Ghalavand, M.; Qamsari, E.S.; Dorostkar, R.; Yasemi, M. Development of T follicular helper cells and their role in disease and immune system. *Biomed. Pharmacother.* **2016**, *84*, 1668–1678. [CrossRef] [PubMed]
87. Qin, L.; Waseem, T.C.; Sahoo, A.; Bieerkehazhi, S.; Zhou, H.; Galkina, E.V.; Nurieva, R. Insights Into the Molecular Mechanisms of T Follicular Helper-Mediated Immunity and Pathology. *Front. Immunol.* **2018**, *9*, 1884. [CrossRef] [PubMed]
88. Gu-Trantien, C.; Loi, S.; Garaud, S.; Equeter, C.; Libin, M.; de Wind, A.; Ravoet, M.; Le Buanec, H.; Sibille, C.; Manfouo-Foutsop, G.; et al. CD4(+) follicular helper T cell infiltration predicts breast cancer survival. *J. Clin. Invest.* **2013**, *123*, 2873–2892. [CrossRef] [PubMed]
89. Bindea, G.; Mlecnik, B.; Tosolini, M.; Kirilovsky, A.; Waldner, M.; Obenauf, A.C.; Angell, H.; Fredriksen, T.; Lafontaine, L.; Berger, A.; et al. Spatiotemporal dynamics of intratumoral immune cells reveal the immune landscape in human cancer. *Immunity* **2013**, *39*, 782–795. [CrossRef]
90. Alshekaili, J.; Chand, R.; Lee, C.E.; Corley, S.; Kwong, K.; Papa, I.; Fulcher, D.A.; Randall, K.L.; Leiding, J.W.; Ma, C.S.; et al. STAT3 regulates cytotoxicity of human CD57+ CD4+ T cells in blood and lymphoid follicles. *Sci. Rep.* **2018**, *8*, 3529. [CrossRef]
91. Ray, J.P.; Marshall, H.D.; Laidlaw, B.J.; Staron, M.M.; Kaech, S.M.; Craft, J. Transcription factor STAT3 and type I interferons are corepressive insulators for differentiation of follicular helper and T helper 1 cells. *Immunity* **2014**, *40*, 367–377. [CrossRef] [PubMed]
92. Wu, H.; Xu, L.L.; Teuscher, P.; Liu, H.; Kaplan, M.H.; Dent, A.L. An Inhibitory Role for the Transcription Factor Stat3 in Controlling IL-4 and Bcl6 Expression in Follicular Helper T Cells. *J. Immunol.* **2015**, *195*, 2080–2089. [CrossRef] [PubMed]
93. Read, K.A.; Powell, M.D.; Baker, C.E.; Sreekumar, B.K.; Ringel-Scaia, V.M.; Bachus, H.; Martin, R.E.; Cooley, I.D.; Allen, I.C.; Ballesteros-Tato, A.; et al. Integrated STAT3 and Ikaros Zinc Finger Transcription Factor Activities Regulate Bcl-6 Expression in CD4(+) Th Cells. *J. Immunol.* **2017**, *199*, 2377–2387. [CrossRef] [PubMed]
94. Chen, W.; Nyuydzefe, M.S.; Weiss, J.M.; Zhang, J.; Waksal, S.D.; Zanin-Zhorov, A. ROCK2, but not ROCK1 interacts with phosphorylated STAT3 and co-occupies TH17/TFH gene promoters in TH17-activated human T cells. *Sci. Rep.* **2018**, *8*, 16636. [CrossRef] [PubMed]
95. Rivera Vargas, T.; Humblin, E.; Vegran, F.; Ghiringhelli, F.; Apetoh, L. TH9 cells in anti-tumor immunity. *Semin. Immunopathol.* **2017**, *39*, 39–46. [CrossRef]
96. Durgeau, A.; Virk, Y.; Corgnac, S.; Mami-Chouaib, F. Recent Advances in Targeting CD8 T-Cell Immunity for More Effective Cancer Immunotherapy. *Front. Immunol.* **2018**, *9*, 14. [CrossRef] [PubMed]
97. Emmerich, J.; Mumm, J.B.; Chan, I.H.; LaFace, D.; Truong, H.; McClanahan, T.; Gorman, D.M.; Oft, M. IL-10 directly activates and expands tumor-resident CD8(+) T cells without de novo infiltration from secondary lymphoid organs. *Cancer Res.* **2012**, *72*, 3570–3581. [CrossRef] [PubMed]
98. Wang, X.; Xin, W.; Zhang, H.; Zhang, F.; Gao, M.; Yuan, L.; Xu, X.; Hu, X.; Zhao, M. Aberrant expression of p-STAT3 in peripheral blood CD4+ and CD8+ T cells related to hepatocellular carcinoma development. *Mol. Med. Rep.* **2014**, *10*, 2649–2656. [CrossRef] [PubMed]

99. Marigo, I.; Dolcetti, L.; Serafini, P.; Zanovello, P.; Bronte, V. Tumor-induced tolerance and immune suppression by myeloid derived suppressor cells. *Immunol. Rev.* **2008**, *222*, 162–179. [CrossRef]
100. Cheng, F.; Wang, H.W.; Cuenca, A.; Huang, M.; Ghansah, T.; Brayer, J.; Kerr, W.G.; Takeda, K.; Akira, S.; Schoenberger, S.P.; et al. A critical role for Stat3 signaling in immune tolerance. *Immunity* **2003**, *19*, 425–436. [CrossRef]
101. Brayer, J.; Cheng, F.; Wang, H.; Horna, P.; Vicente-Suarez, I.; Pinilla-Ibarz, J.; Sotomayor, E.M. Enhanced CD8 T cell cross-presentation by macrophages with targeted disruption of STAT3. *Immunol. Lett.* **2010**, *131*, 126–130. [CrossRef] [PubMed]
102. Kortylewski, M.; Kujawski, M.; Herrmann, A.; Yang, C.; Wang, L.; Liu, Y.; Salcedo, R.; Yu, H. Toll-like receptor 9 activation of signal transducer and activator of transcription 3 constrains its agonist-based immunotherapy. *Cancer Res.* **2009**, *69*, 2497–2505. [CrossRef] [PubMed]
103. Cheng, Z.; Zhang, D.; Gong, B.; Wang, P.; Liu, F. CD163 as a novel target gene of STAT3 is a potential therapeutic target for gastric cancer. *Oncotarget* **2017**, *8*, 87244–87262. [CrossRef] [PubMed]
104. Solis-Martinez, R.; Cancino-Marentes, M.; Hernandez-Flores, G.; Ortiz-Lazareno, P.; Mandujano-Alvarez, G.; Cruz-Galvez, C.; Sierra-Diaz, E.; Rodriguez-Padilla, C.; Jave-Suarez, L.F.; Aguilar-Lemarroy, A.; et al. Regulation of immunophenotype modulation of monocytes-macrophages from M1 into M2 by prostate cancer cell-culture supernatant via transcription factor STAT3. *Immunol. Lett.* **2018**, *196*, 140–148. [CrossRef] [PubMed]
105. Kubala, M.H.; Punj, V.; Placencio-Hickok, V.R.; Fang, H.; Fernandez, G.E.; Sposto, R.; DeClerck, Y.A. Plasminogen Activator Inhibitor-1 Promotes the Recruitment and Polarization of Macrophages in Cancer. *Cell Rep.* **2018**, *25*, 2177–2191. [CrossRef]
106. Ham, S.; Lima, L.G.; Chai, E.P.Z.; Muller, A.; Lobb, R.J.; Krumeich, S.; Wen, S.W.; Wiegmans, A.P.; Moller, A. Breast Cancer-Derived Exosomes Alter Macrophage Polarization via gp130/STAT3 Signaling. *Front. Immunol.* **2018**, *9*, 871. [CrossRef]
107. Fujiwara, Y.; Komohara, Y.; Ikeda, T.; Takeya, M. Corosolic acid inhibits glioblastoma cell proliferation by suppressing the activation of signal transducer and activator of transcription-3 and nuclear factor-kappa B in tumor cells and tumor-associated macrophages. *Cancer Sci.* **2011**, *102*, 206–211. [CrossRef]
108. Fujiwara, Y.; Komohara, Y.; Kudo, R.; Tsurushima, K.; Ohnishi, K.; Ikeda, T.; Takeya, M. Oleanolic acid inhibits macrophage differentiation into the M2 phenotype and glioblastoma cell proliferation by suppressing the activation of STAT3. *Oncol. Rep.* **2011**, *26*, 1533–1537. [PubMed]
109. Andersen, M.N.; Etzerodt, A.; Graversen, J.H.; Holthof, L.C.; Moestrup, S.K.; Hokland, M.; Moller, H.J. STAT3 inhibition specifically in human monocytes and macrophages by CD163-targeted corosolic acid-containing liposomes. *Cancer Immunol. Immunother.* **2019**, *68*, 489–502. [CrossRef]
110. Giurisato, E.; Xu, Q.; Lonardi, S.; Telfer, B.; Russo, I.; Pearson, A.; Finegan, K.G.; Wang, W.; Wang, J.; Gray, N.S.; et al. Myeloid ERK5 deficiency suppresses tumor growth by blocking protumor macrophage polarization via STAT3 inhibition. *Proc. Natl. Acad. Sci. USA* **2018**, *115*, E2801–E2810. [CrossRef]
111. Dominguez-Soto, A.; Sierra-Filardi, E.; Puig-Kroger, A.; Perez-Maceda, B.; Gomez-Aguado, F.; Corcuera, M.T.; Sanchez-Mateos, P.; Corbi, A.L. Dendritic cell-specific ICAM-3-grabbing nonintegrin expression on M2-polarized and tumor-associated macrophages is macrophage-CSF dependent and enhanced by tumor-derived IL-6 and IL-10. *J. Immunol.* **2011**, *186*, 2192–2200. [CrossRef] [PubMed]
112. Hiwatashi, K.; Tamiya, T.; Hasegawa, E.; Fukaya, T.; Hashimoto, M.; Kakoi, K.; Kashiwagi, I.; Kimura, A.; Inoue, N.; Morita, R.; et al. Suppression of SOCS3 in macrophages prevents cancer metastasis by modifying macrophage phase and MCP2/CCL8 induction. *Cancer Lett.* **2011**, *308*, 172–180. [CrossRef] [PubMed]
113. Hasita, H.; Komohara, Y.; Okabe, H.; Masuda, T.; Ohnishi, K.; Lei, X.F.; Beppu, T.; Baba, H.; Takeya, M. Significance of alternatively activated macrophages in patients with intrahepatic cholangiocarcinoma. *Cancer Sci.* **2010**, *101*, 1913–1919. [CrossRef] [PubMed]
114. Lee, J.H.; Lee, G.T.; Woo, S.H.; Ha, Y.S.; Kwon, S.J.; Kim, W.J.; Kim, I.Y. BMP-6 in renal cell carcinoma promotes tumor proliferation through IL-10-dependent M2 polarization of tumor-associated macrophages. *Cancer Res.* **2013**, *73*, 3604–3614. [CrossRef] [PubMed]
115. Kujawski, M.; Kortylewski, M.; Lee, H.; Herrmann, A.; Kay, H.; Yu, H. Stat3 mediates myeloid cell-dependent tumor angiogenesis in mice. *J. Clin. Invest.* **2008**, *118*, 3367–3377. [CrossRef] [PubMed]
116. Laouar, Y.; Welte, T.; Fu, X.Y.; Flavell, R.A. STAT3 is required for Flt3L-dependent dendritic cell differentiation. *Immunity* **2003**, *19*, 903–912. [CrossRef]

117. Kortylewski, M.; Kujawski, M.; Wang, T.; Wei, S.; Zhang, S.; Pilon-Thomas, S.; Niu, G.; Kay, H.; Mule, J.; Kerr, W.G.; et al. Inhibiting Stat3 signaling in the hematopoietic system elicits multicomponent antitumor immunity. *Nat. Med.* **2005**, *11*, 1314–1321. [CrossRef]
118. Herrmann, A.; Kortylewski, M.; Kujawski, M.; Zhang, C.; Reckamp, K.; Armstrong, B.; Wang, L.; Kowolik, C.; Deng, J.; Figlin, R.; et al. Targeting Stat3 in the myeloid compartment drastically improves the in vivo antitumor functions of adoptively transferred T cells. *Cancer Res.* **2010**, *70*, 7455–7464. [CrossRef]
119. Iwata-Kajihara, T.; Sumimoto, H.; Kawamura, N.; Ueda, R.; Takahashi, T.; Mizuguchi, H.; Miyagishi, M.; Takeda, K.; Kawakami, Y. Enhanced cancer immunotherapy using STAT3-depleted dendritic cells with high Th1-inducing ability and resistance to cancer cell-derived inhibitory factors. *J. Immunol.* **2011**, *187*, 27–36. [CrossRef]
120. Sanseverino, I.; Purificato, C.; Varano, B.; Conti, L.; Gessani, S.; Gauzzi, M.C. STAT3-silenced human dendritic cells have an enhanced ability to prime IFNgamma production by both alphabeta and gammadelta T lymphocytes. *Immunobiology* **2014**, *219*, 503–511. [CrossRef]
121. Hoentjen, F.; Sartor, R.B.; Ozaki, M.; Jobin, C. STAT3 regulates NF-kappaB recruitment to the IL-12p40 promoter in dendritic cells. *Blood* **2005**, *105*, 689–696. [CrossRef] [PubMed]
122. Kitamura, H.; Kamon, H.; Sawa, S.; Park, S.J.; Katunuma, N.; Ishihara, K.; Murakami, M.; Hirano, T. IL-6-STAT3 controls intracellular MHC class II alphabeta dimer level through cathepsin S activity in dendritic cells. *Immunity* **2005**, *23*, 491–502. [CrossRef] [PubMed]
123. Ohno, Y.; Kitamura, H.; Takahashi, N.; Ohtake, J.; Kaneumi, S.; Sumida, K.; Homma, S.; Kawamura, H.; Minagawa, N.; Shibasaki, S.; et al. IL-6 down-regulates HLA class II expression and IL-12 production of human dendritic cells to impair activation of antigen-specific CD4(+) T cells. *Cancer Immunol. Immunother.* **2016**, *65*, 193–204. [CrossRef] [PubMed]
124. Li, H.S.; Liu, C.; Xiao, Y.; Chu, F.; Liang, X.; Peng, W.; Hu, J.; Neelapu, S.S.; Sun, S.C.; Hwu, P.; et al. Bypassing STAT3-mediated inhibition of the transcriptional regulator ID2 improves the antitumor efficacy of dendritic cells. *Sci. Signal.* **2016**, *9*, ra94. [CrossRef] [PubMed]
125. Yu, S.; Liu, C.; Su, K.; Wang, J.; Liu, Y.; Zhang, L.; Li, C.; Cong, Y.; Kimberly, R.; Grizzle, W.E.; et al. Tumor exosomes inhibit differentiation of bone marrow dendritic cells. *J. Immunol.* **2007**, *178*, 6867–6875. [CrossRef]
126. Zhang, H.; Nguyen-Jackson, H.; Panopoulos, A.D.; Li, H.S.; Murray, P.J.; Watowich, S.S. STAT3 controls myeloid progenitor growth during emergency granulopoiesis. *Blood* **2010**, *116*, 2462–2471. [CrossRef] [PubMed]
127. Nefedova, Y.; Huang, M.; Kusmartsev, S.; Bhattacharya, R.; Cheng, P.; Salup, R.; Jove, R.; Gabrilovich, D. Hyperactivation of STAT3 is involved in abnormal differentiation of dendritic cells in cancer. *J. Immunol.* **2004**, *172*, 464–474. [CrossRef] [PubMed]
128. Nefedova, Y.; Nagaraj, S.; Rosenbauer, A.; Muro-Cacho, C.; Sebti, S.M.; Gabrilovich, D.I. Regulation of dendritic cell differentiation and antitumor immune response in cancer by pharmacologic-selective inhibition of the janus-activated kinase 2/signal transducers and activators of transcription 3 pathway. *Cancer Res.* **2005**, *65*, 9525–9535. [CrossRef]
129. Hossain, D.M.; Pal, S.K.; Moreira, D.; Duttagupta, P.; Zhang, Q.; Won, H.; Jones, J.; D'Apuzzo, M.; Forman, S.; Kortylewski, M. TLR9-Targeted STAT3 Silencing Abrogates Immunosuppressive Activity of Myeloid-Derived Suppressor Cells from Prostate Cancer Patients. *Clin. Cancer Res.* **2015**, *21*, 3771–3782. [CrossRef]
130. Moreira, D.; Adamus, T.; Zhao, X.; Su, Y.L.; Zhang, Z.; White, S.V.; Swiderski, P.; Lu, X.; DePinho, R.A.; Pal, S.K.; et al. STAT3 Inhibition Combined with CpG Immunostimulation Activates Antitumor Immunity to Eradicate Genetically Distinct Castration-Resistant Prostate Cancers. *Clin. Cancer Res.* **2018**, *24*, 5948–5962. [CrossRef]
131. Zhou, J.; Qu, Z.; Sun, F.; Han, L.; Li, L.; Yan, S.; Stabile, L.P.; Chen, L.F.; Siegfried, J.M.; Xiao, G. Myeloid STAT3 Promotes Lung Tumorigenesis by Transforming Tumor Immunosurveillance into Tumor-Promoting Inflammation. *Cancer Immunol. Res.* **2017**, *5*, 257–268. [CrossRef] [PubMed]
132. Corzo, C.A.; Cotter, M.J.; Cheng, P.; Cheng, F.; Kusmartsev, S.; Sotomayor, E.; Padhya, T.; McCaffrey, T.V.; McCaffrey, J.C.; Gabrilovich, D.I. Mechanism regulating reactive oxygen species in tumor-induced myeloid-derived suppressor cells. *J. Immunol.* **2009**, *182*, 5693–5701. [CrossRef] [PubMed]
133. Chalmin, F.; Ladoire, S.; Mignot, G.; Vincent, J.; Bruchard, M.; Remy-Martin, J.P.; Boireau, W.; Rouleau, A.; Simon, B.; Lanneau, D.; et al. Membrane-associated Hsp72 from tumor-derived exosomes mediates STAT3-dependent immunosuppressive function of mouse and human myeloid-derived suppressor cells. *J. Clin. Invest.* **2010**, *120*, 457–471. [CrossRef] [PubMed]

134. Waight, J.D.; Netherby, C.; Hensen, M.L.; Miller, A.; Hu, Q.; Liu, S.; Bogner, P.N.; Farren, M.R.; Lee, K.P.; Liu, K.; et al. Myeloid-derived suppressor cell development is regulated by a STAT/IRF-8 axis. *J. Clin. Invest.* **2013**, *123*, 4464–4478. [CrossRef] [PubMed]
135. Thorn, M.; Guha, P.; Cunetta, M.; Espat, N.J.; Miller, G.; Junghans, R.P.; Katz, S.C. Tumor-associated GM-CSF overexpression induces immunoinhibitory molecules via STAT3 in myeloid-suppressor cells infiltrating liver metastases. *Cancer Gene Ther.* **2016**, *23*, 188–198. [CrossRef] [PubMed]
136. Vasquez-Dunddel, D.; Pan, F.; Zeng, Q.; Gorbounov, M.; Albesiano, E.; Fu, J.; Blosser, R.L.; Tam, A.J.; Bruno, T.; Zhang, H.; et al. STAT3 regulates arginase-I in myeloid-derived suppressor cells from cancer patients. *J. Clin. Invest.* **2013**, *123*, 1580–1589. [CrossRef]
137. Yu, J.; Du, W.; Yan, F.; Wang, Y.; Li, H.; Cao, S.; Yu, W.; Shen, C.; Liu, J.; Ren, X. Myeloid-derived suppressor cells suppress antitumor immune responses through IDO expression and correlate with lymph node metastasis in patients with breast cancer. *J. Immunol.* **2013**, *190*, 3783–3797. [CrossRef]
138. Kumar, V.; Cheng, P.; Condamine, T.; Mony, S.; Languino, L.R.; McCaffrey, J.C.; Hockstein, N.; Guarino, M.; Masters, G.; Penman, E.; et al. CD45 Phosphatase Inhibits STAT3 Transcription Factor Activity in Myeloid Cells and Promotes Tumor-Associated Macrophage Differentiation. *Immunity* **2016**, *44*, 303–315. [CrossRef]
139. Wu, T.; Wang, C.; Wang, W.; Hui, Y.; Zhang, R.; Qiao, L.; Dai, Y. Embelin impairs the accumulation and activation of MDSCs in colitis-associated tumorigenesis. *OncoImmunology* **2018**, *7*, e1498437. [CrossRef]
140. Kuroda, H.; Mabuchi, S.; Kozasa, K.; Yokoi, E.; Matsumoto, Y.; Komura, N.; Kawano, M.; Hashimoto, K.; Sawada, K.; Kimura, T. PM01183 inhibits myeloid-derived suppressor cells in vitro and in vivo. *Immunotherapy* **2017**, *9*, 805–817. [CrossRef]
141. Yin, T.; Zhao, Z.B.; Guo, J.; Wang, T.; Yang, J.B.; Wang, C.; Long, J.; Ma, S.; Huang, Q.; Zhang, K.; et al. Aurora-A inhibition eliminates myeloid cell-mediated immunosuppression and enhances the efficacy of anti-PD-L1 therapy in breast cancer. *Cancer Res.* **2019**. [CrossRef] [PubMed]
142. Guha, P.; Gardell, J.; Darpolor, J.; Cunetta, M.; Lima, M.; Miller, G.; Espat, N.J.; Junghans, R.P.; Katz, S.C. STAT3 inhibition induces Bax-dependent apoptosis in liver tumor myeloid-derived suppressor cells. *Oncogene* **2019**, *38*, 533–548. [CrossRef] [PubMed]
143. Mills, C.D.; Kincaid, K.; Alt, J.M.; Heilman, M.J.; Hill, A.M. M-1/M-2 macrophages and the Th1/Th2 paradigm. *J. Immunol.* **2000**, *164*, 6166–6173. [CrossRef] [PubMed]
144. Martinez, F.O.; Sica, A.; Mantovani, A.; Locati, M. Macrophage activation and polarization. *Front. Biosci.* **2008**, *13*, 453–461. [CrossRef] [PubMed]
145. Pollard, J.W. Tumour-educated macrophages promote tumour progression and metastasis. *Nat. Rev. Cancer* **2004**, *4*, 71–78. [CrossRef] [PubMed]
146. Sica, A.; Schioppa, T.; Mantovani, A.; Allavena, P. Tumour-associated macrophages are a distinct M2 polarised population promoting tumour progression: Potential targets of anti-cancer therapy. *Eur. J. Cancer* **2006**, *42*, 717–727. [CrossRef]
147. Lewis, C.E.; Pollard, J.W. Distinct role of macrophages in different tumor microenvironments. *Cancer Res.* **2006**, *66*, 605–612. [CrossRef]
148. Jenkins, B.J.; Grail, D.; Inglese, M.; Quilici, C.; Bozinovski, S.; Wong, P.; Ernst, M. Imbalanced gp130-dependent signaling in macrophages alters macrophage colony-stimulating factor responsiveness via regulation of c-fms expression. *Mol. Cell Biol.* **2004**, *24*, 1453–1463. [CrossRef]
149. Sun, Z.; Yao, Z.; Liu, S.; Tang, H.; Yan, X. An oligonucleotide decoy for Stat3 activates the immune response of macrophages to breast cancer. *Immunobiology* **2006**, *211*, 199–209. [CrossRef]
150. Komohara, Y.; Ohnishi, K.; Kuratsu, J.; Takeya, M. Possible involvement of the M2 anti-inflammatory macrophage phenotype in growth of human gliomas. *J. Pathol.* **2008**, *216*, 15–24. [CrossRef]
151. Fu, X.L.; Duan, W.; Su, C.Y.; Mao, F.Y.; Lv, Y.P.; Teng, Y.S.; Yu, P.W.; Zhuang, Y.; Zhao, Y.L. Interleukin 6 induces M2 macrophage differentiation by STAT3 activation that correlates with gastric cancer progression. *Cancer Immunol. Immunother.* **2017**, *66*, 1597–1608. [CrossRef] [PubMed]
152. Li, Y.; Cai, L.; Wang, H.; Wu, P.; Gu, W.; Chen, Y.; Hao, H.; Tang, K.; Yi, P.; Liu, M.; et al. Pleiotropic regulation of macrophage polarization and tumorigenesis by formyl peptide receptor-2. *Oncogene* **2011**, *30*, 3887–3899. [CrossRef] [PubMed]
153. Crowley, M.; Inaba, K.; Steinman, R.M. Dendritic cells are the principal cells in mouse spleen bearing immunogenic fragments of foreign proteins. *J. Exp. Med.* **1990**, *172*, 383–386. [CrossRef] [PubMed]

154. Steinman, R.M. The dendritic cell system and its role in immunogenicity. *Annu. Rev. Immunol.* **1991**, *9*, 271–296. [CrossRef]
155. Park, S.J.; Nakagawa, T.; Kitamura, H.; Atsumi, T.; Kamon, H.; Sawa, S.; Kamimura, D.; Ueda, N.; Iwakura, Y.; Ishihara, K.; et al. IL-6 regulates in vivo dendritic cell differentiation through STAT3 activation. *J. Immunol.* **2004**, *173*, 3844–3854. [CrossRef]
156. Farren, M.R.; Carlson, L.M.; Netherby, C.S.; Lindner, I.; Li, P.K.; Gabrilovich, D.I.; Abrams, S.I.; Lee, K.P. Tumor-induced STAT3 signaling in myeloid cells impairs dendritic cell generation by decreasing PKCbetaII abundance. *Sci. Signal.* **2014**, *7*, ra16. [CrossRef]
157. Wagner, A.H.; Conzelmann, M.; Fitzer, F.; Giese, T.; Gulow, K.; Falk, C.S.; Kramer, O.H.; Dietrich, S.; Hecker, M.; Luft, T. JAK1/STAT3 activation directly inhibits IL-12 production in dendritic cells by preventing CDK9/P-TEFb recruitment to the p35 promoter. *Biochem. Pharmacol.* **2015**, *96*, 52–64. [CrossRef]
158. Cheng, F.; Lienlaf, M.; Wang, H.W.; Perez-Villarroel, P.; Lee, C.; Woan, K.; Rock-Klotz, J.; Sahakian, E.; Woods, D.; Pinilla-Ibarz, J.; et al. A novel role for histone deacetylase 6 in the regulation of the tolerogenic STAT3/IL-10 pathway in APCs. *J. Immunol.* **2014**, *193*, 2850–2862. [CrossRef]
159. Gabrilovich, D.I.; Bronte, V.; Chen, S.H.; Colombo, M.P.; Ochoa, A.; Ostrand-Rosenberg, S.; Schreiber, H. The terminology issue for myeloid-derived suppressor cells. *Cancer Res.* **2007**, *67*, 425. [CrossRef]
160. Tu, S.; Bhagat, G.; Cui, G.; Takaishi, S.; Kurt-Jones, E.A.; Rickman, B.; Betz, K.S.; Penz-Oesterreicher, M.; Bjorkdahl, O.; Fox, J.G.; et al. Overexpression of interleukin-1beta induces gastric inflammation and cancer and mobilizes myeloid-derived suppressor cells in mice. *Cancer Cell* **2008**, *14*, 408–419. [CrossRef]
161. Almand, B.; Clark, J.I.; Nikitina, E.; van Beynen, J.; English, N.R.; Knight, S.C.; Carbone, D.P.; Gabrilovich, D.I. Increased production of immature myeloid cells in cancer patients: A mechanism of immunosuppression in cancer. *J. Immunol.* **2001**, *166*, 678–689. [CrossRef] [PubMed]
162. Diaz-Montero, C.M.; Salem, M.L.; Nishimura, M.I.; Garrett-Mayer, E.; Cole, D.J.; Montero, A.J. Increased circulating myeloid-derived suppressor cells correlate with clinical cancer stage, metastatic tumor burden, and doxorubicin-cyclophosphamide chemotherapy. *Cancer Immunol. Immunother.* **2009**, *58*, 49–59. [CrossRef] [PubMed]
163. Nagaraj, S.; Gupta, K.; Pisarev, V.; Kinarsky, L.; Sherman, S.; Kang, L.; Herber, D.L.; Schneck, J.; Gabrilovich, D.I. Altered recognition of antigen is a mechanism of CD8+ T cell tolerance in cancer. *Nat. Med.* **2007**, *13*, 828–835. [CrossRef] [PubMed]
164. Tcyganov, E.; Mastio, J.; Chen, E.; Gabrilovich, D.I. Plasticity of myeloid-derived suppressor cells in cancer. *Curr. Opin. Immunol.* **2018**, *51*, 76–82. [CrossRef] [PubMed]
165. Yu, H.; Liu, Y.; McFarland, B.C.; Deshane, J.S.; Hurst, D.R.; Ponnazhagan, S.; Benveniste, E.N.; Qin, H. SOCS3 Deficiency in Myeloid Cells Promotes Tumor Development: Involvement of STAT3 Activation and Myeloid-Derived Suppressor Cells. *Cancer Immunol. Res.* **2015**, *3*, 727–740. [CrossRef]
166. Xin, J.; Zhang, Z.; Su, X.; Wang, L.; Zhang, Y.; Yang, R. Epigenetic Component p66a Modulates Myeloid-Derived Suppressor Cells by Modifying STAT3. *J. Immunol.* **2017**, *198*, 2712–2720. [CrossRef]
167. Gabrilovich, D.I.; Nagaraj, S. Myeloid-derived suppressor cells as regulators of the immune system. *Nat. Rev. Immunol.* **2009**, *9*, 162–174. [CrossRef]
168. Mi, T.; Wang, Z.; Bunting, K.D. The Cooperative Relationship between STAT5 and Reactive Oxygen Species in Leukemia: Mechanism and Therapeutic Potential. *Cancers* **2018**, *10*, 359. [CrossRef]
169. Cheng, P.; Corzo, C.A.; Luetteke, N.; Yu, B.; Nagaraj, S.; Bui, M.M.; Ortiz, M.; Nacken, W.; Sorg, C.; Vogl, T.; et al. Inhibition of dendritic cell differentiation and accumulation of myeloid-derived suppressor cells in cancer is regulated by S100A9 protein. *J. Exp. Med.* **2008**, *205*, 2235–2249. [CrossRef]
170. Kyi, C.; Postow, M.A. Immune checkpoint inhibitor combinations in solid tumors: Opportunities and challenges. *Immunotherapy* **2016**, *8*, 821–837. [CrossRef]
171. Giuroiu, I.; Weber, J. Novel Checkpoints and Cosignaling Molecules in Cancer Immunotherapy. *Cancer J.* **2017**, *23*, 23–31. [CrossRef] [PubMed]
172. Austin, J.W.; Lu, P.; Majumder, P.; Ahmed, R.; Boss, J.M. STAT3, STAT4, NFATc1, and CTCF regulate PD-1 through multiple novel regulatory regions in murine T cells. *J. Immunol.* **2014**, *192*, 4876–4886. [CrossRef] [PubMed]
173. Marzec, M.; Zhang, Q.; Goradia, A.; Raghunath, P.N.; Liu, X.; Paessler, M.; Wang, H.Y.; Wysocka, M.; Cheng, M.; Ruggeri, B.A.; et al. Oncogenic kinase NPM/ALK induces through STAT3 expression of immunosuppressive protein CD274 (PD-L1, B7-H1). *Proc. Natl. Acad. Sci. USA* **2008**, *105*, 20852–20857. [CrossRef] [PubMed]

174. Fang, W.; Zhang, J.; Hong, S.; Zhan, J.; Chen, N.; Qin, T.; Tang, Y.; Zhang, Y.; Kang, S.; Zhou, T.; et al. EBV-driven LMP1 and IFN-gamma up-regulate PD-L1 in nasopharyngeal carcinoma: Implications for oncotargeted therapy. *Oncotarget* **2014**, *5*, 12189–12202. [CrossRef] [PubMed]
175. Keremu, A.; Aimaiti, A.; Liang, Z.; Zou, X. Role of the HDAC6/STAT3 pathway in regulating PD-L1 expression in osteosarcoma cell lines. *Cancer Chemother. Pharmacol.* **2019**, *83*, 255–264. [CrossRef] [PubMed]
176. Gowrishankar, K.; Gunatilake, D.; Gallagher, S.J.; Tiffen, J.; Rizos, H.; Hersey, P. Inducible but not constitutive expression of PD-L1 in human melanoma cells is dependent on activation of NF-kappaB. *PLoS ONE* **2015**, *10*, e0123410. [CrossRef]
177. Koh, J.; Jang, J.Y.; Keam, B.; Kim, S.; Kim, M.Y.; Go, H.; Kim, T.M.; Kim, D.W.; Kim, C.W.; Jeon, Y.K.; et al. EML4-ALK enhances programmed cell death-ligand 1 expression in pulmonary adenocarcinoma via hypoxia-inducible factor (HIF)-1alpha and STAT3. *OncoImmunology* **2016**, *5*, e1108514. [CrossRef] [PubMed]
178. Zhang, C.; Li, F.; Li, J.; Xu, Y.; Wang, L.; Zhang, Y. Docetaxel Down-Regulates PD-1 Expression via STAT3 in T Lymphocytes. *Clin. Lung. Cancer* **2018**, *19*, e675–e683. [CrossRef]
179. Li, P.; Huang, T.; Zou, Q.; Liu, D.; Wang, Y.; Tan, X.; Wei, Y.; Qiu, H. FGFR2 Promotes Expression of PD-L1 in Colorectal Cancer via the JAK/STAT3 Signaling Pathway. *J. Immunol.* **2019**. [CrossRef] [PubMed]
180. Zhang, N.; Zeng, Y.; Du, W.; Zhu, J.; Shen, D.; Liu, Z.; Huang, J.A. The EGFR pathway is involved in the regulation of PD-L1 expression via the IL-6/JAK/STAT3 signaling pathway in EGFR-mutated non-small cell lung cancer. *Int. J. Oncol.* **2016**, *49*, 1360–1368. [CrossRef]
181. Abdelhamed, S.; Ogura, K.; Yokoyama, S.; Saiki, I.; Hayakawa, Y. AKT-STAT3 Pathway as a Downstream Target of EGFR Signaling to Regulate PD-L1 Expression on NSCLC cells. *J. Cancer* **2016**, *7*, 1579–1586. [CrossRef] [PubMed]
182. Lamano, J.B.; Lamano, J.B.; Li, Y.D.; DiDomenico, J.D.; Choy, W.; Veliceasa, D.; Oyon, D.E.; Fakurnejad, S.; Ampie, L.; Kesavabhotla, K.; et al. Glioblastoma-Derived IL-6 Induces Immunosuppressive Peripheral Myeloid Cell PD-L1 and Promotes Tumor Growth. *Clin. Cancer Res.* **2019**. [CrossRef] [PubMed]
183. Cheng, Y.; Li, H.; Deng, Y.; Tai, Y.; Zeng, K.; Zhang, Y.; Liu, W.; Zhang, Q.; Yang, Y. Cancer-associated fibroblasts induce PDL1+ neutrophils through the IL6-STAT3 pathway that foster immune suppression in hepatocellular carcinoma. *Cell Death Dis.* **2018**, *9*, 422. [CrossRef] [PubMed]
184. Spary, L.K.; Salimu, J.; Webber, J.P.; Clayton, A.; Mason, M.D.; Tabi, Z. Tumor stroma-derived factors skew monocyte to dendritic cell differentiation toward a suppressive CD14(+) PD-L1(+) phenotype in prostate cancer. *OncoImmunology* **2014**, *3*, e955331. [CrossRef] [PubMed]
185. Kondo, K.; Shaim, H.; Thompson, P.A.; Burger, J.A.; Keating, M.; Estrov, Z.; Harris, D.; Kim, E.; Ferrajoli, A.; Daher, M.; et al. Ibrutinib modulates the immunosuppressive CLL microenvironment through STAT3-mediated suppression of regulatory B-cell function and inhibition of the PD-1/PD-L1 pathway. *Leukemia* **2018**, *32*, 960–970. [CrossRef] [PubMed]
186. Horlad, H.; Ma, C.; Yano, H.; Pan, C.; Ohnishi, K.; Fujiwara, Y.; Endo, S.; Kikukawa, Y.; Okuno, Y.; Matsuoka, M.; et al. An IL-27/Stat3 axis induces expression of programmed cell death 1 ligands (PD-L1/2) on infiltrating macrophages in lymphoma. *Cancer Sci.* **2016**, *107*, 1696–1704. [CrossRef]
187. Song, S.; Yuan, P.; Wu, H.; Chen, J.; Fu, J.; Li, P.; Lu, J.; Wei, W. Dendritic cells with an increased PD-L1 by TGF-beta induce T cell anergy for the cytotoxicity of hepatocellular carcinoma cells. *Int. Immunopharmacol.* **2014**, *20*, 117–123. [CrossRef]
188. Bazhin, A.V.; von Ahn, K.; Fritz, J.; Werner, J.; Karakhanova, S. Interferon-alpha Up-Regulates the Expression of PD-L1 Molecules on Immune Cells Through STAT3 and p38 Signaling. *Front. Immunol.* **2018**, *9*, 2129. [CrossRef]
189. Garcia-Diaz, A.; Shin, D.S.; Moreno, B.H.; Saco, J.; Escuin-Ordinas, H.; Rodriguez, G.A.; Zaretsky, J.M.; Sun, L.; Hugo, W.; Wang, X.; et al. Interferon Receptor Signaling Pathways Regulating PD-L1 and PD-L2 Expression. *Cell Rep.* **2017**, *19*, 1189–1201. [CrossRef]
190. Che, K.F.; Shankar, E.M.; Muthu, S.; Zandi, S.; Sigvardsson, M.; Hinkula, J.; Messmer, D.; Larsson, M. p38 Mitogen-activated protein kinase/signal transducer and activator of transcription-3 pathway signaling regulates expression of inhibitory molecules in T cells activated by HIV-1-exposed dendritic cells. *Mol. Med.* **2012**, *18*, 1169–1182. [CrossRef]
191. Zhang, W.; Zhang, J.; Zhang, Z.; Guo, Y.; Wu, Y.; Wang, R.; Wang, L.; Mao, S.; Yao, X. Overexpression of Indoleamine 2,3-Dioxygenase 1 Promotes Epithelial-Mesenchymal Transition by Activation of the IL-6/STAT3/PD-L1 Pathway in Bladder Cancer. *Transl. Oncol.* **2019**, *12*, 485–492. [CrossRef] [PubMed]

192. Huang, X.; Bai, X.; Cao, Y.; Wu, J.; Huang, M.; Tang, D.; Tao, S.; Zhu, T.; Liu, Y.; Yang, Y.; et al. Lymphoma endothelium preferentially expresses Tim-3 and facilitates the progression of lymphoma by mediating immune evasion. *J. Exp. Med.* **2010**, *207*, 505–520. [CrossRef] [PubMed]
193. Arra, A.; Lingel, H.; Kuropka, B.; Pick, J.; Schnoeder, T.; Fischer, T.; Freund, C.; Pierau, M.; Brunner-Weinzierl, M.C. The differentiation and plasticity of Tc17 cells are regulated by CTLA-4-mediated effects on STATs. *OncoImmunology* **2017**, *6*, e1273300. [CrossRef] [PubMed]
194. Mankan, A.K.; Greten, F.R. Inhibiting signal transducer and activator of transcription 3: Rationality and rationale design of inhibitors. *Expert Opin. Investig. Drugs* **2011**, *20*, 1263–1275. [CrossRef] [PubMed]
195. Shouksmith, A.E.; Gunning, P.T. Targeting Signal Transducer and Activator of Transcription (STAT) 3 with Small Molecules. In *Small-Molecule Transcription Factor Inhibitors in Oncology*; Khondaker, M.R.D.E.T., Ed.; Royal Society of Chemistry: London, UK, 2019; pp. 147–168.

9

STAT5 is Expressed in CD34$^+$/CD38$^-$ Stem Cells and Serves as a Potential Molecular Target in Ph-Negative Myeloproliferative Neoplasms

Emir Hadzijusufovic [1,2,3,*], Alexandra Keller [3], Daniela Berger [1,3], Georg Greiner [4], Bettina Wingelhofer [5], Nadine Witzeneder [4], Daniel Ivanov [1,3], Emmanuel Pecnard [6], Harini Nivarthi [7], Florian K. M. Schur [3], Yüksel Filik [1,3], Christoph Kornauth [3], Heidi A. Neubauer [5], Leonhard Müllauer [8], Gary Tin [9], Jisung Park [9], Elvin D. de Araujo [9], Patrick T. Gunning [9], Gregor Hoermann [4], Fabrice Gouilleux [6,10], Robert Kralovics [7], Richard Moriggl [5] and Peter Valent [1,2]

1 Ludwig Boltzmann Institute for Hematology and Oncology, Medical University of Vienna, 1090 Vienna, Austria; daniela.berger@meduniwien.ac.at (D.B.); daniel.ivanov@meduniwien.ac.at (D.I.); yueksel.filik@onc.lbg.ac.at (Y.F.); peter.valent@meduniwien.ac.at (P.V.)
2 Department/Hospital for Companion Animals and Horses, University Hospital for Small Animals, Internal Medicine Small Animals, University of Veterinary Medicine Vienna, 1210 Vienna, Austria
3 Department of Internal Medicine I, Division of Hematology & Hemostaseology, Medical University of Vienna, 1090 Vienna, Austria; alexandra.keller@meduniwien.ac.at (A.K.); florian.schur@ist.ac.at (F.K.M.S.); christoph.kornauth@meduniwien.ac.at (C.K.)
4 Department of Laboratory Medicine, Medical University of Vienna, 1090 Vienna, Austria; georg.greiner@meduniwien.ac.at (G.G.); nadine.witzeneder@meduniwien.ac.at (N.W.); gregor.hoermann@meduniwien.ac.at (G.H.)
5 Institute of Animal Breeding and Genetics, University of Veterinary Medicine Vienna, 1210 Vienna, Austria; bettina.wingelhofer@manchester.ac.uk (B.W.); heidi.neubauer@vetmeduni.ac.at (H.A.N.); richard.moriggl@vetmeduni.ac.at (R.M.)
6 INSERM, ERI-12, Faculté de Pharmacie, Université de Picardie Jules Verne, 80000 Amiens, France; emmanuel.pecnard@univ-tours.fr (E.P.); fabrice.gouilleux@univ-tours.fr (F.G.)
7 Research Center for Molecular Medicine (CeMM), 1090 Vienna, Austria; harini.nivarthi@meduniwien.ac.at (H.N.); robert.kralovics@meduniwien.ac.at (R.K.)
8 Department of Pathology, Medical University of Vienna, 1090 Vienna, Austria; leonhard.muellauer@meduniwien.ac.at
9 Department of Chemistry, University of Toronto, Toronto, ON M5S 1A1, Canada; gary.tin@mail.utoronto.ca (G.T.); ji.park@mail.utoronto.ca (J.P.); e.dearaujo@mail.utoronto.ca (E.D.d.A.); patrick.gunning@utoronto.ca (P.T.G.)
10 CNRS UMR 6239, GICC, Faculté de Médecine, Université François Rabelais, 37020 Tours, France
* Correspondence: emir.hadzijusufovic@meduniwien.ac.at

Abstract: Janus kinase 2 (JAK2) and signal transducer and activator of transcription-5 (STAT5) play a key role in the pathogenesis of myeloproliferative neoplasms (MPN). In most patients, *JAK2* V617F or *CALR* mutations are found and lead to activation of various downstream signaling cascades and molecules, including STAT5. We examined the presence and distribution of phosphorylated (p) STAT5 in neoplastic cells in patients with MPN, including polycythemia vera (PV, $n = 10$), essential thrombocythemia (ET, $n = 15$) and primary myelofibrosis (PMF, $n = 9$), and in the *JAK2* V617F-positive cell lines HEL and SET-2. As assessed by immunohistochemistry, MPN cells displayed pSTAT5 in all patients examined. Phosphorylated STAT5 was also detected in putative CD34$^+$/CD38$^-$ MPN stem cells (MPN-SC) by flow cytometry. Immunostaining experiments and Western blotting demonstrated pSTAT5 expression in both the cytoplasmic and nuclear compartment of MPN cells. Confirming previous studies, we also found that JAK2-targeting drugs counteract the expression of pSTAT5 and growth in HEL and SET-2 cells. Growth-inhibition of MPN cells was also induced by the

STAT5-targeting drugs piceatannol, pimozide, AC-3-019 and AC-4-130. Together, we show that CD34$^+$/CD38$^-$ MPN-SC express pSTAT5 and that pSTAT5 is expressed in the nuclear and cytoplasmic compartment of MPN cells. Whether direct targeting of pSTAT5 in MPN-SC is efficacious in MPN patients remains unknown.

Keywords: MPN; STAT5; JAK2 V617F; neoplastic stem cells

---

1. Introduction

Classical myeloproliferative neoplasms (MPN) are incurable stem cell disorders characterized by the abnormal expansion of myeloid cells in the bone marrow (BM), elevated blood counts, extramedullary myelopoiesis, and a genetic instability with enhanced risk to transform to secondary acute myeloid leukemia (sAML) [1–6]. In most patients, a mutation in the *calreticulin* (*CALR*) gene or the *Janus kinase 2* (*JAK2*) point mutation V617F is found [3–6]. MPN-related morbidity and mortality are emerging health problems in the Western world. Notably, improved diagnostics and therapy, together with an enhanced life expectancy, have led to an increasing prevalence of MPN. For patients with advanced MPN or sAML, the only curative approach is allogeneic hematopoietic stem cell transplantation [7–9]. However, this therapy can only be offered to a subset of patients. In all other cases, disease management is based on symptom control and the use of growth-inhibitory drugs, including interferon-alpha, anagrelide, hydroxyurea or ruxolitinib [10–15]. However, these drugs have little if any curative potential and in many cases resistance develops during therapy [10–15]. Therefore, current research is seeking new molecular targets and is attempting to develop new targeted drugs for patients with MPN.

Based on the classification of the World Health Organization (WHO), three types of classical MPN have been defined: polycythemia vera (PV), essential thrombocythemia (ET) and primary myelofibrosis (PMF) [3]. Each of these neoplasms exhibits unique clinical, histopathological and molecular features [1–4,6]. However, the three MPN entities share molecular and pathologic characteristics, and in many cases an overlap or transition from one into another type of MPN is seen. In most patients, mutations in the *JAK2*, *CALR* or *thrombopoietin receptor* (*MPL*) gene are found [16–20]. Independent of the disease variant, JAK2 activation leads to a cascade of downstream signaling molecules and pathways in neoplastic cells [21–25]. One of the key downstream signaling molecules is the 'signal transducer and activator of transcription-5' (STAT5) protein [21–27].

Although STAT5 was initially characterized as a key transcription factor in various physiologic and pathologic processes, more recent data suggest that STAT5 also serves as a cytoplasmic signaling molecule that binds to and interacts with other signaling molecules in neoplastic cells to promote oncogenesis. Both the cytoplasmic and the nuclear fractions of STAT5 are considered to critically contribute to leukemogenesis in patients with myeloid neoplasms [28–30].

Similar to other myeloid neoplasms, MPN are considered to develop from transformed myeloid stem cells [31–35]. As only the neoplastic stem cells of an MPN (MPN-SC) can propagate the malignancy for unlimited time periods, they represent an important cellular target of therapy. However, little is known about the phenotype and target expression profiles of neoplastic stem cells in MPN. As in other myeloid neoplasms, MPN-SC are considered to reside within the CD34$^+$/CD38$^-$ population of the clone [32,33,35]. It has also been described that the immature CD34$^+$ cells in MPN patients express *JAK2* V617F [35].

The aims of the present study were to examine MPN cells for expression of phosphorylated (p) STAT5, to study the cellular distribution of pSTAT5 and to analyze the effects of pSTAT5-targeting drugs on MPN cells. Our data show that pSTAT5 is expressed in CD34$^+$/CD38$^-$ MPN stem cells and serves as a potential therapeutic target in MPN.

2. Results

2.1. *Primary MPN Cells Express Nuclear and Cytoplasmic pSTAT5*

As assessed by immunohistochemistry (IHC), primary MPN cells in the BM of patients with PV, ET and PMF expressed pSTAT5 in their nuclear and cytoplasmic compartment (Figure 1A and Table 1). The expression of pSTAT5 in normal BM cells (controls) was similar to that found in MPN BM sections examined by IHC. In all samples tested, megakaryocytes stained clearly positive for pSTAT5 (positive control), whereas erythroid cells stained negative for pSTAT5 (negative control). We were also able to confirm expression of cytoplasmic pSTAT5 in BM cells in patients with various MPN by multi-color flow cytometry (Figure 1B). In these experiments, all myeloid cells tested, including CD15$^+$ granulomonocytic cells, CD14$^+$ monocytes and CD34$^+$ stem and progenitor cells, were found to stain positive for pSTAT5 (Figure 1C). pSTAT5 was identified in BM cells in all three categories of MPN, regardless of expression of *JAK2* V617F and without major differences in staining intensities (Figure 1B, Table 1).

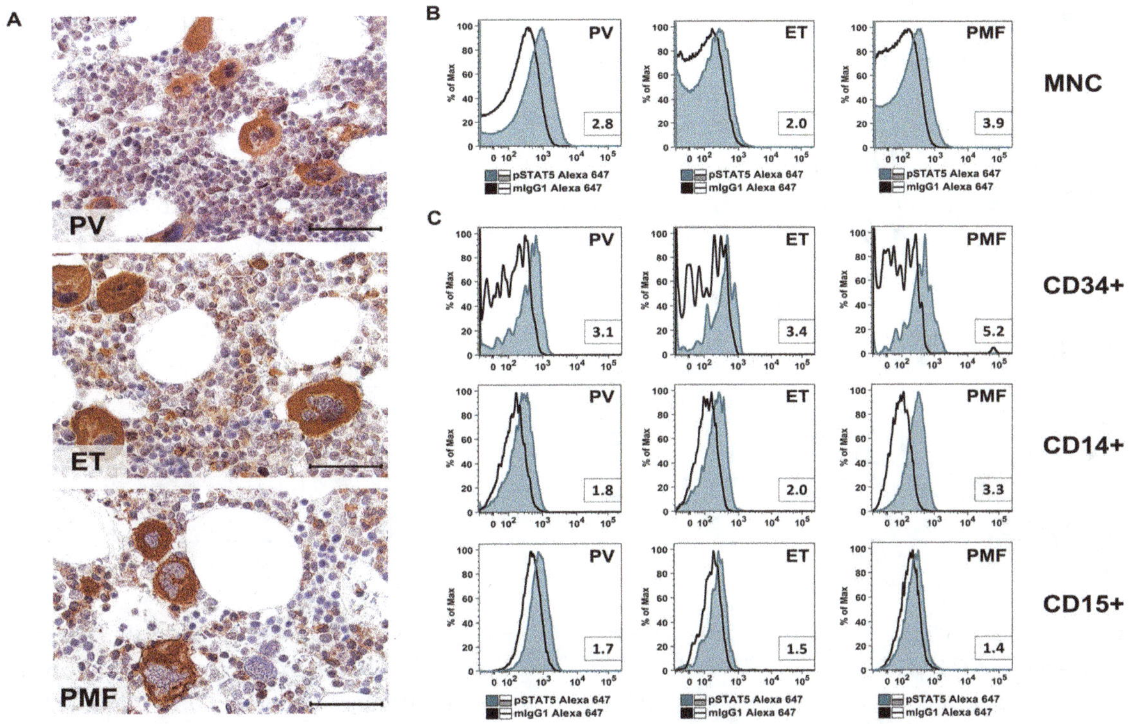

Figure 1. (**A**) Sections prepared from paraffin-embedded bone marrow (iliac crest) of patients with polycythemia vera (PV; patient #06), essential thrombocythemia (ET; patient #34) or primary myelofibrosis (PMF; patient #29) were stained with an anti-phosphorylated signal transducer and activator of transcription-5 (pSTAT5) antibody using immunohistochemistry. Examples of nuclear- and cytoplasmic staining are shown in Figure A1. Scale bar: 30 µm. Patient characteristics are shown in Table A1. (**B**,**C**) Bone marrow (BM) mononuclear cells (MNC) of patients with PV (patient #30), ET (patient #08) or PMF (patient #29) were stained with an anti-pSTAT5 Alexa-647 antibody. Intracellular expression levels of pSTAT5 were analyzed by flow cytometry in total MNC (**B**), or in cell subsets gated for CD34, CD14 or CD15 (**C**). The isotype-matched control antibody is also shown (open black histogram). Numbers in the small boxes represent the staining index defined as the ratio of the median fluorescence intensity (MFI) obtained with the anti-pSTAT5 antibody and MFI obtained with the isotype-matched control antibody (mIgG1).

Table 1. Immunohistochemical detection of pSTAT5 in bone marrow cells of MPN patients and controls.

Diagnosis	PV	PV	PV	PMF	PMF	PMF	ET	ET	ET	nBM	nBM	nBM	nBM
Patient #	18	06	30	20	29	16	34	02	23	46	48	50	51
Megakaryocytes	++	++	++	+	++	++	++	++	+	++	++	++	++
Myeloid prog.	+	+	+	+	+	+	+	+/−	+/−	+	+(+)	+	+
Neutrophil gran.	+	+	+/−	+	+	+	+	−	+/−	+/−	+	−	+/−
Eosinophil gran.	−	−	−	−	−	−	−	−	n.a.	−	−	n.a.	n.a.
Erythroid prog.	−	−	−	−	−	−	−	−	−	−	−	−	−

Score: ++, strong expression in most cells; +, clear expression in the majority of cases; +/-, expressed in subsets of cells or only weakly expressed; −, no expression (below detection limit). Abbreviations: CM, cutaneous mastocytosis; ET, essential thrombocythemia; gran., granulocytes; MPN, myeloproliferative neoplasm; n.a., not analyzed (no cells found by microscopy); nBM, normal bone marrow; NHL, Non-Hodgkin lymphoma; PMF, primary myelofibrosis; prog., progenitors; PV, polycythemia vera.

2.2. Primary CD34$^+$/CD38$^-$ MPN-SC Express pSTAT5

Expression of pSTAT5 in CD34$^+$/CD38$^-$ cells was examined in normal/reactive BM cells and in BM samples obtained from patients with MPN by multi-color flow cytometry. As visible in Figure 2, pSTAT5 was found to be expressed in normal CD34$^+$/CD38$^-$ stem cells as well as in CD34$^+$/CD38$^-$ MPN-SC. We also found that pSTAT5 levels were higher in *JAK2* V617F+ CD34$^+$/CD38$^-$ MPN-SC compared to normal stem cells (p = 0.015) (Figure 2A). In addition, we found that pSTAT5 is expressed at slightly higher levels in CD34$^+$/CD38$^-$ MPN-SC in *JAK2* V617F+ patients compared to *JAK2* V617F- patients, although the difference was not statistically significant (p = 0.073) (Figure 2B). However, no substantial differences in pSTAT5 expression in CD34$^+$/CD38$^-$ MPN cells were found when comparing various subsets of MPN (PV vs. ET vs. PMF) (Figure 2C).

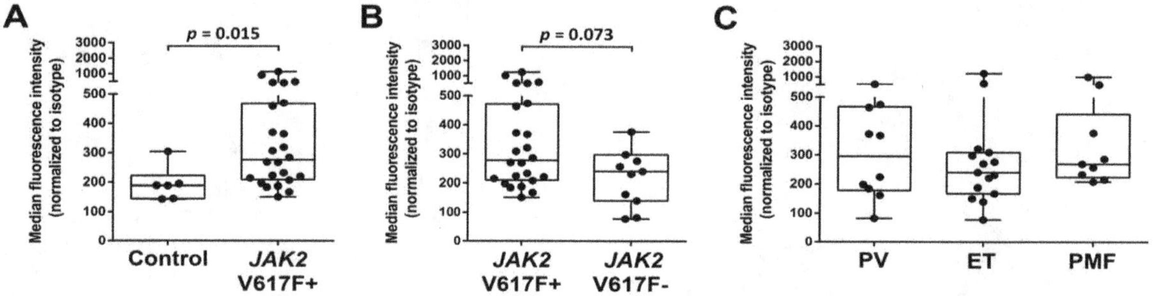

Figure 2. Bone marrow cells from patients with PV, ET or PMF were analyzed for intracellular expression of pSTAT5 in CD34$^+$/CD38$^-$/CD45^{dim} cells using an anti-pSTAT5 Alexa-647 antibody. (**A**) Expression of pSTAT5 in normal/reactive bone marrow (Control, n = 6) and bone marrow of MPN patients (MPN, n = 24). (**B**) Expression of pSTAT5 in CD34$^+$/CD38$^-$/CD45^{dim} bone marrow cells in *JAK2* V617F+ patients (V617F+, n = 24) and patients with wild type *JAK2*, a *CALR* mutation or an *MPL* mutation (V617F−, n = 10). (**C**) Expression of pSTAT5 in CD34$^+$/CD38$^-$/CD45^{dim} bone marrow cells in the three different MPN subgroups (PV, n = 10; ET, n = 15, PMF, n = 9). Boxes indicate the upper and lower quartiles, the median is defined by a horizontal line inside the boxes, and the whiskers show the highest and lowest values.

2.3. Detection of pSTAT5 in HEL and SET-2 Cells

We next examined the *JAK2* V617F+ cell lines HEL and SET-2 by immunocytochemistry (ICC). Confirming previous studies [36,37], we found that both cell lines express pSTAT5. Interestingly, both cell lines expressed pSTAT5 in their nuclear and cytoplasmic compartments (Figure 3A). Intracellular expression of pSTAT5 in these cell lines was also confirmed by flow cytometry (Figure 3B). Preincubation of HEL and SET-2 cells with JAK2-targeting drugs (ruxolitinib [38,39], R763 [40],

TG101348 [41,42], AZD1480 [43,44]) or STAT5-targeting drugs (piceatannol [45], pimozide [46,47], AC-3-019 [48], AC-4-130 [48,49]) resulted in reduced pSTAT5 staining (Figure A2). The characteristics of the STAT5- and JAK2-targeting drugs used in these experiments together with their main targets are depicted in Table A2. We also compared pSTAT5 levels in purified nuclear and cytoplasmic fractions of HEL and SET-2 cells by Western blotting. Total STAT5 (STAT5A and STAT5B) was expressed more abundantly in the cytoplasmic extracts of HEL and SET-2 cells than in nuclear extracts (Figure 3C). Moreover, pSTAT5 was found at higher levels in the cytoplasm of HEL cells compared to nuclear fractions. By contrast, in SET-2 cells, pSTAT5 was found to be expressed more abundantly in the nuclear fractions compared to cytoplasmic fractions (Figure 3C).

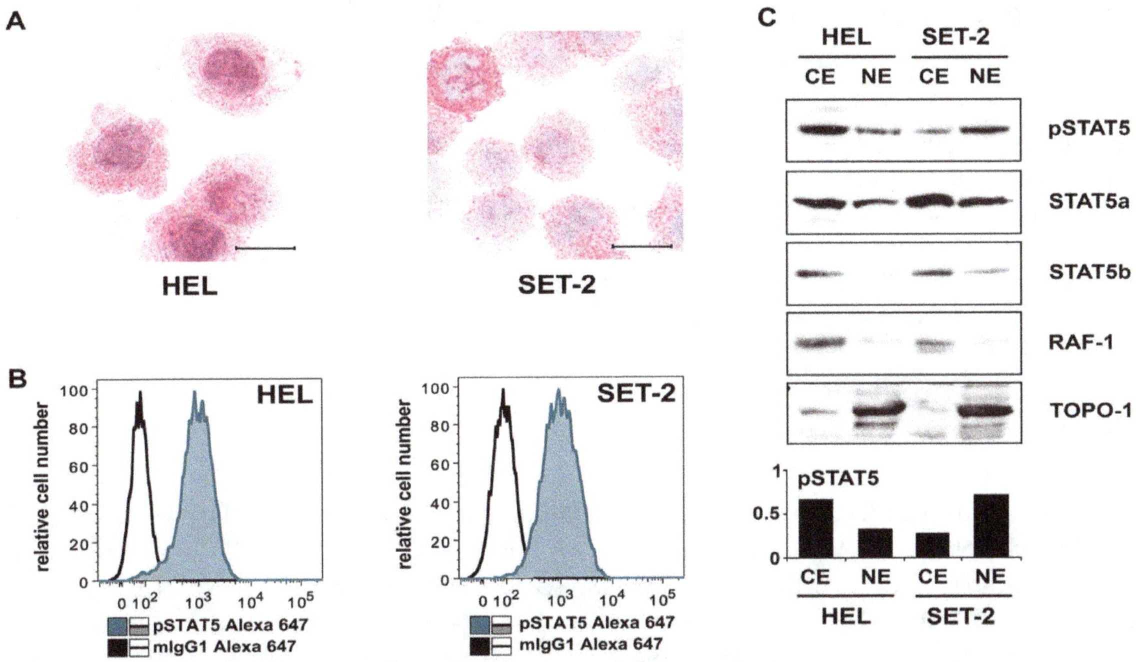

Figure 3. (**A**) Cytospin preparations of HEL cells and SET-2 cells were stained overnight with an anti-pSTAT5 antibody using immunocytochemistry. Scale bar: 20 μM. (**B**) HEL cells and SET-2 cells were stained with an anti-pSTAT5 Alexa-647 antibody for 30 min at room temperature and intracellular expression levels were analyzed by flow cytometry. (**C**) Nuclear (NE) and cytoplasmic (CE) fractions of HEL or SET-2 cells were analyzed for expression of phosphorylated STAT5 (pSTAT5), total STAT5a and total STAT5b by Western blotting. Antibodies against RAF-1 (cytoplasm) and TOPO-1 (nucleus) were used as fraction controls. The columns show the densitometry for pSTAT5. Uncropped blots are shown in Figure S1.

2.4. *Effects of JAK2 V617F and CALR Mutants on Expression of Total STAT5 and pSTAT5 in Ba/F3 Cells*

To explore the mechanism of expression and activation of STAT5 in MPN cells, we expressed *JAK2* V617F and mutated *CALR* in Ba/F3 cells containing human *MPL* (Ba/F3-MPL). As expected, expression of JAK2 V617F was followed by an increase in pSTAT5 levels in these cells (Figure A3). Moreover, we were able to show that drugs targeting STAT5 (piceatannol, pimozide) or JAK2 (AZD1480, TG101348, R763, ruxolitinib) counteract mutant-induced overexpression of pSTAT5 in our Ba/F3-MPL cells (Figure 4).

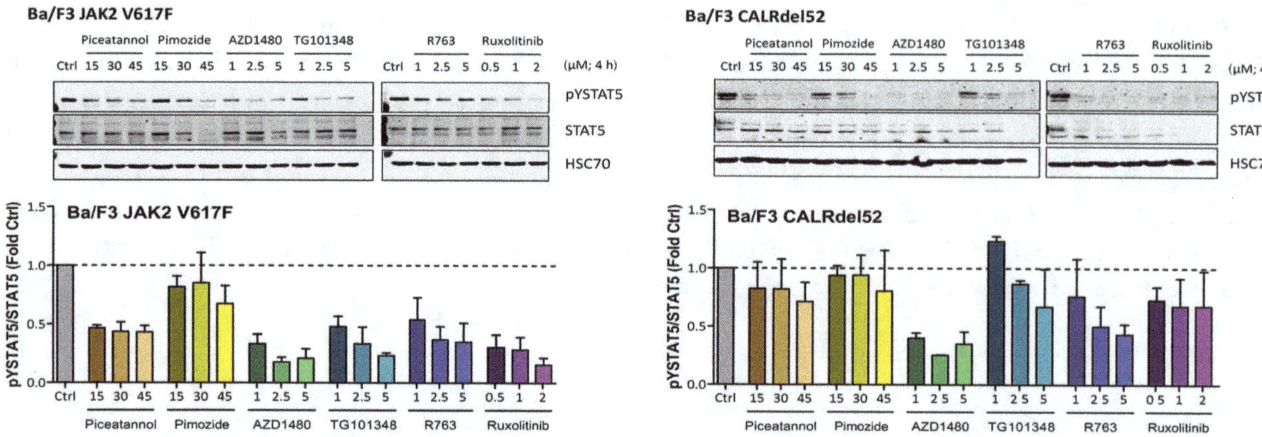

Figure 4. Ba/F3 cells modified to express JAK2 V617F or CALRdel52 were incubated with various JAK2 or STAT5 inhibitors (as indicated) for four hours at 37 °C. Thereafter, the expression of activated STAT5 (pSTAT5), total STAT5 (STAT5) and heat shock cognate 70 (HSC70), which was used as loading control, was analyzed using Western blotting. The results were quantified using densitometry and are expressed as the ratio of activated and total STAT5 normalized to the results obtained with control cells (Ctrl). Uncropped blots are shown in Figure S2.

2.5. *Effects of Targeted Drugs on the Growth and Survival of HEL and SET-2 Cells*

To confirm that pSTAT5 serves as a molecular target in MPN cells, we applied various JAK2-targeting drugs and STAT5-targeting drugs on HEL cells and SET-2 cells. As shown in Figure 5, the JAK2 blockers (ruxolitinib, R763, TG101348, AZD1480) and the STAT5 blockers (piceatannol, pimozide, AC-3-019, AC-4-130) were found to inhibit ^{3}[H]-thymidine uptake and thus proliferation with varying potency. For several drugs, these data confirmed previous studies [50–53]. In our study, the rank order of potency for HEL cells was AZD1480 > TG101348 > ruxolitinib > R763 > AC-4-130 > AC-3-019 > pimozide > piceatannol. The rank order of potency for SET-2 cells was R763 > ruxolitinib > AZD1480 > TG101348 > pimozide > AC-4-130 > AC-3-019 > piceatannol. Next, we examined the effects of various targeted drugs on the survival of MPN cells. In these experiments, we found that the JAK2 and STAT5 blockers examined induce apoptosis in HEL cells and SET-2 cells (Figure A4). In a separate set of experiments, we applied ruxolitinib and AC-4-130 in combination in HEL and SET-2 cells. However, no clear additive or synergistic effects of this drug combination was observed (Data not shown [54]). We also examined the effects of the JAK2 and STAT5 inhibitors on proliferation of two pSTAT5-low/negative solid cancer cell lines, A2780 and A375. As shown in Table A3, these cells were in general less sensitive to these drugs compared to HEL cells or SET2 cells.

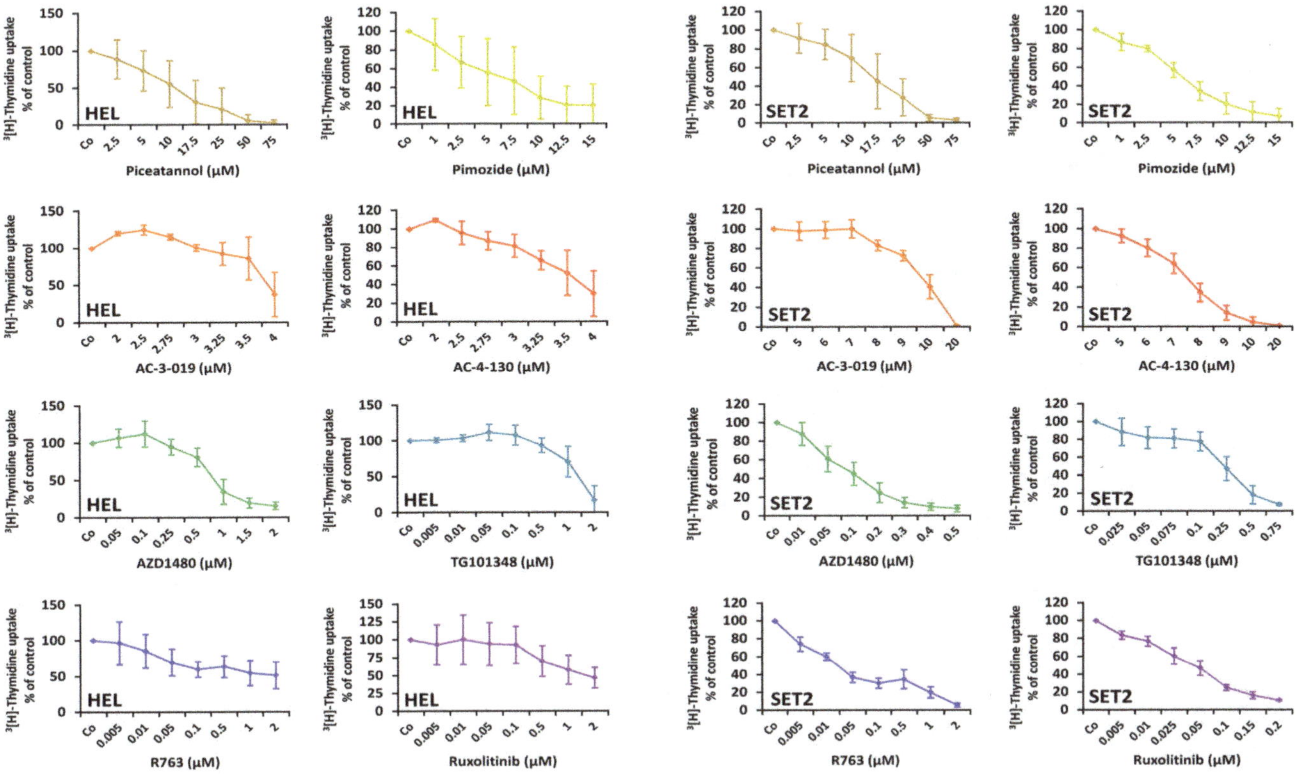

Figure 5. HEL and SET-2 cells were incubated with different concentrations of JAK2 or STAT5 targeting drugs for 48 h at 37 °C. Thereafter, ^{3}[H]-thymidine was added for 16 h and its incorporation was analyzed using a beta counter. The diagrams show the mean ± standard deviation (SD) of at least three independent experiments performed in triplicate.

2.6. *Effects of Targeted Drugs on Primary Human MPN Cells*

In a final step, we examined the effects of various JAK-2-targeting drugs and STAT5-targeting drugs on the growth and survival of primary mononuclear cells (MNC) obtained from the BM of patients with MPN. In these experiments, we found that the JAK-2 blockers and the STAT5 blockers used in this study are capable of inhibiting the proliferation of primary MPN cells (Figure 6A). Moreover, we found that these drugs decrease the relative numbers of primary CD34^{+}/CD38^{-} MPN-SC in vitro (Figure 6B,C). Interestingly, ruxolitinib was found to decrease MPN-SC numbers after 48 h but not after 24 h. All drugs also decreased pSTAT5 levels in MPN-SC, although the downregulating effects of these drugs were rather weak (Figure 6D).

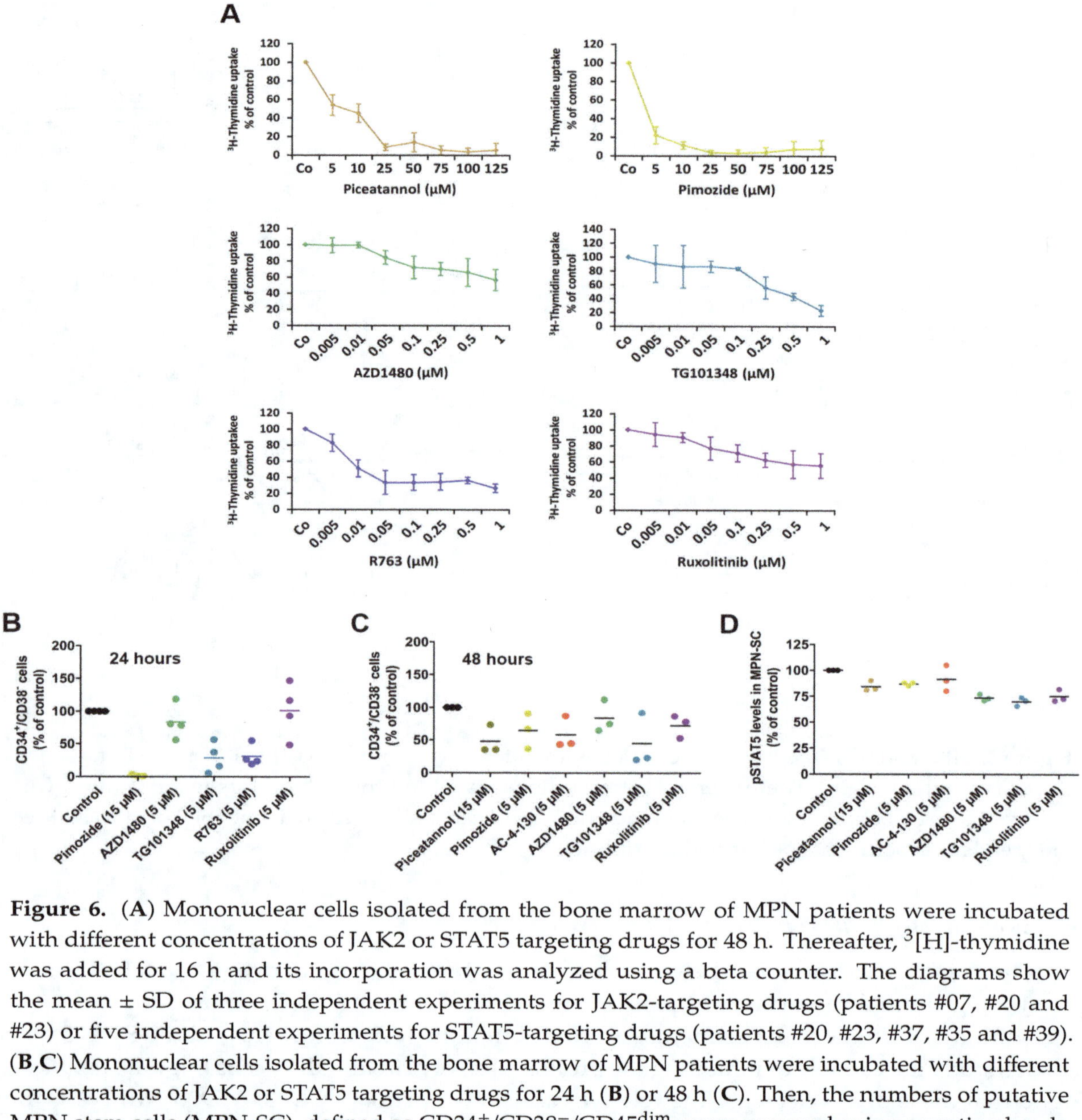

Figure 6. (**A**) Mononuclear cells isolated from the bone marrow of MPN patients were incubated with different concentrations of JAK2 or STAT5 targeting drugs for 48 h. Thereafter, ^{3}[H]-thymidine was added for 16 h and its incorporation was analyzed using a beta counter. The diagrams show the mean ± SD of three independent experiments for JAK2-targeting drugs (patients #07, #20 and #23) or five independent experiments for STAT5-targeting drugs (patients #20, #23, #37, #35 and #39). (**B**,**C**) Mononuclear cells isolated from the bone marrow of MPN patients were incubated with different concentrations of JAK2 or STAT5 targeting drugs for 24 h (**B**) or 48 h (**C**). Then, the numbers of putative MPN stem cells (MPN-SC), defined as CD34^{+}/CD38^{-}/CD45^{dim}, were assessed using counting beads. The graphs show MPN-SC as percent of control in four patients (#14, #29, #30 and #31) in (**B**) and in three patients (#31, #42 and #43) in (**C**). Horizontal lines indicate mean values. (**D**) pSTAT5 levels in CD34^{+}/CD38^{-} MPN-SC determined by flow cytometry (same patients as in (**C**)) after an incubation with targeted drugs (as indicated) for 4 h. Values represent pSTAT5 levels relative to the control. The mean staining index is also shown (horizontal bars). Patient characteristics are shown in Table A1.

3. Discussion

Recent data suggest that STAT5 activation is a critical event triggering oncogenesis and growth of neoplastic cells in various hematologic malignancies [55,56]. It has also been described that leukemia-specific oncoproteins, such as BCR-ABL1, induce activation of STAT5 and thereby contribute to clonal expansion of neoplastic cells [57]. Several studies have shown that phosphorylated STAT5 (pSTAT5) is expressed in the cytoplasm and nuclei of neoplastic cells in patients with chronic myeloid leukemia (CML) and systemic mastocytosis (SM) [28,58]. Our study shows that neoplastic cells in PV and PMF also express nuclear and cytoplasmic pSTAT5 in a constitutive manner. In addition, we found that putative CD34^{+}/CD38^{-} MPN-SC display pSTAT5. Finally, our data show that pharmacologic targeting of STAT5 reduces the growth of MPN cells and the numbers of MPN-SC. Together, these data suggest that the STAT5 pathway may contribute to oncogene-dependent growth of neoplastic cells in MPN. Whether inhibitors of pSTAT5, alone or in combination with other drugs, can exert clinically meaningful effects in MPN patients, remains unknown at present.

Recent data suggest that pSTAT5 is detectable in the cytoplasm of neoplastic cells in patients with AML, CML and SM, and that STAT5 acts as a pro-oncogenic driver in these myeloid neoplasms [28–30,58–60]. An interesting observation has been that the levels of cytoplasmic pSTAT5 often exceed the amounts of pSTAT5 found in the nuclear compartments in these cells [28,58]. In the current study, we found that pSTAT5 is located in both the cytoplasmic and nuclear fractions of primary MPN cells and in the MPN-related cell lines HEL and SET-2. In both cell lines, cytoplasmic and nuclear pSTAT5 were detected by ICC, flow cytometry and Western blotting (Figure 3). As assessed by Western blotting, the cytoplasmic and nuclear fractions of these cells displayed detectable levels of pSTAT5, and total STAT5 was found to be expressed more abundantly in the cytoplasmic fraction. Currently, it remains unknown whether nuclear pSTAT5 or cytoplasmic pSTAT5 plays a more important role in oncogenesis in MPN. Whereas nuclear pSTAT5 is considered to act as a pro-oncogenic transcription factors, cytoplasmic pSTAT5 may be involved in pro-oncogenic signaling involving the PI3 kinase pathway, similar to the situation in AML and SM [29,61].

MPN cells are considered to be organized in a 'stem cell hierarchy' similar to normal hematopoiesis [34]. In addition, MPN cells can undergo differentiation and terminal maturation in the same way as normal myeloid cells. As in normal hematopoiesis, only the most immature neoplastic stem cells (MPN-SC) have the capacity of self-renewal in MPN, a hypothesis that has major implications regarding drug therapy [62,63]. Notably, this model predicts that these cells can propagate the malignancy for unlimited time periods and that anti-neoplastic drugs have curative potential only when eliminating most or all of these neoplastic stem cells in a given neoplasm. So far, only little is known about the phenotype and function of MPN-SC [35,64]. Like in other myeloid neoplasms, these cells are considered to reside in a $CD34^+$ fraction of the clone [31]. In the present study, we were able to show that pSTAT5 is not only expressed in more mature clonal MPN cells, but also in immature $CD34^+/CD38^-$ (putative) MPN-SC (Figures 1 and 2). To the best of our knowledge, our study is the first to demonstrate that $CD34^+/CD38^-$ MPN-SC express pSTAT5. Regarding more mature clonal cells, monocytes, known to play a major role in MPN [65–67], were found to express high levels of pSTAT5, making these cells an additional potential target of STAT5 inhibition. As assessed by flow cytometry, we also found that the levels of pSTAT5 are higher in putative MPN-SC in patients with *JAK2* V617F$^+$ MPN compared to patients with *JAK2* V617F$^-$ MPN or normal $CD34^+/CD38^-$ stem cells. In contrast, no statistically significant difference was observed when comparing patients with *JAK2* V617F$^-$ MPN or normal $CD34^+/CD38^-$ stem cells, although some patients with *JAK2* V617F$^-$ MPN showed higher pSTAT5 levels than normal controls. Interestingly, when testing for pSTAT5 levels by IHC, no differences were found between the BM of MPN patients and normal controls, which seems to be in contrast to our flow cytometry results. However, our flow cytometry staining experiments were performed on stem cells, whereas IHC was performed on the bulk of MPN cells. Moreover, the IHC stain may be less capable of precisely quantifying differences in staining intensities compared to flow cytometry. This hypothesis is supported by the work of Teofili et al. [68], who did not detect differences in pSTAT5 levels between different subsets of MPN when using IHC in bulk cells. By contrast, using a flow cytometry approach, Abba et al. [69], were able to show differences in pSTAT5 levels when comparing $CD34^+$ MPN cells with normal $CD34^+$ cells.

In our study, no differences were seen when comparing pSTAT5 expression levels in $CD34^+/CD38^-$ MPN-SC among the three groups of MPN patients, and in each case, pSTAT5 was homogenously expressed in all MPN-SC in all patients. Collectively, these data suggest that neoplastic stem and progenitor cells in MPN patients express pSTAT5. As mentioned above, our results are also in line with the data published by Abba et al. [69], who showed that pSTAT5 levels are higher in $CD34^+$ MPN cells compared to normal $CD34^+$ cells. However, Abba et al. did not look into the more immature fraction of $CD34^+/CD38^-$ stem cells [69].

A number of previous and more recent studies have shown that STAT5 activation is a critical event triggering oncogenesis in MPN (stem) cells and that mutated forms of JAK2 and CALR can induce STAT5 activation [22–25]. In our study, we were able to show that putative SC in MPN express pSTAT5, but these cells only expressed pSTAT5 in excess over normal stem cells in patients with *JAK2*-mutated MPN. These data suggest that STAT5 may play a particular role in MPN-SC downstream of JAK2. However, more studies are required to define the exact role that STAT5 activation plays in the immature stem cell compartment in MPN.

Inhibitors of JAK2 and STAT5 were found to suppress expression of pSTAT5 in HEL and SET-2 cells (Figure A1). For several of these drugs, our data confirm the available literature [50–53]. An interesting observation was that whereas the JAK2-targeting drugs blocked STAT5 activation and MPN cell growth at relatively low concentrations, much higher concentrations of the STAT5 blockers were required to counteract proliferation in MPN cells (Figure 5). These observations suggest that targeting of STAT5 may be an interesting approach to block oncogenic signaling in MPN cells directly, but more potent and specific STAT5 inhibitors need to be developed to better inhibit MPN cell growth. Indeed, multiple attempts have been made recently to develop selective and potent STAT5 inhibitors. In the present study, we examined the effects of two such novel STAT5 inhibitors, AC-3-019 and AC-4-130 [49]. Similar to piceatannol and pimozide, these selective STAT5-SH2-domain-targeting drugs produced growth inhibition and apoptosis, albeit at relatively high concentrations (Figures 5 and A4). We also observed the effects of these inhibitors and of the other STAT5 or JAK2 blockers on MPN-SC. However, the effects on MPN-SC were weak, so these drugs are not expected to be able to eradicate the disease. One explanation for this result may be that other downstream signaling molecules and pathways are also involved in triggering oncogenesis and neoplastic stem cell growth in MPN. Therefore, we believe that more specific and more potent STAT5 blockers may be a reasonable approach to target MPN cells, and additional drugs or drug combinations, as proposed by Bar-Natan et al. [53] and others, may be required to elicit optimal anti-neoplastic or even curative effects.

4. Materials and Methods

4.1. Patients

Thirty-four patients with MPN, including 10 with PV, 15 with ET and 9 with PMF were examined for levels of pSTAT5 in MPN-SC. MPN variants were diagnosed according to WHO criteria [3]. Patient characteristics are shown in Table A1. Routine staging included physical examination, blood counts, morphologic examination of cells on BM smears, BM histology and immunohistochemistry, and analysis of BM and peripheral blood cells for expression of *JAK2* V617F, *CALR* and *MPL* mutations. Expression of *JAK2* V617F was determined by two PCR assays: the qualitative Ipsogena MutaScreen assay and the quantitative MutaQuant assay. Both assays were applied according to the recommendations of the manufacturer (Qiagen, Venlo, Netherlands). In *JAK2* V617F-negative patients, MPN cells were screened for *CALR* mutations using fluorescence- based PCR, followed by Sanger sequencing of codons 351–404 of *CALR* as described [16]. When no *JAK2* or *CALR* mutations were detected, the patients were analyzed for *MPL* mutations using an allelic discrimination assay as described [20]. In 15 patients (PV, $n = 4$; ET, $n = 5$; PMF, $n = 6$), BM mononuclear cells (MNC) were enriched using Ficoll. These MNC were used to assess drug effects on proliferation and/or survival. In addition, BM cells obtained from eight donors without MPN (control BM samples) were analyzed (Table A4). All investigations were approved by the local ethics committee of the Medical University of Vienna (ethic code: 224/2006; 1184/2014; 1063/2018). Informed consent was obtained from all patients.

4.2. Antibodies (Ab) and Other Reagents

The anti-pSTAT5 alpha (Tyr694) polyclonal Ab was purchased from Invitrogen (order number 71-6900; Carlsbad, CA, USA), anti-pSTAT5 (Y694) Alexa Fluor® 647 monoclonal Ab (mAb) 47 (order number: 612599) and an isotype-matched control antibody (mIgG1-Alexa Fluor® 647, order number: 557783) from BD Biosciences Pharmingen (San Jose, CA, USA), piceatannol (order number: P0453) and pimozide (order number: P1793) from Merck (Darmstadt, Germany), and the JAK2 blockers AZD1480 (order number: CT-A1480), TG101348 (order number: CT-TG101) and ruxolitinib (order number: CT-INCB) from ChemieTek (Indianapolis, IN, USA). The specificity of pSTAT5 (Y694) Alexa Fluor® 647 was confirmed by flow cytometry experiments performed with human cell lines with detectable pSTAT5 (KOPT-K1 and MYLA) or no detectable pSTAT5 (HUT78 and HH). In addition, we employed Ba/F3 cells with IL-3-inducible expression of pSTAT5. In these experiments, the specificity of the antibody was confirmed (Figure A5a,b). pSTAT5 expression in the cell lines tested was confirmed by Western Blotting (Figure A5c,d). Roswell Park Memorial Institute (RPMI) 1640 medium (order number: 10-041-CVR) was purchased from Corning (Manassas, VA, USA) and fetal calf serum (FCS; order number: 10270-106) from Gibco (Karlsbad, CA, USA). The JAK2 and Aurora kinase-targeting drug R763 was kindly provided by Yasumichi Hitoshi (Rigel Pharmaceuticals, San Francisco, CA, USA). The STAT5 inhibitors AC-3-019 and AC-4-130 were produced as described [48]. Stock solutions of drugs were prepared by dissolving in dimethyl sulfoxide (DMSO) (order number: D2650; Merck).

4.3. Cell Lines

A375 were purchased from LGC Standards (Wesel Germany); HEL and SET-2 cell lines were purchased from Deutsche Sammlung von Mikroorganismen und Zellkulturen (Braunschweig, Germany); KOPT-K1 cells were kindly provided by Takaomi Sanda (Cancer Science Institute of Singapore, Singapore); HH, HUT78 and MYLA were kindly provided by Marco Herling (University Hospital Cologne, Cologne, Germany). A2780 cells were purchased from Sigma (St. Louis, MO, USA). All cell lines were cultured in RPMI 1640 medium supplemented with 10% FCS.

4.4. Immunohistochemistry and Immunocytochemistry

Immunohistochemistry was performed on paraffin-embedded, formalin-fixed BM biopsy specimens using the indirect immunoperoxidase staining technique following established protocols [28]. Endogenous peroxidase was blocked by methanol/H_2O_2 and heat-induced epitope retrieval was performed (96 °C, 20 min, pH 9). A polyclonal anti-pSTAT5 antibody was applied at 1:100 for 20 h at 4 °C. Biotinylated goat anti-rabbit IgG (Vector Laboratories, Burlingham, CA, USA, order number: BA-1000) was applied as secondary antibody for 30 min at room temperature. Then, slides were exposed to an avidin/biotinylated peroxidase complex (Vectastain ABC Kit from Vector, order number: PK-6100) for 30 min. The chromogen 3-amino-9-ethylcarabzole (AEC) was then used. Finally, slides were counterstained in Mayer's hematoxylin (Morphisto, Frankfurt am Main, Germany, order number: 10231.01000). In each sample, the specificity of the anti-pSTAT5 stain was controlled by analyzing the internal negative control and positive control. In fact, erythroid cells always stained negative and megakaryocytes always stained positive as reported previously [28]. Immunocytochemistry was performed using HEL and SET-2 cells as described [28]. Cells were spun on cytospin slides and fixed with acetone for 8 min. Slides were pretreated in citrate buffer (pH 6.0) at 95 °C for 20 min and incubated with a polyclonal anti-pSTAT5 antibody (Invitrogen, Carlsbad, CA, USA order number: 71-6900) diluted 1:100, overnight at 4 °C. Slides were incubated with biotinylated goat anti-rabbit IgG (Biocare Medical, Walnut Creek, CA, USA) for 30 min at room temperature (RT) and then with streptavidin AP label (Biocare Medical, Walnut Creek, CA, USA) for 30 min. Neofuchsin (Nichirei, Tokyo, Japan) was used as the chromogen. All slides were counterstained in Mayer´s hematoxylin.

4.5. Flow Cytometry

Expression of cell surface antigens on primary neoplastic stem cells was analyzed by multicolor flow cytometry using antibodies against CD34, CD38 and CD45 as described [70]. Putative stem cells were defined as $CD34^+/CD38^-/CD45^{dim}$. The gating strategy is shown in Figure A6. For assessing the absolute numbers of stem cells by flow cytometry, Absolute Counting Beads (Thermo Fisher Scientific, Waltham, MA, USA, order number: C36950) were used according to the instructions by the manufacturer. For the flow cytometric detection of cytoplasmic pSTAT5, cells were first stained for cell surface antigens and then fixed in formaldehyde (2%). Cells were subsequently permeabilized by exposure to 50% methanol (−20 °C, 10 min), washed in phosphate-buffered saline containing 0.1% bovine serum albumin (order number: A4503; Merck) and stained with the Alexa 647-conjugated anti-pSTAT5 mAb 47 pY694 or an isotype-matched control antibody for 30 min at RT. Cells were then washed and analyzed on a FACSCanto (BD Biosciences). Staining reactions were expressed as median fluorescence intensity (MFI). pSTAT5 expression levels are shown as staining index (SI) defined as MFI produced by anti-pSTAT5 antibody:MFI of the isotype-matched control antibody.

4.6. Western Blot Analysis of Expression of pSTAT5 in Ba/F3 Cells

To confirm the selective effects of JAK2 or STAT5 targeting drugs, Western blot experiments were performed using the pSTAT5 antibody Tyr694 on Ba/F3 and Ba/F3-MPL cells engineered to express *JAK2* V617F and *CALR*del52, respectively. Ba/F3 cells were generated as described [71,72]. Cells were incubated with drugs targeting JAK2 (AZD1480, TG101348, ruxolitinib, R763; 1–5 μM) or STAT5 (piceatannol, pimozide; 10–45 μM) for 4 h. Then, pSTAT5 expression was analyzed by Western blotting essentially as described [49]. Nitrocellulose membranes (0.45 μm Amersham Protran; order number: 10600002; GE Healthcare, Buckinghamshire, UK) were incubated with the following antibodies at the dilution indicated: polyclonal rabbit anti-phospho-STAT5 (Y694) antibody (order number: 71-6900; 1:1000; Invitrogen, Camarillo, CA, USA), monoclonal mouse anti-STAT5 antibody 89/Stat5 (order number: 610191; 1:1000; BD Biosciences), mouse anti-HSC70 monoclonal antibody B-6 (order number: SC-7298; 1:10,000; Santa Cruz, St. Louis, MO, USA), IRDye® 680RD goat anti-rabbit IgG (order number: 925-68071; 1:10000; LI-COR, Lincoln, NE, USA), and IRDye® 800CW goat anti-mouse IgG (order number: 925-32210; 1:10000; LI-COR). pSTAT5 levels were quantified by densitometry and expressed as the pSTAT5/loading control ratio normalized to control (untreated) cells.

4.7. Isolation of the Cytoplasmic and Nuclear Fractions of HEL and SET-2 Cells

HEL and SET-2 cells were lysed in hypotonic buffer (20 mM HEPES, 10 mM KCl, 1 mM ethylenediaminetetraacetic acid, 0.2% NP40, 10% glycerol, 5 μg/mL aprotinin, 5 μg/mL leupeptin, 1 mM phenylmethylsulfonide fluoril, and 1 mM Na_2VO_4). Cell lysates were centrifuged (5 min, 800× *g*) to separate cytoplasmic and nuclear fractions [61]. Supernatants (cytoplasmic fraction) were frozen at −70 °C. Pelleted nuclei were resuspended in hypertonic buffer (hypotonic buffer plus 350 mM NaCl) and protein extracts were prepared by agitation (30 min, 4 °C). After debris was removed by centrifugation, nuclear extracts were frozen at −70 °C. Expression of pSTAT5 was determined by Western blotting and quantified by densitometry as reported [61]. Fractionation of subcellular compartments was controlled by applying anti-RAF-1 (cytoplasmic) and anti-topoisomerase-1 (nuclear) antibodies in parallel. All antibodies were from Santa Cruz.

4.8. Evaluation of Drug Effects on the Growth and Survival of MPN Cells

To further determine the functional role of STAT5 in MPN cells, we applied several targeting drugs: piceatannol, pimozide, AZD1480, TG101348, R763, ruxolitinib, AC-3-019 and AC-4-130 (Table A2). Primary human MPN cells (ET, $n = 2$; PMF, $n = 3$; PV, $n = 2$), HEL cells and SET-2 cells were incubated with increasing drug concentrations at 37 °C for 48 h. Thereafter, ^{3}[H]-thymidine was added, and its uptake was analyzed after 16 h using a beta-counter. For evaluation of apoptosis, HEL and SET-2 cells were incubated in control medium or in various drug concentrations for 24 h and 48 h at 37 °C. The percentage of apoptotic cells was quantified using Annexin V/Propidium Iodide staining as described [73]. In a subset of patients, we examined drug effects on putative $CD34^+/CD38^-$ MPN-SC.

5. Conclusions

STAT5 is a critical molecule in MPN cells that acts downstream of oncogenic JAK2 V617F and mutant CALR. We found that pSTAT5 is expressed abundantly in the nuclear and cytoplasmic compartment of MPN cells and that pSTAT5 is not only present in more mature clonal cells, but also in putative $CD34^+/CD38^-$ MPN-SC. Moreover, we show that STAT5 expression correlates with survival of MPN cells and that drugs targeting STAT5 can block growth and survival of these cells. Since MPN-SC display STAT5, and STAT5 is downstream of both JAK2 V617F and mutant CALR, targeting of STAT5 may be a promising approach to treat MPN.

Author Contributions: Conceptualization, E.H. and P.V.; methodology, validation and formal analysis, E.H., A.K., D.B., G.G., B.W., N.W., D.I., E.P., H.N., F.K.M.S., Y.F., C.K., H.A.N., L.M., G.H., F.G., R.K.; resources, G.T., J.P., E.D.d.A., P.T.G., L.M. R.K., R.M., P.V.; writing—original draft preparation, E.H. and P.V.; writing—review and editing, all authors; supervision, P.V.; project administration, E.H.; funding acquisition, E.H., R.K., H.A.N., P.T.G., R.M., P.V. All authors have read and agreed to the published version of the manuscript.

Acknowledgments: The authors would like to thank Sabine Cerny-Reiterer, Susanne Gamperl and Gabriele Stefanzl for their skillful technical assistance.

Appendix A

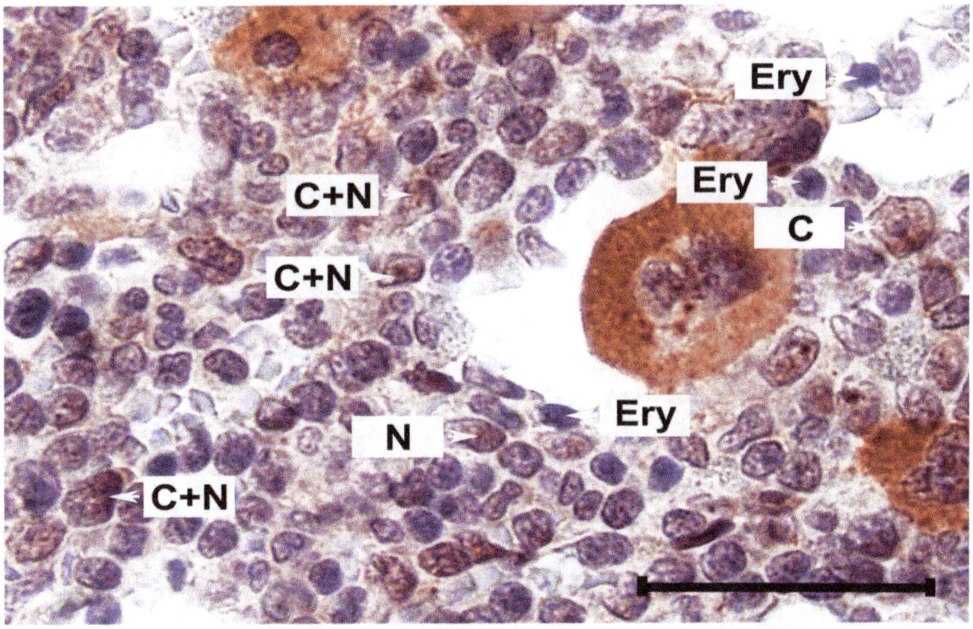

Figure A1. The picture shows an enlarged part of the picture of patient #06 (PV) from Figure 1A. The arrows point at examples of cytoplasmic 'C', nuclear 'N' and cytoplasmic/nuclear 'C+N' staining. 'Ery' marks examples of erythroid cells that were used as internal negative controls. Scale bar: 30 μm.

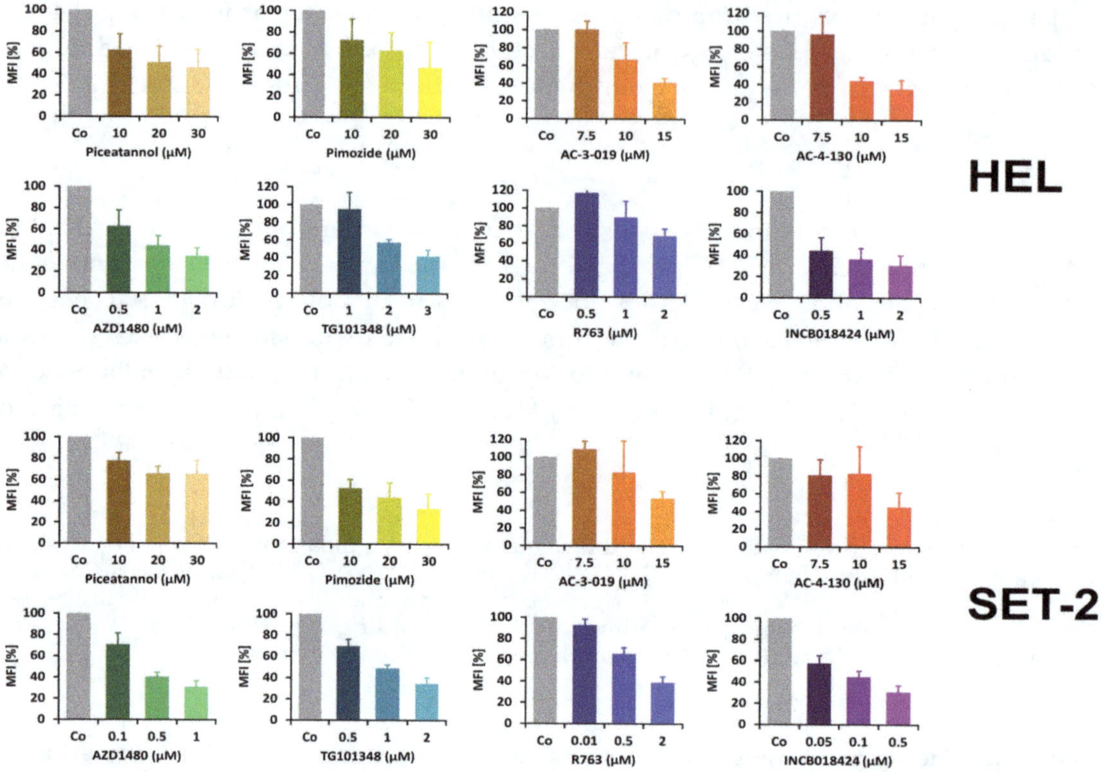

Figure A2. HEL and SET-2 cells were incubated with various concentrations of JAK2-targeting drugs (ruxolitinib, R763, TG101348, AZD1480) or STAT5-targeting drugs (piceatannol, pimozide, AC-3-019, AC-4-130) for 4 h. Thereafter, expression of pSTAT5 was analyzed by multicolor flow cytometry. The levels of pSTAT5 are depicted as median fluorescence index (MFI) values relative to the untreated control (Co).

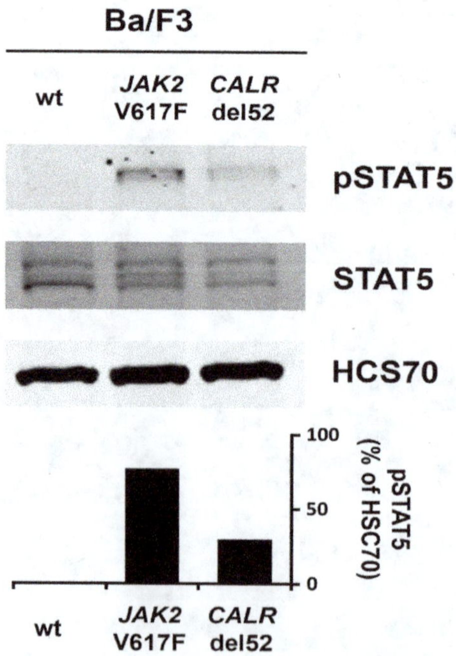

Figure A3. Wild type (wt) Ba/F3 cells or Ba/F3 cells transfected with either *JAK2* V617F or *CALRdel52* were incubated overnight in medium without IL-3. After, cell lysates were subjected to Western blotting using antibodies against pSTAT5, STAT5 and HSC70. The columns show the levels of pSTAT5 in percent of HSC70 as analyzed by densitometry. Uncropped blots are shown in Figure S3.

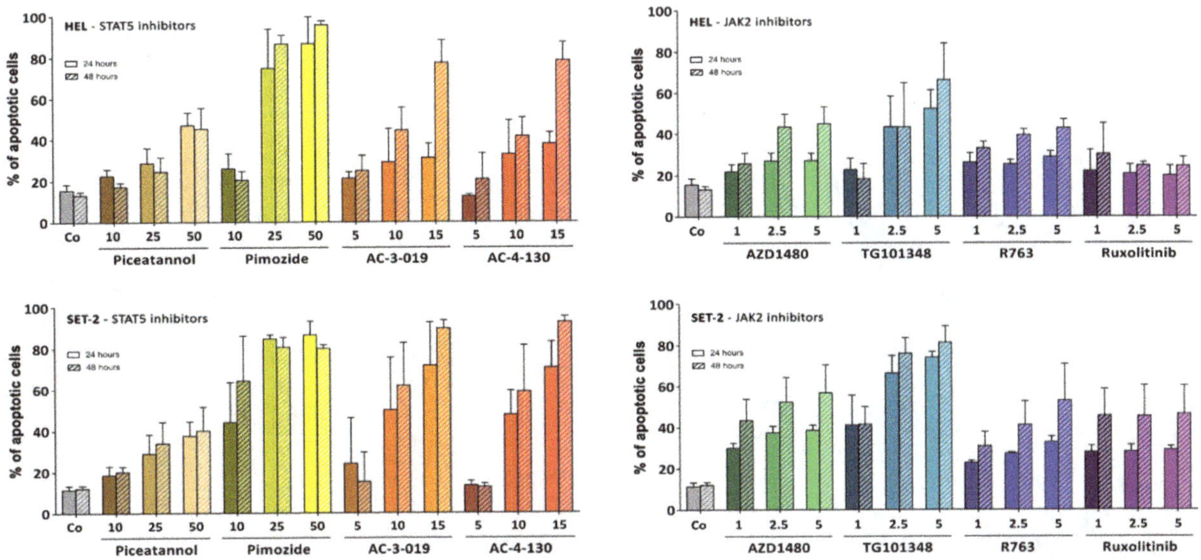

Figure A4. HEL and SET-2 cells (as indicated) were incubated with different concentrations of JAK2 or STAT5 targeting drugs for 24 h or 48 h at 37 °C. Thereafter, apoptosis induction was assessed using Annexin V/propidium iodide (PI) staining. The columns show the sum of cells positive for Annexin V-only, PI-only or Annexin V/PI for each condition and are depicted as mean ± SD of at least three independent experiments.

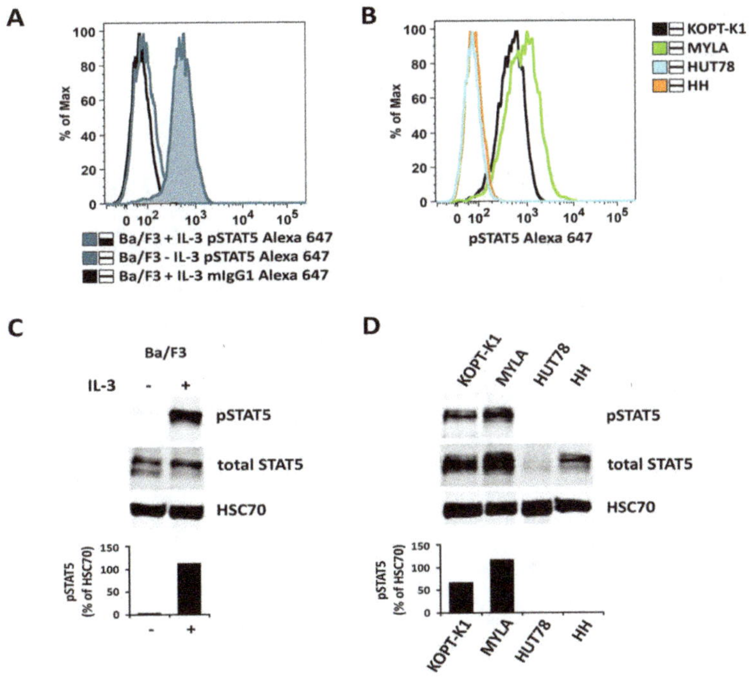

Figure A5. Ba/F3 cells were kept in medium without IL-3 overnight and split in the morning. One half was incubated with 10 ng/mL IL-3 for 40 min (Ba/F3 + IL-3), while the other half was kept in medium without IL-3 (Ba/F3 − IL-3). Thereafter, cells were analyzed for expression of pSTAT5 either by flow cytometry (**A**) or Western blotting (**C**). In (**A**), an Alexa-647-labeled anti-pSTAT5 antibody was used (with IL-3: blue histogram; without IL-3: open blue histogram). mIgG1 Alexa-647 was used as an isotype control (open black histogram) in Ba/F3 + IL-3 cells (**A**). Human lymphoma cell lines with detectable pSTAT5 levels (KOPT-K1 and MYLA) or no detectable pSTAT5 (HUT78 and HH) were also analyzed for pSTAT5 expression using flow cytometry (**B**) and Western blotting (**D**). In Western blot experiments, HSC70 served as a loading control. The columns show the levels of pSTAT5 in percent of HSC70 as analyzed by densitometry. Uncropped blots are shown in Figure S4.

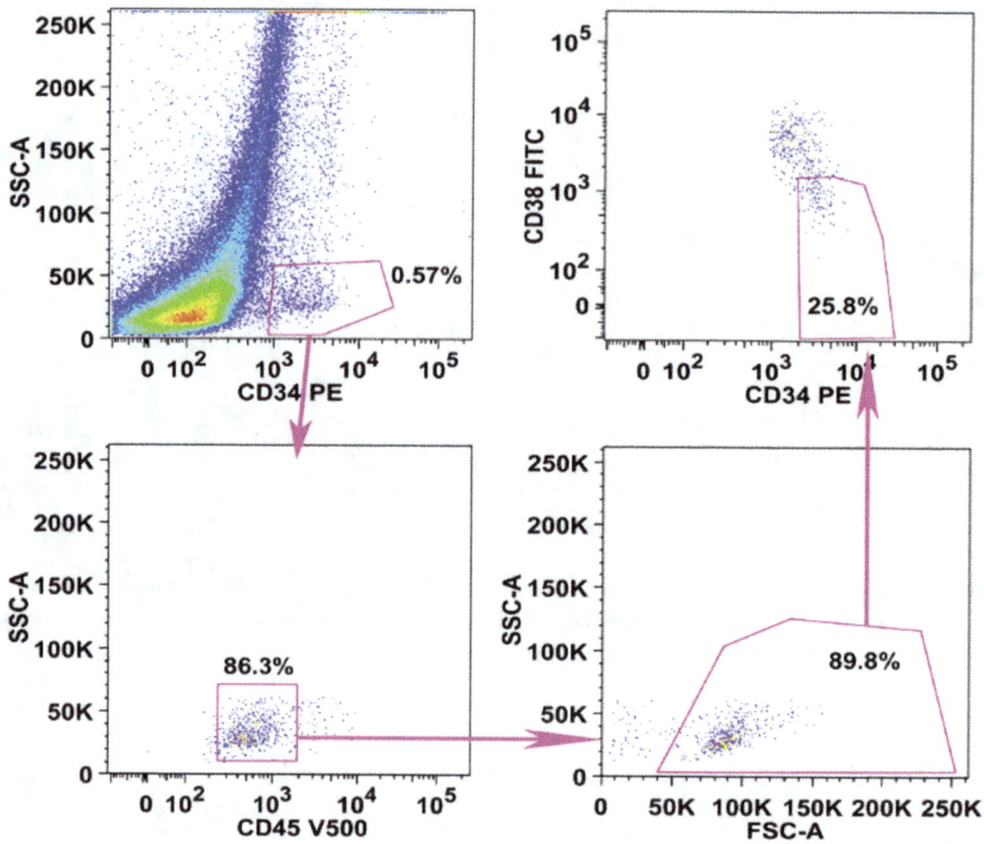

Figure A6. To identify immature CD34$^+$/CD38$^-$ stem cells (SC), we performed a sequential gating algorithm, indicated by pink arrows using FlowJo software. After excluding CD45-negative cells, immature cells were identified by their expression of CD34 (upper left panel) and were then gated as CD45 dim-positive blast cells (lower left panel). Thereafter, viable cells were selected by their light-scatter properties (lower right panel) and were then gated according to the lack (pink gate) of CD38 (upper right panel). The example shows bone marrow cells from patient #23.

Table A1. Patient characteristics.

#	Sex	Age at Sampling	Diagnosis	Mutated *JAK2*, *CALR* or *MPL*	Mutation	pSTAT5 FACS	pSTAT5 IHC	Proliferation	SC Assay	pSTAT5 Regulation
01	f	44	PMF	*JAK2*	V617F	yes	-	-	-	-
02	f	61	ET	none	–	yes	yes	-	-	-
03	f	53	ET	none	–	yes	-	-	-	-
04	f	71	ET	*JAK2*	V617F	yes	-	-	-	-
05	f	76	PV	*JAK2*	V617F	yes	-	-	-	-
06	f	76	PV	*JAK2*	V617F	yes	yes	-	-	-
07	f	53	PV	none	–	yes	-	yes	-	-
08	f	61	ET	*CALR*	ins5: c.1154_1155insTTGTC, p.Lys385Asnfs*47	yes	-	-	-	-
09	f	50	PMF	*JAK2*	V617F	yes	-	-	-	-
10	f	64	PMF	*JAK2*	V617F	yes	-	-	-	-
11	f	74	ET	*JAK2*	V617F	yes	-	-	-	-
12	f	52	PMF	*CALR*	ins5: c.1154_1155insTTGTC, p.Lys385Asnfs*47	yes	-	-	-	-
13	f	50	ET	*MPL*	W515L	yes	-	-	-	-
14	f	71	ET	*JAK2*	V617F	yes	-	-	yes	-
15	m	67	PV	none	–	yes	-	-	-	-
16	m	70	PMF	*CALR*	del52: c.1099_1150del, p. Leu367Thrfs*46	yes	yes	-	-	-
17	f	37	ET	none	–	yes	-	-	-	-
18	f	66	PV	*JAK2*	V617F	yes	yes	-	-	-
19	m	74	PV	*JAK2*	V617F	yes	-	-	-	-
20	m	53	PMF	*JAK2*	V617F	yes	yes	yes	-	-
21	m	71	PV	*JAK2*	V617F	yes	-	-	-	-
22	m	51	PMF	*JAK2*	V617F	yes	-	-	-	-
23	m	43	ET	*JAK2*	V617F	yes	yes	yes	-	-
24	m	59	ET	*CALR*	del52: c.1099_1150del, p. Leu367Thrfs*46	yes	-	-	-	-
25	f	84	ET	none	–	yes	-	-	-	-
26	m	37	ET	*JAK2*	V617F	yes	-	-	-	-
27	f	45	PMF	*JAK2*	V617F	yes	-	-	yes	-
28	f	31	ET	*JAK2*	V617F	yes	-	-	-	-
29	f	85	PMF	*JAK2*	V617F	yes	yes	-	yes	-
30	f	74	PV	*JAK2*	V617F	yes	yes	-	yes	-

Table A1. *Cont.*

#	Sex	Age at Sampling	Diagnosis	Mutated *JAK2*, *CALR* or *MPL*	Mutation	pSTAT5 FACS	pSTAT5 IHC	Proliferation	SC Assay	pSTAT5 Regulation
31	f	80	PV	*JAK2*	V617F	yes	-	-	yes	yes
32	f	72	ET	*JAK2*	V617F	yes	-	-	-	-
33	m	49	PV	*JAK2*	V617F	yes	-	-	-	-
34	m	64	ET	*JAK2*	V617F	yes	yes	-	-	-
35	f	71	PMF	*JAK2*	V617F	-	-	yes	-	-
36	f	68	ET	*JAK2*	V617F	-	-	yes	-	-
37	f	48	PMF	*JAK2*	V617F	-	-	yes	-	-
38	f	34	PV	*JAK2*	V617F	-	-	yes	-	-
39	m	88	PMF	*CALR*	del52: c.1099_1150del, p. Leu367Thrfs*46	-	-	-	yes	-
40	f	42	ET	*JAK2*	V617F	-	-	-	yes	-
41	f	38	ET	*JAK2*	V617F	-	-	-	yes	-
42	f	75	PV	*JAK2*	V617F	-	-	-	yes	yes
43	f	93	PMF	*JAK2*	V617F	-	-	-	yes	yes

CALR, *calreticulin*; ET, essential thrombocythemia; *JAK2*, *Janus kinase 2; MPL*, *MPL proto-oncogene, thrombopoietin receptor*; MPN, myeloproliferative neoplasm; PMF, primary myelofibrosis; Proliferation, effects of drugs on proliferation of MNC isolated from MPN patients; pSTAT5 FACS, sample analyzed for expression of pSTAT5 in $CD34^+/CD38^-$ putative stem cells; pSTAT5 IHC, sample analyzed by immunohistochemistry for expression of pSTAT5 in different bone marrow cells; pSTAT5 regulation, effects of JAK2 or STAT5 targeting drugs on pSTAT5 levels in $CD34^+/CD38^-/CD45^{dim}$ cells; SC assay, effects of JAK2 or STAT5 targeting drugs on relative numbers of $CD34^+/CD38^-/CD45^{dim}$ cells.

Table A2. Specifications of inhibitors used in this study.

Name [Ref]	Known Targets	Result of Target Inhibition (Drug Action)	Clinical Application	C_{max} in μM (at Dose/Day)	Concentration Range (μM) *	Supplier **
R763 [40]	JAK2, aurora kinase A, aurora kinase B, FLT3	G2/M phase arrest, endoreduplication	Phase 1 trial (human): 11.4–85.3 mg/day	0.09 (85.3 mg)	0.005–5	Rigel Pharmaceuticals
TG101348 [41,42]	JAK2, JAK1, JAK3, FLT3, RET, TYK2	proliferation inhibition, apoptosis induction	Phase 1 trial (human): 100–600 mg/day	2.8 (500 mg)	0.005–7.5	ChemieTek
AZD1480 [43,44]	JAK2, JAK1, JAK3, TYK2, FGFR3, STAT3	proliferation inhibition, apoptosis induction	Phase 1 trial (human): 5–80 mg/day	1.7 (30 mg)	0.005–7.5	ChemieTek
Ruxolitinib [38,39]	JAK2, JAK1, JAK3	proliferation inhibition, apoptosis induction	approved (human): PMF, PV (EU, USA)	2.3 (50 mg)	1–20	ChemieTek
Pimozide [46,47]	STAT5, D_2 dopamine receptor, 5-HT_7 receptor, Ca^{2+} channels	proliferation inhibition, apoptosis induction	approved (human): Tourette's Syndrome (EU, USA)	0.007 (2 mg)	0.5–25	Merck
Piceatannol [45]	STAT5, SYK, LCK	proliferation inhibition, apoptosis induction, histamine release blockade	n.a.	8.1 (80.7 mg/kg)	1–75	Merck
AC-3-019 [48]	STAT5	proliferation inhibition, apoptosis induction	n.a.	n.a.	0.05–15	P. Gunning
AC-4-130 [48,49]	STAT5	proliferation inhibition, apoptosis induction	n.a.	n.a.	0.25–15	P. Gunning

C_{max}, peak plasma concentration of a drug after administration; FGFR3, fibroblast growth factor receptor 3; FLT3, fms-like tyrosine kinase 3; JAK, janus kinase; LCK, leukocyte C-terminal SRC kinase; LYN, LCK/YES novel tyrosine kinase; n.a., not applicable; PMF, primary myelofibrosis; PV, polycythemia vera; Ref, Reference; STAT, signal transducer and activator of transcription; SYK, spleen tyrosine kinase; TYK2, tyrosine kinase 2; * Range of concentrations used in this study. ** ChemieTek (Indianapolis, IN, USA); LC Laboratories (Woburn, MA, USA); Merck, (Darmstadt, Germany); Rigel Pharmaceuticals (San Francisco, CA, USA); Patrick Gunning (Department of Chemistry, University of Toronto, Canada).

Table A3. IC_{50} concentrations of JAK2- and STAT5 targeting drugs in pSTAT5 high and low cell lines.

IC_{50} Obtained with Drugs in Various Cell Lines (SI pSTAT5)				
Inhibitor	HEL (13.4)	SET-2 (8.6)	A375 (1.93)	A2780 (1.97)
Piceatannol	10–17.5	10–17.5	>75	17.5–25
Pimozide	5–7.5	5–7.5	12.5–15	12.5–15
AC-3-019	3.5–4	9–10	10–12.5	12.5–15
AC-4-130	3.5–4	7–8	>15	>15
AZD1480	0.5–1	0.05–0.1	>2	0.5–1
TG1010348	1–2	0.1–0.25	>2	1–2
Ruxolitinib	1–2	0.0025–0.05	>2	>2

IC_{50} concentration: half maximal inhibitory concentration; SI: Staining Index (MFI produced by the anti-pSTAT5 antibody:MFI of the isotype-matched control antibody).

Table A4. Characteristics of control bone marrow donors.

#	**Sex**	**Age at Sampling**	**Diagnosis**	**pSTAT5 FACS**	**pSTAT5 IHC**
44	f	33	NHL	yes	-
45	m	37	nBM	yes	-
46	m	40	NHL	yes	yes
47	m	24	B-ALL (CR)	yes	-
48	f	47	CM	yes	yes
49	m	26	NHL	yes	-
50	f	33	NHL	-	yes
51	m	61	NHL	-	yes

B-ALL (CR), b-cell acute lymphoblastic leukemia in complete remission; CM, cutaneous mastocytosis; nBM, normal bone marrow; NHL, non-Hodgkin lymphoma; PMF, primary myelofibrosis; pSTAT5 FACS, sample analyzed for expression of pSTAT5 in $CD34^{+}/CD38^{-}$ putative stem cells; pSTAT5 IHC, sample analyzed by immunohistochemistry for expression of pSTAT5 in different bone marrow cells; PV, polycythemia vera.

References

1. Campbell, P.J.; Green, A.R. The myeloproliferative disorders. *N. Engl. J. Med.* **2006**, *355*, 2452–2466. [CrossRef] [PubMed]
2. Scott, L.M.; Tong, W.; Levine, R.L.; Scott, M.A.; Beer, P.A.; Stratton, M.R.; Futreal, P.A.; Erber, W.N.; McMullin, M.F.; Harrison, C.N.; et al. JAK2 exon 12 mutations in polycythemia vera and idiopathic erythrocytosis. *N. Engl. J. Med.* **2007**, *356*, 459–468. [CrossRef] [PubMed]
3. Arber, D.A.; Orazi, A.; Hasserjian, R.; Thiele, J.; Borowitz, M.J.; Le Beau, M.M.; Bloomfield, C.D.; Cazzola, M.; Vardiman, J.W. The 2016 revision to the World Health Organization classification of myeloid neoplasms and acute leukemia. *Blood* **2016**, *127*, 2391–2405. [CrossRef] [PubMed]
4. Skoda, R.C.; Duek, A.; Grisouard, J. Pathogenesis of myeloproliferative neoplasms. *Exp. Hematol.* **2015**, *43*, 599–608. [CrossRef] [PubMed]
5. Spivak, J.L. Myeloproliferative Neoplasms. *N. Engl. J. Med.* **2017**, *376*, 2168–2181. [CrossRef] [PubMed]
6. Tefferi, A. Primary myelofibrosis: 2012 update on diagnosis, risk stratification, and management. *Am. J. Hematol.* **2011**, *86*, 1017–1026. [CrossRef] [PubMed]
7. Cherington, C.; Slack, J.L.; Leis, J.; Adams, R.H.; Reeder, C.B.; Mikhael, J.R.; Camoriano, J.; Noel, P.; Fauble, V.; Betcher, J.; et al. Allogeneic stem cell transplantation for myeloproliferative neoplasm in blast phase. *Leuk. Res.* **2012**, *36*, 1147–1151. [CrossRef] [PubMed]
8. Deeg, H.J.; Bredeson, C.; Farnia, S.; Ballen, K.; Gupta, V.; Mesa, R.A.; Popat, U.; Hari, P.; Saber, W.; Seftel, M.; et al. Hematopoietic Cell Transplantation as Curative Therapy for Patients with Myelofibrosis: Long-Term Success in all Age Groups. *Biol. Blood Marrow Transpl.* **2015**, *21*, 1883–1887. [CrossRef]
9. Wolf, D.; Rudzki, J.; Gastl, G. Current treatment concepts of Philadelphia-negative MPN. *Curr. Cancer Drug Targets* **2011**, *11*, 44–55. [CrossRef]
10. Barosi, G.; Lupo, L.; Rosti, V. Management of myeloproliferative neoplasms: From academic guidelines to clinical practice. *Curr. Hematol. Malig. Rep.* **2012**, *7*, 50–56. [CrossRef]

11. Emadi, A.; Spivak, J.L. Anagrelide: 20 years later. *Expert Rev. Anticancer Ther.* **2009**, *9*, 37–50. [CrossRef] [PubMed]
12. Harrison, C.; Kiladjian, J.J.; Al-Ali, H.K.; Gisslinger, H.; Waltzman, R.; Stalbovskaya, V.; McQuitty, M.; Hunter, D.S.; Levy, R.; Knoops, L.; et al. JAK inhibition with ruxolitinib versus best available therapy for myelofibrosis. *N. Engl. J. Med.* **2012**, *366*, 787–798. [CrossRef] [PubMed]
13. Kiladjian, J.J.; Giraudier, S.; Cassinat, B. Interferon-alpha for the therapy of myeloproliferative neoplasms: Targeting the malignant clone. *Leukemia* **2016**, *30*, 776–781. [CrossRef] [PubMed]
14. Vannucchi, A.M.; Harrison, C.N. Emerging treatments for classical myeloproliferative neoplasms. *Blood* **2017**, *129*, 693–703. [CrossRef]
15. Verstovsek, S.; Mesa, R.A.; Gotlib, J.; Levy, R.S.; Gupta, V.; DiPersio, J.F.; Catalano, J.V.; Deininger, M.; Miller, C.; Silver, R.T.; et al. A double-blind, placebo-controlled trial of ruxolitinib for myelofibrosis. *N. Engl. J. Med.* **2012**, *366*, 799–807. [CrossRef] [PubMed]
16. Klampfl, T.; Gisslinger, H.; Harutyunyan, A.S.; Nivarthi, H.; Rumi, E.; Milosevic, J.D.; Them, N.C.; Berg, T.; Gisslinger, B.; Pietra, D.; et al. Somatic mutations of calreticulin in myeloproliferative neoplasms. *N. Engl. J. Med.* **2013**, *369*, 2379–2390. [CrossRef]
17. Kralovics, R.; Passamonti, F.; Buser, A.S.; Teo, S.S.; Tiedt, R.; Passweg, J.R.; Tichelli, A.; Cazzola, M.; Skoda, R.C. A gain-of-function mutation of JAK2 in myeloproliferative disorders. *N. Engl. J. Med.* **2005**, *352*, 1779–1790. [CrossRef]
18. Nangalia, J.; Massie, C.E.; Baxter, E.J.; Nice, F.L.; Gundem, G.; Wedge, D.C.; Avezov, E.; Li, J.; Kollmann, K.; Kent, D.G.; et al. Somatic CALR mutations in myeloproliferative neoplasms with nonmutated JAK2. *N. Engl. J. Med.* **2013**, *369*, 2391–2405. [CrossRef]
19. Pardanani, A.D.; Levine, R.L.; Lasho, T.; Pikman, Y.; Mesa, R.A.; Wadleigh, M.; Steensma, D.P.; Elliott, M.A.; Wolanskyj, A.P.; Hogan, W.J.; et al. MPL515 mutations in myeloproliferative and other myeloid disorders: A study of 1182 patients. *Blood* **2006**, *108*, 3472–3476. [CrossRef]
20. Pikman, Y.; Lee, B.H.; Mercher, T.; McDowell, E.; Ebert, B.L.; Gozo, M.; Cuker, A.; Wernig, G.; Moore, S.; Galinsky, I.; et al. MPLW515L is a novel somatic activating mutation in myelofibrosis with myeloid metaplasia. *PLoS Med.* **2006**, *3*, e270. [CrossRef]
21. Funakoshi-Tago, M.; Tago, K.; Abe, M.; Sonoda, Y.; Kasahara, T. STAT5 activation is critical for the transformation mediated by myeloproliferative disorder-associated JAK2 V617F mutant. *J. Biol. Chem.* **2010**, *285*, 5296–5307. [CrossRef] [PubMed]
22. Gibson, S.E.; Schade, A.E.; Szpurka, H.; Bak, B.; Maciejewski, J.P.; Hsi, E.D. Phospho-STAT5 expression pattern with the MPL W515L mutation is similar to that seen in chronic myeloproliferative disorders with JAK2 V617F. *Hum. Pathol.* **2008**, *39*, 1111–1114. [CrossRef] [PubMed]
23. Koschmieder, S.; Mughal, T.I.; Hasselbalch, H.C.; Barosi, G.; Valent, P.; Kiladjian, J.J.; Jeryczynski, G.; Gisslinger, H.; Jutzi, J.S.; Pahl, H.L.; et al. Myeloproliferative neoplasms and inflammation: Whether to target the malignant clone or the inflammatory process or both. *Leukemia* **2016**, *30*, 1018–1024. [CrossRef]
24. O'Sullivan, J.M.; Harrison, C.N. JAK-STAT signaling in the therapeutic landscape of myeloproliferative neoplasms. *Mol. Cell. Endocrinol.* **2017**, *451*, 71–79. [CrossRef] [PubMed]
25. Pasquier, F.; Cabagnols, X.; Secardin, L.; Plo, I.; Vainchenker, W. Myeloproliferative neoplasms: JAK2 signaling pathway as a central target for therapy. *Clin. Lymphoma Myeloma Leuk.* **2014**, *14*, S23–S35. [CrossRef] [PubMed]
26. Walz, C.; Ahmed, W.; Lazarides, K.; Betancur, M.; Patel, N.; Hennighausen, L.; Zaleskas, V.M.; Van Etten, R.A. Essential role for Stat5a/b in myeloproliferative neoplasms induced by BCR-ABL1 and JAK2(V617F) in mice. *Blood* **2012**, *119*, 3550–3560. [CrossRef]
27. Yan, D.; Hutchison, R.E.; Mohi, G. Critical requirement for Stat5 in a mouse model of polycythemia vera. *Blood* **2012**, *119*, 3539–3549. [CrossRef]
28. Baumgartner, C.; Cerny-Reiterer, S.; Sonneck, K.; Mayerhofer, M.; Gleixner, K.V.; Fritz, R.; Kerenyi, M.; Boudot, C.; Gouilleux, F.; Kornfeld, J.W.; et al. Expression of activated STAT5 in neoplastic mast cells in systemic mastocytosis: Subcellular distribution and role of the transforming oncoprotein KIT D816V. *Am. J. Pathol.* **2009**, *175*, 2416–2429. [CrossRef]
29. Harir, N.; Pecquet, C.; Kerenyi, M.; Sonneck, K.; Kovacic, B.; Nyga, R.; Brevet, M.; Dhennin, I.; Gouilleux-Gruart, V.; Beug, H.; et al. Constitutive activation of Stat5 promotes its cytoplasmic localization and association with PI3-kinase in myeloid leukemias. *Blood* **2007**, *109*, 1678–1686. [CrossRef]

30. Weber, A.; Borghouts, C.; Brendel, C.; Moriggl, R.; Delis, N.; Brill, B.; Vafaizadeh, V.; Groner, B. Stat5 Exerts Distinct, Vital Functions in the Cytoplasm and Nucleus of Bcr-Abl+ K562 and Jak2(V617F)+ HEL Leukemia Cells. *Cancers* **2015**, *7*, 503–537. [CrossRef]
31. Angona, A.; Alvarez-Larran, A.; Bellosillo, B.; Longaron, R.; Camacho, L.; Fernandez-Rodriguez, M.C.; Pairet, S.; Besses, C. Characterization of CD34+ hematopoietic progenitor cells in JAK2V617F and CALR-mutated myeloproliferative neoplasms. *Leuk. Res.* **2016**, *48*, 11–15. [CrossRef] [PubMed]
32. Chaligne, R.; James, C.; Tonetti, C.; Besancenot, R.; Le Couedic, J.P.; Fava, F.; Mazurier, F.; Godin, I.; Maloum, K.; Larbret, F.; et al. Evidence for MPL W515L/K mutations in hematopoietic stem cells in primitive myelofibrosis. *Blood* **2007**, *110*, 3735–3743. [CrossRef] [PubMed]
33. Jamieson, C.H.; Gotlib, J.; Durocher, J.A.; Chao, M.P.; Mariappan, M.R.; Lay, M.; Jones, C.; Zehnder, J.L.; Lilleberg, S.L.; Weissman, I.L. The JAK2 V617F mutation occurs in hematopoietic stem cells in polycythemia vera and predisposes toward erythroid differentiation. *Proc. Natl. Acad. Sci. USA* **2006**, *103*, 6224–6229. [CrossRef] [PubMed]
34. Mead, A.J.; Mullally, A. Myeloproliferative neoplasm stem cells. *Blood* **2017**, *129*, 1607–1616. [CrossRef] [PubMed]
35. Staerk, J.; Constantinescu, S.N. The JAK-STAT pathway and hematopoietic stem cells from the JAK2 V617F perspective. *JAK-STAT* **2012**, *1*, 184–190. [CrossRef]
36. Quentmeier, H.; Geffers, R.; Jost, E.; Macleod, R.A.; Nagel, S.; Rohrs, S.; Romani, J.; Scherr, M.; Zaborski, M.; Drexler, H.G. SOCS2: Inhibitor of JAK2V617F-mediated signal transduction. *Leukemia* **2008**, *22*, 2169–2175. [CrossRef]
37. Liu, R.Y.; Fan, C.; Garcia, R.; Jove, R.; Zuckerman, K.S. Constitutive activation of the JAK2/STAT5 signal transduction pathway correlates with growth factor independence of megakaryocytic leukemic cell lines. *Blood* **1999**, *93*, 2369–2379. [CrossRef]
38. Hornakova, T.; Springuel, L.; Devreux, J.; Dusa, A.; Constantinescu, S.N.; Knoops, L.; Renauld, J.C. Oncogenic JAK1 and JAK2-activating mutations resistant to ATP-competitive inhibitors. *Haematologica* **2011**, *96*, 845–853. [CrossRef]
39. Bartalucci, N.; Calabresi, L.; Balliu, M.; Martinelli, S.; Rossi, M.C.; Villeval, J.L.; Annunziato, F.; Guglielmelli, P.; Vannucchi, A.M. Inhibitors of the PI3K/mTOR pathway prevent STAT5 phosphorylation in JAK2V617F mutated cells through PP2A/CIP2A axis. *Oncotarget* **2017**, *8*, 96710–96724. [CrossRef]
40. Peter, B.; Bibi, S.; Eisenwort, G.; Wingelhofer, B.; Berger, D.; Stefanzl, G.; Blatt, K.; Herrmann, H.; Hadzijusufovic, E.; Hoermann, G.; et al. Drug-induced inhibition of phosphorylation of STAT5 overrides drug resistance in neoplastic mast cells. *Leukemia* **2018**, *32*, 1016–1022. [CrossRef]
41. Geron, I.; Abrahamsson, A.E.; Barroga, C.F.; Kavalerchik, E.; Gotlib, J.; Hood, J.D.; Durocher, J.; Mak, C.C.; Noronha, G.; Soll, R.M.; et al. Selective inhibition of JAK2-driven erythroid differentiation of polycythemia vera progenitors. *Cancer Cell* **2008**, *13*, 321–330. [CrossRef] [PubMed]
42. Wernig, G.; Kharas, M.G.; Okabe, R.; Moore, S.A.; Leeman, D.S.; Cullen, D.E.; Gozo, M.; McDowell, E.P.; Levine, R.L.; Doukas, J.; et al. Efficacy of TG101348, a selective JAK2 inhibitor, in treatment of a murine model of JAK2V617F-induced polycythemia vera. *Cancer Cell* **2008**, *13*, 311–320. [CrossRef] [PubMed]
43. Cook, A.M.; Li, L.; Ho, Y.; Lin, A.; Li, L.; Stein, A.; Forman, S.; Perrotti, D.; Jove, R.; Bhatia, R. Role of altered growth factor receptor-mediated JAK2 signaling in growth and maintenance of human acute myeloid leukemia stem cells. *Blood* **2014**, *123*, 2826–2837. [CrossRef] [PubMed]
44. Ioannidis, S.; Lamb, M.L.; Wang, T.; Almeida, L.; Block, M.H.; Davies, A.M.; Peng, B.; Su, M.; Zhang, H.J.; Hoffmann, E.; et al. Discovery of 5-chloro-N2-[(1S)-1-(5-fluoropyrimidin-2-yl)ethyl]-N4-(5-methyl-1H-pyrazol-3-yl)p yrimidine-2,4-diamine (AZD1480) as a novel inhibitor of the Jak/Stat pathway. *J. Med. Chem.* **2011**, *54*, 262–276. [CrossRef] [PubMed]
45. Su, L.; David, M. Distinct mechanisms of STAT phosphorylation via the interferon-alpha/beta receptor. Selective inhibition of STAT3 and STAT5 by piceatannol. *J. Biol. Chem.* **2000**, *275*, 12661–12666. [CrossRef]
46. Nelson, E.A.; Walker, S.R.; Weisberg, E.; Bar-Natan, M.; Barrett, R.; Gashin, L.B.; Terrell, S.; Klitgaard, J.L.; Santo, L.; Addorio, M.R.; et al. The STAT5 inhibitor pimozide decreases survival of chronic myelogenous leukemia cells resistant to kinase inhibitors. *Blood* **2011**, *117*, 3421–3429. [CrossRef]
47. Rondanin, R.; Simoni, D.; Maccesi, M.; Romagnoli, R.; Grimaudo, S.; Pipitone, R.M.; Meli, M.; Cascio, A.; Tolomeo, M. Effects of Pimozide Derivatives on pSTAT5 in K562 Cells. *ChemMedChem* **2017**, *12*, 1183–1190. [CrossRef]

48. Cumaraswamy, A.A.; Lewis, A.M.; Geletu, M.; Todic, A.; Diaz, D.B.; Cheng, X.R.; Brown, C.E.; Laister, R.C.; Muench, D.; Kerman, K.; et al. Nanomolar-Potency Small Molecule Inhibitor of STAT5 Protein. *ACS Med. Chem. Lett.* **2014**, *5*, 1202–1206. [CrossRef]
49. Wingelhofer, B.; Maurer, B.; Heyes, E.C.; Cumaraswamy, A.A.; Berger-Becvar, A.; de Araujo, E.D.; Orlova, A.; Freund, P.; Ruge, F.; Park, J.; et al. Pharmacologic inhibition of STAT5 in acute myeloid leukemia. *Leukemia* **2018**, *32*, 1135–1146. [CrossRef]
50. Szymanska, J.; Smolewski, P.; Majchrzak, A.; Cebula-Obrzut, B.; Chojnowski, K.; Trelinski, J. Pro-Apoptotic Activity of Ruxolitinib Alone and in Combination with Hydroxyurea, Busulphan, and PI3K/mTOR Inhibitors in JAK2-Positive Human Cell Lines. *Adv. Clin. Exp. Med.* **2015**, *24*, 195–202. [CrossRef]
51. Fiskus, W.; Verstovsek, S.; Manshouri, T.; Smith, J.E.; Peth, K.; Abhyankar, S.; McGuirk, J.; Bhalla, K.N. Dual PI3K/AKT/mTOR inhibitor BEZ235 synergistically enhances the activity of JAK2 inhibitor against cultured and primary human myeloproliferative neoplasm cells. *Mol. Cancer Ther.* **2013**, *12*, 577–588. [CrossRef] [PubMed]
52. Bogani, C.; Bartalucci, N.; Martinelli, S.; Tozzi, L.; Guglielmelli, P.; Bosi, A.; Vannucchi, A.M.; Associazione Italiana per la Ricerca sul Cancro, A.G.I.M.M. mTOR inhibitors alone and in combination with JAK2 inhibitors effectively inhibit cells of myeloproliferative neoplasms. *PLoS ONE* **2013**, *8*, e54826. [CrossRef] [PubMed]
53. Bar-Natan, M.; Nelson, E.A.; Walker, S.R.; Kuang, Y.; Distel, R.J.; Frank, D.A. Dual inhibition of Jak2 and STAT5 enhances killing of myeloproliferative neoplasia cells. *Leukemia* **2012**, *26*, 1407–1410. [CrossRef] [PubMed]
54. Emir Hadzijusufovic (Ludwig Boltzmann Institute for Hematology and Oncology, Medical University of Vienna, 1090 Vienna, Austria). *Personal observation*, 2018.
55. Freund, P.; Kerenyi, M.A.; Hager, M.; Wagner, T.; Wingelhofer, B.; Pham, H.T.T.; Elabd, M.; Han, X.; Valent, P.; Gouilleux, F.; et al. O-GlcNAcylation of STAT5 controls tyrosine phosphorylation and oncogenic transcription in STAT5-dependent malignancies. *Leukemia* **2017**, *31*, 2132–2142. [CrossRef]
56. Prestipino, A.; Emhardt, A.J.; Aumann, K.; O'Sullivan, D.; Gorantla, S.P.; Duquesne, S.; Melchinger, W.; Braun, L.; Vuckovic, S.; Boerries, M.; et al. Oncogenic JAK2(V617F) causes PD-L1 expression, mediating immune escape in myeloproliferative neoplasms. *Sci. Transl. Med.* **2018**, *10*. [CrossRef]
57. Reckel, S.; Hamelin, R.; Georgeon, S.; Armand, F.; Jolliet, Q.; Chiappe, D.; Moniatte, M.; Hantschel, O. Differential signaling networks of Bcr-Abl p210 and p190 kinases in leukemia cells defined by functional proteomics. *Leukemia* **2017**, *31*, 1502–1512. [CrossRef]
58. Chatain, N.; Ziegler, P.; Fahrenkamp, D.; Jost, E.; Moriggl, R.; Schmitz-Van de Leur, H.; Muller-Newen, G. Src family kinases mediate cytoplasmic retention of activated STAT5 in BCR-ABL-positive cells. *Oncogene* **2013**, *32*, 3587–3597. [CrossRef]
59. Bibi, S.; Arslanhan, M.D.; Langenfeld, F.; Jeanningros, S.; Cerny-Reiterer, S.; Hadzijusufovic, E.; Tchertanov, L.; Moriggl, R.; Valent, P.; Arock, M. Co-operating STAT5 and AKT signaling pathways in chronic myeloid leukemia and mastocytosis: Possible new targets of therapy. *Haematologica* **2014**, *99*, 417–429. [CrossRef]
60. Bunting, K.D.; Xie, X.Y.; Warshawsky, I.; Hsi, E.D. Cytoplasmic localization of phosphorylated STAT5 in human acute myeloid leukemia is inversely correlated with Flt3-ITD. *Blood* **2007**, *110*, 2775–2776. [CrossRef]
61. Harir, N.; Boudot, C.; Friedbichler, K.; Sonneck, K.; Kondo, R.; Martin-Lanneree, S.; Kenner, L.; Kerenyi, M.; Yahiaoui, S.; Gouilleux-Gruart, V.; et al. Oncogenic Kit controls neoplastic mast cell growth through a Stat5/PI3-kinase signaling cascade. *Blood* **2008**, *112*, 2463–2473. [CrossRef]
62. Schulenburg, A.; Blatt, K.; Cerny-Reiterer, S.; Sadovnik, I.; Herrmann, H.; Marian, B.; Grunt, T.W.; Zielinski, C.C.; Valent, P. Cancer stem cells in basic science and in translational oncology: Can we translate into clinical application? *J. Hematol. Oncol.* **2015**, *8*, 16. [CrossRef] [PubMed]
63. Adorno-Cruz, V.; Kibria, G.; Liu, X.; Doherty, M.; Junk, D.J.; Guan, D.; Hubert, C.; Venere, M.; Mulkearns-Hubert, E.; Sinyuk, M.; et al. Cancer stem cells: Targeting the roots of cancer, seeds of metastasis, and sources of therapy resistance. *Cancer Res.* **2015**, *75*, 924–929. [CrossRef] [PubMed]
64. Delhommeau, F.; Dupont, S.; Tonetti, C.; Masse, A.; Godin, I.; Le Couedic, J.P.; Debili, N.; Saulnier, P.; Casadevall, N.; Vainchenker, W.; et al. Evidence that the JAK2 G1849T (V617F) mutation occurs in a lymphomyeloid progenitor in polycythemia vera and idiopathic myelofibrosis. *Blood* **2007**, *109*, 71–77. [CrossRef] [PubMed]

65. Woods, B.; Chen, W.; Chiu, S.; Marinaccio, C.; Fu, C.; Gu, L.; Bulic, M.; Yang, Q.; Zouak, A.; Jia, S.; et al. Activation of JAK/STAT Signaling in Megakaryocytes Sustains Myeloproliferation In Vivo. *Clin. Cancer Res.* **2019**, *25*, 5901–5912. [CrossRef] [PubMed]
66. Vainchenker, W.; Constantinescu, S.N.; Plo, I. Recent advances in understanding myelofibrosis and essential thrombocythemia. *F1000Research* **2016**, *5*. [CrossRef]
67. Zhang, Y.; Lin, C.H.S.; Kaushansky, K.; Zhan, H. JAK2V617F Megakaryocytes Promote Hematopoietic Stem/Progenitor Cell Expansion in Mice Through Thrombopoietin/MPL Signaling. *Stem Cells* **2018**, *36*, 1676–1684. [CrossRef]
68. Teofili, L.; Martini, M.; Cenci, T.; Petrucci, G.; Torti, L.; Storti, S.; Guidi, F.; Leone, G.; Larocca, L.M. Different STAT-3 and STAT-5 phosphorylation discriminates among Ph-negative chronic myeloproliferative diseases and is independent of the V617F JAK-2 mutation. *Blood* **2007**, *110*, 354–359. [CrossRef]
69. Abba, C.; Campanelli, R.; Catarsi, P.; Villani, L.; Abbonante, V.; Sesta, M.A.; Barosi, G.; Rosti, V.; Massa, M. Constitutive STAT5 phosphorylation in CD34+ cells of patients with primary myelofibrosis: Correlation with driver mutation status and disease severity. *PLoS ONE* **2019**, *14*, e0220189. [CrossRef]
70. Herrmann, H.; Sadovnik, I.; Cerny-Reiterer, S.; Rulicke, T.; Stefanzl, G.; Willmann, M.; Hoermann, G.; Bilban, M.; Blatt, K.; Herndlhofer, S.; et al. Dipeptidylpeptidase IV (CD26) defines leukemic stem cells (LSC) in chronic myeloid leukemia. *Blood* **2014**, *123*, 3951–3962. [CrossRef]
71. Nivarthi, H.; Chen, D.; Cleary, C.; Kubesova, B.; Jager, R.; Bogner, E.; Marty, C.; Pecquet, C.; Vainchenker, W.; Constantinescu, S.N.; et al. Thrombopoietin receptor is required for the oncogenic function of CALR mutants. *Leukemia* **2016**, *30*, 1759–1763. [CrossRef]
72. Milosevic Feenstra, J.D.; Nivarthi, H.; Gisslinger, H.; Leroy, E.; Rumi, E.; Chachoua, I.; Bagienski, K.; Kubesova, B.; Pietra, D.; Gisslinger, B.; et al. Whole-exome sequencing identifies novel MPL and JAK2 mutations in triple-negative myeloproliferative neoplasms. *Blood* **2016**, *127*, 325–332. [CrossRef] [PubMed]
73. Wedeh, G.; Cerny-Reiterer, S.; Eisenwort, G.; Herrmann, H.; Blatt, K.; Hadzijusufovic, E.; Sadovnik, I.; Mullauer, L.; Schwaab, J.; Hoffmann, T.; et al. Identification of bromodomain-containing protein-4 as a novel marker and epigenetic target in mast cell leukemia. *Leukemia* **2015**, *29*, 2230–2237. [CrossRef] [PubMed]

10

Balancing STAT Activity as a Therapeutic Strategy

Kelsey L. Polak [1,†], Noah M. Chernosky [1,†], Jacob M. Smigiel [1], Ilaria Tamagno [1] and Mark W. Jackson [1,2,*]

1 Department of Pathology, Case Western Reserve University, School of Medicine, Cleveland, OH 44106, USA; kxp328@case.edu (K.L.P.); nmc71@case.edu (N.M.C.); jxs1094@case.edu (J.M.S.); ixt64@case.edu (I.T.)

2 Case Comprehensive Cancer Center, Case Western Reserve University, School of Medicine, Cleveland, OH 44106, USA

* Correspondence: mark.w.jackson@case.edu

† These authors contributed equally to this work.

Abstract: Driven by dysregulated IL-6 family member cytokine signaling in the tumor microenvironment (TME), aberrant signal transducer and activator of transcription (STAT3) and (STAT5) activation have been identified as key contributors to tumorigenesis. Following transformation, persistent STAT3 activation drives the emergence of mesenchymal/cancer-stem cell (CSC) properties, important determinants of metastatic potential and therapy failure. Moreover, STAT3 signaling within tumor-associated macrophages and neutrophils drives secretion of factors that facilitate metastasis and suppress immune cell function. Persistent STAT5 activation is responsible for cancer cell maintenance through suppression of apoptosis and tumor suppressor signaling. Furthermore, STAT5-mediated CD4+/CD25+ regulatory T cells (T_{regs}) have been implicated in suppression of immunosurveillance. We discuss these roles for STAT3 and STAT5, and weigh the attractiveness of different modes of targeting each cancer therapy. Moreover, we discuss how anti-tumorigenic STATs, including STAT1 and STAT2, may be leveraged to suppress the pro-tumorigenic functions of STAT3/STAT5 signaling.

Keywords: STAT3; STAT5; cancer progression; cancer-stem cell; cytokine; therapy resistance; metastasis; immunosuppression; tumor microenvironment; proliferation

1. Introduction

A complex milieu of both cellular and non-cellular components creates a heterogeneous tumor and microenvironment [1–8]. As a tumor becomes more heterogeneous, the risk of metastasis and therapy failure increases [9–12]. Cancer cells, pericytes, immune cells, fibroblasts, and endothelial cells are just some of the cellular components of the tumor [13,14]. A highly dysregulated network of cytokines and growth factors, emanating from cancer and stromal tumor microenvironment (TME) cells, contributes to the evolution of cancer cells, and often, suppression of immune cell function. Many of these cytokines and growth factors result in the phosphorylation and activation of signal transducers and activators of transcription (STAT) proteins, which can drive cell-specific changes in gene expression. STAT3 and STAT5 activity is often elevated in aggressive subtypes of cancer and serve as prognostic indicators [15–24]. Here, we discuss the impact of microenvironmental signals on STAT3/STAT5 activation during cancer development and progression. Elevated STAT3 activity promotes epithelial-mesenchymal transition (EMT) and a stem cell program in cancer cells, while also suppressing the function of immune cells within the tumor, all of which are important steps that underlie metastasis and therapy failure [25–30]. Likewise, persistent STAT5 activity induces (i) transformation, (ii) proliferation, and (iii) anti-apoptotic signals that contribute to hematological malignancies, while also suppressing anti-tumor immunity by expanding CD4+/CD25+ regulatory T cells (T_{regs}) [28,31–36]. We will discuss options for targeting STAT3/5 in cancer, either directly or indirectly through the inhibition of upstream kinases, receptors and/or ligands. In addition, we will discuss how STAT1/2 activity can counter the more aggressive phenotypes induced by STAT3/5. We propose that balancing STAT-activated cytokine signaling in the TME may serve as an effective therapeutic strategy.

2. Activating STAT3 and STAT5

The STAT family of transcription factors is comprised of seven different members, STAT1, -2, -3, -4, -5a, -5b, and -6. Hereafter, when discussing the overlapping functions of STAT5A and STAT5B, we will refer to them as "STAT5". STAT proteins transduce signals from the cell membrane to the nucleus, bypassing the need for second messengers [37–39]. STATs are phosphorylated by Janus Kinases (JAK1, 2, 3) or Tyrosine Kinase 2 (Tyk2), which are recruited to ligand-activated receptors, including cytokine, growth factor, or g-protein associated receptors. Most important of the STAT3/5 activators are the IL-6 family members, which include IL-6, IL-11, ciliary neurotrophic factor (CNTF), leukemia inhibitory factor (LIF), oncostatin-m (OSM), cardiotrophin 1 (CT-1), cardiotrophin-like cytokine (CLC), and IL-27. IL-6 family cytokines form a heterodimeric complex consisting of gp130 and a cytokine specific subunit (IL-6Rα, IL-11Rα, CNTFRα, gp130, LIFR, and OSMR), recruiting and activating the JAKs or Tyk2. Once phosphorylated, STATs dimerize and translocate to the nucleus, where they bind to short stretches of DNA and act as transcription factors to induce the expression of genes implicated in cell proliferation, survival, differentiation, motility, apoptosis, and metabolism (Figure 1) [37,40–43].

The crucial role STATs play in these normal physiological processes was first demonstrated in STAT-deficient mouse models. The generation of tissue-specific STAT3 knockout models have identified STAT3 as a key component in a wide variety of processes, including, but not limited to: T-cell proliferation, suppression of apoptosis, epidermal regeneration during wound healing, macrophage and neutrophil anti-inflammatory responses, and mammary gland involution [44–46]. Deletion of STAT5 in mice demonstrated high incidence of perinatal lethality, prevented the appropriate development of B-cells and T-cells, and inhibited the function of hematopoietic stem cells [47]. Under normal conditions, JAK/STAT activation is tightly regulated by protein inhibitors of activated STATs (PIAS), tyrosine phosphatases, and suppressors of cytokine signaling (SOCS) proteins that inhibit JAK catalytic activity [48,49]. In cancer however, STAT3 and STAT5 activity becomes dysregulated, resulting in elevated STAT3/5-driven responses in tumor, stromal, and immune cells.

Advances in sequencing technologies have allowed scientists to investigate the frequency of mutations in the JAK/STAT signaling pathway, resulting in the identification of mutations that constitutively activate STAT3, STAT5, and JAK2. The majority of STAT mutations occur in the SH2 and C-terminal domains of STAT3 and STAT5B and associate with leukemias and lymphomas [50,51]. STAT3 is the most frequently mutated member of the STAT family, with high incidence of mutation in T-cell large granular lymphocytic leukemias and NK lymphoproliferative disorders [52,53]. STAT5B mutations were similarly identified in these diseases, but with lower frequency. In addition, sequencing of STAT3 exons in diffuse large B-cell lymphoma patients identified a missense point mutation (M206K) in the coiled-coil domain that affected SH2 domain function and drove robust proliferation [54,55]. Furthermore, JAK2 V617F, a constitutively active JAK2 mutant, phosphorylates both STAT3 and STAT5 proteins and has high frequency in patients with hematopoietic stem cell diseases, such as myeloproliferative diseases, essential thrombocythemia, polycythemia vera (PV), and idiopathic myelofibrosis (IMF) [56]. In addition, JAK2 V617F mutations have transformation potential in in vivo bone marrow transplantation assays and induce persistent activation of STAT5 and a PV phenotype [57]. While persistent activation of both STAT3 and STAT5 has been implicated in the transformation process, the greater impact of dysregulated STAT3/5 appears to be their influence on the induction of aggressive cancer cell properties and immunosuppression. The impacts of both cell-intrinsic reprogramming and immune dysfunction are discussed below.

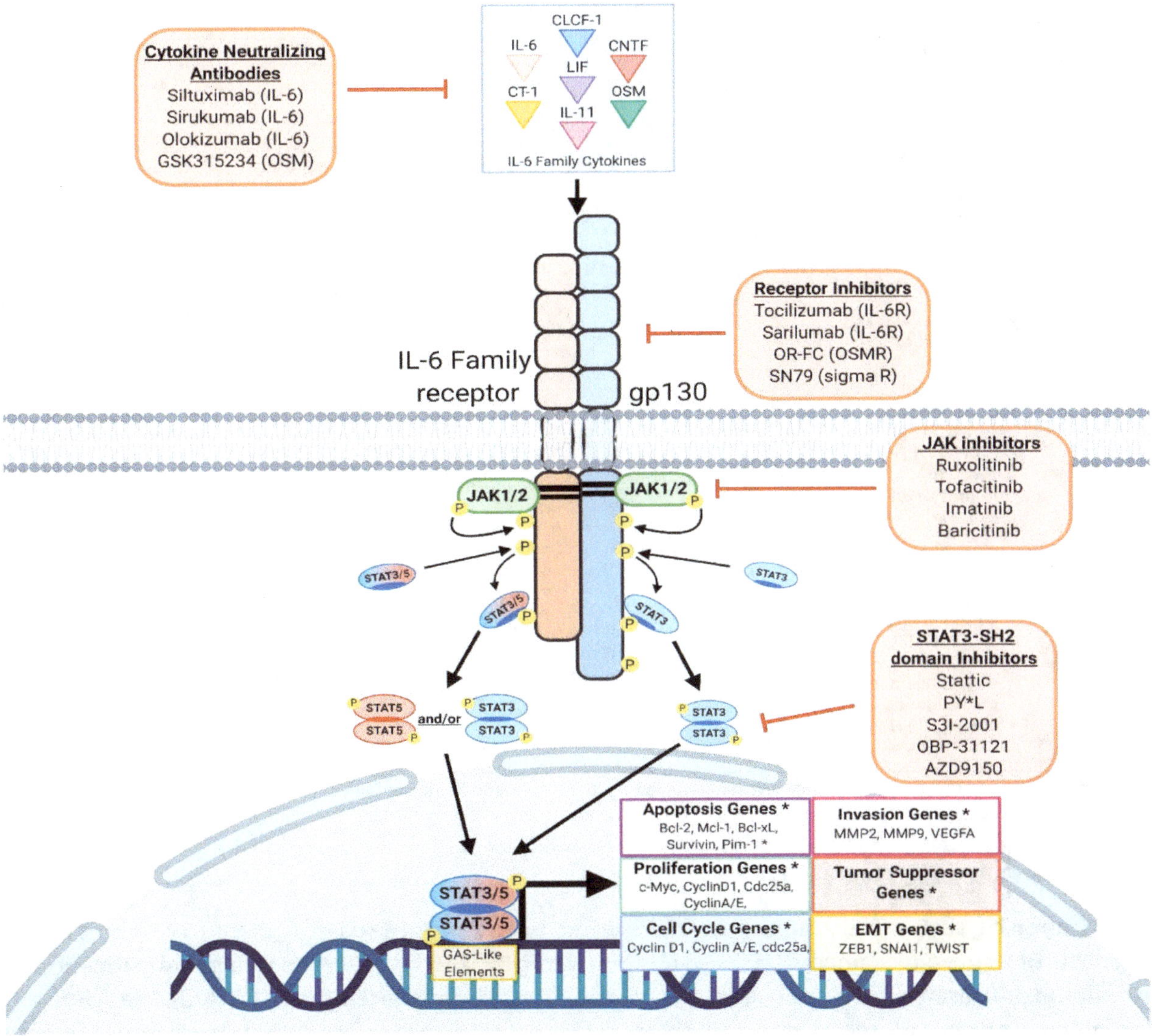

Figure 1. STAT3/5 Signaling Cascades and Therapy Targets. Schematic representation of canonical activation of signal transducer and activator of transcription-3 (STAT3) and STAT5 by IL-6 family member cytokines. IL-6 family cytokines drive receptor heterodimerization and subsequent Janus Kinase (JAK activation). JAKs phosphorylate tyrosine residues along the cytoplasmic domain of the receptor dimer, which recruits STAT proteins and facilitates their binding to interferon-gamma activation site-like (GAS-like) elements and regulation of large sets of genes. Asterisks (*) denote that additional info can be found in Table 1.

Table 1. Summary of the Roles of STAT3 and STAT5 in Cancer and Strategies for their Inhibition.

STAT-Family Protein	pYSTAT3/5-Activating Cytokines and Growth Factors	Normal Immune Function	Pro-Tumorigenic Genes Activated	Pro-Tumorigenic Effects	Therapies and Drugs in Development
STAT3	**Growth Factors:** EGFs, FGFs, HGFs, Leptin (REF), PDGFs **Lymphoid Cytokines:** IL-4, IL-13 **Myeloid Cytokines:** G-CSF, IL-10 **Ubiquitous Cytokines:** CNTF, LIF, IL-6, OSM	Development of Mature Neutrophils [58] Neutrophil Mobilization from Bone Marrow [59]	**Apoptosis:** BCL2, BCL-XL, MCL1, PIM1 **Cell Cycle:** Cyclin A, Cyclin D1, CDC25A **EMT:** ZEB1, SNAI1, TWIST, CDH2, Vimentin **Migration/Invasion:** MMP2, MMP9, VEGFA **Proliferation:** cMYC, NOTCH4 **Stem Cell:** SOX2, NANOG, OCT4 **Tumor Suppressor:** p53	Transformation Activation of Anti-Apoptotic Proteins EMT M2 Polarization N2 Polarization Enhanced Metastasis Therapy Resistance	Imatinib (JAK1/2) Ruxolitinib (JAK1/2) Tofacitinib (JAK1/2) *Siltuximab* (IL-6) *Tocilizumab* (IL-6R) *GSK315234* (OSM) *OS-FC* (OSMR) *PY*L* (SH2 Domain) *S3I-2001* (SH2 Domain) *SN79* (Sigma Receptor) IFNβ

Table 1. *Cont.*

STAT-Family Protein	pYSTAT3/5-Activating Cytokines and Growth Factors	Normal Immune Function	Pro-Tumorigenic Genes Activated	Pro-Tumorigenic Effects	Therapies and Drugs in Development
STAT3	**Growth Factors:** EGFs, FGFs, HGFs, Leptin (REF), PDGFs **Lymphoid Cytokines:** IL-4, IL-13 **Myeloid Cytokines:** G-CSF, IL-10 **Ubiquitous Cytokines:** CNTF, LIF, IL-6, OSM	Development of Mature Neutrophils [58] Neutrophil Mobilization from Bone Marrow [59]	**Apoptosis:** BCL2, BCL-XL, MCL1, PIM1 **Cell Cycle:** Cyclin A, Cyclin D1, CDC25A **EMT:** ZEB1, SNAI1, TWIST, CDH2, Vimentin **Migration/Invasion:** MMP2, MMP9, VEGFA **Proliferation:** cMYC, NOTCH4 **Stem Cell:** SOX2, NANOG, OCT4 **Tumor Suppressor:** p53	Transformation Activation of Anti-Apoptotic Proteins EMT M2 Polarization N2 Polarization Enhanced Metastasis Therapy Resistance	Imatinib (JAK1/2) Ruxolitinib (JAK1/2) Tofacitinib (JAK1/2) *Siltuximab* (IL-6) *Tocilizumab* (IL-6R) *GSK315234* (OSM) *OS-FC* (OSMR) *PY*L* (SH2 Domain) *S3I-2001* (SH2 Domain) *SN79* (Sigma Receptor) IFNβ
STAT5	**Growth Factors:** EGFs, FGFs, FLT3L, Leptin [60], PDGFs, Prolactin, SCF **Lymphoid Cytokines:** IL-2, IL-4, IL-7 [61], IL-9 [62], IL-13, IL-15, Thymic Stromal Lymphopoietin [63] **Myeloid Cytokines:** Erythropoietin [64], G-CSF, GM-CSF, IL-3, IL-5, IL-10, Thrombopoietin [65] **Ubiquitous Cytokines:** IL-21 [66], IL-31 [67], OSM	Differentiation, Survival, and Lineage Expansion of NK and NKT Cells Dendritic Cell Function [68] T Cell Differentiation and Expansion Effector Memory CD8+ T Cell-Mediated Cancer Cell Clearance [69] Myeloid Cell Differentiation and Survival [70]	**Apoptosis:** BCL-2, BCL-XL, MCL1, PIM1, Survivin **Cell Cycle:** Cyclin D1, Cyclin E **Immune Function:** PRDM1, BCL-6 **Migration/Invasion:** MMP2, MMP9, VEGFA **Proliferation:** AKT1, cMYC, PI3K **Tumor Suppressor:** p53	Transformation Activation of Anti-Apoptotic Proteins T_{reg} Population Expansion M2 Polarization [71] Megakaryopoeisis [72] Erythropoeisis [73]	Imatinib (JAK1/2) Ruxolitinib (JAK1/2) Tofacitinib (JAK1/2) *Siltuximab* (IL-6) *Tocilizumab* (IL-6R) *GSK315234* (OSM) *OS-FC* (OSMR) *AC-4-130* (SH2 Domain) [74] *BP-1-107* (SH2 Domain) [75] *BP-1-108* (SH2 Domain) [75] *Pomstafib-2* (SH2 Domain) [76] *SF-1-087* (SH2 Domain) [75] *SF-1-088* (SH2 Domain) [75] IFNβ

Therapies included in the far right column are listed by their respective name followed by their biological target in parentheses. Italicized font denotes therapies that are not currently approved by the FDA as cancer therapies.

3. IL-6 Family Cytokine Dysregulation in the TME

A number of IL-6 family members have long been recognized for their involvement in the pathogenesis of aggressive cancers [19,77–81]. For example, IL-6 levels serve as a prognostic biomarker and predictor of therapeutic response in pancreatic ductal adenocarcinoma (PDAC), bladder, gastric, lung adenocarcinoma, colorectal, cervical, liver, and breast cancers: all of which have a high incidence of metastasis and resistance [77,82–86]. This is due to the pro-tumor effects of IL-6 in tumor cells and stromal components. In tumor cells, IL-6 can drive EMT, therapy resistance, and invasive characteristics [87–89]. Concurrently, IL-6 can shift the anti-tumor immune responses towards immunosuppression via recruitment of myeloid-derived suppressor cells (MDSCs) and expansion of FoxP3+ T_{regs} [90–92]. Furthermore, IL-6 secretion by certain stromal components (cancer-associated fibroblasts, macrophages, and neutrophils) drives EMT in associated tumor populations, which is supported by immunohistochemical staining at the invasive edge of patient breast tumors, where levels of phosphorylated STAT3 and IL-6 is elevated [93,94].

Interestingly, IL-6 activation of STAT3 functions in a positive feed-forward loop to drive the secretion of new IL-6 into the TME, which then interacts with IL-6R/gp130 to further activate JAK/STAT signaling [93,95]. OSM also potently activates a feed-forward loop, resulting in the de novo production of additional OSM and OSMR by tumor and immune cells [96]. Interestingly, OSM was first identified to play a tumor suppressive role and inhibited the proliferation of melanoma cell models [97]. However, later studies correlated OSM-OSMR signaling with robust STAT3 and STAT5 activation and more aggressive tumor phenotypes [98–106]. Like IL-6, OSM feed-forward signaling is observed in aggressive cancers with limited-therapeutic options, including glioblastoma (GBM), non-small cell lung carcinoma (NSCLC), PDAC, and triple negative breast cancer (TNBC) [107–111]. Elevated signaling through the OSM/OSMR axis induces high levels of an 'inflammatory module', which includes IL-6, CCL2, IL-1, CXCL1, CXCL9, CXCL10, and CXCL11—all of which have been implicated in migration, invasion, therapy failure, and dedifferentiation to a cancer stem cell (CSC) program. Importantly, neutralization of OSM by treatment with an Fc-tagged soluble OSMR suppresses this inflammatory module suggesting that the OSM/OSMR feed-forward loop may be critical for the long-term maintenance of inflammatory signaling [112,113].

IL-11 similarly engages in an autocrine feed-forward mechanism to drive persistent JAK2/STAT3 activation, which can promote resistance to platinum-based therapies [114]. Furthermore, IL-11 and LIF both contribute to tumorigenesis by enhancing tumor cell survival through STAT3-mediated activation of anti-apoptotic proteins, Bcl-2 and Survivin, and the inhibition of tumor suppressor p53 [114–116]. IL-11 and LIF also contribute to cancer progression by driving EMT through STAT3 and Akt/mTOR signaling, thereby conferring an enhanced migratory capacity [81,117,118]. The impact of CT-1, CLC, CNTF, and IL-27 on cancer progression is currently understudied. While IL-6 family cytokines are important mediators of STAT3 activation, other cancer-associated receptors can also activate STAT3. STAT3-driven tumor progression can also be achieved by epidermal growth factor receptors (both wild-type EGFR and EGFRvIII), fibroblast growth factor receptors (FGFR), insulin-like growth factor receptor (IGFR), hepatocyte growth factor (HGFR, also known as MET), platelet-derived growth factor receptor (PDGFR), vascular endothelial growth factor receptor (VEGFR), v-src, and Bcr-Abl [119–127]. Interestingly, acetylation of STAT3 also induces tumor progression through enhanced pro-tumorigenic IL-17A secretion [128,129]. These examples demonstrate the abundance of mechanisms through which STAT3 can become activated.

4. STAT3 Activation of a Mesenchymal/CSC Program in Cancer Cells

The majority of cancers have constitutive activation of STAT3 [130–132]. STAT3 was first termed oncogenic when its persistent activation was discovered in v-src transformed mouse embryonic fibroblasts [133]. Subsequent studies demonstrated that expression of a constitutively active STAT3 isoform (STAT3-C) can drive transformation of pre-malignant human mammary epithelial cells (HMEC) and MCF-10A cells to malignant breast cancer [134]. In addition, Ras-induced transformation in bladder and breast carcinoma models exhibit mitochondrial accumulation of STAT3 and more robust cellular glycolysis, a characteristic of cancer cells [135]. In PDAC, STAT3 is required for both the development of pre-malignant pancreatic interepithelial neoplasias (PanINs), as well as the progression of PanINs to PDAC [136]. While STAT3 has been strongly implicated as a driver of oncogenesis, evidence suggests that persistent cytokine activation of STAT3 in pre-malignant lesions, engages a tumor suppressive senescence response. In non-transformed HMEC models, OSM engages senescence through a direct STAT3 interaction with mothers against decapentaplegic-3 (SMAD3). However, downstream constitutive expression of c-Myc could overcome OSM-induced senescence and drive EMT and invasion [137]. Beyond the genetic events that occur as a normal cell becomes transformed, cancer progression relies heavily on an evolving microenvironment, which impacts both the cancer cells and the immune system, ultimately influencing patient outcomes. In cancer cells, increased STAT3 activity induces EMT-driving transcription factors, such as ZEB1, SNAIL, and Twist, which initiate the repression of epithelial markers and expression of mesenchymal markers (N-cadherin, Vimentin) [138–141]. In addition, STAT3 induces the expression of matrix metalloproteinases (MMP), which can also contribute to the loss of cell-cell contacts [142–144].

While EMT is important in normal physiology to allow cells to migrate during development and wound healing, inappropriate EMT and the loss of cell-cell interactions contributes to aggressive cancer cell behaviors, including metastasis and resistance to therapy. In TNBC, the loss of E-cadherin or gain of Vimentin, N-Cadherin, or Snail expression, typically at the tumor's edge, correlates with poor clinical outcome [145–149]. Likewise, the presence and abundance of circulating tumor cells (CTC) that express mesenchymal markers have been referred to as the "silent predictors of metastasis" because they correlate with tumor cell dissemination [150]. Moreover, mesenchymal CTC can be used to track a patient's response to therapy, with increasing numbers correlating with increased risk of relapse [151–155].

Likewise, the emergence of CSC properties, which are often defined experimentally as using tumorsphere- or tumor-initiating assays, frequently occur concomitantly with a mesenchymal phenotype [156–163]. STAT3 has been identified as an essential driver of the de novo reprogramming to a CSC state through activation of Sox2, Nanog, and Oct4 [164–170]. Further evidence linking EMT and a CSC phenotype is provided by the observation that a subset of CTC, responsible for initiating metastasis termed the metastasis-initiating cells, express high levels of the STAT3-driven CSC marker CD44 [151–153,171–174]

The importance of mesenchymal/CSC reprogramming in metastasis and therapy failure continues to emerge. For example, single-cell analysis identified a predominantly mesenchymal/CSC program in early-stage TNBC micro-metastases, in contrast to late-stage metastases [154]. The findings are consistent with the idea that mesenchymal/CSC initiate metastatic outgrowth at a secondary site, followed by differentiation. Single cell RNA sequencing (scRNA-seq) confirmed that EMT in primary tumors proceeds through distinct, hybrid states, ranging from completely epithelial to completely mesenchymal [155]. The epithelial-mesenchymal hybrids, which harbor the greatest level of phenotypic plasticity, are more efficient at intravasating, surviving in circulation, extravasating to the lungs, and forming metastases [175]. Acute exposure to Adriamycin or Taxanes drives the adaptive emergence of therapy-resistant, $CD44^{HIGH}$ CSC in both breast tumor explants and breast cancer cell lines [176]. scRNA-seq determined that chemo-resistant cells activate an EMT program, which was not evident before treatment [177]. In mouse models, the ability to undergo EMT is important for therapeutic resistance [178,179]. These findings suggest that potent mesenchymal/CSC programming has significant consequences that allow cancer cells to adapt to chemotherapy and survive, ultimately contributing to therapy failure.

Indeed, STAT3 has also been implicated in acquired therapy resistance in many cancers including NSCLC, GBM, PDAC, melanoma, and breast cancer [107,180–185]. Elevated STAT3 phosphorylation in ovarian cancer is associated with paclitaxel resistance and increased tumor cell invasion post-therapy, consistent with the elevated expression of mesenchymal/CSC genes and increased tumor initiating potential [176,186,187]. In Trastuzumab-resistant HER2+ breast cancer, STAT3 feed-forward loops generate a TME rich with STAT3-activating cytokines that promote and maintain the mesenchymal/CSC phenotypes. Inhibition of the STAT3 feed-forward activation diminished tumor growth and metastasis and resensitized cells to therapy [188]. In cancer cells driven by diverse receptor tyrosine kinases (RTKs) (EGFR, HER2, ALK, and MET), MEK inhibitors drive feedback activation of STAT3 through FGFR and JAKs, resulting in therapy failure [189]. Likewise, in NSCLC cells resistant to molecularly-targeted therapies (EGFR-TKI, ALK inhibitor Crizotinib, and MEK inhibitor Selumetinib), OSM/JAK1/STAT3–signaling protects cells from targeted drug-induced apoptosis [190]. JAK/STAT3 signaling also interacts with numerous other growth, proliferative, and survival pathways, such as PI3K/Akt, MAPK, NF-kB, Notch, Wnt/β-Catenin, and TGF-β, among others [191–196]. Tamoxifen-resistant breast cancers have elevated STAT3 and Notch4 expression associated with metastasis and tumorigenicity. Interestingly, inhibition of Notch4 was able to reduce the phosphorylation of STAT3 and suppress metastasis, suggesting STAT3 and Notch4 cooperate to promote therapy resistance [197]. In addition, a STAT3/NF-kB complex promotes cisplatin resistance in malignant mesothelioma, and targeted inhibition of this complex inhibits the growth of refractory tumors [198]. Such evidence suggests STAT3 may not be solely responsible for therapy failure. Instead, STAT3-mediated cross-talk with additional signaling effectors may coordinate resistance [140,199–201]. Nonetheless, the common theme appears to be a STAT3-activated, mesenchymal/CSC program.

5. A STAT3-Generated Pro-Metastatic Immune Microenvironment

An important and rapidly emerging area of research is the impact of the immune microenvironment on metastasis and therapy failure. Beyond its impact on tumor cells, STAT3 has an important role in restricting immune cell functions and producing immunosuppressive factors. STAT3-induced cytokines are important mediators of the crosstalk between tumor cells, tumor-associated macrophages (TAMs), and tumor-associated neutrophils (TANs), which are responsible for generating a pro-metastatic and pro-angiogenic TME [202]. In the TME, macrophages and neutrophils are exposed to a host of STAT3-induced cytokines, such as IL-4, IL-6, IL-10, IL-13, VEGFA, and TGF-β that drive their polarization to a pro-tumorigenic M2 (macrophages) or N2 (neutrophils) state [203,204]. Conversely, robust STAT3 signaling activity in M2-TAMs and N2-TANs correlates with the production of factors able to drive cancer cell EMT (OSM, IL-6, TGF-β) and angiogenesis (VEGF, TGF-β, PDGF, and FGF) [205–208].

Importantly, because of their localization at the invasive edge of tumors, the contribution of M2-TAMs and N2-TANs to metastasis is increasingly being recognized. For example, TAMs have been demonstrated to form simultaneous physical contacts with tumor cells and endothelial cells that result in the formation of invadopodia, which assist cancer cells in transendothelial migration and escape into the circulatory system. These sites of cancer cell intravasation are called "tumor microenvironment of metastasis (TMEM)" and have been validated as prognostic markers of metastasis. Chemotherapy increases TMEM in breast cancer patients, thereby potentially facilitating metastasis [209,210]. STAT3 inhibition in TAM populations re-sensitizes breast cancer cells to paclitaxel, further suggesting tumor and TAM crosstalk is an essential component in STAT3-driven therapy resistance [205,211]. TANs, on the other hand, were found to function as circulatory escorts of CTC and promote their proliferation, survival, and seeding of secondary sites [212–214]. Importantly, OSM and IL-6 were two of the 4 most frequent cytokines secreted by neutrophils found clustered with CTC. These cytokines interact with OSMR and IL-6R, which are expressed on cancer cells [212]. The neutrophil/CTC cross-talk promotes the cell cycle progression in CTC, thereby expanding their metastatic potential.

Following the classical events of the metastatic cascade, after a tumor cell intravasates into circulation, it extravasates to establish secondary sites. An emerging concept in the metastatic cascade is the role of myeloid cells- such as basophils, neutrophils, eosinophils, monocytes, and macrophages- in the establishment of a pre-metastatic niche [215]. Although the exact TME components required for colonization of secondary sites remain a mystery, the activation of a STAT3-sphingosine 1-phosphate receptor-1 (S1PR1) axis in tumor cells, and secretion of IL-6 and IL-10, was observed to persistently activate STAT3 at distant, pre-metastatic sites. At these pre-metastatic sites, persistent STAT3 phosphorylation was associated with myeloid cell migration from the primary tumor to the secondary site. Subsequent targeting of STAT3 in myeloid cells disrupted metastatic tumor outgrowth, suggesting STAT3 plays an integral role in priming distant metastatic sites for tumor cell outgrowth [216].

6. STAT5 in Cancer Cells

As previously mentioned, cells produce two different STAT5 proteins, STAT5A and STAT5B, which share greater than 90% sequence homology [217]. However, evidence suggests STAT5A and STAT5B play different functional roles in normal and cancer cell systems. Genetic deletion of STAT5 in pure mouse backgrounds are embryonic lethal, due to the essential roles of STAT5 in erythropoiesis and iron metabolism [218–220]. While the distinct roles of STAT5A and STAT5B remain understudied, data from mammary gland-specific knockouts suggest that STAT5A is required for lactogenesis in the mammary gland, while STAT5B is imperative for mammary gland differentiation and development [221]. The function of STAT5A and STAT5B appear to be cell-specific. They can have either synergistic or opposing effects, such as in memory B-cell differentiation, which may be due to (i) the formation of STAT5A/STAT5B homo- or hetero-dimers, and/or (ii) differences in nuclear shuttling mechanisms [222–224]. Furthermore, genetic tuning models depleting STAT5A and/or STAT5B have demonstrated a critical role for STAT5 in the accumulation and development of innate lymphoid cells, such as NK cells [225–227].

Given its role in lymphoid cell development and differentiation, it is not surprising that STAT5 activity contributes to hematologic malignancies. Deletion of STAT5 prevents transformation by the Abl oncogene, thereby preventing leukemia development [228]. Genetic and pharmacologic inhibition of STAT5 activity decreases expression of apoptosis inhibitors MCL1 and BCL2 and inhibits leukemogenesis of BCR-ABL1+ acute lymphoblastic leukemia (ALL), both in cell lines and newly diagnosed and relapsed/TKI-resistant ALL patients [229]. Likewise, a new, STAT5 inhibitor suppressed the proliferation of human acute myeloid leukemia (AML) cell lines and primary FLT3-ITD+ AML patient cells [74]. Combined inhibition of STAT3 and STAT5 by shRNAs also suppressed growth in chronic myeloid leukemia, suggesting that combinatorial suppression of STAT3 and STAT5 may be efficacious in treating hematological malignancies [230].

STAT5 activation has also been implicated in the progression of solid tumor malignancies. Deletion of STAT5 in the mammary gland, hepatocytes, and prostate cells delays the development of mammary, liver, and prostate cancer [32,231,232]. Like STAT3, experimental evidence implicates STAT5B as a driver of tumorigenesis, as it can drive EMT and increased invasiveness in hepatocellular carcinoma (HCC) [233]. Moreover, in mammary epithelial cells, thymocytes, and epithelial prostate cancer cells, persistent activation of STAT5 is sufficient to drive transformation [234–236]. Furthermore, the function of STAT5 in solid tumors extends beyond oncogenesis as evidence has emerged that STAT5 signaling can induce a metastatic cascade. For example, STAT5 inhibition in colorectal cancer induces G1 cell cycle arrest and reduces cancer cell migration, demonstrating the role of STAT5 in proliferation and metastasis [237]. Additional studies demonstrate that STAT5A/B signaling in prostate cancer and squamous cell carcinoma of the head and neck drive EMT programming, which results in enhanced cell migration, invasion, and formation of metastases [238,239].

An increasing number of reports demonstrate that STAT5 drives tumorigenesis and cancer progression through cooperation with other intracellular signaling cascades and activation of additional feed-forward loops. STAT5 activates transcription of AKT1 and PI3K, and, in turn, Akt1 phosphorylates STAT5 to induce cell survival [240,241]. Furthermore, STAT5-dependent Akt restores cyclin D expression, which promotes proliferation [241]. Once cells aberrantly proliferate, apoptosis suppressors Bcl-xL and Bcl-2 are activated via persistent STAT5 signaling, driving tumor cell survival [16,234,242–244]. BCL-XL expression is also enhanced via formation of a transcription factor complex comprised of phosphorylated STAT5 and nuclear EGFRvIII. This transcription factor complex binds to the BCL-XL promoter to induce its transcription and promote anti-apoptotic signaling [245]. Similar to STAT3, STAT5 translocates to tumor cell mitochondria, suggesting an interaction with the mitochondrial genome to promote aerobic glycolysis (the Warburg Effect), a defining characteristic of cancer cells [246]. Collectively, this data demonstrates that STAT5 mediates crosstalk between cancer cell survival, and proliferation, and metabolism signaling pathways.

Surprisingly, STAT5 in certain model systems has been demonstrated to function in a tumor suppressive manner. Human breast cancers infrequently (~7%) show signs of STAT5 activation (compared to 40% of STAT3 activation). This elevated STAT5 activity trends with more differentiated and lower grade tumors, suggesting that STAT5 does not induce the aggressive cancer cell program initiated by STAT3, at least in breast cancer [247]. STAT5 expression in these models stabilizes E-cadherin surface marker expression and reverses the undifferentiated mesenchymal phenotype [248]. In normal human fibroblasts, aberrant activation of STAT5A induces a senescence response concurrent with accumulation of p53 and DNA damaged foci. Furthermore, knockdown DNA-repair kinase, ATM, and tumor suppressor, retinoblastoma protein did not eliminate damaged foci, providing evidence for the persistence of DNA damage in pre-malignant lesions [249]. Interestingly in HCC models, liver specific STAT5 knockout results in tumor formation through the enhanced activation of TGFβ/STAT3 signaling [20]. Physiologically, STAT proteins have been identified as drivers of erythropoiesis. STAT5A/B double knockout mice in a mixed genetic background (Sv129 x C57Bl/6) results in mild hematopoietic phenotypes, due to compensatory activation and enhanced DNA-binding of STAT1/3 [218].

7. STAT5 in T_{reg}-Associated Immunosuppression

In addition to its impact on cancer cells, activated STAT5 dampens anti-tumor immune function. This immunosuppressive function is largely driven by CD4+/CD25+ T_{regs}, a subset of T cells that contribute to tumor progression and metastasis [250] and correlates with poor patient prognosis [251,252]. Sustained STAT5 phosphorylation in progenitor T cells induces the differentiation to a T_{reg} population that, in turn, significantly diminishes the function of cytotoxic and helper T cells [253–255]. Experimental depletion of T_{regs} from the TME results in enhanced infiltration of mature CD4+ and CD8+ T cells into the tumor, leading to tumor rejection [256,257]. Furthermore, STAT5-mediated T_{reg} expansion increases IL-10, IL-4, and IL-13, which skew TAMs to an M2 immunosuppressive phenotype. M2 macrophages are immunosuppressive because they release elevated levels of IL-10 and transforming growth factor-β (TGF-β) and restrict secretion of immune stimulatory cytokines via NF-kB repression [258,259]. STAT5-induced T_{regs} and M2 macrophage populations secrete VEGF-A, which, along with TGF-β, promotes angiogenesis [255,260,261].

Tumor clearance mechanisms are also suppressed by T_{reg} expansion through impediment of B cell development and maturation [262]. STAT5-activated T_{regs} result in a decrease in follicular helper T (T_{fh}) cell populations via Blimp-1, which severely hampers germinal center formation in lymph nodes [263]. This reduction in germinal centers diminishes the number of B cells that can be recruited and primed to aid in an anti-tumor immune response. Interestingly, the differentiation and self-renewal of memory B cells are respectively influenced by STAT5A-mediated repression and STAT5B-mediated induction of BCL-6. Immunosuppression driven by the expansion of T_{regs}, relies on STAT5-mediated alteration in T-cell metabolism. Mature effector T cells preferentially undergo glycolysis and require a de novo fatty acid synthesis reliant on acetyl-coA carboxylase 1 whereas T_{regs} undergo lipid-oxidation and readily synthesize fatty acids because of a structural reconfiguration of mitochondrial cristae [264–266]. Accumulation of intracellular lipids impairs autophagy, providing a mechanism for T_{reg}-mediated immunosuppression [267,268]. Just as STAT5 function in the mitochondria impacts tumor cell functions, as described earlier, mitochondrial STAT5 activation drives metabolic shifts in the immune compartment, inducing an expansion of T_{regs}.

However, while the suppression of T_{regs} increases tumor immunity, provided STAT5 remains functional, the overall impact of suppressing STAT5 signaling in the remaining immune cells of the TME remains open to debate. Mouse models deficient in STAT5 have depleted CD8+ T cell, NK cell, and T_{reg} populations, suggesting STAT5 plays an integral role in the proper development of multiple immune cell types [269]. STAT5 signaling contributes to the differentiation of naive CD4+ T cells into CD8+ T cells, T_h1, T_h2, T_h9, T_hGM, and T_{regs}, while inhibition of STAT5 is required for the generation of T_h17 and T_{fh} cells [270,271]. Importantly, STAT5 is heavily involved in the development, survival, and lytic function of NK cells. Knock-out or suppression of STAT5 in NK populations sparked the secretion of VEGF-A, a growth factor that supports tumor-associated angiogenesis in melanoma and leukemia models [269,272]. Taken together, these findings suggest that targeting STAT5 may threaten the integrity of anti-tumor immune functions and drive worse outcome in patients [269,272].

8. Targeting STAT Activity

Given the roles of STAT3 and STAT5 in tumor progression and immunosuppression discussed above (Figure 2), multiple methods of inhibiting their activity are being pursued. Successful inhibition of STAT3 would prevent the acquisition of, and potentially revert, a mesenchymal/CSC program, making cancer cells less invasive and more sensitive to therapy. Moreover, STAT3 inhibition would help activate anti-tumor immunity by reducing immunosuppressive factors and increasing the infiltration of immune cells into the TME. Likewise, suppressing STAT5 in cancer cells, particularly leukemia, halts proliferation and induces apoptosis, suggesting that STAT5 may be a valuable therapeutic target [74]. However, due to STAT5's controversial roles in tumor progression and immune cell maturation and differentiation, further studies are required to elucidate the effects of targeting STAT5 in cancer patients. [273]. Generally speaking, the majority of small molecule inhibitors are designed to have high affinity for the catalytic domain of an enzyme; the ATP binding site for example, which STAT proteins lack. Therefore, direct inhibition of STAT3 relies on disruption of binding motifs necessary for downstream signal transduction. A series of STAT3 phospho-ester SH-2 domain inhibitors have been developed, with the intent to inhibit dimerization of activated STAT3 (PY*L, S3I-2001, OPB-31121, etc.). While these approaches are promising, the compounds continue to be refined [274–277]. An alternative approach would involve targeting the upstream activator of STAT3, which could include neutralizing antibodies for specific IL-6 family cytokines, competitive antibodies hindering cytokine-receptor interactions, and JAK inhibitors.

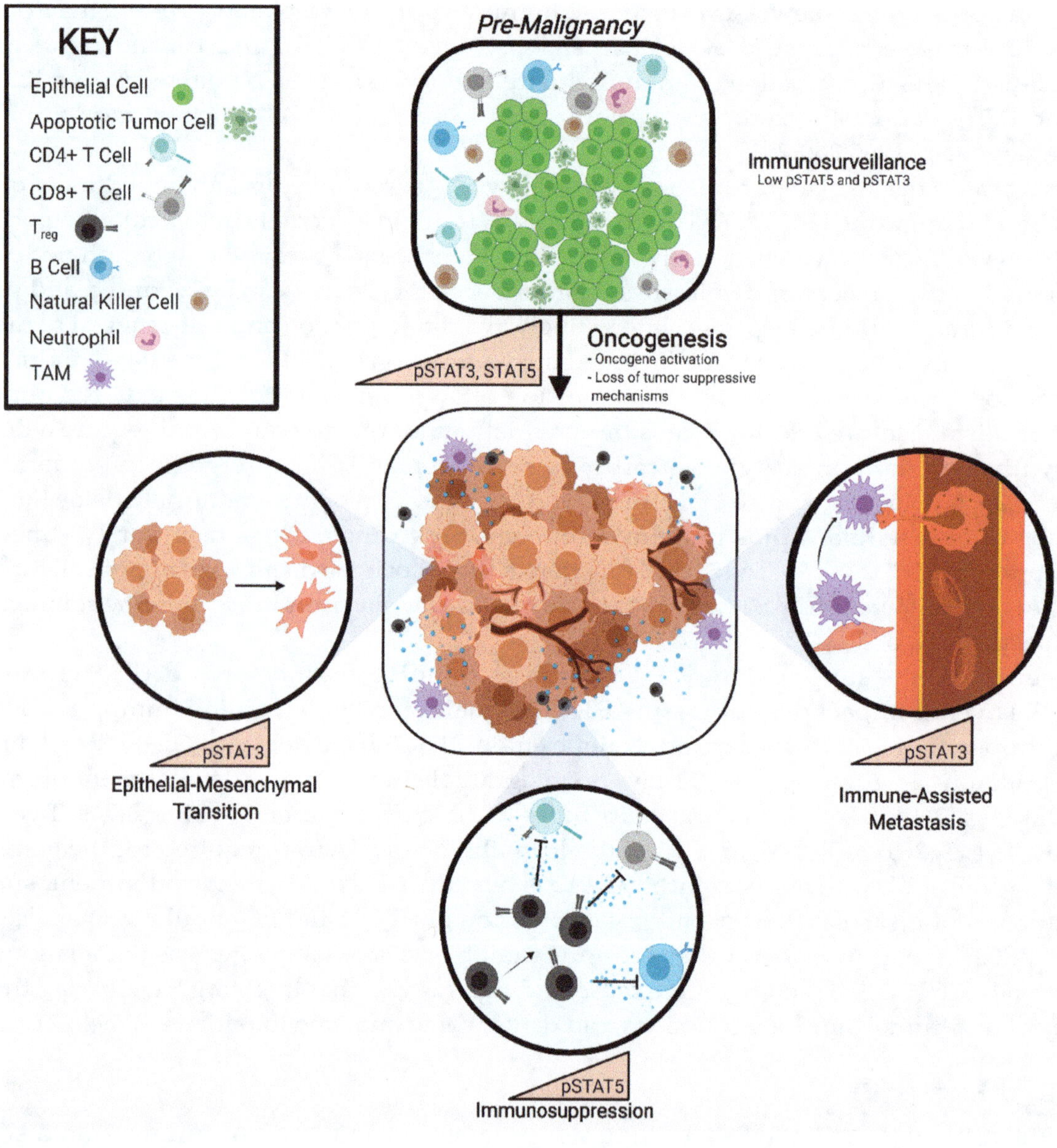

Figure 2. Biological Impact of STAT3 and STAT5 Activation. Pre-malignant cell populations, in which apoptotic signaling and immunosurveillance are functional, exhibit low levels of phosphorylated STAT3 (pSTAT3) and STAT5 (pSTAT5). Elevated activity of pSTAT3 and/or pSTAT5 accompanies tumorigenesis, leading to the inhibition of apoptotic pathways and repression of immune cell recognition of a burgeoning tumor. pSTAT3 is utilized by malignant cell populations to drive epithelial-mesenchymal transition (EMT) and by tumor-associated macrophages (TAMs) and tumor-associated neutrophils (TANs) to drive metastasis. pSTAT5 activity in progenitor T-cells drives expansion of a Treg population that then secretes factors that inhibit the function of CD4+ and CD8+ T-cells as well as B-cells.

One of the first IL-6 monoclonal antibodies generated was Tocilizumab, which inhibits IL-6 signaling by preventing IL-6 binding to both the soluble and transmembrane forms of IL-6R [278,279]. Pre-clinical studies demonstrated strong anti-tumor cell activity in multiple myeloma and therapeutic efficacy in Castelman's disease, rheumatoid arthritis, and cytokine release syndrome, however, Tocilizumab is not currently FDA-approved for cancer treatments [280–283]. Clinical trials using Tocilizumab in combination with other monoclonal antibodies, chemotherapies, and immunotherapies to treat cancers such as HER2+ breast cancer, B-cell Non-Hodgkin Lymphoma, metastatic NSCLC, and recurrent metastatic colorectal adenocarcinoma are ongoing [284]. In addition to Tocilizumab, Siltuximab is an IL-6 specific neutralizing antibody that has emerged as another promising therapy. Pre-clinical studies support Siltuximab use in KRAS-mutant lung cancer, particularly in tumors with elevated stromal production of IL-6 [285]. Similar to Tocilizumab, Siltuximab is undergoing clinical trials for patients with malignant solid tumors in cancers with elevated stromal presence, such as ovarian, pancreatic, colorectal, head and neck, and lung neoplasms [286]. Furthermore, phase II studies of combination therapy with Siltuximab have demonstrated anti-tumor effects for patients diagnosed with metastatic prostate cancer, suggesting clinical efficacy of targeting the IL-6-STAT signaling axis with combination therapies [287].

Our lab has focused on OSM, given its potent activity at inducing numerous inflammatory cytokines that promote mesenchymal/CSC reprogramming in cancer cells and generate a pro-tumor immune microenvironment [106,288–290]. Neither OSM nor OSMR protein are abundantly expressed in normal tissues in the absence of inflammation, in contrast to JAK1, JAK2, and STAT3 (key OSM effectors) [109]. This finding is supported by the observation that knocking out OSM or OSMR from mice results in only mild phenotypes [291]. Moreover, OSMR has characteristics unique from other IL-6 family co-receptors, resulting in distinct signaling and biological effects [43,292,293]. For example, OSMR strongly recruits SHC, resulting in the hyper-activation of the MAPK signaling cascade [293]. Other gp130 co-receptors fail to do this, and rely solely on the gp130-mediated SHP-2 recruitment for MAPK activation, which is less robust than the gp130/OSMR heterodimer [43]. Therefore, suppressing the OSM signaling axis may have benefits in aggressive subtypes of cancer. Anti-OSM antibody (GSK315234) and OSMR-fusion protein (OR-FC) were first examined in pre-clinical studies in chronic inflammatory disease models, such as rheumatoid arthritis and inflammatory heart disease [294,295]. Antibodies suppressing OSM signaling ameliorate these pathological conditions, suggesting that OSM is a driver of these chronic hyper-inflamed states. More recently, OSM signaling was identified as a driver of inflammatory bowel disease (IBD), especially in patients who fail to respond to anti-tumor necrosis factor-α (TNF-α) antibodies. Neutralization of OSM in IBD models suppresses a cadre of inflammatory cytokines and reduces colitis severity, further supporting the OSM feed-forward loop as a critical mediator in the long-term maintenance of inflammatory signaling, a state common in the TME [112].

Another recent study investigating the effects of an anti-OSM antibody in a murine model of lupus nephritis demonstrated that OSM-driven EMT and extracellular matrix secretion, leading to renal fibrosis, could be suppressed, concomitant with the suppression of JAK/STAT3 activation [296]. More recently, a clinical grade OSM neutralizing antibody was used to treat pre-clinical models of squamous cell carcinoma. Again, OSM neutralizing antibodies suppressed the STAT3 feed forward signaling, resulting in reduced invasion and metastasis [96,297]. Disrupting cell surface receptor activation of STAT3 by inhibiting OSMR signaling was recently described in a study of an OSMR/gp130 antagonist (SN79), which prevents STAT3 phosphorylation in astrogliosis [298]. While these studies demonstrate the potential of OSM and OSMR inhibition as a therapeutic strategy, a number of ligand/receptors activate STAT3 and STAT5, as described above. Therefore, additional studies will be needed to define whether single ligand-receptor inhibitors can sufficiently impact STAT3 activation, thus suppressing tumor growth.

Currently, JAK inhibitors are the most promising inhibitors of STAT-driven phenotypes. Commonly used JAK 1/2 inhibitor, Ruxolitinib, has been shown to robustly block both STAT3 and STAT5 activation.

Yet, while JAK inhibitors can reduce STAT3 activation, there is conflicting data on the impact of JAK inhibitors. Some studies find that JAK inhibition suppresses tumor growth [93], while other studies find that they ultimately enhance metastasis, likely because they also suppress the positive influence of JAK activity on other STAT proteins (including STAT5 and STAT1/2, as discussed below) [299]. In addition, side effects of JAK inhibitors may be more pronounced, as JAKs activate other pathways, such as MAPK and PI3K in normal cells as well as cancer [43].

9. Balancing Opposing STAT-Activated Cytokine Signaling as a Therapeutic Strategy

Though STAT proteins are grouped together based on their structural similarities and common functions as transcription factors, individual STAT proteins can have diverse functions. We have focused extensively on STAT3 and STAT5 and their described roles in cancer progression, however this is not the universal effect among all STATs. For example, Interferon-β (IFNβ) induces the phosphorylation and activation of STAT1/2, which form a complex with IRF9 to create the transcription factor complex ISGF3. IFNβ/P-ISGF3 signaling induces interferon-stimulated genes (ISG), mesenchymal-epithelial transition (MET), and the differentiation of CSC into a less aggressive epithelial, non-CSC state with reduced migratory potential and reduced tumorsphere forming capabilities [111,300,301]. Importantly, the IFNβ and OSM/STAT3 signaling pathways strongly oppose one another. OSM represses transcription of IFNβ, thereby eliminating autocrine and paracrine IFNβ-mediated activation of P-ISGF3 and repressing ISG expression in both cancer cells and immune cells [301].

In addition to the impact of IFNβ on cancer cells, increasing rationale supports developing methods for the delivery of P-ISGF3 activators (or Type I IFN-agonists more generally) directly to the TME. First, favorable responses to frontline chemotherapy correlate with robust IFN signaling in both mouse and human studies [111,302–304]. Elevated IFN signaling in the tumor correlates with immunologically "hot" tumors harboring elevated numbers of tumor infiltrating lymphocytes (TILs), activated immune surveillance, increased tumor antigen cross presentation, and diminished numbers of immunosuppressive cells including MDSCs and T_{regs} [111,302,305–307]. Second, loss of Type I IFN signaling correlates with metastasis and decreased survival. Restoration of Type I IFN signaling significantly decreases metastasis and improves survival outcome [303,304]. Third, in contrast to STAT3 activators (which promote a pro-tumorigenic M2 state), addition of type I IFN inhibits macrophage polarization to an M2 state [308,309]. Type I IFNs also induce the differentiation of neutrophils into anti-tumor N1s [310]. Fourth, administration of IFNβ prior to surgical resection significantly improves response rates to immunotherapies such as anti-PD1/anti-PDL-1 [311]. Therefore, we propose balancing pro-tumor STAT3 activation with anti-tumor STAT1/STAT2 activation as a novel therapeutic approach. This STAT3/STAT1 balancing would (i) reprogram mesenchymal/CSC to a non-CSC state, making them more susceptible to chemotherapy and (ii) enhance anti-tumor immunity, thereby facilitating immune cell-mediated tumor cell killing. Yet, while IFN treatment is currently approved to treat hematological malignancies and some solid tumors (melanoma), the high doses of IFNs needed to inhibit cancer cell proliferation or induce cell death result in side-effects that limit its effectiveness [311–313]. We suggest tumor targeting antibodies (or nanobodies) linked to IFNβ. Generation of an oncogenic cytokine or receptor antibody conjugated to an IFNβ first demonstrated success in limiting resistance to EGFR inhibitors in breast cancer [314]. The designed therapy sought to re-activate innate and adaptive immune components, while simultaneously targeting the oncogenic receptor EGFR [303]. IFNβ-conjugated antibodies show immense promise. They would limit toxicity by using tumor-associated receptors to target IFNs to the TME and suppress STAT3 activation, while simultaneously, activating STAT1/2 in both tumor cells and immune cells [315].

10. Conclusions

As discussed throughout this review, STAT3 and STAT5 have emerged as essential components involved in regulating tumor progression. Cytokines and cytokine receptors of the IL-6 family are some of the most widely recognized STAT activators and are abundantly expressed on cancer cells as well as tumor-infiltrating immune cells. The role of STAT3 in promoting molecular programs in cancer cells that induce tumor metastasis and therapy resistance mechanisms continue to emerge, as does the impact of STAT3 as a suppressor of immune cell function in the TME. These findings suggest that specifically suppressing STAT3 activation would be beneficial to patients. Targeting STAT5 in hematological malignancies is gaining traction, and the clinical successes of JAK and tyrosine kinase inhibitors in disrupting STAT3 and STAT5 activation, provide strong support for the development of direct STAT3 and STAT5 inhibitors, summarized in Table 1. Specific suppression of STAT5 in immune-suppressive T_{regs} could also prove beneficial, but STAT5 is essential for many other immune cells as well. Thus, systemic suppression of STAT5 activity could undermine tumor immunity and promote tumor progression, as recently reported for STAT5 knock-out from NK cells [272]. However, reducing the aberrant activation of STAT5 without complete ablation may have therapeutic efficacy upon combination with other vulnerabilities. We conclude that targeting STAT3, either directly by disrupting STAT3-homodimer formation or indirectly by suppressing the activation of receptors responsible for persistent STAT3 phosphorylation, would reverse the cellular programs driving metastasis and therapy failure. Furthermore, by activating STAT1/2 within TME cells, the programs that prevent metastasis and enhance therapeutic efficacy could be re-engaged. This STAT balancing would improve outcomes for patients, particularly those with aggressive cancers that may currently have limited therapeutic options.

Acknowledgments: Both Figures 1 and 2 were created with BioRender.

References

1. Lin, E.Y.; Nguyen, A.V.; Russell, R.G.; Pollard, J.W. Colony-stimulating factor 1 promotes progression of mammary tumors to malignancy. *J. Exp. Med.* **2001**, *193*, 727–740. [CrossRef]
2. Vaupel, P. Tumor microenvironmental physiology and its implications for radiation oncology. *Semin. Radiat. Oncol.* **2004**, *14*, 198–206. [CrossRef]
3. Jimenez-Sanchez, A.; Memon, D.; Pourpe, S.; Veeraraghavan, H.; Li, Y.; Vargas, H.A.; Gill, M.B.; Park, K.J.; Zivanovic, O.; Konner, J.; et al. Heterogeneous Tumor-Immune Microenvironments among Differentially Growing Metastases in an Ovarian Cancer Patient. *Cell* **2017**, *170*, 927–938.e920. [CrossRef]
4. Johnson, B.E.; Mazor, T.; Hong, C.; Barnes, M.; Aihara, K.; McLean, C.Y.; Fouse, S.D.; Yamamoto, S.; Ueda, H.; Tatsuno, K.; et al. Mutational analysis reveals the origin and therapy-driven evolution of recurrent glioma. *Science* **2014**, *343*, 189–193. [CrossRef]
5. De Bruin, E.C.; McGranahan, N.; Mitter, R.; Salm, M.; Wedge, D.C.; Yates, L.; Jamal-Hanjani, M.; Shafi, S.; Murugaesu, N.; Rowan, A.J.; et al. Spatial and temporal diversity in genomic instability processes defines lung cancer evolution. *Science* **2014**, *346*, 251–256. [CrossRef]
6. McGranahan, N.; Favero, F.; de Bruin, E.C.; Birkbak, N.J.; Szallasi, Z.; Swanton, C. Clonal status of actionable driver events and the timing of mutational processes in cancer evolution. *Sci. Transl. Med.* **2015**, *7*, 283ra254. [CrossRef]
7. Natrajan, R.; Sailem, H.; Mardakheh, F.K.; Arias Garcia, M.; Tape, C.J.; Dowsett, M.; Bakal, C.; Yuan, Y. Microenvironmental Heterogeneity Parallels Breast Cancer Progression: A Histology-Genomic Integration Analysis. *PLoS Med.* **2016**, *13*, e1001961. [CrossRef]
8. Azizi, E.; Carr, A.J.; Plitas, G.; Cornish, A.E.; Konopacki, C.; Prabhakaran, S.; Nainys, J.; Wu, K.; Kiseliovas, V.; Setty, M. Single-Cell Map of Diverse Immune Phenotypes in the Breast Tumor Microenvironment. *Cell* **2018**, *174*, 1293–1308.e1236. [CrossRef]
9. Rybinski, B.; Yun, K. Addressing intra-tumoral heterogeneity and therapy resistance. *Oncotarget* **2016**, *7*, 72322–72342. [CrossRef]
10. Mroz, E.A.; Tward, A.D.; Pickering, C.R.; Myers, J.N.; Ferris, R.L.; Rocco, J.W. High intratumor genetic heterogeneity is related to worse outcome in patients with head and neck squamous cell carcinoma. *Cancer* **2013**, *119*, 3034–3042. [CrossRef]

11. Caswell, D.R.; Swanton, C. The role of tumour heterogeneity and clonal cooperativity in metastasis, immune evasion and clinical outcome. *BMC Med.* **2017**, *15*, 133. [CrossRef]
12. Jamal-Hanjani, M.; Quezada, S.A.; Larkin, J.; Swanton, C. Translational implications of tumor heterogeneity. *Clin. Cancer Res.* **2015**, *21*, 1258–1266. [CrossRef]
13. Plava, J.; Cihova, M.; Burikova, M.; Matuskova, M.; Kucerova, L.; Miklikova, S. Recent advances in understanding tumor stroma-mediated chemoresistance in breast cancer. *Mol. Cancer* **2019**, *18*, 67. [CrossRef]
14. Marusyk, A.; Almendro, V.; Polyak, K. Intra-tumour heterogeneity: A looking glass for cancer? *Nat. Rev. Cancer* **2012**, *12*, 323. [CrossRef]
15. Wagner, K.U.; Rui, H. Jak2/Stat5 signaling in mammogenesis, breast cancer initiation and progression. *J. Mammary Gland. Biol. Neoplasia* **2008**, *13*, 93–103. [CrossRef]
16. Ahonen, T.J.; Xie, J.; LeBaron, M.J.; Zhu, J.; Nurmi, M.; Alanen, K.; Rui, H.; Nevalainen, M.T. Inhibition of transcription factor Stat5 induces cell death of human prostate cancer cells. *J. Biol. Chem.* **2003**, *278*, 27287–27292. [CrossRef]
17. Tan, S.H.; Dagvadorj, A.; Shen, F.; Gu, L.; Liao, Z.; Abdulghani, J.; Zhang, Y.; Gelmann, E.P.; Zellweger, T.; Culig, Z.; et al. Transcription factor Stat5 synergizes with androgen receptor in prostate cancer cells. *Cancer Res.* **2008**, *68*, 236–248. [CrossRef]
18. Leong, P.L.; Xi, S.; Drenning, S.D.; Dyer, K.F.; Wentzel, A.L.; Lerner, E.C.; Smithgall, T.E.; Grandis, J.R. Differential function of STAT5 isoforms in head and neck cancer growth control. *Oncogene* **2002**, *21*, 2846–2853. [CrossRef]
19. Grivennikov, S.; Karin, E.; Terzic, J.; Mucida, D.; Yu, G.Y.; Vallabhapurapu, S.; Scheller, J.; Rose-John, S.; Cheroutre, H.; Eckmann, L.; et al. IL-6 and Stat3 are required for survival of intestinal epithelial cells and development of colitis-associated cancer. *Cancer Cell* **2009**, *15*, 103–113. [CrossRef]
20. Hosui, A.; Kimura, A.; Yamaji, D.; Zhu, B.M.; Na, R.; Hennighausen, L. Loss of STAT5 causes liver fibrosis and cancer development through increased TGF-{beta} and STAT3 activation. *J. Exp. Med.* **2009**, *206*, 819–831. [CrossRef]
21. Lesina, M.; Kurkowski, M.U.; Ludes, K.; Rose-John, S.; Treiber, M.; Klöppel, G.; Yoshimura, A.; Reindl, W.; Sipos, B.; Akira, S.; et al. Stat3/Socs3 activation by IL-6 transsignaling promotes progression of pancreatic intraepithelial neoplasia and development of pancreatic cancer. *Cancer Cell* **2011**, *19*, 456–469. [CrossRef] [PubMed]
22. Burke, W.M.; Jin, X.; Lin, H.J.; Huang, M.; Liu, R.; Reynolds, R.K.; Lin, J. Inhibition of constitutively active Stat3 suppresses growth of human ovarian and breast cancer cells. *Oncogene* **2001**, *20*, 7925–7934. [CrossRef] [PubMed]
23. Wu, P.; Wu, D.; Zhao, L.; Huang, L.; Shen, G.; Huang, J.; Chai, Y. Prognostic role of STAT3 in solid tumors: A systematic review and meta-analysis. *Oncotarget* **2016**, *7*, 19863–19883. [CrossRef] [PubMed]
24. Mao, Y.L.; Li, Z.W.; Lou, C.J.; Pang, D.; Zhang, Y.Q. Phospho-STAT5 expression is associated with poor prognosis of human colonic adenocarcinoma. *Pathol. Oncol. Res.* **2011**, *17*, 333–339. [CrossRef] [PubMed]
25. Ma, J.H.; Qi, J.; Lin, S.Q.; Zhang, C.Y.; Liu, F.Y.; Xie, W.D.; Li, X. STAT3 targets ERR-alpha to promote epithelial-mesenchymal transition, migration and invasion in triple negative breast cancer cells. *Mol. Cancer Res.* **2019**. [CrossRef] [PubMed]
26. Xie, T.X.; Huang, F.J.; Aldape, K.D.; Kang, S.H.; Liu, M.; Gershenwald, J.E.; Xie, K.; Sawaya, R.; Huang, S. Activation of stat3 in human melanoma promotes brain metastasis. *Cancer Res.* **2006**, *66*, 3188–3196. [CrossRef] [PubMed]
27. Abdulghani, J.; Gu, L.; Dagvadorj, A.; Lutz, J.; Leiby, B.; Bonuccelli, G.; Lisanti, M.P.; Zellweger, T.; Alanen, K.; Mirtti, T.; et al. Stat3 promotes metastatic progression of prostate cancer. *Am. J. Pathol.* **2008**, *172*, 1717–1728. [CrossRef]
28. Klupp, F.; Diers, J.; Kahlert, C.; Neumann, L.; Halama, N.; Franz, C.; Schmidt, T.; Lasitschka, F.; Warth, A.; Weitz, J.; et al. Expressional STAT3/STAT5 Ratio is an Independent Prognostic Marker in Colon Carcinoma. *Ann. Surg. Oncol.* **2015**, *22* (Suppl. 3), S1548–S1555. [CrossRef]
29. Real, P.J.; Sierra, A.; De Juan, A.; Segovia, J.C.; Lopez-Vega, J.M.; Fernandez-Luna, J.L. Resistance to chemotherapy via Stat3-dependent overexpression of Bcl-2 in metastatic breast cancer cells. *Oncogene* **2002**, *21*, 7611–7618. [CrossRef]

30. Fan, Q.M.; Jing, Y.Y.; Yu, G.F.; Kou, X.R.; Ye, F.; Gao, L.; Li, R.; Zhao, Q.D.; Yang, Y.; Lu, Z.H.; et al. Tumor-associated macrophages promote cancer stem cell-like properties via transforming growth factor-beta1-induced epithelial-mesenchymal transition in hepatocellular carcinoma. *Cancer Lett.* **2014**, *352*, 160–168. [CrossRef]
31. Baskiewicz-Masiuk, M.; Machalinski, B. The role of the STAT5 proteins in the proliferation and apoptosis of the CML and AML cells. *Eur. J. Haematol.* **2004**, *72*, 420–429. [CrossRef] [PubMed]
32. Morcinek, J.C.; Weisser, C.; Geissinger, E.; Schartl, M.; Wellbrock, C. Activation of STAT5 triggers proliferation and contributes to anti-apoptotic signalling mediated by the oncogenic Xmrk kinase. *Oncogene* **2002**, *21*, 1668–1678. [CrossRef] [PubMed]
33. Mahmud, S.A.; Manlove, L.S.; Farrar, M.A. Interleukin-2 and STAT5 in regulatory T cell development and function. *JAKSTAT* **2013**, *2*, e23154. [CrossRef] [PubMed]
34. Rani, A.; Murphy, J.J. STAT5 in Cancer and Immunity. *J. Interferon Cytokine Res.* **2016**, *36*, 226–237. [CrossRef] [PubMed]
35. Han, S.; Toker, A.; Liu, Z.Q.; Ohashi, P.S. Turning the Tide Against Regulatory T Cells. *Front. Oncol.* **2019**, *9*, 279. [CrossRef]
36. Shou, J.; Zhang, Z.; Lai, Y.; Chen, Z.; Huang, J. Worse outcome in breast cancer with higher tumor-infiltrating FOXP3+ Tregs: A systematic review and meta-analysis. *BMC Cancer* **2016**, *16*, 687. [CrossRef]
37. Lim, C.P.; Cao, X. Structure, function, and regulation of STAT proteins. *Mol. Biosyst.* **2006**, *2*, 536–550. [CrossRef]
38. Bromberg, J. Stat proteins and oncogenesis. *J. Clin. Investig.* **2002**, *109*, 1139–1142. [CrossRef]
39. Clevenger, C.V. Roles and Regulation of Stat Family Transcription Factors in Human Breast Cancer. *Am. J. Pathol.* **2004**, *165*, 1449–1460. [CrossRef]
40. Decker, T.; Kovarik, P.; Meinke, A. GAS elements: A few nucleotides with a major impact on cytokine-induced gene expression. *J. Interferon Cytokine Res.* **1997**, *17*, 121–134. [CrossRef]
41. Rawlings, J.S.; Rosler, K.M.; Harrison, D.A. The JAK/STAT signaling pathway. *J. Cell Sci.* **2004**, *117*, 1281–1283. [CrossRef] [PubMed]
42. Murakami, M.; Kamimura, D.; Hirano, T. Pleiotropy and Specificity: Insights from the Interleukin 6 Family of Cytokines. *Immunity* **2019**, *50*, 812–831. [CrossRef] [PubMed]
43. Heinrich, P.C.; Behrmann, I.; Haan, S.; Hermanns, H.M.; Muller-Newen, G.; Schaper, F. Principles of interleukin (IL)-6-type cytokine signalling and its regulation. *Biochem. J.* **2003**, *374*, 1–20. [CrossRef] [PubMed]
44. Raz, R.; Lee, C.K.; Cannizzaro, L.A.; d'Eustachio, P.; Levy, D.E. Essential role of STAT3 for embryonic stem cell pluripotency. *Proc. Natl. Acad. Sci. USA* **1999**, *96*, 2846–2851. [CrossRef] [PubMed]
45. Kirito, K.; Osawa, M.; Morita, H.; Shimizu, R.; Yamamoto, M.; Oda, A.; Fujita, H.; Tanaka, M.; Nakajima, K.; Miura, Y.; et al. A functional role of Stat3 in in vivo megakaryopoiesis. *Blood* **2002**, *99*, 3220–3227. [CrossRef] [PubMed]
46. Akira, S. Roles of STAT3 defined by tissue-specific gene targeting. *Oncogene* **2000**, *19*, 2607–2611. [CrossRef]
47. Yao, Z.; Cui, Y.; Watford, W.T.; Bream, J.H.; Yamaoka, K.; Hissong, B.D.; Li, D.; Durum, S.K.; Jiang, Q.; Bhandoola, A.; et al. Stat5a/b are essential for normal lymphoid development and differentiation. *Proc. Natl. Acad. Sci. USA* **2006**, *103*, 1000–1005. [CrossRef]
48. Wu, M.; Song, D.; Li, H.; Yang, Y.; Ma, X.; Deng, S.; Ren, C.; Shu, X. Negative regulators of STAT3 signaling pathway in cancers. *Cancer Manag. Res.* **2019**, *11*, 4957–4969. [CrossRef]
49. Kershaw, N.J.; Murphy, J.M.; Lucet, I.S.; Nicola, N.A.; Babon, J.J. Regulation of Janus kinases by SOCS proteins. *Biochem. Soc. Trans.* **2013**, *41*, 1042–1047. [CrossRef]
50. Wingelhofer, B.; Neubauer, H.A.; Valent, P.; Han, X.; Constantinescu, S.N.; Gunning, P.T.; Muller, M.; Moriggl, R. Implications of STAT3 and STAT5 signaling on gene regulation and chromatin remodeling in hematopoietic cancer. *Leukemia* **2018**, *32*, 1713–1726. [CrossRef]
51. Orlova, A.; Wingelhofer, B.; Neubauer, H.A.; Maurer, B.; Berger-Becvar, A.; Keseru, G.M.; Gunning, P.T.; Valent, P.; Moriggl, R. Emerging therapeutic targets in myeloproliferative neoplasms and peripheral T-cell leukemia and lymphomas. *Expert Opin. Targets* **2018**, *22*, 45–57. [CrossRef] [PubMed]
52. Forbes, S.A.; Beare, D.; Boutselakis, H.; Bamford, S.; Bindal, N.; Tate, J.; Cole, C.G.; Ward, S.; Dawson, E.; Ponting, L.; et al. COSMIC: Somatic cancer genetics at high-resolution. *Nucleic Acids Res.* **2017**, *45*, D777–D783. [CrossRef] [PubMed]

53. Shahmarvand, N.; Nagy, A.; Shahryari, J.; Ohgami, R.S. Mutations in the signal transducer and activator of transcription family of genes in cancer. *Cancer Sci.* **2018**, *109*, 926–933. [CrossRef] [PubMed]
54. Zhang, T.; Kee, W.H.; Seow, K.T.; Fung, W.; Cao, X. The coiled-coil domain of Stat3 is essential for its SH2 domain-mediated receptor binding and subsequent activation induced by epidermal growth factor and interleukin-6. *Mol. Cell Biol.* **2000**, *20*, 7132–7139. [CrossRef] [PubMed]
55. Hu, G.; Witzig, T.E.; Gupta, M. A novel missense (M206K) STAT3 mutation in diffuse large B cell lymphoma deregulates STAT3 signaling. *PLoS ONE* **2013**, *8*, e67851. [CrossRef]
56. Levine, R.L.; Wadleigh, M.; Cools, J.; Ebert, B.L.; Wernig, G.; Huntly, B.J.; Boggon, T.J.; Wlodarska, I.; Clark, J.J.; Moore, S.; et al. Activating mutation in the tyrosine kinase JAK2 in polycythemia vera, essential thrombocythemia, and myeloid metaplasia with myelofibrosis. *Cancer Cell* **2005**, *7*, 387–397. [CrossRef]
57. James, C.; Ugo, V.; Le Couedic, J.P.; Staerk, J.; Delhommeau, F.; Lacout, C.; Garcon, L.; Raslova, H.; Berger, R.; Bennaceur-Griscelli, A.; et al. A unique clonal JAK2 mutation leading to constitutive signalling causes polycythaemia vera. *Nature* **2005**, *434*, 1144–1148. [CrossRef]
58. Panopoulos, A.D.; Zhang, L.; Snow, J.W.; Jones, D.M.; Smith, A.M.; El Kasmi, K.C.; Liu, F.; Goldsmith, M.A.; Link, D.C.; Murray, P.J.; et al. STAT3 governs distinct pathways in emergency granulopoiesis and mature neutrophils. *Blood* **2006**, *108*, 3682–3690. [CrossRef]
59. Kang, S.; Tanaka, T.; Narazaki, M.; Kishimoto, T. Targeting Interleukin-6 Signaling in Clinic. *Immunity* **2019**, *50*, 1007–1023. [CrossRef]
60. Mutze, J.; Roth, J.; Gerstberger, R.; Hubschle, T. Nuclear translocation of the transcription factor STAT5 in the rat brain after systemic leptin administration. *Neurosci. Lett.* **2007**, *417*, 286–291. [CrossRef]
61. Ribeiro, D.; Melao, A.; van Boxtel, R.; Santos, C.I.; Silva, A.; Silva, M.C.; Cardoso, B.A.; Coffer, P.J.; Barata, J.T. STAT5 is essential for IL-7-mediated viability, growth, and proliferation of T-cell acute lymphoblastic leukemia cells. *Blood Adv.* **2018**, *2*, 2199–2213. [CrossRef] [PubMed]
62. Demoulin, J.B.; Uyttenhove, C.; Lejeune, D.; Mui, A.; Groner, B.; Renauld, J.C. STAT5 activation is required for interleukin-9-dependent growth and transformation of lymphoid cells. *Cancer Res.* **2000**, *60*, 3971–3977. [PubMed]
63. Rochman, Y.; Kashyap, M.; Robinson, G.W.; Sakamoto, K.; Gomez-Rodriguez, J.; Wagner, K.U.; Leonard, W.J. Thymic stromal lymphopoietin-mediated STAT5 phosphorylation via kinases JAK1 and JAK2 reveals a key difference from IL-7-induced signaling. *Proc. Natl. Acad. Sci. USA* **2010**, *107*, 19455–19460. [CrossRef] [PubMed]
64. Okutani, Y.; Kitanaka, A.; Tanaka, T.; Kamano, H.; Ohnishi, H.; Kubota, Y.; Ishida, T.; Takahara, J. Src directly tyrosine-phosphorylates STAT5 on its activation site and is involved in erythropoietin-induced signaling pathway. *Oncogene* **2001**, *20*, 6643–6650. [CrossRef] [PubMed]
65. Kirito, K.; Watanabe, T.; Sawada, K.; Endo, H.; Ozawa, K.; Komatsu, N. Thrombopoietin regulates Bcl-xL gene expression through Stat5 and phosphatidylinositol 3-kinase activation pathways. *J. Biol. Chem.* **2002**, *277*, 8329–8337. [CrossRef]
66. Scheeren, F.A.; Diehl, S.A.; Smit, L.A.; Beaumont, T.; Naspetti, M.; Bende, R.J.; Blom, B.; Karube, K.; Ohshima, K.; van Noesel, C.J.; et al. IL-21 is expressed in Hodgkin lymphoma and activates STAT5: Evidence that activated STAT5 is required for Hodgkin lymphomagenesis. *Blood* **2008**, *111*, 4706–4715. [CrossRef]
67. Maier, E.; Mittermeir, M.; Ess, S.; Neuper, T.; Schmiedlechner, A.; Duschl, A.; Horejs-Hoeck, J. Prerequisites for Functional Interleukin 31 Signaling and Its Feedback Regulation by Suppressor of Cytokine Signaling 3 (SOCS3). *J. Biol. Chem.* **2015**, *290*, 24747–24759. [CrossRef]
68. Toniolo, P.A.; Liu, S.; Yeh, J.E.; Moraes-Vieira, P.M.; Walker, S.R.; Vafaizadeh, V.; Barbuto, J.A.; Frank, D.A. Inhibiting STAT5 by the BET bromodomain inhibitor JQ1 disrupts human dendritic cell maturation. *J. Immunol.* **2015**, *194*, 3180–3190. [CrossRef]
69. Tripathi, P.; Kurtulus, S.; Wojciechowski, S.; Sholl, A.; Hoebe, K.; Morris, S.C.; Finkelman, F.D.; Grimes, H.L.; Hildeman, D.A. STAT5 is critical to maintain effector CD8+ T cell responses. *J. Immunol.* **2010**, *185*, 2116–2124. [CrossRef]
70. Kieslinger, M.; Woldman, I.; Moriggl, R.; Hofmann, J.; Marine, J.C.; Ihle, J.N.; Beug, H.; Decker, T. Antiapoptotic activity of Stat5 required during terminal stages of myeloid differentiation. *Genes Dev.* **2000**, *14*, 232–244.
71. Kuroda, E.; Ho, V.; Ruschmann, J.; Antignano, F.; Hamilton, M.; Rauh, M.J.; Antov, A.; Flavell, R.A.; Sly, L.M.; Krystal, G. SHIP represses the generation of IL-3-induced M2 macrophages by inhibiting IL-4 production from basophils. *J. Immunol.* **2009**, *183*, 3652–3660. [CrossRef] [PubMed]

72. Park, H.J.; Li, J.; Hannah, R.; Biddie, S.; Leal-Cervantes, A.I.; Kirschner, K.; Flores Santa Cruz, D.; Sexl, V.; Gottgens, B.; Green, A.R. Cytokine-induced megakaryocytic differentiation is regulated by genome-wide loss of a uSTAT transcriptional program. *EMBO J.* **2016**, *35*, 580–594. [CrossRef] [PubMed]
73. Kim, A.R.; Ulirsch, J.C.; Wilmes, S.; Unal, E.; Moraga, I.; Karakukcu, M.; Yuan, D.; Kazerounian, S.; Abdulhay, N.J.; King, D.S.; et al. Functional Selectivity in Cytokine Signaling Revealed Through a Pathogenic EPO Mutation. *Cell* **2017**, *168*, 1053–1064 e1015. [CrossRef] [PubMed]
74. Wingelhofer, B.; Maurer, B.; Heyes, E.C.; Cumaraswamy, A.A.; Berger-Becvar, A.; de Araujo, E.D.; Orlova, A.; Freund, P.; Ruge, F.; Park, J.; et al. Pharmacologic inhibition of STAT5 in acute myeloid leukemia. *Leukemia* **2018**, *32*, 1135–1146. [CrossRef]
75. Page, B.D.; Khoury, H.; Laister, R.C.; Fletcher, S.; Vellozo, M.; Manzoli, A.; Yue, P.; Turkson, J.; Minden, M.D.; Gunning, P.T. Small molecule STAT5-SH2 domain inhibitors exhibit potent antileukemia activity. *J. Med. Chem.* **2012**, *55*, 1047–1055. [CrossRef]
76. Elumalai, N.; Berg, A.; Rubner, S.; Blechschmidt, L.; Song, C.; Natarajan, K.; Matysik, J.; Berg, T. Rational development of Stafib-2: A selective, nanomolar inhibitor of the transcription factor STAT5b. *Sci. Rep.* **2017**, *7*, 819. [CrossRef]
77. Unver, N.; McAllister, F. IL-6 family cytokines: Key inflammatory mediators as biomarkers and potential therapeutic targets. *Cytokine Growth Factor Rev.* **2018**, *41*, 10–17. [CrossRef]
78. Sullivan, N.J.; Sasser, A.K.; Axel, A.E.; Vesuna, F.; Raman, V.; Ramirez, N.; Oberyszyn, T.M.; Hall, B.M. Interleukin-6 induces an epithelial-mesenchymal transition phenotype in human breast cancer cells. *Oncogene* **2009**, *28*, 2940–2947. [CrossRef]
79. Putoczki, T.L.; Ernst, M. IL-11 signaling as a therapeutic target for cancer. *Immunotherapy* **2015**, *7*, 441–453. [CrossRef]
80. Lu, J.; Ksendzovsky, A.; Yang, C.; Mehta, G.U.; Yong, R.L.; Weil, R.J.; Park, D.M.; Mushlin, H.M.; Fang, X.; Balgley, B.M.; et al. CNTF receptor subunit alpha as a marker for glioma tumor-initiating cells and tumor grade: Laboratory investigation. *J. Neurosurg.* **2012**, *117*, 1022–1031. [CrossRef]
81. Li, X.; Yang, Q.; Yu, H.; Wu, L.; Zhao, Y.; Zhang, C.; Yue, X.; Liu, Z.; Wu, H.; Haffty, B.G.; et al. LIF promotes tumorigenesis and metastasis of breast cancer through the AKT-mTOR pathway. *Oncotarget* **2014**, *5*, 788–801. [CrossRef] [PubMed]
82. Liao, W.C.; Lin, J.T.; Wu, C.Y.; Huang, S.P.; Lin, M.T.; Wu, A.S.; Huang, Y.J.; Wu, M.S. Serum interleukin-6 level but not genotype predicts survival after resection in stages II and III gastric carcinoma. *Clin. Cancer Res.* **2008**, *14*, 428–434. [CrossRef] [PubMed]
83. Jiang, X.P.; Yang, D.C.; Elliott, R.L.; Head, J.F. Reduction in serum IL-6 after vacination of breast cancer patients with tumour-associated antigens is related to estrogen receptor status. *Cytokine* **2000**, *12*, 458–465. [CrossRef] [PubMed]
84. Chung, Y.-C.; Chang, Y.-F. Serum interleukin-6 levels reflect the disease status of colorectal cancer. *J. Surg. Oncol.* **2003**, *83*, 222–226. [CrossRef] [PubMed]
85. Tawara, K.; Oxford, J.T.; Jorcyk, C.L. Clinical significance of interleukin (IL)-6 in cancer metastasis to bone: Potential of anti-IL-6 therapies. *Cancer Manag. Res.* **2011**, *3*, 177–189. [CrossRef] [PubMed]
86. Komoda, H.; Tanaka, Y.; Honda, M.; Matsuo, Y.; Hazama, K.; Takao, T. Interleukin-6 levels in colorectal cancer tissues. *World J. Surg.* **1998**, *22*, 895–898. [CrossRef]
87. Ebbing, E.A.; van der Zalm, A.P.; Steins, A.; Creemers, A.; Hermsen, S.; Rentenaar, R.; Klein, M.; Waasdorp, C.; Hooijer, G.K.J.; Meijer, S.L.; et al. Stromal-derived interleukin 6 drives epithelial-to-mesenchymal transition and therapy resistance in esophageal adenocarcinoma. *Proc. Natl. Acad. Sci. USA* **2019**, *116*, 2237–2242. [CrossRef]
88. Yadav, A.; Kumar, B.; Datta, J.; Teknos, T.N.; Kumar, P. IL-6 promotes head and neck tumor metastasis by inducing epithelial-mesenchymal transition via the JAK-STAT3-SNAIL signaling pathway. *Mol. Cancer Res.* **2011**, *9*, 1658–1667. [CrossRef]
89. Gyamfi, J.; Lee, Y.H.; Eom, M.; Choi, J. Interleukin-6/STAT3 signalling regulates adipocyte induced epithelial-mesenchymal transition in breast cancer cells. *Sci. Rep.* **2018**, *8*, 8859. [CrossRef]
90. Jiang, M.; Chen, J.; Zhang, W.; Zhang, R.; Ye, Y.; Liu, P.; Yu, W.; Wei, F.; Ren, X.; Yu, J. Interleukin-6 Trans-Signaling Pathway Promotes Immunosuppressive Myeloid-Derived Suppressor Cells via Suppression of Suppressor of Cytokine Signaling 3 in Breast Cancer. *Front. Immunol.* **2017**, *8*, 1840. [CrossRef]

91. Liu, Q.; Yu, S.; Li, A.; Xu, H.; Han, X.; Wu, K. Targeting interlukin-6 to relieve immunosuppression in tumor microenvironment. *Tumour Biol.* **2017**, *39*, 1010428317712445. [CrossRef] [PubMed]
92. Kato, T.; Noma, K.; Ohara, T.; Kashima, H.; Katsura, Y.; Sato, H.; Komoto, S.; Katsube, R.; Ninomiya, T.; Tazawa, H.; et al. Cancer-Associated Fibroblasts Affect Intratumoral CD8(+) and FoxP3(+) T Cells Via IL6 in the Tumor Microenvironment. *Clin. Cancer Res.* **2018**, *24*, 4820–4833. [CrossRef] [PubMed]
93. Chang, Q.; Bournazou, E.; Sansone, P.; Berishaj, M.; Gao, S.P.; Daly, L.; Wels, J.; Theilen, T.; Granitto, S.; Zhang, X.; et al. The IL-6/JAK/Stat3 feed-forward loop drives tumorigenesis and metastasis. *Neoplasia* **2013**, *15*, 848–862. [CrossRef] [PubMed]
94. Wu, X.; Tao, P.; Zhou, Q.; Li, J.; Yu, Z.; Wang, X.; Li, J.; Li, C.; Yan, M.; Zhu, Z.; et al. IL-6 secreted by cancer-associated fibroblasts promotes epithelial-mesenchymal transition and metastasis of gastric cancer via JAK2/STAT3 signaling pathway. *Oncotarget* **2017**, *8*, 20741–20750. [CrossRef] [PubMed]
95. Chang, Q.; Daly, L.; Bromberg, J. The IL-6 feed-forward loop: A driver of tumorigenesis. *Semin. Immunol.* **2014**, *26*, 48–53. [CrossRef] [PubMed]
96. Smigiel, J.; Parvani, J.G.; Tamagno, I.; Polak, K.; Jackson, M.W. Breaking the oncostatin M feed-forward loop to suppress metastasis and therapy failure. *J. Pathol.* **2018**, *245*, 6–8. [CrossRef]
97. Zarling, J.M.; Shoyab, M.; Marquardt, H.; Hanson, M.B.; Lioubin, M.N.; Todaro, G.J. Oncostatin M: A growth regulator produced by differentiated histiocytic lymphoma cells. *Proc. Natl. Acad. Sci. USA* **1986**, *83*, 9739–9743. [CrossRef]
98. Auguste, P.; Guillet, C.; Fourcin, M.; Olivier, C.; Veziers, J.; Pouplard-Barthelaix, A.; Gascan, H. Signaling of type II oncostatin M receptor. *J. Biol. Chem.* **1997**, *272*, 15760–15764. [CrossRef]
99. Mirmohammadsadegh, A.; Hassan, M.; Bardenheuer, W.; Marini, A.; Gustrau, A.; Nambiar, S.; Tannapfel, A.; Bojar, H.; Ruzicka, T.; Hengge, U.R. STAT5 phosphorylation in malignant melanoma is important for survival and is mediated through SRC and JAK1 kinases. *J. Investig. Derm.* **2006**, *126*, 2272–2280. [CrossRef]
100. Lacreusette, A.; Nguyen, J.M.; Pandolfino, M.C.; Khammari, A.; Dreno, B.; Jacques, Y.; Godard, A.; Blanchard, F. Loss of oncostatin M receptor β in metastatic melanoma cells. *Oncogene* **2006**, *26*, 881–892. [CrossRef]
101. Hassel, J.C.; Winnemoller, D.; Schartl, M.; Wellbrock, C. STAT5 contributes to antiapoptosis in melanoma. *Melanoma Res.* **2008**, *18*, 378–385. [CrossRef] [PubMed]
102. West, N.R.; Murray, J.I.; Watson, P.H. Oncostatin-M promotes phenotypic changes associated with mesenchymal and stem cell-like differentiation in breast cancer. *Oncogene* **2014**, *33*, 1485–1494. [CrossRef] [PubMed]
103. Lapeire, L.; Hendrix, A.; Lambein, K.; Van Bockstal, M.; Braems, G.; Van Den Broecke, R.; Limame, R.; Mestdagh, P.; Vandesompele, J.; Vanhove, C.; et al. Cancer-associated adipose tissue promotes breast cancer progression by paracrine oncostatin M and Jak/STAT3 signaling. *Cancer Res.* **2014**, *74*, 6806–6819. [CrossRef] [PubMed]
104. Kim, M.S.; Louwagie, J.; Carvalho, B.; Terhaar Sive Droste, J.S.; Park, H.L.; Chae, Y.K.; Yamashita, K.; Liu, J.; Ostrow, K.L.; Ling, S.; et al. Promoter DNA methylation of oncostatin m receptor-beta as a novel diagnostic and therapeutic marker in colon cancer. *PLoS ONE* **2009**, *4*, e6555. [CrossRef] [PubMed]
105. Queen, M.M.; Ryan, R.E.; Holzer, R.G.; Keller-Peck, C.R.; Jorcyk, C.L. Breast cancer cells stimulate neutrophils to produce oncostatin M: Potential implications for tumor progression. *Cancer Res.* **2005**, *65*, 8896–8904. [CrossRef]
106. Junk, D.J.; Bryson, B.L.; Smigiel, J.M.; Parameswaran, N.; Bartel, C.A.; Jackson, M.W. Oncostatin M promotes cancer cell plasticity through cooperative STAT3-SMAD3 signaling. *Oncogene* **2017**, *36*, 4001–4013. [CrossRef]
107. Jahani-Asl, A.; Yin, H.; Soleimani, V.D.; Haque, T.; Luchman, H.A.; Chang, N.C.; Sincennes, M.-C.; Puram, S.V.; Scott, A.M.; Lorimer, I.A.J.; et al. Control of glioblastoma tumorigenesis by feed-forward cytokine signaling. *Nat. Neurosci.* **2016**, *19*, 798–806. [CrossRef]
108. Shien, K.; Papadimitrakopoulou, V.A.; Ruder, D.; Behrens, C.; Shen, L.; Kalhor, N.; Song, J.; Lee, J.J.; Wang, J.; Tang, X.; et al. JAK1/STAT3 Activation through a Proinflammatory Cytokine Pathway Leads to Resistance to Molecularly Targeted Therapy in Non-Small Cell Lung Cancer. *Mol. Cancer* **2017**, *16*, 2234–2245. [CrossRef]
109. Smigiel, J.M.; Parameswaran, N.; Jackson, M.W. Potent EMT and CSC Phenotypes Are Induced By Oncostatin-M in Pancreatic Cancer. *Mol. Cancer Res.* **2017**, *15*, 478–488. [CrossRef]
110. Tawara, K.; Bolin, C.; Koncinsky, J.; Kadaba, S.; Covert, H.; Sutherland, C.; Bond, L.; Kronz, J.; Garbow, J.R.; Jorcyk, C.L. OSM potentiates preintravasation events, increases CTC counts, and promotes breast cancer metastasis to the lung. *Breast Cancer Res.* **2018**, *20*, 53. [CrossRef]

111. Doherty, M.R.; Cheon, H.; Junk, D.J.; Vinayak, S.; Varadan, V.; Telli, M.L.; Ford, J.M.; Stark, G.R.; Jackson, M.W. Interferon-beta represses cancer stem cell properties in triple-negative breast cancer. *Proc. Natl. Acad. Sci. USA* **2017**, *114*, 13792–13797. [CrossRef] [PubMed]
112. West, N.R.; Hegazy, A.N.; Owens, B.M.J.; Bullers, S.J.; Linggi, B.; Buonocore, S.; Coccia, M.; Gortz, D.; This, S.; Stockenhuber, K.; et al. Oncostatin M drives intestinal inflammation and predicts response to tumor necrosis factor-neutralizing therapy in patients with inflammatory bowel disease. *Nat. Med.* **2017**, *23*, 579–589. [CrossRef] [PubMed]
113. Diveu, C.; Venereau, E.; Froger, J.; Ravon, E.; Grimaud, L.; Rousseau, F.; Chevalier, S.; Gascan, H. Molecular and functional characterization of a soluble form of oncostatin M/interleukin-31 shared receptor. *J. Biol. Chem.* **2006**, *281*, 36673–36682. [CrossRef] [PubMed]
114. Tao, L.; Huang, G.; Wang, R.; Pan, Y.; He, Z.; Chu, X.; Song, H.; Chen, L. Cancer-associated fibroblasts treated with cisplatin facilitates chemoresistance of lung adenocarcinoma through IL-11/IL-11R/STAT3 signaling pathway. *Sci. Rep.* **2016**, *6*, 38408. [CrossRef]
115. Putoczki, T.L.; Thiem, S.; Loving, A.; Busuttil, R.A.; Wilson, N.J.; Ziegler, P.K.; Nguyen, P.M.; Preaudet, A.; Farid, R.; Edwards, K.M.; et al. Interleukin-11 is the dominant IL-6 family cytokine during gastrointestinal tumorigenesis and can be targeted therapeutically. *Cancer Cell* **2013**, *24*, 257–271. [CrossRef]
116. Yu, H.; Yue, X.; Zhao, Y.; Li, X.; Wu, L.; Zhang, C.; Liu, Z.; Lin, K.; Xu-Monette, Z.Y.; Young, K.H.; et al. LIF negatively regulates tumour-suppressor p53 through Stat3/ID1/MDM2 in colorectal cancers. *Nat. Commun.* **2014**, *5*, 5218. [CrossRef]
117. Yuan, J.H.; Yang, F.; Wang, F.; Ma, J.Z.; Guo, Y.J.; Tao, Q.F.; Liu, F.; Pan, W.; Wang, T.T.; Zhou, C.C.; et al. A long noncoding RNA activated by TGF-beta promotes the invasion-metastasis cascade in hepatocellular carcinoma. *Cancer Cell* **2014**, *25*, 666–681. [CrossRef]
118. Yue, X.; Zhao, Y.; Zhang, C.; Li, J.; Liu, Z.; Liu, J.; Hu, W. Leukemia inhibitory factor promotes EMT through STAT3-dependent miR-21 induction. *Oncotarget* **2016**, *7*, 3777–3790. [CrossRef]
119. Bohrer, L.R.; Chuntova, P.; Bade, L.K.; Beadnell, T.C.; Leon, R.P.; Brady, N.J.; Ryu, Y.; Goldberg, J.E.; Schmechel, S.C.; Koopmeiners, J.S.; et al. Activation of the FGFR-STAT3 pathway in breast cancer cells induces a hyaluronan-rich microenvironment that licenses tumor formation. *Cancer Res.* **2014**, *74*, 374–386. [CrossRef]
120. Quintanal-Villalonga, A.; Ojeda-Marquez, L.; Marrugal, A.; Yague, P.; Ponce-Aix, S.; Salinas, A.; Carnero, A.; Ferrer, I.; Molina-Pinelo, S.; Paz-Ares, L. The FGFR4-388arg Variant Promotes Lung Cancer Progression by N-Cadherin Induction. *Sci. Rep.* **2018**, *8*, 2394. [CrossRef]
121. Yao, C.; Su, L.; Shan, J.; Zhu, C.; Liu, L.; Liu, C.; Xu, Y.; Yang, Z.; Bian, X.; Shao, J.; et al. IGF/STAT3/NANOG/Slug Signaling Axis Simultaneously Controls Epithelial-Mesenchymal Transition and Stemness Maintenance in Colorectal Cancer. *Stem Cells* **2016**, *34*, 820–831. [CrossRef] [PubMed]
122. Ding, X.; Ji, J.; Jiang, J.; Cai, Q.; Wang, C.; Shi, M.; Yu, Y.; Zhu, Z.; Zhang, J. HGF-mediated crosstalk between cancer-associated fibroblasts and MET-unamplified gastric cancer cells activates coordinated tumorigenesis and metastasis. *Cell Death Dis.* **2018**, *9*, 867. [CrossRef] [PubMed]
123. Cheng, C.C.; Liao, P.N.; Ho, A.S.; Lim, K.H.; Chang, J.; Su, Y.W.; Chen, C.G.; Chiang, Y.W.; Yang, B.L.; Lin, H.C.; et al. STAT3 exacerbates survival of cancer stem-like tumorspheres in EGFR-positive colorectal cancers: RNAseq analysis and therapeutic screening. *J. Biomed. Sci.* **2018**, *25*, 60. [CrossRef] [PubMed]
124. Zhao, D.; Pan, C.; Sun, J.; Gilbert, C.; Drews-Elger, K.; Azzam, D.J.; Picon-Ruiz, M.; Kim, M.; Ullmer, W.; El-Ashry, D.; et al. VEGF drives cancer-initiating stem cells through VEGFR-2/Stat3 signaling to upregulate Myc and Sox2. *Oncogene* **2015**, *34*, 3107–3119. [CrossRef]
125. Ando, T.; Kudo, Y.; Iizuka, S.; Tsunematsu, T.; Umehara, H.; Shrestha, M.; Matsuo, T.; Kubo, T.; Shimose, S.; Arihiro, K.; et al. Ameloblastin induces tumor suppressive phenotype and enhances chemosensitivity to doxorubicin via Src-Stat3 inactivation in osteosarcoma. *Sci. Rep.* **2017**, *7*, 40187. [CrossRef]
126. Ma, L.; Xu, Z.; Wang, J.; Zhu, Z.; Lin, G.; Jiang, L.; Lu, X.; Zou, C. Matrine inhibits BCR/ABL mediated ERK/MAPK pathway in human leukemia cells. *Oncotarget* **2017**, *8*, 108880–108889. [CrossRef]
127. Puram, S.V.; Yeung, C.M.; Jahani-Asl, A.; Lin, C.; de la Iglesia, N.; Konopka, G.; Jackson-Grusby, L.; Bonni, A. STAT3-iNOS Signaling Mediates EGFRvIII-Induced Glial Proliferation and Transformation. *J. Neurosci.* **2012**, *32*, 7806–7818. [CrossRef]
128. Yuan, Z.L.; Guan, Y.J.; Chatterjee, D.; Chin, Y.E. Stat3 dimerization regulated by reversible acetylation of a single lysine residue. *Science* **2005**, *307*, 269–273. [CrossRef]

129. Limagne, E.; Thibaudin, M.; Euvrard, R.; Berger, H.; Chalons, P.; Vegan, F.; Humblin, E.; Boidot, R.; Rebe, C.; Derangere, V.; et al. Sirtuin-1 Activation Controls Tumor Growth by Impeding Th17 Differentiation via STAT3 Deacetylation. *Cell Rep.* **2017**, *19*, 746–759. [CrossRef]
130. Johnston, P.A.; Grandis, J.R. STAT3 signaling: Anticancer strategies and challenges. *Mol. Interv.* **2011**, *11*, 18–26. [CrossRef]
131. Bromberg, J.F.; Wrzeszczynska, M.H.; Devgan, G.; Zhao, Y.; Pestell, R.G.; Albanese, C.; Darnell, J.E. Stat3 as an Oncogene. *Cell* **1999**, *98*, 295–303. [CrossRef]
132. Avalle, L.; Pensa, S.; Regis, G.; Novelli, F.; Poli, V. STAT1 and STAT3 in tumorigenesis: A matter of balance. *JAKSTAT* **2012**, *1*, 65–72. [CrossRef] [PubMed]
133. Bromberg, J.F.; Horvath, C.M.; Besser, D.; Lathem, W.W.; Darnell, J.E., Jr. Stat3 activation is required for cellular transformation by v-src. *Mol. Cell Biol.* **1998**, *18*, 2553–2558. [CrossRef] [PubMed]
134. Dechow, T.N.; Pedranzini, L.; Leitch, A.; Leslie, K.; Gerald, W.L.; Linkov, I.; Bromberg, J.F. Requirement of matrix metalloproteinase-9 for the transformation of human mammary epithelial cells by Stat3-C. *Proc. Natl. Acad. Sci. USA* **2004**, *101*, 10602–10607. [CrossRef]
135. Gough, D.J.; Corlett, A.; Schlessinger, K.; Wegrzyn, J.; Larner, A.C.; Levy, D.E. Mitochondrial STAT3 supports Ras-dependent oncogenic transformation. *Science* **2009**, *324*, 1713–1716. [CrossRef]
136. Fukuda, A.; Wang, S.C.; Morris, J.P.t.; Folias, A.E.; Liou, A.; Kim, G.E.; Akira, S.; Boucher, K.M.; Firpo, M.A.; Mulvihill, S.J.; et al. Stat3 and MMP7 contribute to pancreatic ductal adenocarcinoma initiation and progression. *Cancer Cell* **2011**, *19*, 441–455. [CrossRef]
137. Bryson, B.L.; Junk, D.J.; Cipriano, R.; Jackson, M.W. STAT3-mediated SMAD3 activation underlies Oncostatin M-induced Senescence. *Cell Cycle* **2017**, *16*, 319–334. [CrossRef]
138. Rokavec, M.; Oner, M.G.; Li, H.; Jackstadt, R.; Jiang, L.; Lodygin, D.; Kaller, M.; Horst, D.; Ziegler, P.K.; Schwitalla, S.; et al. IL-6R/STAT3/miR-34a feedback loop promotes EMT-mediated colorectal cancer invasion and metastasis. *J. Clin. Investig.* **2014**, *124*, 1853–1867. [CrossRef]
139. Cho, K.H.; Jeong, K.J.; Shin, S.C.; Kang, J.; Park, C.G.; Lee, H.Y. STAT3 mediates TGF-beta1-induced TWIST1 expression and prostate cancer invasion. *Cancer Lett.* **2013**, *336*, 167–173. [CrossRef]
140. Xiong, H.; Hong, J.; Du, W.; Lin, Y.-w.; Ren, L.-l.; Wang, Y.-c.; Su, W.-y.; Wang, J.-l.; Cui, Y.; Wang, Z.-h.; et al. Roles of STAT3 and ZEB1 proteins in E-cadherin down-regulation and human colorectal cancer epithelial-mesenchymal transition. *J. Biol. Chem.* **2012**, *287*, 5819–5832. [CrossRef]
141. Singh, A.; Settleman, J. EMT, cancer stem cells and drug resistance: An emerging axis of evil in the war on cancer. *Oncogene* **2010**, *29*, 4741–4751. [CrossRef] [PubMed]
142. Xie, T.X.; Wei, D.; Liu, M.; Gao, A.C.; Ali-Osman, F.; Sawaya, R.; Huang, S. Stat3 activation regulates the expression of matrix metalloproteinase-2 and tumor invasion and metastasis. *Oncogene* **2004**, *23*, 3550–3560. [CrossRef] [PubMed]
143. Jia, Z.H.; Jia, Y.; Guo, F.J.; Chen, J.; Zhang, X.W.; Cui, M.H. Phosphorylation of STAT3 at Tyr705 regulates MMP-9 production in epithelial ovarian cancer. *PLoS ONE* **2017**, *12*, e0183622. [CrossRef] [PubMed]
144. Lin, C.Y.; Tsai, P.H.; Kandaswami, C.C.; Lee, P.P.; Huang, C.J.; Hwang, J.J.; Lee, M.T. Matrix metalloproteinase-9 cooperates with transcription factor Snail to induce epithelial-mesenchymal transition. *Cancer Sci.* **2011**, *102*, 815–827. [CrossRef] [PubMed]
145. Doyle, S.; Evans, A.J.; Rakha, E.A.; Green, A.R.; Ellis, I.O. Influence of E-cadherin expression on the mammographic appearance of invasive nonlobular breast carcinoma detected at screening. *Radiology* **2009**, *253*, 51–55. [CrossRef]
146. Rakha, E.A.; Abd El Rehim, D.; Pinder, S.E.; Lewis, S.A.; Ellis, I.O. E-cadherin expression in invasive non-lobular carcinoma of the breast and its prognostic significance. *Histopathology* **2005**, *46*, 685–693. [CrossRef]
147. Rakha, E.A.; Patel, A.; Powe, D.G.; Benhasouna, A.; Green, A.R.; Lambros, M.B.; Reis-Filho, J.S.; Ellis, I.O. Clinical and biological significance of E-cadherin protein expression in invasive lobular carcinoma of the breast. *Am. J. Surg. Pathol.* **2010**, *34*, 1472–1479. [CrossRef]
148. Liu, T.; Zhang, X.; Shang, M.; Zhang, Y.; Xia, B.; Niu, M.; Liu, Y.; Pang, D. Dysregulated expression of Slug, vimentin, and E-cadherin correlates with poor clinical outcome in patients with basal-like breast cancer. *J. Surg. Oncol.* **2013**, *107*, 188–194. [CrossRef]
149. Markiewicz, A.; Welnicka-Jaskiewicz, M.; Seroczynska, B.; Skokowski, J.; Majewska, H.; Szade, J.; Zaczek, A.J. Epithelial-mesenchymal transition markers in lymph node metastases and primary breast tumors—Relation to dissemination and proliferation. *Am. J. Transl. Res.* **2014**, *6*, 793–808.

150. Zhou, L.; Dicker, D.T.; Matthew, E.; El-Deiry, W.S.; Alpaugh, R.K. Circulating tumor cells: Silent predictors of metastasis. *F1000Research* **2017**, *6*. [CrossRef]
151. Yu, M.; Bardia, A.; Wittner, B.S.; Stott, S.L.; Smas, M.E.; Ting, D.T.; Isakoff, S.J.; Ciciliano, J.C.; Wells, M.N.; Shah, A.M.; et al. Circulating breast tumor cells exhibit dynamic changes in epithelial and mesenchymal composition. *Science* **2013**, *339*, 580–584. [CrossRef] [PubMed]
152. Wu, S.; Liu, S.; Liu, Z.; Huang, J.; Pu, X.; Li, J.; Yang, D.; Deng, H.; Yang, N.; Xu, J. Classification of circulating tumor cells by epithelial-mesenchymal transition markers. *PLoS ONE* **2015**, *10*, e0123976. [CrossRef] [PubMed]
153. Satelli, A.; Mitra, A.; Brownlee, Z.; Xia, X.; Bellister, S.; Overman, M.J.; Kopetz, S.; Ellis, L.M.; Meng, Q.H.; Li, S. Epithelial-mesenchymal transitioned circulating tumor cells capture for detecting tumor progression. *Clin. Cancer Res.* **2015**, *21*, 899–906. [CrossRef] [PubMed]
154. Lawson, D.A.; Bhakta, N.R.; Kessenbrock, K.; Prummel, K.D.; Yu, Y.; Takai, K.; Zhou, A.; Eyob, H.; Balakrishnan, S.; Wang, C.Y.; et al. Single-cell analysis reveals a stem-cell program in human metastatic breast cancer cells. *Nature* **2015**, *526*, 131–135. [CrossRef] [PubMed]
155. Doherty, M.R.; Smigiel, J.M.; Junk, D.J.; Jackson, M.W. Cancer Stem Cell Plasticity Drives Therapeutic Resistance. *Cancers* **2016**, *8*, 8. [CrossRef]
156. Reya, T.; Morrison, S.J.; Clarke, M.F.; Weissman, I.L. Stem cells, cancer, and cancer stem cells. *Nature* **2001**, *414*, 105–111. [CrossRef]
157. Kim, C.F.; Jackson, E.L.; Woolfenden, A.E.; Lawrence, S.; Babar, I.; Vogel, S.; Crowley, D.; Bronson, R.T.; Jacks, T. Identification of bronchioalveolar stem cells in normal lung and lung cancer. *Cell* **2005**, *121*, 823–835. [CrossRef]
158. O'Brien, C.A.; Pollett, A.; Gallinger, S.; Dick, J.E. A human colon cancer cell capable of initiating tumour growth in immunodeficient mice. *Nature* **2007**, *445*, 106–110. [CrossRef]
159. Collins, A.T.; Berry, P.A.; Hyde, C.; Stower, M.J.; Maitland, N.J. Prospective identification of tumorigenic prostate cancer stem cells. *Cancer Res.* **2005**, *65*, 10946–10951. [CrossRef]
160. Hayashida, T.; Jinno, H.; Kitagawa, Y.; Kitajima, M. Cooperation of cancer stem cell properties and epithelial-mesenchymal transition in the establishment of breast cancer metastasis. *J. Oncol.* **2011**, *2011*, 591427. [CrossRef]
161. Choi, S.; Yu, J.; Park, A.; Dubon, M.J.; Do, J.; Kim, Y.; Nam, D.; Noh, J.; Park, K.S. BMP-4 enhances epithelial mesenchymal transition and cancer stem cell properties of breast cancer cells via Notch signaling. *Sci. Rep.* **2019**, *9*, 11724. [CrossRef]
162. Hung, J.J.; Kao, Y.S.; Huang, C.H.; Hsu, W.H. Overexpression of Aiolos promotes epithelial-mesenchymal transition and cancer stem cell-like properties in lung cancer cells. *Sci. Rep.* **2019**, *9*, 2991. [CrossRef] [PubMed]
163. Reiman, J.M.; Knutson, K.L.; Radisky, D.C. Immune promotion of epithelial-mesenchymal transition and generation of breast cancer stem cells. *Cancer Res.* **2010**, *70*, 3005–3008. [CrossRef] [PubMed]
164. Kashyap, V.; Rezende, N.C.; Scotland, K.B.; Shaffer, S.M.; Persson, J.L.; Gudas, L.J.; Mongan, N.P. Regulation of stem cell pluripotency and differentiation involves a mutual regulatory circuit of the NANOG, OCT4, and SOX2 pluripotency transcription factors with polycomb repressive complexes and stem cell microRNAs. *Stem Cells Dev.* **2009**, *18*, 1093–1108. [CrossRef] [PubMed]
165. Loh, Y.H.; Wu, Q.; Chew, J.L.; Vega, V.B.; Zhang, W.; Chen, X.; Bourque, G.; George, J.; Leong, B.; Liu, J.; et al. The Oct4 and Nanog transcription network regulates pluripotency in mouse embryonic stem cells. *Nat. Genet.* **2006**, *38*, 431–440. [CrossRef]
166. Zhou, J.; Wulfkuhle, J.; Zhang, H.; Gu, P.; Yang, Y.; Deng, J.; Margolick, J.B.; Liotta, L.A.; Petricoin, E., 3rd; Zhang, Y. Activation of the PTEN/mTOR/STAT3 pathway in breast cancer stem-like cells is required for viability and maintenance. *Proc. Natl. Acad. Sci. USA* **2007**, *104*, 16158–16163. [CrossRef]
167. Kim, S.Y.; Kang, J.W.; Song, X.; Kim, B.K.; Yoo, Y.D.; Kwon, Y.T.; Lee, Y.J. Role of the IL-6-JAK1-STAT3-Oct-4 pathway in the conversion of non-stem cancer cells into cancer stem-like cells. *Cell Signal* **2013**, *25*, 961–969. [CrossRef]
168. Bareiss, P.M.; Paczulla, A.; Wang, H.; Schairer, R.; Wiehr, S.; Kohlhofer, U.; Rothfuss, O.C.; Fischer, A.; Perner, S.; Staebler, A.; et al. SOX2 expression associates with stem cell state in human ovarian carcinoma. *Cancer Res.* **2013**, *73*, 5544–5555. [CrossRef]
169. Jiang, J.; Li, Z.; Yu, C.; Chen, M.; Tian, S.; Sun, C. MiR-1181 inhibits stem cell-like phenotypes and suppresses SOX2 and STAT3 in human pancreatic cancer. *Cancer Lett.* **2015**, *356*, 962–970. [CrossRef]

170. Yin, X.; Zhang, B.H.; Zheng, S.S.; Gao, D.M.; Qiu, S.J.; Wu, W.Z.; Ren, Z.G. Coexpression of gene Oct4 and Nanog initiates stem cell characteristics in hepatocellular carcinoma and promotes epithelial-mesenchymal transition through activation of Stat3/Snail signaling. *J. Hematol. Oncol.* **2015**, *8*, 23. [CrossRef]
171. Van den Hoogen, C.; van der Horst, G.; Cheung, H.; Buijs, J.T.; Lippitt, J.M.; Guzman-Ramirez, N.; Hamdy, F.C.; Eaton, C.L.; Thalmann, G.N.; Cecchini, M.G.; et al. High aldehyde dehydrogenase activity identifies tumor-initiating and metastasis-initiating cells in human prostate cancer. *Cancer Res.* **2010**, *70*, 5163–5173. [CrossRef] [PubMed]
172. Liu, C.; Kelnar, K.; Liu, B.; Chen, X.; Calhoun-Davis, T.; Li, H.; Patrawala, L.; Yan, H.; Jeter, C.; Honorio, S.; et al. The microRNA miR-34a inhibits prostate cancer stem cells and metastasis by directly repressing CD44. *Nat. Med.* **2011**, *17*, 211–215. [CrossRef] [PubMed]
173. Pascual, G.; Avgustinova, A.; Mejetta, S.; Martin, M.; Castellanos, A.; Attolini, C.S.; Berenguer, A.; Prats, N.; Toll, A.; Hueto, J.A.; et al. Targeting metastasis-initiating cells through the fatty acid receptor CD36. *Nature* **2017**, *541*, 41–45. [CrossRef] [PubMed]
174. Mimeault, M.; Batra, S.K. Hypoxia-inducing factors as master regulators of stemness properties and altered metabolism of cancer- and metastasis-initiating cells. *J. Cell Mol. Med.* **2013**, *17*, 30–54. [CrossRef]
175. Pastushenko, I.; Brisebarre, A.; Sifrim, A.; Fioramonti, M.; Revenco, T.; Boumahdi, S.; Van Keymeulen, A.; Brown, D.; Moers, V.; Lemaire, S.; et al. Identification of the tumour transition states occurring during EMT. *Nature* **2018**, *556*, 463–468. [CrossRef]
176. Goldman, A.; Majumder, B.; Dhawan, A.; Ravi, S.; Goldman, D.; Kohandel, M.; Majumder, P.K.; Sengupta, S. Temporally sequenced anticancer drugs overcome adaptive resistance by targeting a vulnerable chemotherapy-induced phenotypic transition. *Nat. Commun.* **2015**, *6*, 6139. [CrossRef]
177. Kim, C.; Gao, R.; Sei, E.; Brandt, R.; Hartman, J.; Hatschek, T.; Crosetto, N.; Foukakis, T.; Navin, N.E. Chemoresistance Evolution in Triple-Negative Breast Cancer Delineated by Single-Cell Sequencing. *Cell* **2018**, *173*, 879–893 e813. [CrossRef]
178. Zheng, X.; Carstens, J.L.; Kim, J.; Scheible, M.; Kaye, J.; Sugimoto, H.; Wu, C.C.; LeBleu, V.S.; Kalluri, R. Epithelial-to-mesenchymal transition is dispensable for metastasis but induces chemoresistance in pancreatic cancer. *Nature* **2015**, *527*, 525–530. [CrossRef]
179. Fischer, K.R.; Durrans, A.; Lee, S.; Sheng, J.; Li, F.; Wong, S.T.; Choi, H.; El Rayes, T.; Ryu, S.; Troeger, J.; et al. Epithelial-to-mesenchymal transition is not required for lung metastasis but contributes to chemoresistance. *Nature* **2015**, *527*, 472–476. [CrossRef]
180. Zhu, X.; Shen, H.; Yin, X.; Long, L.; Chen, X.; Feng, F.; Liu, Y.; Zhao, P.; Xu, Y.; Li, M.; et al. IL-6R/STAT3/miR-204 feedback loop contributes to cisplatin resistance of epithelial ovarian cancer cells. *Oncotarget* **2017**, *8*, 39154–39166. [CrossRef]
181. Ganguly, D.; Fan, M.; Yang, C.H.; Zbytek, B.; Finkelstein, D.; Roussel, M.F.; Pfeffer, L.M. The critical role that STAT3 plays in glioma-initiating cells: STAT3 addiction in glioma. *Oncotarget* **2018**, *9*, 22095–22112. [CrossRef] [PubMed]
182. Liu, F.; Cao, J.; Wu, J.; Sullivan, K.; Shen, J.; Ryu, B.; Xu, Z.; Wei, W.; Cui, R. Stat3-targeted therapies overcome the acquired resistance to vemurafenib in melanomas. *J. Investig. Derm.* **2013**, *133*, 2041–2049. [CrossRef] [PubMed]
183. Nagathihalli, N.S.; Castellanos, J.A.; Lamichhane, P.; Messaggio, F.; Shi, C.; Dai, X.; Rai, P.; Chen, X.; VanSaun, M.N.; Merchant, N.B. Inverse Correlation of STAT3 and MEK Signaling Mediates Resistance to RAS Pathway Inhibition in Pancreatic Cancer. *Cancer Res.* **2018**, *78*, 6235–6246. [CrossRef] [PubMed]
184. Zhang, X.; Ren, D.; Wu, X.; Lin, X.; Ye, L.; Lin, C.; Wu, S.; Zhu, J.; Peng, X.; Song, L. miR-1266 Contributes to Pancreatic Cancer Progression and Chemoresistance by the STAT3 and NF-kappaB Signaling Pathways. *Mol. Nucleic Acids* **2018**, *11*, 142–158. [CrossRef]
185. Kettner, N.M.; Vijayaraghavan, S.; Durak, M.G.; Bui, T.; Kohansal, M.; Ha, M.J.; Liu, B.; Rao, X.; Wang, J.; Yi, M.; et al. Combined Inhibition of STAT3 and DNA Repair in Palbociclib-Resistant ER-Positive Breast Cancer. *Clin. Cancer Res.* **2019**, *25*, 3996–4013. [CrossRef]
186. Wang, L.; Zhang, F.; Cui, J.Y.; Chen, L.; Chen, Y.T.; Liu, B.W. CAFs enhance paclitaxel resistance by inducing EMT through the IL6/JAK2/STAT3 pathway. *Oncol. Rep.* **2018**, *39*, 2081–2090. [CrossRef]
187. Gupta, P.B.; Fillmore, C.M.; Jiang, G.; Shapira, S.D.; Tao, K.; Kuperwasser, C.; Lander, E.S. Stochastic state transitions give rise to phenotypic equilibrium in populations of cancer cells. *Cell* **2011**, *146*, 633–644. [CrossRef]

188. Korkaya, H.; Kim, G.I.; Davis, A.; Malik, F.; Henry, N.L.; Ithimakin, S.; Quraishi, A.A.; Tawakkol, N.; D'Angelo, R.; Paulson, A.K.; et al. Activation of an IL6 inflammatory loop mediates trastuzumab resistance in HER2+ breast cancer by expanding the cancer stem cell population. *Mol. Cell* **2012**, *47*, 570–584. [CrossRef]
189. Lee, H.J.; Zhuang, G.; Cao, Y.; Du, P.; Kim, H.J.; Settleman, J. Drug resistance via feedback activation of Stat3 in oncogene-addicted cancer cells. *Cancer Cell* **2014**, *26*, 207–221. [CrossRef]
190. Simon, G.R.; Somaiah, N. A tabulated summary of targeted and biologic therapies for non-small-cell lung cancer. *Clin. Lung Cancer* **2014**, *15*, 21–51. [CrossRef]
191. Abell, K.; Watson, C.J. The Jak/Stat pathway: A novel way to regulate PI3K activity. *Cell Cycle* **2005**, *4*, 897–900. [CrossRef] [PubMed]
192. Avila, M.A.; Kagan, P.; Sultan, M.; Tachlytski, I.; Safran, M.; Ben-Ari, Z. Both MAPK and STAT3 signal transduction pathways are necessary for IL-6-dependent hepatic stellate cells activation. *PLoS ONE* **2017**, *12*. [CrossRef]
193. Fan, Y.; Mao, R.; Yang, J. NF-kappaB and STAT3 signaling pathways collaboratively link inflammation to cancer. *Protein Cell* **2013**, *4*, 176–185. [CrossRef] [PubMed]
194. Kamakura, S.; Oishi, K.; Yoshimatsu, T.; Nakafuku, M.; Masuyama, N.; Gotoh, Y. Hes binding to STAT3 mediates crosstalk between Notch and JAK-STAT signalling. *Nat. Cell Biol.* **2004**, *6*, 547–554. [CrossRef] [PubMed]
195. Fragoso, M.A.; Patel, A.K.; Nakamura, R.E.; Yi, H.; Surapaneni, K.; Hackam, A.S. The Wnt/beta-catenin pathway cross-talks with STAT3 signaling to regulate survival of retinal pigment epithelium cells. *PLoS ONE* **2012**, *7*, e46892. [CrossRef]
196. Tang, L.Y.; Heller, M.; Meng, Z.; Yu, L.R.; Tang, Y.; Zhou, M.; Zhang, Y.E. Transforming Growth Factor-beta (TGF-beta) Directly Activates the JAK1-STAT3 Axis to Induce Hepatic Fibrosis in Coordination with the SMAD Pathway. *J. Biol. Chem.* **2017**, *292*, 4302–4312. [CrossRef]
197. Bui, Q.T.; Im, J.H.; Jeong, S.B.; Kim, Y.M.; Lim, S.C.; Kim, B.; Kang, K.W. Essential role of Notch4/STAT3 signaling in epithelial-mesenchymal transition of tamoxifen-resistant human breast cancer. *Cancer Lett.* **2017**, *390*, 115–125. [CrossRef]
198. Canino, C.; Luo, Y.; Marcato, P.; Blandino, G.; Pass, H.I.; Cioce, M. A STAT3-NFkB/DDIT3/CEBPbeta axis modulates ALDH1A3 expression in chemoresistant cell subpopulations. *Oncotarget* **2015**, *6*, 12637–12653. [CrossRef]
199. Alt-Holland, A.; Sowalsky, A.G.; Szwec-Levin, Y.; Shamis, Y.; Hatch, H.; Feig, L.A.; Garlick, J.A. Suppression of E-cadherin function drives the early stages of Ras-induced squamous cell carcinoma through upregulation of FAK and Src. *J. Investig. Derm.* **2011**, *131*, 2306–2315. [CrossRef]
200. Onder, T.T.; Gupta, P.B.; Mani, S.A.; Yang, J.; Lander, E.S.; Weinberg, R.A. Loss of E-cadherin promotes metastasis via multiple downstream transcriptional pathways. *Cancer Res.* **2008**, *68*, 3645–3654. [CrossRef]
201. D'Amico, S.; Shi, J.; Martin, B.L.; Crawford, H.C.; Petrenko, O.; Reich, N.C. STAT3 is a master regulator of epithelial identity and KRAS-driven tumorigenesis. *Genes Dev.* **2018**, *32*, 1175–1187. [CrossRef] [PubMed]
202. Aras, S.; Zaidi, M.R. TAMeless traitors: Macrophages in cancer progression and metastasis. *Br. J. Cancer* **2017**, *117*, 1583–1591. [CrossRef] [PubMed]
203. Qian, B.Z.; Li, J.; Zhang, H.; Kitamura, T.; Zhang, J.; Campion, L.R.; Kaiser, E.A.; Snyder, L.A.; Pollard, J.W. CCL2 recruits inflammatory monocytes to facilitate breast-tumour metastasis. *Nature* **2011**, *475*, 222–225. [CrossRef]
204. Wu, L.; Saxena, S.; Awaji, M.; Singh, R.K. Tumor-Associated Neutrophils in Cancer: Going Pro. *Cancers* **2019**, *11*, 564. [CrossRef]
205. Yang, C.; He, L.; He, P.; Liu, Y.; Wang, W.; He, Y.; Du, Y.; Gao, F. Increased drug resistance in breast cancer by tumor-associated macrophages through IL-10/STAT3/bcl-2 signaling pathway. *Med. Oncol.* **2015**, *32*, 352. [CrossRef]
206. Webb, N.J.; Myers, C.R.; Watson, C.J.; Bottomley, M.J.; Brenchley, P.E. Activated human neutrophils express vascular endothelial growth factor (VEGF). *Cytokine* **1998**, *10*, 254–257. [CrossRef] [PubMed]
207. Li, S.; Cong, X.; Gao, H.; Lan, X.; Li, Z.; Wang, W.; Song, S.; Wang, Y.; Li, C.; Zhang, H.; et al. Tumor-associated neutrophils induce EMT by IL-17a to promote migration and invasion in gastric cancer cells. *J. Exp. Clin. Cancer Res.* **2019**, *38*, 6. [CrossRef] [PubMed]

208. Liu, C.Y.; Xu, J.Y.; Shi, X.Y.; Huang, W.; Ruan, T.Y.; Xie, P.; Ding, J.L. M2-polarized tumor-associated macrophages promoted epithelial-mesenchymal transition in pancreatic cancer cells, partially through TLR4/IL-10 signaling pathway. *Lab. Investig.* **2013**, *93*, 844–854. [CrossRef]
209. Pignatelli, J.; Bravo-Cordero, J.J.; Roh-Johnson, M.; Gandhi, S.J.; Wang, Y.; Chen, X.; Eddy, R.J.; Xue, A.; Singer, R.H.; Hodgson, L.; et al. Macrophage-dependent tumor cell transendothelial migration is mediated by Notch1/MenaINV-initiated invadopodium formation. *Sci. Rep.* **2016**, *6*. [CrossRef]
210. Pignatelli, J.; Goswami, S.; Jones, J.G.; Rohan, T.E.; Pieri, E.; Chen, X.; Adler, E.; Cox, D.; Maleki, S.; Bresnick, A.; et al. Invasive breast carcinoma cells from patients exhibit MenaINV- and macrophage-dependent transendothelial migration. *Sci. Signal* **2014**, *7*, ra112. [CrossRef]
211. Yang, J.; Liao, D.; Chen, C.; Liu, Y.; Chuang, T.H.; Xiang, R.; Markowitz, D.; Reisfeld, R.A.; Luo, Y. Tumor-associated macrophages regulate murine breast cancer stem cells through a novel paracrine EGFR/Stat3/Sox-2 signaling pathway. *Stem Cells* **2013**, *31*, 248–258. [CrossRef] [PubMed]
212. Szczerba, B.M.; Castro-Giner, F.; Vetter, M.; Krol, I.; Gkountela, S.; Landin, J.; Scheidmann, M.C.; Donato, C.; Scherrer, R.; Singer, J.; et al. Neutrophils escort circulating tumour cells to enable cell cycle progression. *Nature* **2019**, *566*, 553–557. [CrossRef] [PubMed]
213. Spicer, J.D.; McDonald, B.; Cools-Lartigue, J.J.; Chow, S.C.; Giannias, B.; Kubes, P.; Ferri, L.E. Neutrophils Promote Liver Metastasis via Mac-1–Mediated Interactions with Circulating Tumor Cells. *Cancer Res.* **2012**, *72*, 3919–3927. [CrossRef] [PubMed]
214. Wculek, S.K.; Malanchi, I. Neutrophils support lung colonization of metastasis-initiating breast cancer cells. *Nature* **2015**, *528*, 413–417. [CrossRef]
215. Psaila, B.; Lyden, D. The metastatic niche: Adapting the foreign soil. *Nat. Rev. Cancer* **2009**, *9*, 285–293. [CrossRef]
216. Deng, J.; Liu, Y.; Lee, H.; Herrmann, A.; Zhang, W.; Zhang, C.; Shen, S.; Priceman, S.J.; Kujawski, M.; Pal, S.K.; et al. S1PR1-STAT3 signaling is crucial for myeloid cell colonization at future metastatic sites. *Cancer Cell* **2012**, *21*, 642–654. [CrossRef]
217. Kanai, T.; Seki, S.; Jenks, J.A.; Kohli, A.; Kawli, T.; Martin, D.P.; Snyder, M.; Bacchetta, R.; Nadeau, K.C. Identification of STAT5A and STAT5B target genes in human T cells. *PLoS ONE* **2014**, *9*, e86790. [CrossRef]
218. Grebien, F.; Kerenyi, M.A.; Kovacic, B.; Kolbe, T.; Becker, V.; Dolznig, H.; Pfeffer, K.; Klingmuller, U.; Muller, M.; Beug, H.; et al. Stat5 activation enables erythropoiesis in the absence of EpoR and Jak2. *Blood* **2008**, *111*, 4511–4522. [CrossRef]
219. Zhu, B.M.; McLaughlin, S.K.; Na, R.; Liu, J.; Cui, Y.; Martin, C.; Kimura, A.; Robinson, G.W.; Andrews, N.C.; Hennighausen, L. Hematopoietic-specific Stat5-null mice display microcytic hypochromic anemia associated with reduced transferrin receptor gene expression. *Blood* **2008**, *112*, 2071–2080. [CrossRef]
220. Kerenyi, M.A.; Grebien, F.; Gehart, H.; Schifrer, M.; Artaker, M.; Kovacic, B.; Beug, H.; Moriggl, R.; Mullner, E.W. Stat5 regulates cellular iron uptake of erythroid cells via IRP-2 and TfR-1. *Blood* **2008**, *112*, 3878–3888. [CrossRef]
221. Barash, I. Stat5 in the mammary gland: Controlling normal development and cancer. *J. Cell Physiol.* **2006**, *209*, 305–313. [CrossRef] [PubMed]
222. Cella, N.; Groner, B.; Hynes, N.E. Characterization of Stat5a and Stat5b homodimers and heterodimers and their association with the glucocortiocoid receptor in mammary cells. *Mol. Cell Biol.* **1998**, *18*, 1783–1792. [CrossRef] [PubMed]
223. Zeng, R.; Aoki, Y.; Yoshida, M.; Arai, K.; Watanabe, S. Stat5B shuttles between cytoplasm and nucleus in a cytokine-dependent and -independent manner. *J. Immunol.* **2002**, *168*, 4567–4575. [CrossRef] [PubMed]
224. Meinke, A.; Barahmand-Pour, F.; Wohrl, S.; Stoiber, D.; Decker, T. Activation of different Stat5 isoforms contributes to cell-type-restricted signaling in response to interferons. *Mol. Cell Biol.* **1996**, *16*, 6937–6944. [CrossRef] [PubMed]
225. Villarino, A.V.; Sciumè, G.; Davis, F.P.; Iwata, S.; Zitti, B.; Robinson, G.W.; Hennighausen, L.; Kanno, Y.; O'Shea, J.J. Subset- and tissue-defined STAT5 thresholds control homeostasis and function of innate lymphoid cells. *J. Exp. Med.* **2017**, *214*, 2999–3014. [CrossRef]
226. Maurer, B.; Farlik, M.; Sexl, V. It is a differentiation game: STAT5 in a new role. *Cell Death Differ.* **2017**, *24*, 953–954. [CrossRef]
227. Heltemes-Harris, L.M.; Farrar, M.A. The role of STAT5 in lymphocyte development and transformation. *Curr. Opin. Immunol.* **2012**, *24*, 146–152. [CrossRef]

228. Hoelbl, A.; Kovacic, B.; Kerenyi, M.A.; Simma, O.; Warsch, W.; Cui, Y.; Beug, H.; Hennighausen, L.; Moriggl, R.; Sexl, V. Clarifying the role of Stat5 in lymphoid development and Abelson-induced transformation. *Blood* **2006**, *107*, 4898–4906. [CrossRef]
229. Minieri, V.; De Dominici, M.; Porazzi, P.; Mariani, S.A.; Spinelli, O.; Rambaldi, A.; Peterson, L.F.; Porcu, P.; Nevalainen, M.T.; Calabretta, B. Targeting STAT5 or STAT5-Regulated Pathways Suppresses Leukemogenesis of Ph+ Acute Lymphoblastic Leukemia. *Cancer Res.* **2018**, *78*, 5793–5807. [CrossRef]
230. Gleixner, K.V.; Schneeweiss, M.; Eisenwort, G.; Berger, D.; Herrmann, H.; Blatt, K.; Greiner, G.; Byrgazov, K.; Hoermann, G.; Konopleva, M.; et al. Combined targeting of STAT3 and STAT5: A novel approach to overcome drug resistance in chronic myeloid leukemia. *Haematologica* **2017**, *102*, 1519–1529. [CrossRef]
231. Kaltenecker, D.; Themanns, M.; Mueller, K.M.; Spirk, K.; Golob-Schwarzl, N.; Friedbichler, K.; Kenner, L.; Haybaeck, J.; Moriggl, R. STAT5 deficiency in hepatocytes reduces diethylnitrosamine-induced liver tumorigenesis in mice. *Cytokine* **2018**. [CrossRef] [PubMed]
232. Boutillon, F.; Pigat, N.; Sala, L.S.; Reyes-Gomez, E.; Moriggl, R.; Guidotti, J.E.; Goffin, V. STAT5a/b Deficiency Delays, but does not Prevent, Prolactin-Driven Prostate Tumorigenesis in Mice. *Cancers* **2019**, *11*, 929. [CrossRef] [PubMed]
233. Lee, T.K.; Man, K.; Poon, R.T.P.; Lo, C.M.; Yuen, A.P.; Ng, I.O.; Ng, K.T.; Leonard, W.; Fan, S.T. Signal Transducers and Activators of Transcription 5b Activation Enhances Hepatocellular Carcinoma Aggressiveness through Induction of Epithelial-Mesenchymal Transition. *Cancer Res.* **2006**, *66*, 9948–9956. [CrossRef] [PubMed]
234. Johnston, A.N.; Bu, W.; Hein, S.; Garcia, S.; Camacho, L.; Xue, L.; Qin, L.; Nagi, C.; Hilsenbeck, S.G.; Kapali, J.; et al. Hyperprolactinemia-inducing antipsychotics increase breast cancer risk by activating JAK-STAT5 in precancerous lesions. *Breast Cancer Res.* **2018**, *20*, 42. [CrossRef]
235. Vafaizadeh, V.; Klemmt, P.; Brendel, C.; Weber, K.; Doebele, C.; Britt, K.; Grez, M.; Fehse, B.; Desrivieres, S.; Groner, B. Mammary epithelial reconstitution with gene-modified stem cells assigns roles to Stat5 in luminal alveolar cell fate decisions, differentiation, involution, and mammary tumor formation. *Stem Cells* **2010**, *28*, 928–938. [CrossRef]
236. Bessette, K.; Lang, M.L.; Fava, R.A.; Grundy, M.; Heinen, J.; Horne, L.; Spolski, R.; Al-Shami, A.; Morse, H.C., 3rd; Leonard, W.J.; et al. A Stat5b transgene is capable of inducing CD8+ lymphoblastic lymphoma in the absence of normal TCR/MHC signaling. *Blood* **2008**, *111*, 344–350. [CrossRef]
237. Xiong, H.; Su, W.Y.; Liang, Q.C.; Zhang, Z.G.; Chen, H.M.; Du, W.; Chen, Y.X.; Fang, J.Y. Inhibition of STAT5 induces G1 cell cycle arrest and reduces tumor cell invasion in human colorectal cancer cells. *Lab. Investig.* **2009**, *89*, 717–725. [CrossRef]
238. Koppikar, P.; Lui, V.W.; Man, D.; Xi, S.; Chai, R.L.; Nelson, E.; Tobey, A.B.; Grandis, J.R. Constitutive activation of signal transducer and activator of transcription 5 contributes to tumor growth, epithelial-mesenchymal transition, and resistance to epidermal growth factor receptor targeting. *Clin. Cancer Res.* **2008**, *14*, 7682–7690. [CrossRef]
239. Talati, P.G.; Gu, L.; Ellsworth, E.M.; Girondo, M.A.; Trerotola, M.; Hoang, D.T.; Leiby, B.; Dagvadorj, A.; McCue, P.A.; Lallas, C.D.; et al. Jak2-Stat5a/b Signaling Induces Epithelial-to-Mesenchymal Transition and Stem-Like Cell Properties in Prostate Cancer. *Am. J. Pathol.* **2015**, *185*, 2505–2522. [CrossRef]
240. Creamer, B.A.; Sakamoto, K.; Schmidt, J.W.; Triplett, A.A.; Moriggl, R.; Wagner, K.U. Stat5 promotes survival of mammary epithelial cells through transcriptional activation of a distinct promoter in Akt1. *Mol. Cell Biol.* **2010**, *30*, 2957–2970. [CrossRef]
241. Schmidt, J.W.; Wehde, B.L.; Sakamoto, K.; Triplett, A.A.; Anderson, S.M.; Tsichlis, P.N.; Leone, G.; Wagner, K.U. Stat5 regulates the phosphatidylinositol 3-kinase/Akt1 pathway during mammary gland development and tumorigenesis. *Mol. Cell Biol.* **2014**, *34*, 1363–1377. [CrossRef] [PubMed]
242. Tsuruyama, T.; Hiratsuka, T.; Jin, G.; Imai, Y.; Takeuchi, H.; Maruyama, Y.; Kanaya, K.; Ozeki, M.; Takakuwa, T.; Haga, H.; et al. Murine leukemia retrovirus integration induces the formation of transcription factor complexes on palindromic sequences in the signal transducer and activator of transcription factor 5a gene during the development of pre-B lymphomagenesis. *Am. J. Pathol.* **2011**, *178*, 1374–1386. [CrossRef] [PubMed]
243. Chen, Y.; Zhou, Q.; Zhang, L.; Zhong, Y.; Fan, G.; Zhang, Z.; Wang, R.; Jin, M.; Qiu, Y.; Kong, D. Stellettin B induces apoptosis in human chronic myeloid leukemia cells via targeting PI3K and Stat5. *Oncotarget* **2017**, *8*, 28906–28921. [CrossRef] [PubMed]

244. Dagvadorj, A.; Collins, S.; Jomain, J.B.; Abdulghani, J.; Karras, J.; Zellweger, T.; Li, H.; Nurmi, M.; Alanen, K.; Mirtti, T.; et al. Autocrine prolactin promotes prostate cancer cell growth via Janus kinase-2-signal transducer and activator of transcription-5a/b signaling pathway. *Endocrinology* **2007**, *148*, 3089–3101. [CrossRef] [PubMed]
245. Latha, K.; Li, M.; Chumbalkar, V.; Gururaj, A.; Hwang, Y.; Dakeng, S.; Sawaya, R.; Aldape, K.; Cavenee, W.K.; Bogler, O.; et al. Nuclear EGFRvIII-STAT5b complex contributes to glioblastoma cell survival by direct activation of the Bcl-XL promoter. *Int. J. Cancer* **2013**, *132*, 509–520. [CrossRef]
246. Chueh, F.-Y.; Leong, K.-F.; Yu, C.-L. Mitochondrial translocation of signal transducer and activator of transcription 5 (STAT5) in leukemic T cells and cytokine-stimulated cells. *Biochem. Biophys. Res. Commun.* **2010**, *402*, 778–783. [CrossRef]
247. Walker, S.R.; Xiang, M.; Frank, D.A. Distinct roles of STAT3 and STAT5 in the pathogenesis and targeted therapy of breast cancer. *Mol. Cell Endocrinol.* **2014**, *382*, 616–621. [CrossRef]
248. Sultan, A.S.; Xie, J.; LeBaron, M.J.; Ealley, E.L.; Nevalainen, M.T.; Rui, H. Stat5 promotes homotypic adhesion and inhibits invasive characteristics of human breast cancer cells. *Oncogene* **2005**, *24*, 746–760. [CrossRef]
249. Mallette, F.A.; Gaumont-Leclerc, M.F.; Ferbeyre, G. The DNA damage signaling pathway is a critical mediator of oncogene-induced senescence. *Genes Dev.* **2007**, *21*, 43–48. [CrossRef]
250. Nishikawa, H.; Sakaguchi, S. Regulatory T cells in cancer immunotherapy. *Curr. Opin. Immunol.* **2014**, *27*, 1–7. [CrossRef]
251. Knol, A.C.; Nguyen, J.M.; Quereux, G.; Brocard, A.; Khammari, A.; Dreno, B. Prognostic value of tumor-infiltrating Foxp3+ T-cell subpopulations in metastatic melanoma. *Exp. Derm.* **2011**, *20*, 430–434. [CrossRef] [PubMed]
252. Sasada, T.; Kimura, M.; Yoshida, Y.; Kanai, M.; Takabayashi, A. CD4+CD25+ regulatory T cells in patients with gastrointestinal malignancies: Possible involvement of regulatory T cells in disease progression. *Cancer* **2003**, *98*, 1089–1099. [CrossRef] [PubMed]
253. Zhao, P.; Li, J.; Tian, Y.; Mao, J.; Liu, X.; Feng, S.; Li, J.; Bian, Q.; Ji, H.; Zhang, L. Restoring Th17/Treg balance via modulation of STAT3 and STAT5 activation contributes to the amelioration of chronic obstructive pulmonary disease by Bufei Yishen formula. *J. Ethnopharmacol.* **2018**, *217*, 152–162. [CrossRef] [PubMed]
254. Burchill, M.A.; Yang, J.; Vogtenhuber, C.; Blazar, B.R.; Farrar, M.A. IL-2 receptor beta-dependent STAT5 activation is required for the development of Foxp3+ regulatory T cells. *J. Immunol.* **2007**, *178*, 280–290. [CrossRef]
255. O'Shea, J.J.; Paul, W.E. Mechanisms underlying lineage commitment and plasticity of helper CD4+ T cells. *Science* **2010**, *327*, 1098–1102. [CrossRef]
256. Li, X.; Kostareli, E.; Suffner, J.; Garbi, N.; Hammerling, G.J. Efficient Treg depletion induces T-cell infiltration and rejection of large tumors. *Eur. J. Immunol.* **2010**, *40*, 3325–3335. [CrossRef]
257. Fisher, S.A.; Aston, W.J.; Chee, J.; Khong, A.; Cleaver, A.L.; Solin, J.N.; Ma, S.; Lesterhuis, W.J.; Dick, I.; Holt, R.A.; et al. Transient Treg depletion enhances therapeutic anti-cancer vaccination. *Immun. Inflamm. Dis.* **2017**, *5*, 16–28. [CrossRef]
258. Schmidt, A.; Zhang, X.M.; Joshi, R.N.; Iqbal, S.; Wahlund, C.; Gabrielsson, S.; Harris, R.A.; Tegner, J. Human macrophages induce CD4(+)Foxp3(+) regulatory T cells via binding and re-release of TGF-beta. *Immunol. Cell Biol.* **2016**, *94*, 747–762. [CrossRef]
259. Goswami, K.K.; Ghosh, T.; Ghosh, S.; Sarkar, M.; Bose, A.; Baral, R. Tumor promoting role of anti-tumor macrophages in tumor microenvironment. *Cell Immunol.* **2017**, *316*, 1–10. [CrossRef]
260. Müller-Hermelink, N.; Braumüller, H.; Pichler, B.; Wieder, T.; Mailhammer, R.; Schaak, K.; Ghoreschi, K.; Yazdi, A.; Haubner, R.; Sander, C.A.; et al. TNFR1 Signaling and IFN-γ Signaling Determine whether T Cells Induce Tumor Dormancy or Promote Multistage Carcinogenesis. *Cancer Cell* **2008**, *13*, 507–518. [CrossRef]
261. Edwards, J.P.; Thornton, A.M.; Shevach, E.M. Release of active TGF-beta1 from the latent TGF-beta1/GARP complex on T regulatory cells is mediated by integrin beta8. *J. Immunol.* **2014**, *193*, 2843–2849. [CrossRef] [PubMed]
262. Wang, Y.; Schafer, C.C.; Hough, K.P.; Tousif, S.; Duncan, S.R.; Kearney, J.F.; Ponnazhagan, S.; Hsu, H.C.; Deshane, J.S. Myeloid-Derived Suppressor Cells Impair B Cell Responses in Lung Cancer through IL-7 and STAT5. *J. Immunol.* **2018**, *201*, 278–295. [CrossRef] [PubMed]
263. Nurieva, R.I.; Podd, A.; Chen, Y.; Alekseev, A.M.; Yu, M.; Qi, X.; Huang, H.; Wen, R.; Wang, J.; Li, H.S.; et al. STAT5 protein negatively regulates T follicular helper (Tfh) cell generation and function. *J. Biol. Chem.* **2012**, *287*, 11234–11239. [CrossRef] [PubMed]

264. Buck, M.D.; O'Sullivan, D.; Klein Geltink, R.I.; Curtis, J.D.; Chang, C.H.; Sanin, D.E.; Qiu, J.; Kretz, O.; Braas, D.; van der Windt, G.J.; et al. Mitochondrial Dynamics Controls T Cell Fate through Metabolic Programming. *Cell* **2016**, *166*, 63–76. [CrossRef]
265. Berod, L.; Friedrich, C.; Nandan, A.; Freitag, J.; Hagemann, S.; Harmrolfs, K.; Sandouk, A.; Hesse, C.; Castro, C.N.; Bahre, H.; et al. De novo fatty acid synthesis controls the fate between regulatory T and T helper 17 cells. *Nat. Med.* **2014**, *20*, 1327–1333. [CrossRef]
266. Michalek, R.D.; Gerriets, V.A.; Jacobs, S.R.; Macintyre, A.N.; MacIver, N.J.; Mason, E.F.; Sullivan, S.A.; Nichols, A.G.; Rathmell, J.C. Cutting edge: Distinct glycolytic and lipid oxidative metabolic programs are essential for effector and regulatory CD4+ T cell subsets. *J. Immunol.* **2011**, *186*, 3299–3303. [CrossRef]
267. Galluzzi, L.; Baehrecke, E.H.; Ballabio, A.; Boya, P.; Bravo-San Pedro, J.M.; Cecconi, F.; Choi, A.M.; Chu, C.T.; Codogno, P.; Colombo, M.I.; et al. Molecular definitions of autophagy and related processes. *EMBO J.* **2017**, *36*, 1811–1836. [CrossRef]
268. Singh, R.; Kaushik, S.; Wang, Y.; Xiang, Y.; Novak, I.; Komatsu, M.; Tanaka, K.; Cuervo, A.M.; Czaja, M.J. Autophagy regulates lipid metabolism. *Nature* **2009**, *458*, 1131–1135. [CrossRef]
269. Lin, J.X.; Li, P.; Liu, D.; Jin, H.T.; He, J.; Ata Ur Rasheed, M.; Rochman, Y.; Wang, L.; Cui, K.; Liu, C.; et al. Critical Role of STAT5 transcription factor tetramerization for cytokine responses and normal immune function. *Immunity* **2012**, *36*, 586–599. [CrossRef]
270. Owen, D.L.; Farrar, M.A. STAT5 and CD4 (+) T Cell Immunity. *F1000Research* **2017**, *6*, 32. [CrossRef]
271. Grange, M.; Buferne, M.; Verdeil, G.; Leserman, L.; Schmitt-Verhulst, A.M.; Auphan-Anezin, N. Activated STAT5 promotes long-lived cytotoxic CD8+ T cells that induce regression of autochthonous melanoma. *Cancer Res.* **2012**, *72*, 76–87. [CrossRef] [PubMed]
272. Gotthardt, D.; Putz, E.M.; Grundschober, E.; Prchal-Murphy, M.; Straka, E.; Kudweis, P.; Heller, G.; Bago-Horvath, Z.; Witalisz-Siepracka, A.; Cumaraswamy, A.A.; et al. STAT5 Is a Key Regulator in NK Cells and Acts as a Molecular Switch from Tumor Surveillance to Tumor Promotion. *Cancer Discov.* **2016**, *6*, 414–429. [CrossRef] [PubMed]
273. Wolf, D.; Sopper, S.; Pircher, A.; Gastl, G.; Wolf, A.M. Treg(s) in Cancer: Friends or Foe? *J. Cell Physiol.* **2015**, *230*, 2598–2605. [CrossRef] [PubMed]
274. Turkson, J.; Kim, J.S.; Zhang, S.; Yuan, J.; Huang, M.; Glenn, M.; Haura, E.; Sebti, S.; Hamilton, A.D.; Jove, R. Novel peptidomimetic inhibitors of signal transducer and activator of transcription 3 dimerization and biological activity. *Mol. Cancer* **2004**, *3*, 261–269.
275. Fontaine, F.; Overman, J.; Francois, M. Pharmacological manipulation of transcription factor protein-protein interactions: Opportunities and obstacles. *Cell Regen.* **2015**, *4*, 2. [CrossRef]
276. Siddiquee, K.; Zhang, S.; Guida, W.C.; Blaskovich, M.A.; Greedy, B.; Lawrence, H.R.; Yip, M.L.; Jove, R.; McLaughlin, M.M.; Lawrence, N.J.; et al. Selective chemical probe inhibitor of Stat3, identified through structure-based virtual screening, induces antitumor activity. *Proc. Natl. Acad. Sci. USA* **2007**, *104*, 7391–7396. [CrossRef]
277. Siddiquee, K.A.; Gunning, P.T.; Glenn, M.; Katt, W.P.; Zhang, S.; Schrock, C.; Sebti, S.M.; Jove, R.; Hamilton, A.D.; Turkson, J. An oxazole-based small-molecule Stat3 inhibitor modulates Stat3 stability and processing and induces antitumor cell effects. *ACS Chem. Biol.* **2007**, *2*, 787–798. [CrossRef]
278. Sato, K.; Tsuchiya, M.; Saldanha, J.; Koishihara, Y.; Ohsugi, Y.; Kishimoto, T.; Bendig, M.M. Reshaping a human antibody to inhibit the interleukin 6-dependent tumor cell growth. *Cancer Res.* **1993**, *53*, 851–856.
279. Mihara, M.; Kasutani, K.; Okazaki, M.; Nakamura, A.; Kawai, S.; Sugimoto, M.; Matsumoto, Y.; Ohsugi, Y. Tocilizumab inhibits signal transduction mediated by both mIL-6R and sIL-6R, but not by the receptors of other members of IL-6 cytokine family. *Int. Immunopharmacol.* **2005**, *5*, 1731–1740. [CrossRef]
280. Nishimoto, N.; Sasai, M.; Shima, Y.; Nakagawa, M.; Matsumoto, T.; Shirai, T.; Kishimoto, T.; Yoshizaki, K. Improvement in Castleman's disease by humanized anti-interleukin-6 receptor antibody therapy. *Blood* **2000**, *95*, 56–61. [CrossRef]
281. Nishimoto, N.; Yoshizaki, K.; Miyasaka, N.; Yamamoto, K.; Kawai, S.; Takeuchi, T.; Hashimoto, J.; Azuma, J.; Kishimoto, T. Treatment of rheumatoid arthritis with humanized anti-interleukin-6 receptor antibody: A multicenter, double-blind, placebo-controlled trial. *Arthritis Rheum.* **2004**, *50*, 1761–1769. [CrossRef] [PubMed]
282. Dhillon, S. Intravenous Tocilizumab: A Review of Its Use in Adults with Rheumatoid Arthritis. *BioDrugs* **2013**, *28*, 75–106. [CrossRef] [PubMed]

283. Le, R.Q.; Li, L.; Yuan, W.; Shord, S.S.; Nie, L.; Habtemariam, B.A.; Przepiorka, D.; Farrell, A.T.; Pazdur, R. FDA Approval Summary: Tocilizumab for Treatment of Chimeric Antigen Receptor T Cell-Induced Severe or Life-Threatening Cytokine Release Syndrome. *Oncologist* **2018**, *23*, 943–947. [CrossRef] [PubMed]
284. Dambacher, J.; Beigel, F.; Seiderer, J.; Haller, D.; Goke, B.; Auernhammer, C.J.; Brand, S. Interleukin 31 mediates MAP kinase and STAT1/3 activation in intestinal epithelial cells and its expression is upregulated in inflammatory bowel disease. *Gut* **2007**, *56*, 1257–1265. [CrossRef] [PubMed]
285. Song, L.; Smith, M.A.; Doshi, P.; Sasser, K.; Fulp, W.; Altiok, S.; Haura, E.B. Antitumor efficacy of the anti-interleukin-6 (IL-6) antibody siltuximab in mouse xenograft models of lung cancer. *J. Thorac. Oncol.* **2014**, *9*, 974–982. [CrossRef] [PubMed]
286. Chen, R.; Chen, B. Siltuximab (CNTO 328): A promising option for human malignancies. *Drug Des. Devel.* **2015**, *9*, 3455–3458. [CrossRef] [PubMed]
287. Fizazi, K.; De Bono, J.S.; Flechon, A.; Heidenreich, A.; Voog, E.; Davis, N.B.; Qi, M.; Bandekar, R.; Vermeulen, J.T.; Cornfeld, M.; et al. Randomised phase II study of siltuximab (CNTO 328), an anti-IL-6 monoclonal antibody, in combination with mitoxantrone/prednisone versus mitoxantrone/prednisone alone in metastatic castration-resistant prostate cancer. *Eur. J. Cancer* **2012**, *48*, 85–93. [CrossRef]
288. Takata, F.; Dohgu, S.; Matsumoto, J.; Machida, T.; Sakaguchi, S.; Kimura, I.; Yamauchi, A.; Kataoka, Y. Oncostatin M-induced blood-brain barrier impairment is due to prolonged activation of STAT3 signaling in vitro. *J. Cell Biochem.* **2018**, *119*, 9055–9063. [CrossRef]
289. Jorcyk, C.L.; Holzer, R.G.; Ryan, R.E. Oncostatin M induces cell detachment and enhances the metastatic capacity of T-47D human breast carcinoma cells. *Cytokine* **2006**, *33*, 323–336. [CrossRef]
290. Sterbova, S.; Karlsson, T.; Persson, E. Oncostatin M induces tumorigenic properties in non-transformed human prostate epithelial cells, in part through activation of signal transducer and activator of transcription 3 (STAT3). *Biochem. Biophys. Res. Commun.* **2018**, *498*, 769–774. [CrossRef]
291. Richards, C.D. The enigmatic cytokine oncostatin m and roles in disease. *ISRN Inflamm.* **2013**, *2013*, 512103. [CrossRef] [PubMed]
292. Hintzen, C.; Evers, C.; Lippok, B.E.; Volkmer, R.; Heinrich, P.C.; Radtke, S.; Hermanns, H.M. Box 2 region of the oncostatin M receptor determines specificity for recruitment of Janus kinases and STAT5 activation. *J. Biol. Chem.* **2008**, *283*, 19465–19477. [CrossRef]
293. Hermanns, H.M.; Radtke, S.; Schaper, F.; Heinrich, P.C.; Behrmann, I. Non-redundant signal transduction of interleukin-6-type cytokines. The adapter protein Shc is specifically recruited to rhe oncostatin M receptor. *J. Biol. Chem.* **2000**, *275*, 40742–40748. [CrossRef] [PubMed]
294. Choy, E.H.; Bendit, M.; McAleer, D.; Liu, F.; Feeney, M.; Brett, S.; Zamuner, S.; Campanile, A.; Toso, J. Safety, tolerability, pharmacokinetics and pharmacodynamics of an anti- oncostatin M monoclonal antibody in rheumatoid arthritis: Results from phase II randomized, placebo-controlled trials. *Arthritis Res.* **2013**, *15*, R132. [CrossRef] [PubMed]
295. Poling, J.; Gajawada, P.; Richter, M.; Lorchner, H.; Polyakova, V.; Kostin, S.; Shin, J.; Boettger, T.; Walther, T.; Rees, W.; et al. Therapeutic targeting of the oncostatin M receptor-beta prevents inflammatory heart failure. *Basic Res. Cardiol.* **2014**, *109*, 396. [CrossRef] [PubMed]
296. Liu, Q.; Du, Y.; Li, K.; Zhang, W.; Feng, X.; Hao, J.; Li, H.; Liu, S. Anti-OSM Antibody Inhibits Tubulointerstitial Lesion in a Murine Model of Lupus Nephritis. *Mediat. Inflamm.* **2017**, *2017*, 3038514. [CrossRef] [PubMed]
297. Kucia-Tran, J.A.; Tulkki, V.; Scarpini, C.G.; Smith, S.; Wallberg, M.; Paez-Ribes, M.; Araujo, A.M.; Botthoff, J.; Feeney, M.; Hughes, K.; et al. Anti-oncostatin M antibody inhibits the pro-malignant effects of oncostatin M receptor overexpression in squamous cell carcinoma. *J. Pathol.* **2018**, *244*, 283–295. [CrossRef] [PubMed]
298. Robson, M.J.; Turner, R.C.; Naser, Z.J.; McCurdy, C.R.; O'Callaghan, J.P.; Huber, J.D.; Matsumoto, R.R. SN79, a sigma receptor antagonist, attenuates methamphetamine-induced astrogliosis through a blockade of OSMR/gp130 signaling and STAT3 phosphorylation. *Exp. Neurol.* **2014**, *254*, 180–189. [CrossRef]
299. Bottos, A.; Gotthardt, D.; Gill, J.W.; Gattelli, A.; Frei, A.; Tzankov, A.; Sexl, V.; Wodnar-Filipowicz, A.; Hynes, N.E. Decreased NK-cell tumour immunosurveillance consequent to JAK inhibition enhances metastasis in breast cancer models. *Nat. Commun.* **2016**, *7*, 12258. [CrossRef]
300. Doherty, M.R.; Jackson, M.W. Using interferon-beta to combat cancer stem cell properties in triple negative breast cancer. *Oncoscience* **2018**, *5*, 169–171. [CrossRef]
301. Doherty, M.R.; Parvani, J.G.; Tamagno, I.; Junk, D.J.; Bryson, B.L.; Cheon, H.J.; Stark, G.R.; Jackson, M.W.

The opposing effects of interferon-beta and oncostatin-M as regulators of cancer stem cell plasticity in triple-negative breast cancer. *Breast Cancer Res.* **2019**, *21*, 54. [CrossRef] [PubMed]

302. Sistigu, A.; Yamazaki, T.; Vacchelli, E.; Chaba, K.; Enot, D.P.; Adam, J.; Vitale, I.; Goubar, A.; Baracco, E.E.; Remedios, C.; et al. Cancer cell-autonomous contribution of type I interferon signaling to the efficacy of chemotherapy. *Nat. Med.* **2014**, *20*, 1301–1309. [CrossRef] [PubMed]
303. Yang, X.; Zhang, X.; Fu, M.L.; Weichselbaum, R.R.; Gajewski, T.F.; Guo, Y.; Fu, Y.X. Targeting the tumor microenvironment with interferon-beta bridges innate and adaptive immune responses. *Cancer Cell* **2014**, *25*, 37–48. [CrossRef] [PubMed]
304. Ling, X.; Marini, F.; Konopleva, M.; Schober, W.; Shi, Y.; Burks, J.; Clise-Dwyer, K.; Wang, R.Y.; Zhang, W.; Yuan, X.; et al. Mesenchymal Stem Cells Overexpressing IFN-beta Inhibit Breast Cancer Growth and Metastases through Stat3 Signaling in a Syngeneic Tumor Model. *Cancer Microenviron.* **2010**, *3*, 83–95. [CrossRef]
305. Burstein, M.D.; Tsimelzon, A.; Poage, G.M.; Covington, K.R.; Contreras, A.; Fuqua, S.A.; Savage, M.I.; Osborne, C.K.; Hilsenbeck, S.G.; Chang, J.C.; et al. Comprehensive genomic analysis identifies novel subtypes and targets of triple-negative breast cancer. *Clin. Cancer Res.* **2015**, *21*, 1688–1698. [CrossRef]
306. Bidwell, B.N.; Slaney, C.Y.; Withana, N.P.; Forster, S.; Cao, Y.; Loi, S.; Andrews, D.; Mikeska, T.; Mangan, N.E.; Samarajiwa, S.A.; et al. Silencing of Irf7 pathways in breast cancer cells promotes bone metastasis through immune escape. *Nat. Med.* **2012**, *18*, 1224–1231. [CrossRef]
307. Liu, S.; Lachapelle, J.; Leung, S.; Gao, D.; Foulkes, W.D.; Nielsen, T.O. CD8+ lymphocyte infiltration is an independent favorable prognostic indicator in basal-like breast cancer. *Breast Cancer Res.* **2012**, *14*, R48. [CrossRef]
308. Xie, C.; Liu, C.; Wu, B.; Lin, Y.; Ma, T.; Xiong, H.; Wang, Q.; Li, Z.; Ma, C.; Tu, Z. Effects of IRF1 and IFN-beta interaction on the M1 polarization of macrophages and its antitumor function. *Int. J. Mol. Med.* **2016**, *38*, 148–160. [CrossRef]
309. Moreira-Teixeira, L.; Sousa, J.; McNab, F.W.; Torrado, E.; Cardoso, F.; Machado, H.; Castro, F.; Cardoso, V.; Gaifem, J.; Wu, X.; et al. Type I IFN Inhibits Alternative Macrophage Activation during Mycobacterium tuberculosis Infection and Leads to Enhanced Protection in the Absence of IFN-gamma Signaling. *J. Immunol.* **2016**, *197*, 4714–4726. [CrossRef]
310. Pylaeva, E.; Lang, S.; Jablonska, J. The Essential Role of Type I Interferons in Differentiation and Activation of Tumor-Associated Neutrophils. *Front. Immunol.* **2016**, *7*, 629. [CrossRef]
311. Brockwell, N.K.; Owen, K.L.; Zanker, D.; Spurling, A.; Rautela, J.; Duivenvoorden, H.M.; Baschuk, N.; Caramia, F.; Loi, S.; Darcy, P.K.; et al. Neoadjuvant Interferons: Critical for Effective PD-1-Based Immunotherapy in TNBC. *Cancer Immunol. Res.* **2017**, *5*, 871–884. [CrossRef] [PubMed]
312. Parker, B.S.; Rautela, J.; Hertzog, P.J. Antitumour actions of interferons: Implications for cancer therapy. *Nat. Rev. Cancer* **2016**, *16*, 131–144. [CrossRef] [PubMed]
313. Essers, M.A.; Offner, S.; Blanco-Bose, W.E.; Waibler, Z.; Kalinke, U.; Duchosal, M.A.; Trumpp, A. IFNalpha activates dormant haematopoietic stem cells in vivo. *Nature* **2009**, *458*, 904–908. [CrossRef] [PubMed]
314. Ma, H.; Jin, S.; Yang, W.; Zhou, G.; Zhao, M.; Fang, S.; Zhang, Z.; Hu, J. Interferon-alpha enhances the antitumour activity of EGFR-targeted therapies by upregulating RIG-I in head and neck squamous cell carcinoma. *Br. J. Cancer* **2018**, *118*, 509–521. [CrossRef] [PubMed]
315. Cheon, H.; Holvey-Bates, E.G.; Schoggins, J.W.; Forster, S.; Hertzog, P.; Imanaka, N.; Rice, C.M.; Jackson, M.W.; Junk, D.J.; Stark, G.R. IFNbeta-dependent increases in STAT1, STAT2, and IRF9 mediate resistance to viruses and DNA damage. *EMBO J.* **2013**, *32*, 2751–2763. [CrossRef]

11

STAT3 Mutation is Associated with STAT3 Activation in CD30⁺ ALK⁻ ALCL

Emma I. Andersson [1,2,3,†], Oscar Brück [1,2,†], Till Braun [4], Susanna Mannisto [5], Leena Saikko [6], Sonja Lagström [7], Pekka Ellonen [7], Sirpa Leppä [5], Marco Herling [4], Panu E. Kovanen [6] and Satu Mustjoki [1,2,*]

1 Hematology Research Unit Helsinki, Department of Hematology, University of Helsinki and Helsinki University Hospital Comprehensive Cancer Center, 00290 Helsinki, Finland; emma.andersson@hus.fi (E.I.A.); oscar.bruck@helsinki.fi (O.B.)

2 Translational Immunology Research program and Department of Clinical Chemistry and Hematology, University of Helsinki, 00014 Helsinki, Finland

3 HUSLAB, Laboratory of Genetics, Helsinki University Hospital, 00290 Helsinki, Finland

4 Department I of Internal Medicine, CMMC, CECAD, CIO-ABCD, University of Cologne, 50931 Cologne, Germany; till.braun@uk-koeln.de (T.B.); marco.herling@uk-koeln.de (M.H.)

5 Department of Oncology, Comprehensive Cancer Center, Helsinki University Hospital, 00290 Helsinki, Finland; susanna.mannisto@hus.fi (S.M.); sirpa.leppa@hus.fi (S.L.)

6 Department of Pathology, HUSLAB, Helsinki University Central Hospital and University of Helsinki, 00290 Helsinki, Finland; leena.saikko@helsinki.fi (L.S.); panu.kovanen@helsinki.fi (P.E.K.)

7 Institute for Molecular Medicine Finland (FIMM), University of Helsinki, 00014 Helsinki, Finland; sonja.lagstrom@kreftregisteret.no (S.L.); pekka.ellonen@helsinki.fi (P.E.)

* Correspondence: satu.mustjoki@helsinki.fi

† These authors contributed equally to this work.

Abstract: Peripheral T-cell lymphomas (PTCL) are a heterogeneous, and often aggressive group of non-Hodgkin lymphomas. Recent advances in the molecular and genetic characterization of PTCLs have helped to delineate differences and similarities between the various subtypes, and the JAK/STAT pathway has been found to play an important oncogenic role. Here, we aimed to characterize the JAK/STAT pathway in PTCL subtypes and investigate whether the activation of the pathway correlates with the frequency of *STAT* gene mutations. Patient samples from AITL (n = 30), ALCL (n = 21) and PTCL-NOS (n = 12) cases were sequenced for *STAT3, STAT5B, JAK1, JAK3,* and *RHOA* mutations using amplicon sequencing and stained immunohistochemically for pSTAT3, pMAPK, and pAKT. We discovered *STAT3* mutations in 13% of AITL, 13% of ALK⁺ ALCL, 38% of ALK⁻ ALCL and 17% of PTCL-NOS cases. However, no *STAT5B* mutations were found and *JAK* mutations were only present in ALK⁻ ALCL (15%). Concurrent mutations were found in all subgroups except ALK⁺ ALCL where *STAT3* mutations were always seen alone. High pY-STAT3 expression was observed especially in AITL and ALCL samples. When studying JAK-STAT pathway mutations, pY-STAT3 expression was highest in PTCLs harboring either *JAK1* or *STAT3* mutations and CD30⁺ phenotype representing primarily ALK⁻ ALCLs. Further investigation is needed to elucidate the molecular mechanisms of JAK-STAT pathway activation in PTCL.

Keywords: lymphoma; T-cells; STAT3; RHOA; NGS

---

1. Introduction

Peripheral T-cell lymphomas (PTCLs) form a heterogeneous, uncommon, and often aggressive group of non-Hodgkin's lymphomas (NHL) representing approximately 10–15% of all new NHL diagnoses [1]. The most prevalent PTLCs are PTCL not otherwise specified (NOS), angioimmunoblastic

T-cell lymphoma (AITL), anaplastic lymphoma kinase–negative (ALK^- ALCL), and anaplastic lymphoma kinase-positive anaplastic large cell lymphoma (ALK^+ ALCL) [2,3].

Despite generally favorable response rates to chemotherapy, remissions are often not durable, and as such the natural history of PTCL is characterized by relapses and refractory disease. For this reason, upfront hematopoietic stem cell transplantation (HSCT) is often recommended in first remission for patients who are fit and have chemo-sensitive disease [4]. For patients who are not suitable for transplantation, chances of long-term disease control are very limited, with an average progression-free survival (PFS) of 5.5 months [5]. In this setting, optimal therapeutic approaches remain undefined representing an unmet clinical need.

Recent advances in the molecular and genetic characterization of PTCL have helped to delineate differences and similarities between the various subtypes [6]. Several recurrent mutations have been identified in small subsets of patients potentially enabling more accurate disease classification and guide treatment decisions. In AITL, the three most commonly identified genetic lesions occur in the Tet methylcytosine dioxygenase 2 gene (*TET2*), the Ras homolog gene family, member A (*RHOA*), and the isocitrate dehydrogenase 2 gene (*IDH2*). Besides AITL, *TET2* mutations can be seen with a high frequency also in PTCL-NOS with a T follicular helper cell phenotype [7]. RHOA, a small GTPase participating in T-cell activation and polarization, has recently been found to have a specific G17V mutation in 68% of AITL cases [8], predominantly in the background of *TET2* mutations. The overwhelming majority of *IDH2* mutations in PTCL affect the R172 residue [9]. However, *STAT3* mutations are relatively uncommon (5%) in AITL [10].

In ALK^+ ALCL, the ALK chimeras activate STAT3, thus maintaining the neoplastic phenotype in ALK^+ ALCL. In concordance with this, gene expression profiling has revealed a transcriptional gene signature including *ALK*, *TNFRSF8* (*CD30*), *MUC1*, Th17-associated genes (*IL-17A*, *IL-17F*, and *ROR-γ*), a small group of immunoregulatory cytokines and receptors regulating STAT3 pathway [11].

A systematic characterization of the genetic alterations driving ALCL was recently undertaken using sequencing strategies. Activating mutations of *JAK1* and *STAT3* genes were found in 20% of ALK^- ALCLs, 38% of which displayed double lesions [12]. As the JAK/STAT pathway has a critical role in hematopoietic development, it is not surprising that it plays, when deregulated, an important oncogenic role in lymphoproliferative malignancies [13]. Many cancers and hematologic malignancies have been associated with the constitutive activation of the STAT family of proteins, which depends on JAK-mediated tyrosine phosphorylation for transcriptional activation [14]. In particular, activated JAK1/STAT3 and JAK2/STAT5 have been shown to facilitate T-cell transformation [15,16]. Activating mutations of *JAK1-3* and *STAT3-5* have also been found in a subset of NK/T-cell lymphomas, non-hepatosplenic gamma-delta T-cell lymphoma, large granular lymphocytic leukemia and T-cell prolymphocytic leukemia [10,17–22].

Here, we aimed to further characterize the JAK/STAT pathway in PTCL by investigating whether the activation of the pathway quantified with immunohistochemistry correlates with the frequency of *JAK*, *STAT*, and *RHOA* mutations. In addition, we associated JAK-STAT pathway activation with prognosis and essential clinical and pathological parameters. Finally, we identified novel therapeutic approaches for patients with high STAT3 phosphorylation using Reverse Phase Protein Array and drug sensitivity data from the Broad Institute Cancer Cell Line Encyclopedia (CCLE).

2. Results

2.1. *STAT3 Mutations Are Frequent in PTCLs*

As STAT3 is constitutively expressed in both AITLs and ALCLs, we sequenced for *STAT3* and *STAT5B* mutations. The entire *STAT3* gene and the hotspot SH2-domain of *STAT5B* were screened by targeted amplicon sequencing in 63 patients with T-cell lymphoma. We discovered that 13% of AITL and ALK^+ ALCL cases harbored *STAT3* mutations, while 17% of PTCL-NOS cases were found to harbor *STAT3* mutations (Table 1). The highest frequency of *STAT3* mutations was found in the ALK^- ALCL subgroup (38%). The frequency of *STAT3* mutations in the entire patient cohort was 19%. While most mutations were found in the SH2-domain of *STAT3*, we observed one K290T mutation in the coiled coil domain and three patients harbored a P715L mutation in the transactivation domain (Figure 1 and Table S1). The most prevalent mutation type was the P715L mutation and the E616 deletion, which were identified in three patients each. No *STAT5B* SH2-domain mutations were identified in this cohort. *JAK1* mutations were found in two ALK⁻ ALCL patients (15%). Both mutations (G902R and G1097C) were seen in the protein tyrosine kinase domain of *JAK1*. No *JAK3* mutations were detected in any subgroup.

Table 1. *STAT3, JAK1/3,* and *RHOA* mutation frequencies in PTCLs.

PTCL Subtype	*n*	*STAT3* Mutation Frequency	*JAK1/3* Mutation Frequency	*RHOA* Mutation Frequency	Co-Occuring Mutations
AITL	30	13%	0%	70%	10%
NOS	12	17%	0%	17%	8%
ALK^+ ALCL	8	13%	0%	0%	None
ALK^- ALCL	13	38%	15%	0%	8%
All	63	19%	3%	37%	8%

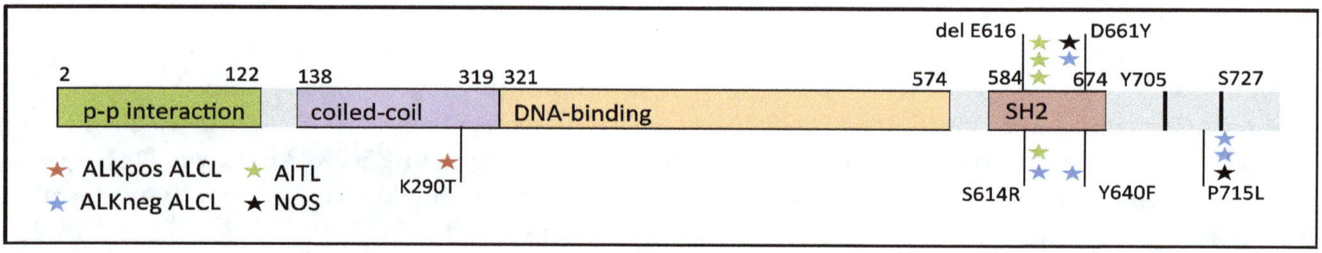

Figure 1. *STAT3* structure and mutation sites in ALCL, AITL, and PTCL-NOS patients of the study cohort.

As *RHOA* mutations are highly prevalent in AITL and have been found to cause activation of the MAPK/PI3K/AKT pathway and T cell receptor signaling, the hotspot mutation G17V was also screened [23,24]. The results showed that these mutations were frequent in AITL (70%) and PTCL-NOS (17%) but remained absent in ALCLs (Table 1). Some cases harbored both *STAT3* and *RHOA* mutations (10%). DNA samples from nodular lymphocyte predominant Hodgkin lymphoma with abundant follicular T helper cells ($n = 13$), were also available for *STAT3/STAT5B* and *RHOA* screening but no mutations were detected in these samples.

2.2. STAT3 Phosphorylation Levels Are Highest in ALK^+ and ALK^- ALCL Cases

To characterize JAK-STAT pathway activation, we stained for pY-STAT3, pMAPK, and pAKT in AITL ($n = 29$), ALCL ($n = 20$) and PTCL-NOS ($n = 12$) patients and control lymph nodes ($n = 4$) using immunohistochemistry (Supplementary Figure S1). The differences between disease groups were significant notably for phosphorylation of pY-STAT3 and recapitulated well previous reports [25]. Further post-hoc analysis showed that pY-STAT3 was shown to be more frequently phosphorylated in AITL (mean = 43.7%) and ALCL (ALK^-: mean = 62.3%, ALK^+: mean = 79.7%) patients compared to control lymph nodes (mean 12.6%; Figure 2).

MAPK phosphorylation was significantly elevated in AITL patients (mean 10.5%) followed by ALK^- ALCL (mean 6.8%) and PTCL NOS (5.2%) when compared to control lymph node (Figure 2). No significant difference in pAKT levels between PTCL patients and control lymph nodes was observed.

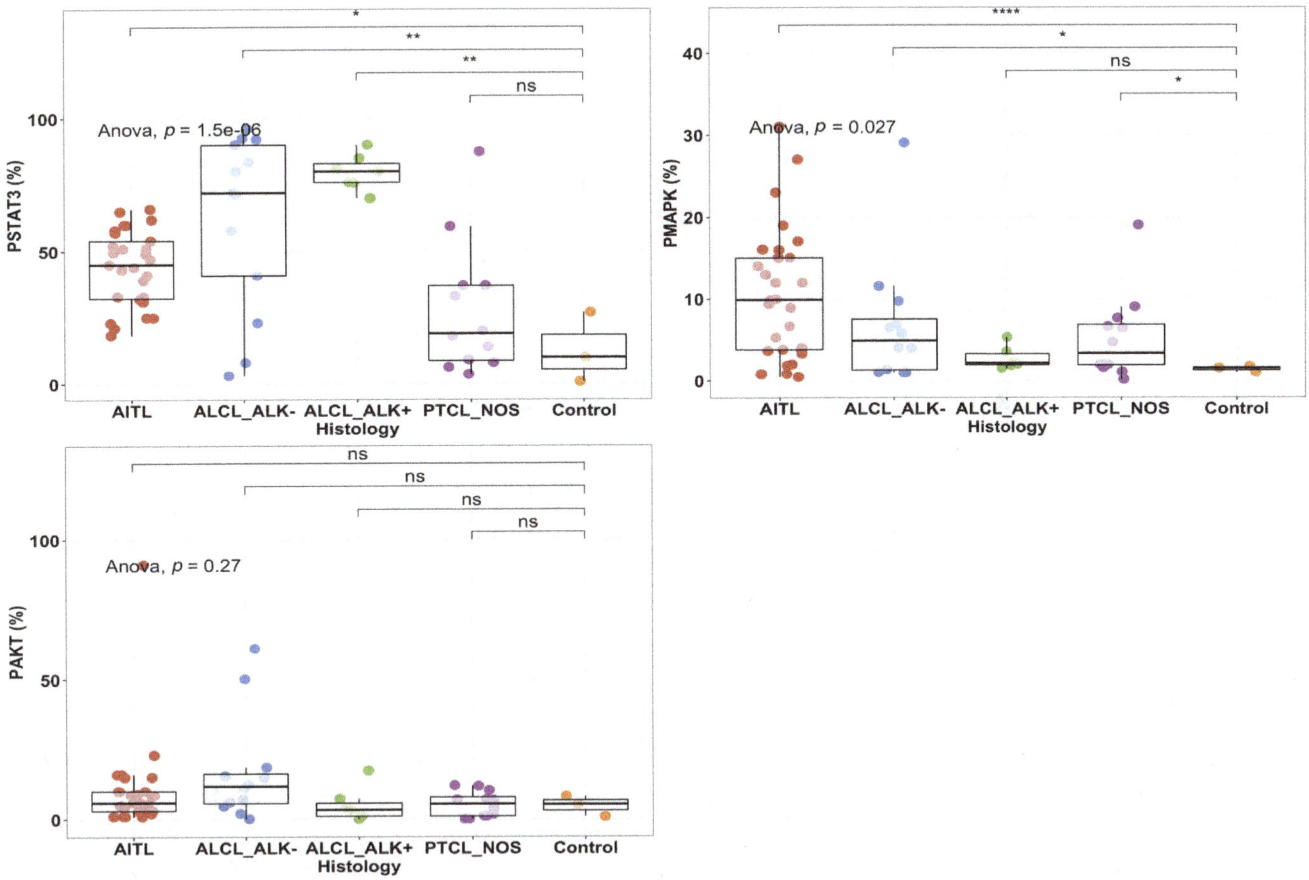

Figure 2. Phosphorylation percentage of pY-STAT3, MAPK, and AKT in PTCL subgroups and healthy controls (n = 2–3) analyzed by immunohistochemistry. Individual dots represent the proportion of positive cells for pSTAT3, pMAPK, and pAKT. Boxplots represent the median and interquartile range of protein phosphorylation levels. The antibodies used were specific for Tyr705 (pStat3), Thr202/Tyr204 (pMAPK), and Thr450 (pAKT). Comparison was analyzed with ANOVA and post-hoc tests between disease groups and healthy controls. *: $p < 0.05$; **: $p < 0.01$, ****: $p < 0.0001$; ns: not significant.

To confirm the findings and study STAT3 activation in other T cell malignancies, we measured STAT3 and pY-STAT3 levels by Western blotting in ALCL, acute T-lymphoblastic leukemia (T-ALL), NK/T-cell lymphoma (NKT), T-cell large granular lymphocyte leukemia (T-LGL), and PTCL cell lines (Figure 3). We confirmed high phosphorylation of pY-STAT3 (Tyr705) in ALCL but not in other T cell malignancies. Total STAT3 was most prominent in PTCL, ALCL and T-ALL cell lines. High JAK3 phosphorylation was observed in SupM2, Karpas299 and TLRB1 (ALCL) as well as NKL (NKT) cell lines and was not associated with pY-STAT3 phosphorylation.

To further investigate the association of protein expression to transcriptome data, we compared the *JAK1, JAK3, AKT,* and *MAPK* RNA level expression with *STAT3* RNA level expression and $pSTAT3^{Tyr705}$ phosphorylation defined with *reverse phase protein arrays* (RPPA) from the CCLE database (Figure S2). Both *STAT3* expression (535 vs. 198 CPM $p = 0.003$, t-test) and phosphorylation (3.6 vs. −0.10 RPPA unit, $p < 0.001$) were observed to be superior in ALCL than non-ALCL malignant T-cells as shown in Figure 2. Higher *JAK3* expression was noted in ALCL over non-ALCL lines (364 vs. 53 CPM, $p < 0.001$), and correlated with *STAT3* expression ($r = 0.60$, $p = 0.01$). Moreover, higher *MAPK* expression was detected in ALCL over non-ALCL cell lines (127 vs. 68, $p = 0.05$), which correlated with *STAT3* expression ($r = 0.65$, $p = 0.006$). No correlation between *STAT3* and *JAK1* or *AKT* expression was observed.

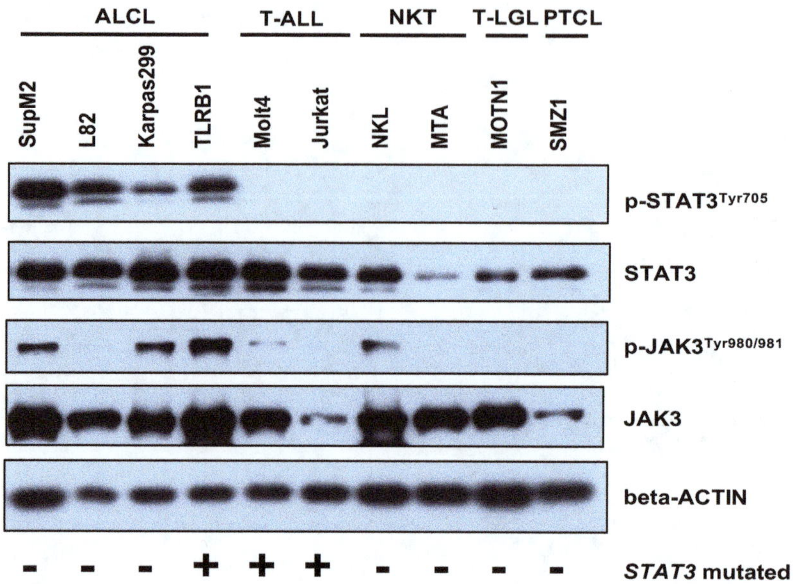

Figure 3. Western blot of p-STAT3 (Tyr705), STAT3, p-JAK3 (Tyr980/981), and JAK3 was characterized in T cell malignancy cell lines. Beta-ACTIN is used as a reference protein.

2.3. STAT3 Phosphorylation Is Associated with JAK1/STAT3 Mutation Status in CD30$^+$ ALK$^-$ ALCLs

Next, we studied whether *STAT3* mutations would be associated with STAT3, MAPK, and AKT phosphorylation. No association between *STAT3* mutation status and pY-STAT3, pMAPK, or pAKT (%) expression was noted when studying all PTCL subtypes (Figure 4A). No association with pY-STAT3 phosphorylation was noted even after adjusting with tumor proportion (mean pSTAT3 77% vs. 66% in STAT3 mutated vs. non-mutated PTCLs). Most of the mutations were noted in relatively low variant allele frequencies (VAF 5–9%), which might in part explain the lack of correlation. Further evidence for this observation was found from cell line data, as the four ALCL cell lines in Figure 2 exhibit high pY-STAT3 phosphorylation but only one of the cell lines harbored a *JAK/STAT* mutation (Table S1). The TLBR1 cell line represents ALK$^-$ ALCL and harbors a known activating *STAT3* missense mutation S614R in the SH2 domain [26]. The other ALCL cell lines expressed ALK, which explains the constitutive STAT3 activation. Both T-ALL cell lines MOLT4 and Jurkat also harbor missense *STAT3/5B* mutations but conversely, the cell lines did not exhibit any pY-STAT3 phosphorylation. This could be explained by the mutations being localized elsewhere than in the activating SH2-domain.

Some PTCL cases harbored both *STAT3* and *RHOA* mutations (8%). Our results showed that the MAPK phosphorylation degree was higher in patients with *RHOA* mutations than patients without *RHOA* mutations (*RHOA*-positive mean = 12.4% vs. *RHOA*-negative mean 5.7%, p = 0.005, t-test; Figure 4B). Yet, *RHOA* mutation was not observed to be associated with STAT3 or AKT phosphorylation.

Phosphorylated STAT3 has been shown to induce CD30 expression in PTCL [27]. In addition, *STAT3* mutations are more frequent in CD30$^+$ than CD30$^-$ T-cell lymphomas [28]. Therefore, we sought to investigate the interaction between mutations in the JAK-STAT pathway, CD30 phenotype and pY-STAT3 phosphorylation. Positive CD30 tumor phenotype was associated with higher STAT3 and AKT phosphorylation, but not with pMAPK (Figure S3A). Interestingly, pSTAT3 expression was highest in samples with CD30$^+$ tumors and simultaneous mutation in *STAT3* or *JAK1* (Figure 4C). This phenotype was represented primarily by the ALK$^-$ ALCL subtype ($p < 0.001$, chi^2 test, Figure 4D), and their pSTAT3 expression (mean 68.7%) to stand above the mean of ALK$^-$ (62.3%) but below ALK$^+$ ALCL (79.7%). We observed that 50% (6/12) of CD30$^+$ ALK$^-$ ALCLs harbored a mutation in *JAK1* or *STAT3*. Higher *JAK1/STAT3* VAF trended for higher pY-STAT3 phosphorylation but the result remained non-significant possibly due to sample size (81.3% vs. 61.1% mean pSTAT3 expression in tumors with high (n = 4) vs. low (n = 4) *JAK1/STAT3* VAF p = 0.22, t-test). Unexpectedly, lowest STAT3 phosphorylation was observed in CD30⁻ patients with a *STAT3* gene mutation. Interestingly, all three in-frame E616 deletions were found in CD30⁻ AITL cases.

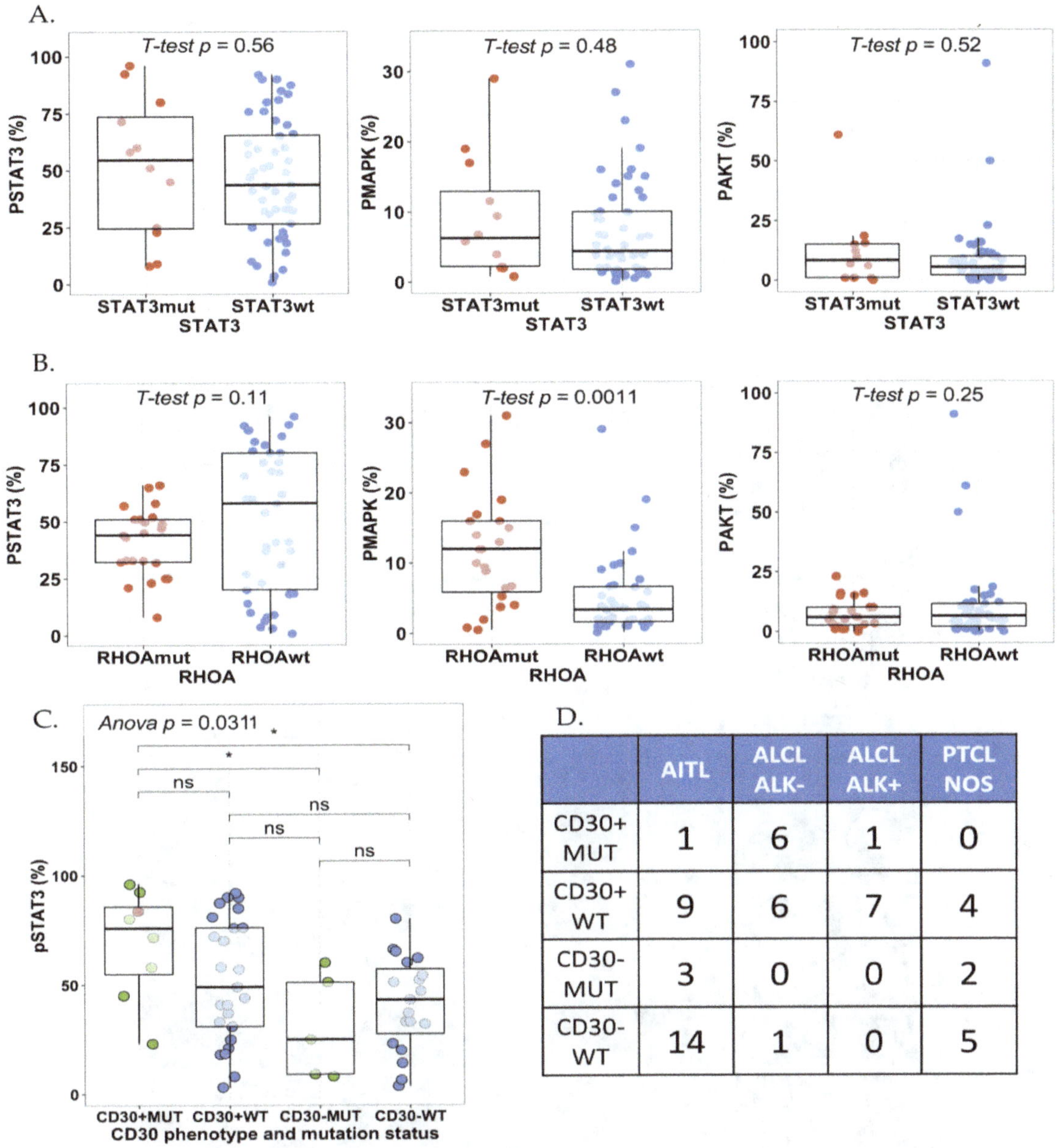

	AITL	ALCL ALK-	ALCL ALK+	PTCL NOS
CD30+ MUT	1	6	1	0
CD30+ WT	9	6	7	4
CD30- MUT	3	0	0	2
CD30- WT	14	1	0	5

Figure 4. Comparison of the phosphorylation level of (**A**) STAT3, MAPK, and AKT by *STAT3* mutation status and by (**B**) *RHOA* mutation status (*t*-test). The phosphorylation level of pStat3 (Tyr705), pMAPK (Thr202/Tyr204) and pAKT (Thr450) was measured by immunohistochemistry. (**C**) Combinatory effect of CD30 phenotype and *JAK1* or *STAT3* mutation status on pSTAT3 expression was studied with one-way ANOVA and post-hoc correction. Green dots correspond to patients with *STAT3* mutations, the red dot correspond to a patient with *JAK1* mutation and blue dots correspond to samples without mutations in *JAK1* or *STAT3*. (**D**) Frequency table of patients by CD30 phenotype and *JAK1* or *STAT3* mutation status (rows) and different PTCL histologies (columns). *: $p < 0.05$; ns: not significant.

EBV status has been shown to be associated with STAT3 activation in B cell lymphomas [29]. No associations between STAT3, MAPK, and AKT phosphorylation and EBV⁺ tumors could be observed in our PTCL cohort (Figure S3B).

As fixation rate differs in samples of various origin and size, we investigated their association with STAT3, MAPK, and AKT phosphorylation. The sample cohort included 9 biopsy samples and 52 excised tumors. Biopsy samples were associated with higher pY-STAT3 but not with MAPK or AKT phosphorylation (Figure S4A). Moreover, correlation between pY-STAT3 and sample size remained non-significant (Figure S4B). Therefore, we hypothesize the difference to be due primarily to biological rather than technical reasons. Except for four samples, the sample cohort consisted of lymph node tissue samples. AKT phosphorylation was higher in lymph node samples, while no difference was observed between pY-STAT3 and MAPK phosphorylation levels (Figure S4B).

To further elucidate the spatial localization of STAT3 phosphorylation, 6 T-cell lymphoma samples (5 AITL, and 1 ALCL) and 2 NLPHL samples were stained for pY-STAT3, PD1, CD4, and CD8 using multiplex immunohistochemistry. Of the 5 AITL samples, two harbored *STAT3* mutations at 5% and 7% VAF, respectively. We found that the staining pattern or level of pY-STAT3 phosphorylation was not associated with *STAT3* mutation status (Figure 5).

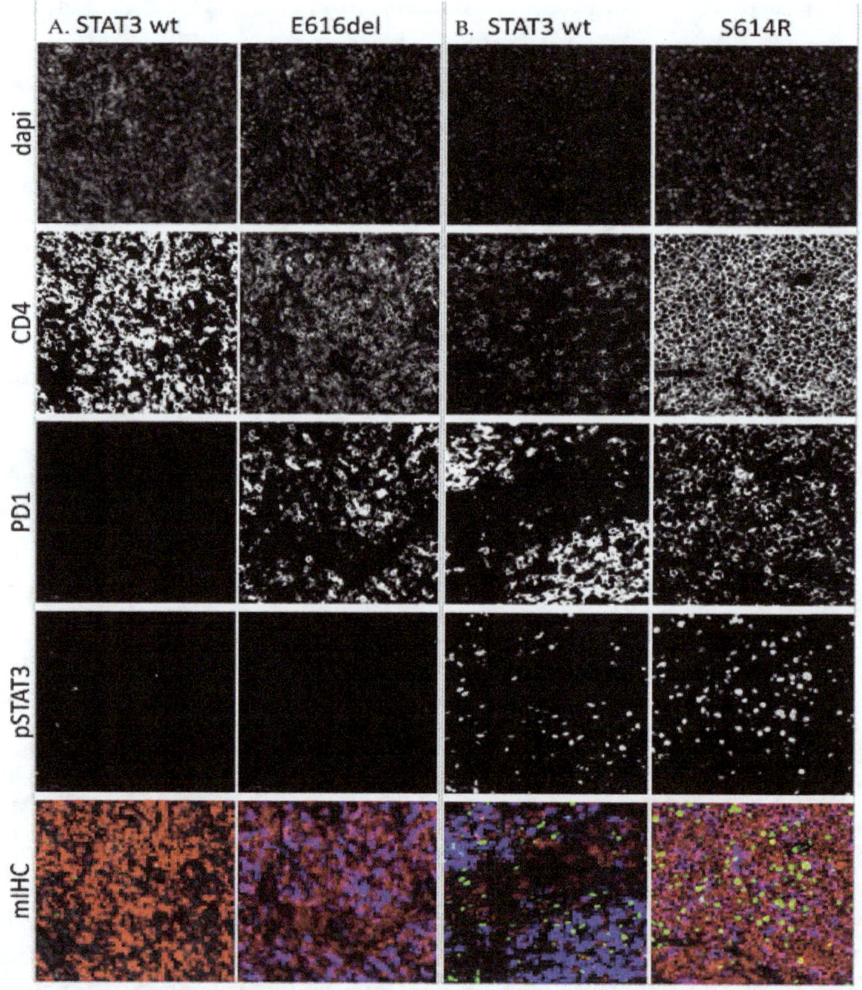

Figure 5. IHC stainings of four angioimmunoblastic T-cell lymphoma (AITL) lymph node samples. (**A**). Samples containing low amount of pSTAT3. (**B**). Samples containing high amounts of pSTAT3. Each slide has been digitalized with a 20× lens and similar exposure time per channel. Images have been further magnified 30× for visualization purposes. The first four rows of images represent single stainings of dapi counterstain, CD4, PD1, and pSTAT3 (Tyr705), respectively, and the last figure their composite image. Staining: red = CD4, blue = PD1, green = pSTAT3.

2.4. High pY-STAT3 Expression Is Associated with $CD3^-$ $CD5^-$ $CD7^-$ $CD30^+$ Immunophenotype Common to ALCL

To understand the association of JAK-STAT signaling pathway activity with clinical determinants, we combined pY-STAT3, pMAPK, and pAKT proportion defined by IHC with information on PTCL disease histology, stage, peripheral blood lactate dehydrogenase (LD) level at diagnosis, survival status, *STAT3* and *RHOA* mutation status (Figure 6). We noted that pY-STAT3, pMAPK, and pAKT expression did not correlate with each other. High pY-STAT3 expression was noted to be associated with ALCL histology as presented before (Figure 2). No association with survival status ($p = 0.17$, *t*-test), disease stage ($p = 0.40$, one-way ANOVA), LD level ($r = -0.13$, $p = 0.31$, Pearson correlation), *STAT3* ($p = 0.56$, *t*-test) or *RHOA* mutation status ($p = 0.11$, *t*-test) was noted.

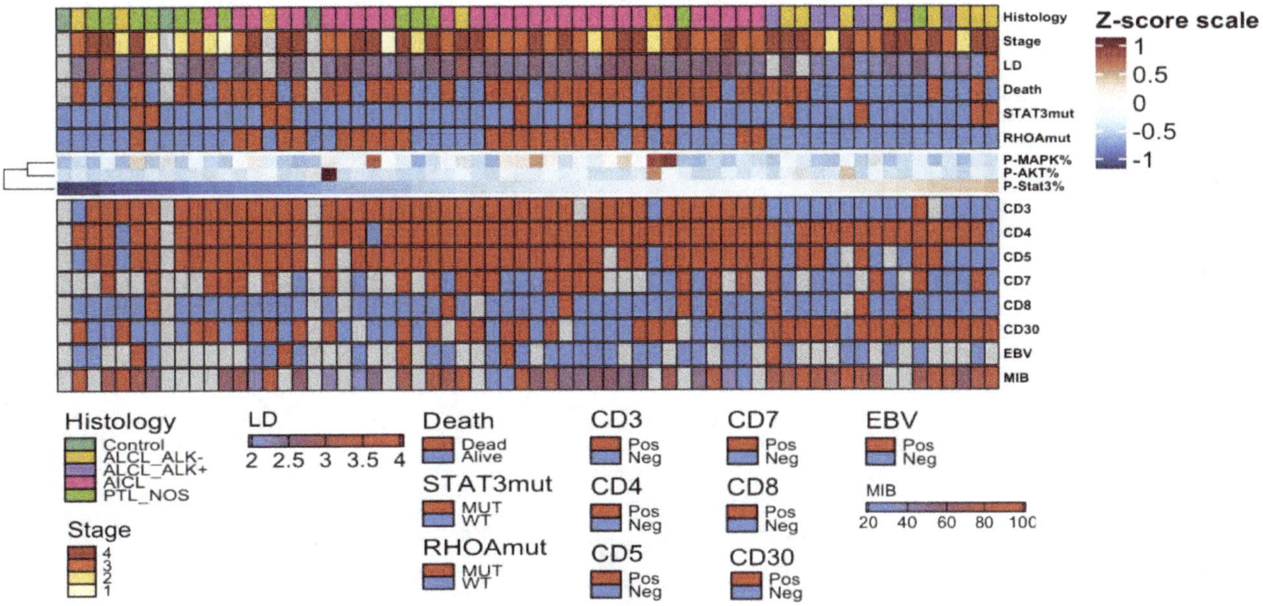

Figure 6. Heatmap visualizing the quantity of pY-STAT3, pMAPK, and pAKT and their association with clinicopathological parameters. The amount of phosphorylated STAT3, MAPK, and AKT have been median-centered and max-scaled, and organized columnwise by pY-STAT3 quantity and rowwise by hierarchical clustering using Spearman correlation distance and Ward linkage (ward.D2) method. Red color denotes higher and blue color lower proportion. Clinical parameters denoting disease histology, disease stage, log10-transformed lactate dehydrogenase (LD) level, survival status, and STAT3 and RHOA mutation status are added as annotations over the heatmap. CD3, CD4, CD5, CD7, CD8, and CD30 immunophenotype status classified as positive or negative, EBV seropositivity and the MIB proliferation index (%) are presented below the heatmap.

To correlate the expression of the JAK-STAT signaling pathway with immunohistochemical and serological factors of disease pathology, we investigated EBV seropositivity, and expression of immunophenotype markers as defined with IHC (Figure 6). Lower pY-STAT3 expression was associated with negative CD3 (37.7% and 75.4% mean pSTAT3 expression, $p < 0.001$, *t*-test), CD5 (42.8% and 68.4%, $p = 0.03$, *t*-test), CD7 (45.2% and 64.6%, $p = 0.01$) and positive CD30 phenotype (Figure S4A) designating ALCL immunophenotype as reported in Figure 2 [30]. No association with EBV seropositivity (Figure S4B), CD4 ($p = 0.86$, *t*-test) or CD8 ($p = 0.35$, *t*-test) immunophenotype nor MIB proliferation index ($r = 0.20$, $p = 0.19$, Pearson correlation) was noted.

2.5. Novel Potential Inhibitors of STAT3 Activation

In myeloproliferative neoplasms the JAK-STAT signaling pathway can be inhibited with the JAK1/JAK2 inhibitor ruxolitinib and in rheumatoid arthritis with less selective JAK inhibitors such as tofacitinib and baricitinib [31]. Several other pharmacological compounds affecting the JAK-STAT pathway are currently investigated in clinical trials [31]. We hypothesized that drugs investigated for other indications might induce differential sensitivity in cancer cell lines with active JAK-STAT signaling. By comparing cytotoxicity measured by the area under the curve (AUC) of 265 investigational and accepted compounds in pSTAT3 high ($n = 27$) and low ($n = 583$) cancer cell lines reported in the Sanger

GDSC and CCLE databases respectively, we identified the JAK-STAT inhibitor ruxolitinib to be more potent in pSTAT3 high cell lines (Figure 7). Interestingly, we discovered also the cell cycle checkpoint kinase Chk1/2 inhibitor AZD7762, the poly ADP ribose polymerase (PARP) inhibitor talazoparib and the nucleoside analog gemcitabine to exhibit most sensitivity in pSTAT3 cell lines.

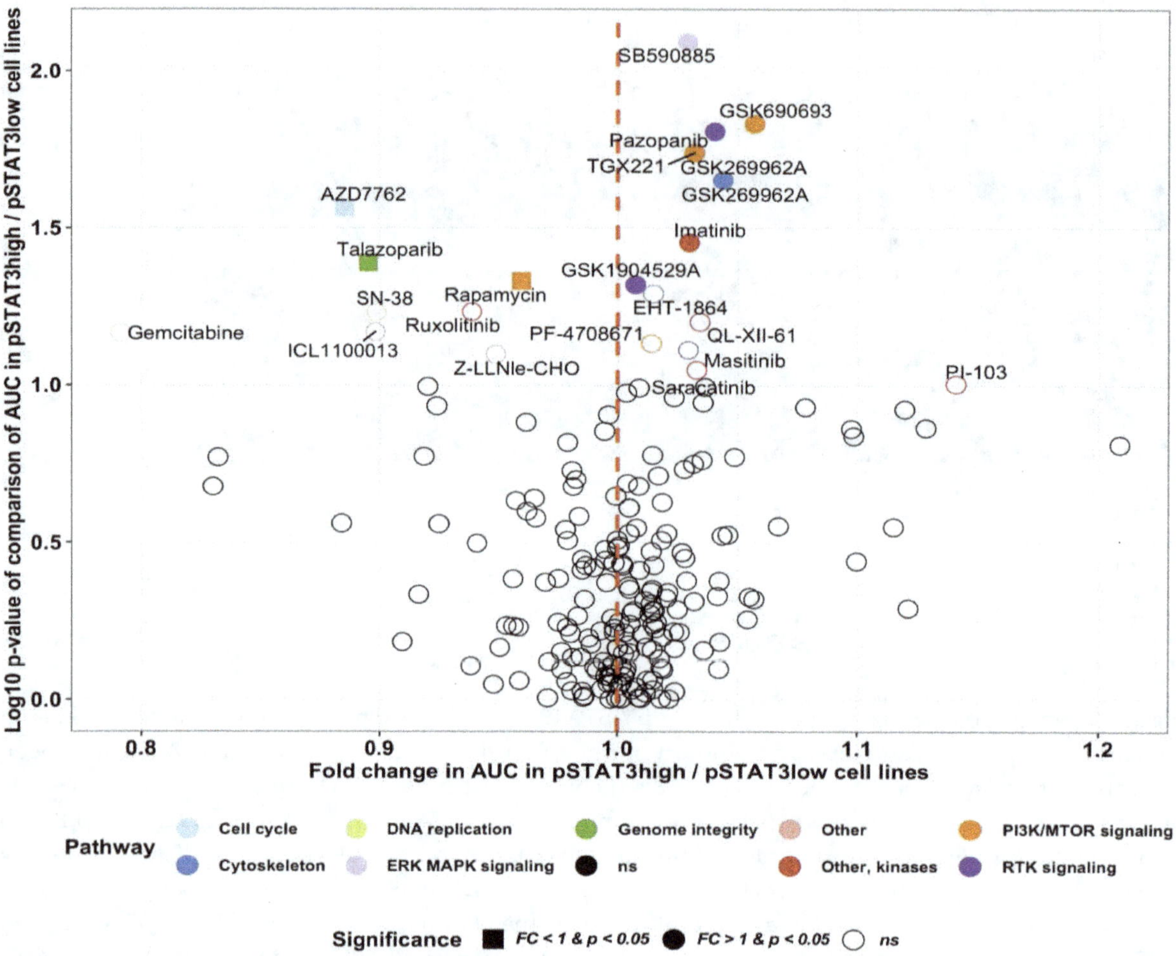

Figure 7. Differential drug sensitivity in pSTAT3 high ($n = 27$) and low ($n = 583$) cancer cell lines. The pSTAT3 phosphorylation level has been quantified with reverse phase protein array (RPPA, cut-off $\text{pSTAT3}^{\text{Tyr705}} = 1$). The drug sensitivity data represent the area under the curve (AUC) response of 265 different phamacological compounds, and has been retrieved from the Sanger GDSC dataset. The RPPA data are derived from the Broad Institute the Cancer Cell Line Encyclopedia (CCLE) database. Differential drug sensitivity has been computed with multiple T-tests, and the fold change defined as the mean AUC ratio in pSTAT3 high-to-low cell lines. Drugs with a fold change (FC) less than 1.0 are more sensitive in pSTAT3 high cell lines. The target pathway of the top pharmacological hits have been color-labeled.

3. Discussion

PTCL patients face unfavorable prognosis as chemotherapy results in poor 5-year overall survival rates [32]. Targeted treatment options only exist for ALK$^+$ ALCL, but are urgently needed for other PTCL entities. Using targeted sequencing, we demonstrated that *STAT3* alterations are prevalent in all PTCL subgroups. We discovered that 13% of AITL and ALK$^+$ ALCL cases and 17% of PTCL-NOS cases harbored *STAT3* mutations. The highest prevalence of *STAT3* mutations was seen in ALK$^-$ ALCL (38%). The mutations were found mostly in the SH2-domain of *STAT3* but also in the coiled coil (K290T) and transactivation domains (P715L). While we observed no association between overall *STAT3* mutation and pY-STAT3 phosphorylation, pY-STAT3 phosphorylation was most elevated in PTCL patients with combined CD30$^+$ tumor phenotype and mutations in either *STAT3* or *JAK1* representing primarily ALK$^-$ ALCLs and suggesting heterogenous mechanisms of STAT3 activation. Unexpectedly, PTCLs with CD30$^-$ phenotype and *STAT3* mutation were associated with lowest pY-STAT3 phosphorylation. As CD30 transcription is regulated by pSTAT3, the result might be explained by non-activating mutations or interference in the JAK-STAT pathway [27].

JAK/STAT mutations have been previously reported in PTCL-NOS, ALCL, and AITL [12,33,34], supporting the results of our study. The frequency of *JAK/STAT* mutations in different cohorts of PTCL has been reported to be around 20% which compares well to the mutation frequency seen in this study. In the whole cohort one of the most prevalent *STAT3* mutation was an in-frame deletion of E616, which was identified in three AITL patients. The E616 deletion has been shown to induce myeloid malignancy in a mouse bone marrow transplantation model [19]. The mutation has been observed previously in AITL, but also in adult T-cell lymphoma [10,35]. The *STAT3* mutation P715L observed in two ALK$^-$ ALCLs and one PTCL-NOS case has been observed in NKTL previously [36].

Some AITL and PTCL-NOS cases harbored concurrent *STAT3* and *RHOA* mutations (3/30 AITL and 1/12 PTCL-NOS). The incidence of *RHOA* mutations in our AITL cohort was 70%, which is somewhat higher than the incidence seen in previous AITL cohorts (68% and 53%) [8,23]. In PTCL-NOS the mutation incidence was 17% (2/12). Our results also showed that the MAPK phosphorylation degree correlated with *RHOA* mutations in our PTCL cohort.

Although this study included limited number of patients representing various PTCLs subtypes, our results suggest that pY-STAT3 is frequently constitutively phosphorylated in PTCL, especially in ALCLs and AITLs, but this was associated with *STAT3* mutations in only a fraction of PTCL samples. Previous studies have reported mechanisms underlying the constitutive activation of STAT3 independent of *STAT3* mutations. Gain-of–function mutations involving *JAK* genes have been implicated in activating STAT3 and contributing to the pathogenesis of hematologic malignancies and solid tumors [37,38]. Various cytokines (e.g., IL-6, IL-10, and IL-11) that are released into the microenvironment by tumor cells have also been shown to activate STAT3 [39]. Another mechanism of STAT3 activation is possible through the deregulation of suppressors of the JAK/STAT pathway such as SOCS3 [40] leading to constitutive STAT activation and oncogenesis. In addition, further studies are needed to combine any association with JAK-STAT pathway activation and expression of essential transcription factors such as GATA3 and Tbet, which define new subclasses of PTCL-NOS with prognostic consequences, where GATA3 signatures are associated with worse prognosis [41,42].

In our cohort high pSTAT3 expression correlated with the CD3$^-$ CD5$^-$ CD7$^-$ CD30$^+$ immunophenotype typical for ALCL. No association with neither immunophenotype markers nor essential clinical variables such as survival status, disease stage, MIB proliferation index or LD level was seen.

By comparing cytotoxicity measured by the area under the curve (AUC) of 265 investigational and accepted compounds in pSTAT3 high and low cancer cell lines, we identified novel potential inhibitors of STAT3 activation. The JAK-inhibitor ruxolitinib was among the top candidates. Ruxolitinib, a selective JAK1/2 inhibitor approved by the FDA for myeloproliferative neoplasms, is being studied in relapsed B-cell lymphoma and PTCL (NCT01431209).

Among compounds exhibiting most sensitivity in pSTAT3 high cell lines were the cell cycle checkpoint kinase Chk1/2 inhibitor AZD7762, the poly ADP ribose polymerase (PARP) inhibitor talazoparib, and the nucleoside analog gemcitabine. In phase II studies, gemcitabine monotherapy has shown activity against T-cell lymphomas. Zinzani et al. reported a 70% response rate in a phase II study of 44 pretreated patients with mycosis fungoides or cutaneous PTCL-unspecified [43]. In another phase II study, gemcitabine was given in combination with romidepsin to relapsed/refractory PTCL patients but the synergy observed in preclinical phase did not improve clinical outcomes [44]. Moreover, gemcitabine has been tested in combination with cisplatin and methylprednisolone as both upfront treatment and in relapsed/refractory PTCL, but did not significantly improve OS [45,46].

4. Materials and Methods

4.1. Patients and Cell Lines

Samples from 63 patients with PTCL were collected. Of these samples 30 were AITL, 12 PTCL-NOS and 21 ALCL (13 ALK^- and 8 ALK^+). Four control samples from normal lymph nodes were also collected. The study was undertaken in compliance with the principles of the Helsinki Declaration and was approved by the ethics committee in the Helsinki University Hospital (Finland). As the samples studied were older diagnostic samples, the ethics committee required no written informed consent (TEO 5326/04/046/06, Valvira 9115/05.01.00.06/2011, HUS 302/E0/2006, HUS/1230/2017). The clinical and pathological characteristics of our study objects are summarized in Table S2.

4.2. Cell Lines and Cell Culture Conditions

The T-cell lines were cultured in RMPI-1640 medium including L-glutamine (Gibco, Grand Island, NY, USA) supplemented with 10% (L82, Karpas299, TLRB1, Molt4, Jurkat, and NKL cell line) or 20% (SupM2, MTA, MOTN1, and SMZ1 cell line) fetal bovine serum (FBS, Gibco) and Penicillin/Streptomycin (100 U/l, Gibco). IL2 (10ng/mL, MedChemExpress, Monmouth Junction, NJ, USA) was added for culturing of TLRB1 and NKL cells. Suspension cells were maintained at a density of 2.0–8.0 × 10^5. Culturing was done in an incubator at 37 °C and 5% CO_2 with 90% humidity.

4.3. Sample Preparation

According to standard clinical procedure, fresh tissue samples consisting mostly of lymph nodes (LN) were fixated in formalin and embedded in paraffin (FFPE) in the central pathology laboratory of Helsinki University Hospital (HUCH), Finland. Consequently, we cut 3.5 μm whole-tissue sections on Superfrost objective slides (Kindler O Gmbh, Freiburg, Germany).

4.4. DNA Extraction

DNA was extracted from FFPE tissue blocks. Ten 10 μm sections were cut with standard microtome (Leica SM2000 R Sliding Microtome, Wetzlar, Germany) using disposable blades. Excess paraffin was trimmed off and the sections were collected into sterile 1.5 mL microcentrifuge tubes. The sections were then deparaffinized with three pre-warmed (55 C) xylene washes followed by 95%, 75%, and 50% ethanol rinses. The tissue pellets were dried briefly at 37 °C to remove traces of ethanol. The pellets were then digested with 20 μL proteinase K (20 mg/mL proteinase K, Roche Diagnostics GmbH, (Mannheim, Germany) and 180 μL digestion buffer (10 mM Tris-HCl, pH 8.0 100 mM EDTA, pH 8.0 50 mM NaCl, and 0.5% SDS). Samples were incubated at 55 °C with mild agitation for 3 to 72 h. Fresh Proteinase K was added every 24 h followed by heat inactivation at 90 °C for 1 h after the tissue had been fully dissolved. For phenol-chloroform extraction, equal volume of phenol (Amresco, Solon, OH, USA) was added and vortexed. After spinning for 3 min at 14,000 rpm, the aqueous layer was transferred to a new tube. Then, an equal volume of phenol-chloroform-isoamyl alcohol (25:25:1) (Invitrogen, Carlsbad, CA, USA) was added, and the solution was vortexed and spun for 5 min at 14,000 rpm in a microcentrifuge. The aqueous layer was again transferred to a new tube and treated with RNase A at 100 μg/mL for 1 h at 37 °C. To remove any remaining RNase A phenol and phenol-chloroform-isoamyl alcohol steps were repeated. The aqueous layer was transferred to a new tube and the DNA was precipitated with 1/10 volume of 3 M sodium acetate and 1 volume of isopropanol. After thorough mixing, the solution was placed in a freezer for 30 min then spun at 14,000 rpm at 4 °C in a microcentrifuge for 10 min. The supernatant was discarded, and the pellet was washed with 1 mL 70% cold ethanol and spun at 14,000 rpm for 10 min at 4 °C. The supernatant was carefully discarded, and the pellet dried and finally suspended with 50 μL dH_2O.

4.5. Targeted Deep Amplicon Sequencing

Locus-specific primers were designed for *STAT3, STAT5B, JAK1, JAK3,* and *RHOA* mutation hotspots using Primer3 with user-defined parameters (http://primer3.wi.mit.edu/). After designing the locus-specific primer sequences (Table S3), sequence tails corresponding to the Illumina adapter sequences, were added to the 5′ end of the forward and reverse locus-specific primers, respectively. All oligonucleotides were ordered from Sigma-Aldrich (St. Louis, MO, USA). Deep targeted amplicon sequencing of known recurrent somatic mutations in the genes *STAT3, STAT5B, JAK1, JAK3,* and *RHOA* was performed with the Illumina MiSeq platform (San Diego, CA, USA)as previously described [47]. The data were analyzed with a bioinformatics pipeline, which is based on calling of variants with certain count/frequency of reads and filtering out false positives using the estimated error rate and quality data of amplicon reads.

4.6. Immunohistochemistry

4.6.1. Single Color Immunohistochemistry

Tissue sections were deparaffinized, rehydrated in graded ethanol series and then subjected to heat-induced epitope retrieval in Tris-HCl (10 mM Tris, pH 8.5, 25 min; for Phospho-MAPK and Phospho-AKT) or in EDTA buffer (10 mM EDTA, pH 8.0, 20 min; for Phospho-Stat3 and -5) in a Pre-Treatment module (DAKO/Agilent Technologies, Waltham, MA, USA). Samples were stained using LabVision autostainer (Thermo Fisher Scientific, Fremont, CA, USA). The endogenous peroxidase activity was blocked with Peroxidase-Blocking Solution (Dako/Agilent Tehnologies). The samples were treated with primary antibody for 1 h at RT. The antibodies used were rabbit monoclonal antibodies from Cell Signaling (Leiden, the Netherlands): clone Tyr705 for pY-STAT3 (1:300), clone Thr202/Tyr204 for Phospho-p44/42MAPK (1:300) and Thr450 for Phospho-AKT (1:100). BrightVision polymerisation technology was utilized to prepare polymeric HRP-linker antibody conjugates (ImmunoLogic, Duiven, the Netherlands) and 3,3-diaminobenzidine (DAB) was used as chromogen. Sections were counterstained with Mayer's hematoxylin (Dako/Agilent Tehnologies) and mounted with Eukitt (Honeywell Fluka, Frankfurt, Germany).

Protein expression was defined by visual examination. Five representative 400×-magnified high-power field-of-view (FOV) were selected, and protein expression (%) was estimated as the proportion of positive cells of 100 cells analyzed by FOV. Finally, the mean proportion of positive cells was calculated and used for statistical analyses.

4.6.2. Multiplex Immunohistochemistry

All phases were performed in room temperature (if not otherwise specified) and protein blocking as well as antibody incubations were performed in a humid chamber. The slides were washed with 0.1% Tween-20 (Thermo Fisher Scientific) diluted in 10 mM Tris-HCL buffered saline pH 7.4 (TBS) three times after peroxide block, each antibody staining, and fluorochrome reaction. Antibodies were tested with normal lymph node and pY-STAT3 was validated with tissue samples from a patient with large granular lymphocyte leukemia (Figure S5).

The slides were deparaffinized in xylene and rehydrated with graded series of ethanol and H2O. HIER was performed in 10 mM Tris-HCl - 1 mM EDTA buffer (pH 9) in +99 °C for 20 min (PT Module, Thermo Fisher Scientific). The peroxide activity was then blocked in 0.9% H2O2 solution for 15 min, and 10% normal goat serum was subsequently applied (TBS-NGS) for 15 min. We applied the primary antibody anti-PD1 (1:5000; clone PDCD1; LsBio, Seattle, WA, USA) diluted in TBS-NGS for 1 h 45 min, and then anti-mouse horseradish peroxidase (HRP) conjugated secondary antibodies (Immunologic) diluted 1:2 in washing buffer for 45 min. Then, we applied tyramide signal amplification (TSA) Alexa Fluor 488 (PerkinElmer, Boston, MA, USA) diluted 1:50 in TBS on the slides for 10 min. In order to multiplex antibodies, we denatured the primary antibody and quenched the enzymatic activity of HRP by repeating HIER as well as performing peroxide and protein block similarly as above. We applied the primary antibody against pY-STAT3 (Tyr705; 1:2500; clone D3A7; CellSignaling) overnight in +4 °C, anti-mouse HRP-conjugated secondary antibody diluted 1:5 in washing buffer for 45 min, and TSA Alexa Fluor 555 (PerkinElmer) for 10 min. We repeated HIER, peroxide block and protein block as above. Next, we applied anti-CD4 (1:150; clone EPR6855; Abcam, Cambridge, UK) diluted in TBS-NGS for 3 h and later AlexaFluor647-conjugated secondary antibody (1:300; Thermo Fisher Scientific) and Hoechst 33,342 (1 μg/mL; Sigma-Aldrich) counterstain diluted in washing buffer for 45 min. Finally, we applied ProLong Gold (Thermo Fisher Scientific) to mount the slides.

The tissue slides were scanned with 20x magnification with the Panoramic P250 Flash II whole slide scanner (3DHistech, Budapest, Hungary). We used DAPI, FITC, Cy3, and Cy5 filters and visually-optimized exposure times.

4.7. Western Blot

Immunoblots were performed on whole-cell protein lysates according to standard techniques. All primary antibodies (pJAK3$^{Tyr980/981}$, clone D44E3; JAK3, clone D7B12; pY-STAT3^{Tyr705}, clone D3A7; STAT3, clone 124H6; beta-ACTIN, clone 13E5) were ordered from Cell Signaling Technology and used at 1:1000 dilutions. Anti-mouse and anti-rabbit, both from Dianova, were used as secondary HRP-coupled antibodies in a 1:5000 dilution. Development of the immunoblots was performed by using Western Bright ECL (Advansta, Menlo Park, CA, USA). The original blots and densitometry readings of each band is available in the Supplementary Materials (Figure S6 and Table S4).

4.8. CCLE and DepMap Data

All CCLE pre-processed data were downloaded from the CCLE data portal (https://portals.broadinstitute.org/ccle/data). RPPA data dated 3 October2018, RNA-seq gene count data dated 29 September 2018, cell line annotation dated 26 December 2018, and mutation data dated 18 July 2018 were used. Gene counts were converted to CPM values using the edgeR and the TMM normalization method without log transformation. The cut-off for high vs. low STAT3 phosphorylation was set to pSTAT3^{Tyr705} = 1 (RPPA unit) based on the shape of the pSTAT3^{Tyr705} frequency histogram.

Area under the curve (AUC) drug sensitivity data annotated as "Sanger GDSC v17.3" and dated March 2018 were downloaded from the Cancer Dependency Map portal (https://depmap.org/portal/download/). Drugs not characterized in both pSTAT3 high and low cell line groups were removed from the analysis. Cell lines with no pSTAT3 RPPA data were removed from the analysis.

4.9. Statistical Analysis

Comparison of continuous variables between two groups was computed with unpaired *t*-test and between multiple groups with one-way ANOVA and post-hoc correction between disease groups and healthy controls.

Overall survival was defined as the time from diagnosis to death or last follow-up. Patients alive at the last follow-up date were censored. The log-rank test was used to compute Cox proportional-hazards.

Differential drug sensitivity was computed using t-test between pSTAT3 high (n = 27) and low (n = 583) cancer cell lines. The fold change in drug sensitivity was defined as the mean AUC ratio in pSTAT3 high-to-low cell lines. Drugs with a fold change (FC) less than 1.0 are more sensitive in pSTAT3 high cell lines.

R 3.5.1. [48] and Prism 6.0 was used for statistical analyses. R packages edgeR 3.24.0, forestplot 1.7.2, survminer 0.4.3, ggplot2 3.2.1, and ComplexHeatmap 2.3.2 were used.

5. Conclusions

In summary, this study discovered that pY-STAT3 phosphorylation was associated with both ALK$^+$ ALCLs and *JAK1/STAT3* mutated CD30$^+$ ALK$^-$ ALCLs suggesting a subgroup potentially benefitting of JAK/STAT targeted therapy.

Supplementary Materials:
Figure S1: pMAPK, pAKT and pSTAT3 staining of PTCLs, Figure S2: *STAT3* expression correlation with *JAK1, JAK3, AKT* and *MAPK* expression in T-cell neoplasia cell lines from the CCLE dataset, Figure S3: Association of STAT3, MAPK and AKT phosphorylation with CD30 phenotype and EBV status, Figure S4: Association of STAT3, MAPK and AKT phosphorylation with sample type and organ origin, Figure S5: Multiplex immunohistochemistry staining of $pSTAT3^{Tyr705}$ in $CD8^{+}$ LGL-leukemia as a positive control stain for pSTAT3 antibody, Figure S6: Full western blot of p-STAT3 (Tyr705), STAT3, p-JAK3 (Tyr980/981), and JAK3 in T cell malignancy cell lines, Table S1: Cell lines and *JAK/STAT* mutation status, Table S2: Clinical and pathological characteristics of PTCL patients, Table S3: Locus-specific primers for *STAT3* and *STAT5B* exons and *RHOA* G17V mutation hotspot, Table S4: Densitometry readings of Western blot stainings.

Author Contributions: conceptualization, S.M. (Satu Mustjoki), P.E.K., O.B. and E.I.A.; methodology, L.S., S.L. (Sonja Lagström) and P.E.; validation, E.I.A., T.B. and O.B.; formal analysis, E.I.A. and O.B.; data curation, S.M. (Susanna Mannisto); writing—original draft preparation, E.I.A. and O.B.; writing—review and editing, S.M. (Satu Mustjoki), P.E.K., S.L. (Sirpa Leppä) and M.H. All authors have read and agreed to the published version of the manuscript.

Acknowledgments: The personnel at the Hematology Research Unit Helsinki, HUSLAB Laboratory of Genetics (Soili Kytölä), and FIMM (Suvi Kyttänen and Tiina Hannunen) are acknowledged for their expert clinical and technical assistance. The authors thank Annabrita Schoonenberg from the Digital and Molecular Pathology Unit supported by Helsinki University and Biocenter Finland. Raphael Koch is acknowledged for providing cell lines. The authors thank Heidi Neubauer and Helena Sorger for valuable comments to the manuscript.

References

1. Project, T.N.-H.L.C. A Clinical Evaluation of the International Lymphoma Study Group Classification of Non-Hodgkin's Lymphoma. *Blood* **1997**, *89*, 3909–3918.
2. Ellin, F.; Landström, J.; Jerkeman, M.; Relander, T. Real-world data on prognostic factors and treatment in peripheral T-cell lymphomas: A study from the Swedish Lymphoma Registry. *Blood* **2014**, *124*, 1570–1577. [CrossRef]
3. International T-Cell Lymphoma Project; Vose, J.; Armitage, J.; Weisenburger, D. International Peripheral T-Cell and Natural Killer/T-Cell Lymphoma Study: Pathology Findings and Clinical Outcomes. *J. Clin. Oncol.* **2008**, *26*, 4124–4130. [CrossRef]
4. D'Amore, F.; Relander, T.; Lauritzsen, G.F.; Jantunen, E.; Hagberg, H.; Anderson, H.; Holte, H.; Osterborg, A.; Merup, M.; Brown, P.; et al. Up-Front Autologous Stem-Cell Transplantation in Peripheral T-Cell Lymphoma: NLG-T-01. *J. Clin. Oncol.* **2012**, *30*, 3093–3099. [CrossRef]
5. Mak, V.; Hamm, J.; Chhanabhai, M.; Shenkier, T.; Klasa, R.; Sehn, L.H.; Villa, D.; Gascoyne, R.D.; Connors, J.M.; Savage, K.J. Survival of Patients With Peripheral T-Cell Lymphoma After First Relapse or Progression: Spectrum of Disease and Rare Long-Term Survivors. *J. Clin. Oncol.* **2013**, *31*, 1970–1976. [CrossRef]
6. Iqbal, J.; Wilcox, R.; Naushad, H.; Rohr, J.; Heavican, T.B.; Wang, C.; Bouska, A.; Fu, K.; Chan, W.C.; Vose, J.M.; et al. Genomic signatures in T-cell lymphoma: How can these improve precision in diagnosis and inform prognosis? *Blood Rev.* **2016**, *30*, 89–100. [CrossRef]
7. Lemonnier, F.; Couronné, L.; Parrens, M.; Jaïs, J.-P.; Travert, M.; Lamant, L.; Tournillac, O.; Rousset, T.; Fabiani, B.; Cairns, R.A.; et al. Recurrent TET2 mutations in peripheral T-cell lymphomas correlate with TFH-like features and adverse clinical parameters. *Blood* **2012**, *120*, 1466–1469. [CrossRef]
8. Sakata-Yanagimoto, M.; Enami, T.; Yoshida, K.; Shiraishi, Y.; Ishii, R.; Miyake, Y.; Muto, H.; Tsuyama, N.; Sato-Otsubo, A.; Okuno, Y.; et al. Somatic RHOA mutation in angioimmunoblastic T cell lymphoma. *Nat. Genet.* **2014**, *46*, 171–175. [CrossRef]
9. Palomero, T.; Couronné, L.; Khiabanian, H.; Kim, M.-Y.; Ambesi-Impiombato, A.; Perez-Garcia, A.; Carpenter, Z.; Abate, F.; Allegretta, M.; Haydu, J.E.; et al. Recurrent mutations in epigenetic regulators, RHOA and FYN kinase in peripheral T cell lymphomas. *Nat. Genet.* **2014**, *46*, 166–170. [CrossRef]
10. Odejide, O.; Weigert, O.; Lane, A.A.; Toscano, D.; Lunning, M.A.; Kopp, N.; Kim, S.S.; Van Bodegom, D.; Bolla, S.; Schatz, J.H.; et al. A targeted mutational landscape of angioimmunoblastic T-cell lymphoma. *Blood* **2014**, *123*, 1293–1296. [CrossRef]
11. Iqbal, J.; Weisenburger, D.D.; Greiner, T.C.; Vose, J.M.; McKeithan, T.; Küçük, C.; Geng, H.; Deffenbacher, K.; Smith, L.; Dybkær, K.; et al. Molecular signatures to improve diagnosis in peripheral T-cell lymphoma and prognostication in angioimmunoblastic T-cell lymphoma. *Blood* **2010** *115*, 1026–1036. [CrossRef]

10. Odejide, O.; Weigert, O.; Lane, A.A.; Toscano, D.; Lunning, M.A.; Kopp, N.; Kim, S.S.; Van Bodegom, D.; Bolla, S.; Schatz, J.H.; et al. A targeted mutational landscape of angioimmunoblastic T-cell lymphoma. *Blood* **2014**, *123*, 1293–1296. [CrossRef]
11. Iqbal, J.; Weisenburger, D.D.; Greiner, T.C.; Vose, J.M.; McKeithan, T.; Küçük, C.; Geng, H.; Deffenbacher, K.; Smith, L.; Dybkær, K.; et al. Molecular signatures to improve diagnosis in peripheral T-cell lymphoma and prognostication in angioimmunoblastic T-cell lymphoma. *Blood* **2010**, *115*, 1026–1036. [CrossRef]
12. Crescenzo, R.; Abate, F.; Lasorsa, E.; Tabbo', F.; Gaudiano, M.; Chiesa, N.; Di Giacomo, F.; Spaccarotella, E.; Barbarossa, L.; Ercole, E.; et al. Convergent mutations and kinase fusions lead to oncogenic STAT3 activation in anaplastic large cell lymphoma. *Cancer Cell* **2015**, *27*, 516–532. [CrossRef]
13. Pencik, J.; Pham, H.T.T.; Schmoellerl, J.; Javaheri, T.; Schlederer, M.; Culig, Z.; Merkel, O.; Moriggl, R.; Grebien, F.; Kenner, L. JAK-STAT signaling in cancer: From cytokines to non-coding genome. *Cytokine* **2016**, *87*, 26–36. [CrossRef]
14. Vainchenker, W.; Constantinescu, S.N. JAK/STAT signaling in hematological malignancies. *Oncogene* **2012**, *32*, 2601–2613. [CrossRef]
15. Migone, T.; Lin, J.; Cereseto, A.; Mulloy, J.; O'Shea, J.; Franchini, G.; Leonard, W. Constitutively activated Jak-STAT pathway in T cells transformed with HTLV-I. *Science* **1995**, *269*, 79–81. [CrossRef]
16. Heinrich, T.; Rengstl, B.; Muik, A.; Petkova, M.; Schmid, F.; Wistinghausen, R.; Warner, K.; Crispatzu, G.; Hansmann, M.-L.; Herling, M.; et al. Mature T-cell Lymphomagenesis Induced by Retroviral Insertional Activation of Janus Kinase 1. *Mol. Ther.* **2013**, *21*, 1160–1168. [CrossRef]
17. Nicolae, A.; Xi, L.; Pittaluga, S.; Abdullaev, Z.; Pack, S.D.; Chen, J.; Waldmann, T.A.; Jaffe, E.S.; Raffeld, M. Frequent STAT5B mutations in $\gamma\delta$ hepatosplenic T-cell lymphomas. *Leukemia* **2014**, *28*, 2244–2248. [CrossRef] [PubMed]
18. Bamford, S.; Dawson, E.; Forbes, S.; Clements, J.; Pettett, R.; Dogan, A.; Flanagan, A.; Teague, J.; Futreal, P.A.; Stratton, M.R.; et al. The COSMIC (Catalogue of Somatic Mutations in Cancer) database and website. *Br. J. Cancer* **2004**, *91*, 355–358. [CrossRef]
19. Couronné, L.; Scourzic, L.; Pilati, C.; Della Valle, V.; Duffourd, Y.; Solary, E.; Vainchenker, W.; Merlio, J.-P.; Beylot-Barry, M.; Damm, F.; et al. STAT3 mutations identified in human hematologic neoplasms induce myeloid malignancies in a mouse bone marrow transplantation model. *Haematological* **2013**, *98*, 1748–1752. [CrossRef]
20. Jerez, A.; Clemente, M.J.; Makishima, H.; Rajala, H.; Gómez-Seguí, I.; Olson, T.; McGraw, K.; Przychodzen, B.; Kulasekararaj, A.; Afable, M.; et al. STAT3 mutations indicate the presence of subclinical T-cell clones in a subset of aplastic anemia and myelodysplastic syndrome patients. *Blood* **2013**, *122*, 2453–2459. [CrossRef]
21. Morin, R.D.; Mendez-Lago, M.; Mungall, A.J.; Goya, R.; Mungall, K.L.; Corbett, R.D.; Johnson, N.A.; Severson, T.M.; Chiu, R.; Field, M.A.; et al. Frequent mutation of histone-modifying genes in non-Hodgkin lymphoma. *Nature* **2011**, *476*, 298–303. [CrossRef] [PubMed]
22. Schrader, A.; Crispatzu, G.; Oberbeck, S.; Mayer, P.; Pützer, S.; Von Jan, J.; Vasyutina, E.; Warner, K.; Weit, N.; Pflug, N.; et al. Actionable perturbations of damage responses by TCL1/ATM and epigenetic lesions form the basis of T-PLL. *Nat. Commun.* **2018**, *9*, 697. [CrossRef] [PubMed]
23. Yoo, H.Y.; Sung, M.; Lee, S.H.; Kim, S.; Lee, H.; Park, S.; Kim, S.C.; Lee, B.; Rho, K.; Lee, W.T.; et al. A recurrent inactivating mutation in RHOA GTPase in angioimmunoblastic T cell lymphoma. *Nat. Genet.* **2014**, *46*, 371–375. [CrossRef] [PubMed]
24. Fujisawa, M.; Sakata-Yanagimoto, M.; Nishizawa, S.; Komori, D.; Gershon, P.; Kiryu, M.; Tanzima, S.; Fukumoto, K.; Enami, T.; Muratani, M.; et al. Activation of RHOA–VAV1 signaling in angioimmunoblastic T-cell lymphoma. *Leukemia* **2017**, *32*, 694–702. [CrossRef]
25. Han, J.J.; O'Byrne, M.; Stenson, M.J.; Maurer, M.; Wellik, L.E.; Feldman, A.L.; McPhail, E.D.; Witzig, T.E.; Gupta, M. Prognostic and therapeutic significance of phosphorylated STAT3 and protein tyrosine phosphatase-6 in peripheral-T cell lymphoma. *Blood Cancer J.* **2018**, *8*, 110. [CrossRef]
26. Chen, J.; Zhang, Y.; Petrus, M.N.; Xiao, W.; Nicolae, A.; Raffeld, M.; Pittaluga, S.; Bamford, R.N.; Nakagawa, M.; Ouyang, S.T.; et al. Cytokine receptor signaling is required for the survival of ALK−anaplastic large cell lymphoma, even in the presence of JAK1/STAT3 mutations. *Proc. Natl. Acad. Sci. USA* **2017**, *114*, 3975–3980. [CrossRef]
27. Chiarle, R.; Voena, C.; Ambrogio, C.; Piva, R.; Inghirami, G. The anaplastic lymphoma kinase in the pathogenesis of cancer. *Nat. Rev. Cancer* **2008**, *8*, 11–23. [CrossRef]

28. Ohgami, R.S.; Ma, L.; Merker, J.D.; Martinez, B.; Zehnder, J.L.; A Arber, D. STAT3 mutations are frequent in CD30+ T-cell lymphomas and T-cell large granular lymphocytic leukemia. *Leukemia* **2013**, *27*, 2244–2247. [CrossRef]
29. Shair, K.H.Y.; Bendt, K.M.; Edwards, R.H.; Bedford, E.C.; Nielsen, J.N.; Raab-Traub, N. EBV Latent Membrane Protein 1 Activates Akt, NFκB, and Stat3 in B Cell Lymphomas. *PLOS Pathog.* **2007**, *3*, e166. [CrossRef]
30. Montes-Mojarro, I.; Steinhilber, J.; Bonzheim, I.; Quintanilla-Martinez, L.; Fend, F. The Pathological Spectrum of Systemic Anaplastic Large Cell Lymphoma (ALCL). *Cancers* **2018**, *10*, 107. [CrossRef]
31. Schwartz, D.M.; Kanno, Y.; Villarino, A.; Ward, M.; Gadina, M.; O'Shea, J.J. JAK inhibition as a therapeutic strategy for immune and inflammatory diseases. *Nat. Rev. Drug Discov.* **2018**, *17*, 78. [CrossRef] [PubMed]
32. Armitage, J.O. The aggressive peripheral T-cell lymphomas: 2017. *Am. J. Hematol.* **2017**, *92*, 706–715. [CrossRef] [PubMed]
33. Schatz, J.H.; Horwitz, S.; Teruya-Feldstein, J.; A Lunning, M.; Viale, A.; Huberman, K.; Socci, N.D.; Lailler, N.; Heguy, A.; Dolgalev, I.; et al. Targeted mutational profiling of peripheral T-cell lymphoma not otherwise specified highlights new mechanisms in a heterogeneous pathogenesis. *Leukemia* **2014**, *29*, 237–241. [CrossRef] [PubMed]
34. Manso, R.; Sánchez-Beato, M.; González-Rincón, J.; Gómez, S.; Rojo, F.; Mollejo, M.; García-Cosio, M.; Menárguez, J.; Piris, M.A.; Rodríguez-Pinilla, S.M. Mutations in the JAK/STAT pathway genes and activation of the pathway, a relevant finding in nodal Peripheral T-cell lymphoma. *Br. J. Haematol.* **2017**, *183*, 497–501. [CrossRef] [PubMed]
35. Kataoka, K.; Nagata, Y.; Kitanaka, A.; Shiraishi, Y.; Shimamura, T.; Yasunaga, J.-I.; Totoki, Y.; Chiba, K.; Sato-Otsubo, A.; Nagae, G.; et al. Integrated molecular analysis of adult T cell leukemia/lymphoma. *Nat. Genet.* **2015**, *47*, 1304–1315. [CrossRef]
36. Song, T.L.; Nairismägi, M.-L.; Laurensia, Y.; Lim, J.Q.; Tan, J.; Li, Z.-M.; Pang, W.-L.; Kizhakeyil, A.; Wijaya, G.-C.; Huang, D.; et al. Oncogenic activation of the STAT3 pathway drives PD-L1 expression in natural killer/T-cell lymphoma. *Blood* **2018**, *132*, 1146–1158. [CrossRef]
37. Kiel, M.J.; Velusamy, T.; Rolland, D.; Sahasrabuddhe, A.; Chung, F.; Bailey, N.G.; Schrader, A.; Li, B.; Li, J.Z.; Ozel, A.B.; et al. Integrated genomic sequencing reveals mutational landscape of T-cell prolymphocytic leukemia. *Blood* **2014**, *124*, 1460–1472. [CrossRef]
38. Gäbler, K.; Behrmann, I.; Haan, C. JAK2 mutants (e.g., JAK2V617F) and their importance as drug targets in myeloproliferative neoplasms. *JAK-STAT* **2013**, *2*, e25025. [CrossRef]
39. Fukuda, A.; Wang, S.; Morris, J.P.; Folias, A.E.; Liou, A.; Kim, G.E.; Akira, S.; Boucher, K.; Firpo, M.A.; Mulvihill, S.J.; et al. Stat3 and MMP7 Contribute to Pancreatic Ductal Adenocarcinoma Initiation and Progression. *Cancer Cell* **2011**, *19*, 441–455. [CrossRef]
40. Alexander, W.; Hilton, D.S. The Role of Suppressors of Cytokine Signaling (SOCS) Proteins in Regulation of the Immune Response. *Annu. Rev. Immunol.* **2004**, *22*, 503–529. [CrossRef]
41. Amador, C.; Greiner, T.; Heavican, T.B.; Smith, L.M.; Galvis, K.T.; Lone, W.G.; Bouska, A.; D'Amore, F.; Pedersen, M.B.; Pileri, S.A.; et al. Reproducing the Molecular Subclassification of Peripheral T-cell Lymphoma-NOS by Immunohistochemistry. *Blood* **2019**, *134*, 2159–2170. [CrossRef]
42. Heavican, T.B.; Bouska, A.; Yu, J.; Lone, W.; Amador, C.; Gong, Q.; Zhang, W.; Li, Y.; Dave, B.J.; Nairismägi, M.-L.; et al. Genetic drivers of oncogenic pathways in molecular subgroups of peripheral T-cell lymphoma. *Blood* **2019**, *133*, 1664–1676. [CrossRef] [PubMed]
43. Zinzani, P.L.; Baliva, G.; Magagnoli, M.; Bendandi, M.; Modugno, G.; Gherlinzoni, F.; Orcioni, G.F.; Ascani, S.; Simoni, R.; Pileri, S.A.; et al. Gemcitabine Treatment in Pretreated Cutaneous T-Cell Lymphoma: Experience in 44 Patients. *J. Clin. Oncol.* **2000**, *18*, 2603–2606. [CrossRef] [PubMed]
44. Pellegrini, C.; Dodero, A.; Chiappella, A.; Monaco, F.; Degl'Innocenti, D.; Salvi, F.; Vitolo, U.; Argnani, L.; Corradini, P.; Zinzani, P.L.; et al. A phase II study on the role of gemcitabine plus romidepsin (GEMRO regimen) in the treatment of relapsed/refractory peripheral T-cell lymphoma patients. *J. Hematol. Oncol.* **2016**, *9*, 1–7. [CrossRef] [PubMed]
45. Arkenau, H.-T.; Chong, G.; Cunningham, D.; Watkins, D.; Sirohi, B.; Chau, I.; Wotherspoon, A.; Norman, A.; Horwich, A.; Matutes, E. Gemcitabine, cisplatin and methylprednisolone for the treatment of patients with peripheral T-cell lymphoma: The Royal Marsden Hospital experience. *Haematology* **2007**, *92*, 271–272. [CrossRef] [PubMed]

46. Mahadevan, D.; Unger, J.M.; Spier, C.M.; Persky, D.O.; Young, F.; Leblanc, M.; Fisher, R.I.; Miller, T.P. Phase 2 trial of combined cisplatin, etoposide, gemcitabine, and methylprednisolone (PEGS) in peripheral T-cell non-Hodgkin lymphoma: Southwest Oncology Group Study S0350. *Cancer* **2012**, *119*, 371–379. [CrossRef] [PubMed]
47. Rajala, H.L.M.; Eldfors, S.; Kuusanmäki, H.; Van Adrichem, A.J.; Olson, T.; Lagström, S.; I Andersson, E.; Jerez, A.; Clemente, M.J.; Yan, Y.; et al. Discovery of somatic STAT5b mutations in large granular lymphocytic leukemia. *Blood* **2013**, *121*, 4541–4550. [CrossRef]
48. Team, R. *RStudio: Integrated Development for R*; RStudio: Boston, MA, USA, 2015.

12

Direct Targeting Options for STAT3 and STAT5 in Cancer

Anna Orlova [1], Christina Wagner [1], Elvin D. de Araujo [2,3], Dávid Bajusz [4], Heidi A. Neubauer [1], Marco Herling [5], Patrick T. Gunning [2,3], György M. Keserű [4] and Richard Moriggl [1,*]

1 Institute of Animal Breeding and Genetics, University of Veterinary Medicine, 1210 Vienna, Austria; anna.orlova@vetmeduni.ac.at (A.O.); Christina-Maria.Wagner@vetmeduni.ac.at (C.W.); Heidi.Neubauer@vetmeduni.ac.at (H.A.N.)

2 Department of Chemical and Physical Sciences, University of Toronto Mississauga, Mississauga, ON L5L 1C6, Canada; e.dearaujo@mail.utoronto.ca (E.D.d.A.); patrick.gunning@utoronto.ca (P.T.G.)

3 Centre for Medicinal Chemistry, University of Toronto Mississauga, Mississauga, ON L5L 1C6, Canada

4 Medicinal Chemistry Research Group, Research Centre for Natural Sciences, H-1117 Budapest, Hungary; bajusz.david@ttk.mta.hu (D.B.); keseru.gyorgy@ttk.mta.hu (G.M.K.)

5 Department I of Internal Medicine, Center for Integrated Oncology (CIO), Excellence Cluster for Cellular Stress Response and Aging-Associated Diseases (CECAD), and Center for Molecular Medicine Cologne (CMMC), Cologne University, 50937 Cologne, Germany; marco.herling@uk-koeln.de

* Correspondence: richard.moriggl@vetmeduni.ac.at

Abstract: Signal transducer and activator of transcription (STAT)3 and STAT5 are important transcription factors that are able to mediate or even drive cancer progression through hyperactivation or gain-of-function mutations. Mutated STAT3 is mainly associated with large granular lymphocytic T-cell leukemia, whereas mutated STAT5B is associated with T-cell prolymphocytic leukemia, T-cell acute lymphoblastic leukemia and $\gamma\delta$ T-cell-derived lymphomas. Hyperactive STAT3 and STAT5 are also implicated in various hematopoietic and solid malignancies, such as chronic and acute myeloid leukemia, melanoma or prostate cancer. Classical understanding of STAT functions is linked to their phosphorylated parallel dimer conformation, in which they induce gene transcription. However, the functions of STAT proteins are not limited to their phosphorylated dimerization form. In this review, we discuss the functions and the roles of unphosphorylated STAT3/5 in the context of chromatin remodeling, as well as the impact of STAT5 oligomerization on differential gene expression in hematopoietic neoplasms. The central involvement of STAT3/5 in cancer has made these molecules attractive targets for small-molecule drug development, but currently there are no direct STAT3/5 inhibitors of clinical grade available. We summarize the development of inhibitors against the SH2 domains of STAT3/5 and discuss their applicability as cancer therapeutics.

Keywords: STAT3; STAT5; cancer; small-molecule inhibitors

---

1. Introduction

The Janus kinase/Signal transducer and activator of transcription (JAK-STAT) pathway is one of the core cancer pathways that integrates signals from cytokines, hormones and growth factors to induce or repress gene expression in cells [1]. The pathway consists of four JAK kinases (JAK1, JAK2, JAK3 and TYK2) and seven STAT transcription factors (STAT1, STAT2, STAT3, STAT4, STAT5A, STAT5B and STAT6). Despite conserved structure and a common mechanism of action, STAT family members show distinct and even opposite functions in tumor biology.

STAT1 is generally not associated with promoting tumor growth and mostly mediates tumor-suppressive and pro-apoptotic functions [2,3]. Consistently, STAT1$^{-/-}$ mice are more prone to tumor development and *STAT1* deletion in leukemic cells decreases MHC class I expression [4,5]. Surprisingly, in a *v-abl*-driven model of STAT1$^{-/-}$ leukemic cells initially harboring low MHC class I, enhanced MHC class I expression was gained during the disease progression, thereby reducing tumor recognition by NK cells [6]. As an exception, STAT1 was shown to be an oncogenic driver in T-cell acute lymphoblastic leukemia (T-ALL) and ALK$^+$ anaplastic large cell lymphoma (ALCL), and STAT1 is associated with the JAK2 exon 12 mutation in the progression of myeloproliferative neoplasms (MPNs) [7–9]. Reports on direct involvements of STAT2, STAT4 and STAT6 in cancerous processes are scarce and are not discussed here further [10]. Associations of STAT3 and STAT5 with cancer progression are well established and heavily studied, and hence, are the main focus of this review.

2. Role of STAT3 and STAT5 in Cancer

STAT3 and STAT5 proteins are of particular interest in cancer research, as their hyperactivation was reported in processes ranging from inflammation and autoimmunity to infection and cancer. Within the latter, these proteins have been implicated in tumor initiation, as well as in metastasis or in conferring drug resistance mechanisms [10–12]. Constitutive hyperactivation of STAT3 and STAT5, as a result of their gain-of-function mutations or via enhanced signaling from upstream drivers, promotes tumor cell growth and survival [3].

STAT3 is the best-studied family member of the JAK-STAT pathway in cancer, and is a known oncogene in various types of solid malignancies, like melanoma or lung cancer [13–15]. Furthermore, both STAT3 and STAT5 are reported to play a major role in the progression and pathogenesis of prostate cancer [16–18]. Hyperactivation of STAT3 and STAT5 is commonly associated with an upstream oncogenic driver, such as hyperactive mutated tyrosine kinases, for example, JAK2^{V617F} or FLT3-ITD, or fusion proteins such as BCR-ABL, TEL-JAK2 or TEL-ABL1 [3,19–21]. The role of STAT5 in the transformation process induced by BCR-ABL p210 fusion protein has been particularly well-studied. It was shown that the absence of STAT5 diminishes the ability of cells to transform even upon harboring potent oncogenes such as BCR-ABL. Inducible deletion of STAT5 arrests and kills chronic myeloid leukemia (CML) cell lines, defining STAT5 as a therapeutic cancer target [22]. Hyperactivation of STAT3 and STAT5 can also occur via direct mutation in these genes, which is also associated with cancer progression in patients [1]. Interestingly, mutated STAT3 is mainly associated with large granular lymphocytic T-cell leukemia (T-LGLL), whereas mutated STAT5B is found in patients with T-cell prolymphocytic leukemia (T-PLL), T-ALL, $\gamma\delta$ T-cell-derived lymphoma and monomorphic epitheliotropic intestinal T-cell lymphoma (MEITL) [23–25].

Inhibitors of kinases upstream of STAT3/5 are available, but patients often relapse by developing drug resistance through persistent signaling or enhanced upregulation of STAT3 or STAT5 expression [21,26]. Targeting STAT3 and STAT5 directly or in combination with tyrosine kinase inhibitors might be an attractive way to overcome these resistance mechanisms [27].

3. Non-Canonical Functions of STAT3 and STAT5

STAT proteins share similar structural architecture including five domains: an N-terminal domain, a coiled-coil domain, a DNA-binding domain, an SH2 domain and a C-terminal transactivation domain [11] (Figure 1a). Upon phosphorylation, STAT5 undergoes a conformational change and forms parallel dimers via the SH2 domain (Figure 1b). This conformation allows the dimers to be recognized by importins and facilitates transport into the nucleus, where they bind GAS consensus sequences to induce target gene transcription. Such dramatic conformational rearrangements are possible due to the flexible linkers that are connecting the core fragment of STAT5 with its N- and C-terminus [28–30]. The complex approach of molecular dynamic simulations and bioinformatic analyses identified three distinct interaction surfaces within the dimer unique to STAT5, which include intramolecular interactions between the SH2 domain and the phosphotyrosine motif [28,31].

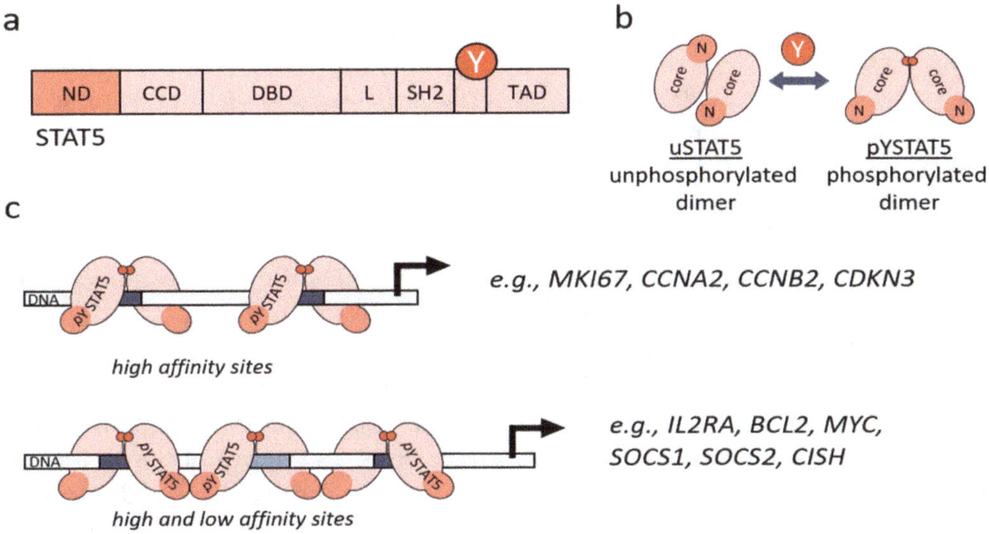

Figure 1. Functions of STAT5. (**a**) Domain structure of STAT5. Position of the critical activating tyrosine phosphorylation site is depicted with Y. ND—N-domain; CCD—coiled-coil domain; DBD—DNA-binding domain; L—linker; SH2—SH2 domain; TAD—transactivation domain. (**b**) Conformational changes of STAT5 from an unphosphorylated antiparallel dimer (uSTAT5) to a phosphorylated parallel dimer (pYSTAT5). (**c**) Dimer and oligomer conformations of STAT5 result in binding to GAS sites on DNA with different affinities, resulting in expression of different genes. Examples of dimer versus tetramer target genes are incorporated from [32,33].

Interestingly, the SH2 domain of the hyperactivated gain-of-function variant STAT5B^{N642H} was also crystallized and compared to wild type human STAT5B. The crystal structure revealed two conformations of the mutant SH2 domain: one conformation is more closed, potentially allowing longer tyrosine phosphorylation lifetimes by blocking phosphatase attack. The other conformation, preserved in the crystal structure, revealed a more open conformation, which could facilitate phospho-peptide or protein interactions leading to hyperactivation [34].

Interestingly, the functions of STAT proteins are not limited to their state as phosphorylated dimers. Unphosphorylated STAT dimers (uSTAT), as well as tetramer/oligomer conformations, are involved in the functionality of some STATs [32,35]. Two phosphorylated dimers can form tetramers via their N-terminal oligomerization domains. This interaction stabilizes DNA binding and allows attraction of the tetramers to low-affinity sites, thereby providing altered binding selectivity and fine-tuning of transcriptional responses [36] (Figure 1c).

STAT5 is particularly known for forming oligomers, a function shared with STAT1 and STAT4. In contrast, STAT3 shows weaker tetramer formation upon activation. STAT2 and STAT6 were not reported to form oligomers in cellulo [32,37–39]. However, yeast hybridization assays showed that recombinant N-domains of all STATs are able to self-dimerize [40]. Interestingly, this interaction is clearly homotypic, which might facilitate individual functions of different STATs. In addition, recombinant STAT2 and STAT6 N-domains can form oligomers with the same affinity as other STAT members, but this was not observed in cellulo [40].

The N-terminus also plays an important role in the function of STAT3: it mediates dimerization of uSTAT3, whereas for phosphorylated STAT3 (pYSTAT3) it can enable tetramerization [41,42]. Interestingly, oligomerization of STAT3 is not commonly observed in cellulo. Still, expression of certain genes like A2M (α2-macroglobulin) was shown to depend on an N-domain interaction of STAT3 [42].

Hu et al. showed that in STAT3$^{-/-}$ MEFs, exogenous expression of an N-terminally truncated STAT3 protein leads to a decrease in expression of a small subset of genes, compared to expression of wild type STAT3 [43]. Not surprisingly, mutated STAT3^{Y705F}, which is unable to become phosphorylated and to form parallel dimers, significantly affected global gene expression. However, certain genes (e.g., *MRAS, MET*) were still activated even by uSTAT3 [44]. Interestingly, $STAT3^{Y705F}$ was able to weakly bind to selected promoters and to induce gene expression, thereby promoting an anti-viral, anti-proliferative effect in response to interferon stimulation. It would be interesting to determine if this activity is connected to the heterodimerization of STAT3 with STAT1 or if it is fully mediated through uSTAT3 [45]. uSTAT3 was also reported to be involved in interactions and complex formation with unphosphorylated nuclear factor kappa-light-chain-enhancer of activated B cells (NF-κB), which resulted in activation of a subset of NF-κB-dependent genes. Of note, the authors showed an additional subset of uSTAT3-dependent, but NF-κB-independent genes [46].

Timofeeva et al. showed that uSTAT3 plays a repressive role in the apoptosis of cancer cells and that inhibition of STAT3 N-domain functions can abolish this repressive effect. Treatment with the STAT3 N-domain peptidomimetic, ST3-H2A2, hindered STAT3 binding to the regulatory domains of various genes, including the gene for the proapoptotic C/EBP-homologous protein (CHOP). This, in turn, led to a decrease in the heterochromatin mark H3K9me3 in the promoter region of this gene [47].

uSTAT5 is mostly localized in the cytoplasm in the form of anti-parallel dimers. In mammalian cells, cytoplasmic uSTAT5 was shown to associate with and stabilize the Golgi apparatus [48]. On the other hand, a smaller proportion of uSTAT5 was also found in the nucleus where it colocalizes with the transcriptional repressor CTCF, thereby diminishing megakaryocyte differentiation via competition for DNA binding with the transcription factor ERG [35]. Additionally, there is evidence that uSTAT5 can migrate into the nucleus and bind heterochromatin protein 1α (HP1α) to promote the formation of heterochromatin. This leads to repression of various genes, among which many are found to be involved in cancer development [49].

One function of the STAT5 N-terminal domain involves docking of STAT5 to receptors. For example, it was shown that STAT5 interacts via the N-terminal domain with the glucocorticoid receptor [50]. The N-domain of STAT5 has an O-GlcNAc modification site on threonine 92. For STAT5A, it was shown that the presence of this glucose-derived modification within the N-domain is essential for full activation, suggesting cross-talk between the N- and C-domains and involvement of the N-domain in the regulation of metabolic functions in cells [51].

Another function of the STAT5 N-domain is mediating STAT5 tetramerization. Tetramerization was shown to be essential for proper T-cell development and was also found to be associated with enhanced activity of STAT5 as an oncogene [32]. STAT5 tetramers can bind to different motifs compared with STAT5 dimers, to induce or repress gene expression (Figure 1c) [52]. It was shown that deletion of the N-domain of STAT5 results in an absence of *c-MYC*, *BCL-2* and *cyclin D2* expression upon stimulation, indicating that oligomers can induce a different subset of genes than dimers [32]. Extensive studies by Lin et al., using a mutated STAT5 N-domain that is unable to form oligomers in vivo, defined the oligomer-dependent subset of genes as well as the importance of oligomerization in NK cell maturation [33,52].

The STAT5 N-domain was shown to be essential for leukemogenic transformation. Deletion of the N-domain or mutation of the O-GlcNAc-modified residue (T92A) abolished the initiation of the leukemic disease driven by gain-of-function STAT5A [32,51,53]. This suggests an important function of the STAT5 N-domain in oncogenic transformation and it proposes that the N-domain can serve as a novel targeting interface of STAT5.

4. Role of STAT3/5 in Chromatin Landscape

Over the last years, it was shown that STAT3 and STAT5 transcription factors can influence gene expression not only directly by binding to gene promoters but also through recruiting various chromatin remodelers and influencing gene expression and chromatin states on the global level. STAT3/5 can change the chromatin landscape in a cell by recruiting various chromatin-remodeling or DNA-modifying enzymes to the DNA, such as histone acetyltransferases (HATs), histone deacetylases (HDACs), as well as ten-eleven translocation methylcytosine dioxygenase 1/2 (TET1/2) or DNA (cytosine-5)-methyltransferase 1 (DNMT1) [54–57] (Figure 2a,b). These interactions influence eu- or hetero-chromatin formation or DNA methylation, thereby activating or repressing transcription. The STATs themselves can also be post-translationally modified by these enzymes: for example, methylation of STAT3 by the enhancer of zeste homolog 2/polycomb repressive complex 2 (EZH2/PRC2), or acetylation of STAT3 and STAT5 by CREB-binding protein (CBP)/p300 [1].

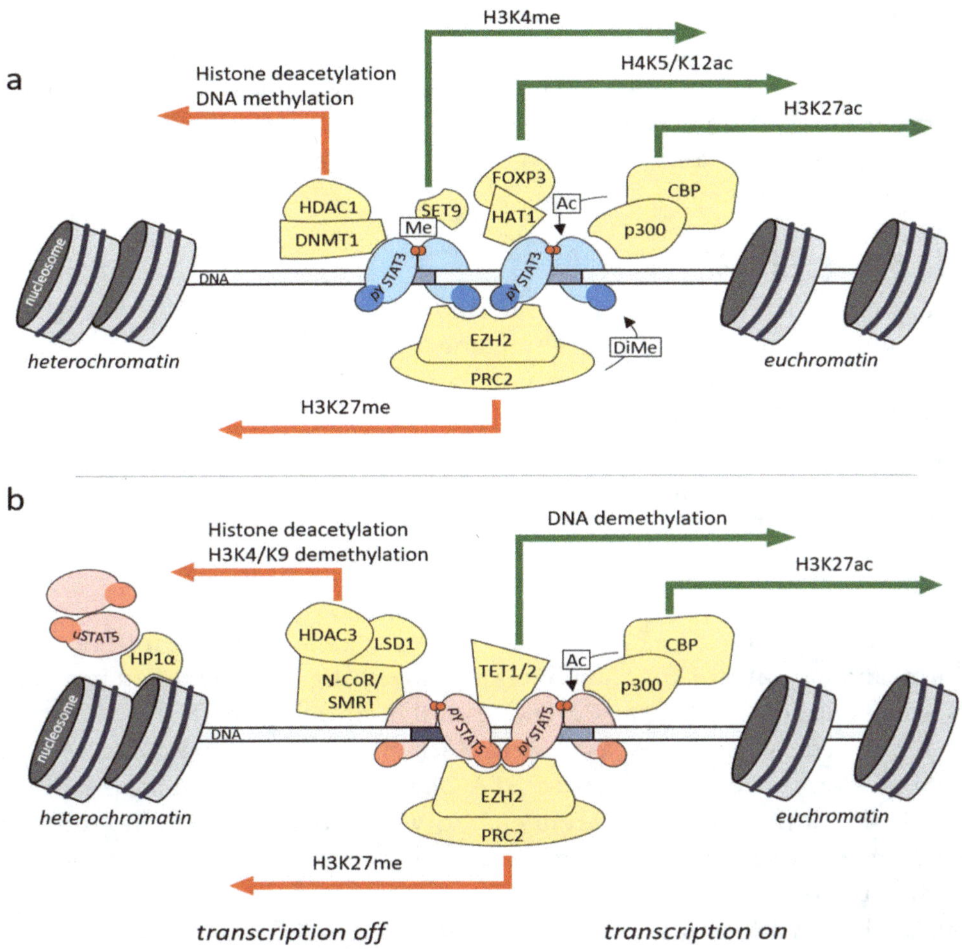

Figure 2. Role of STAT3/5 in regulating the chromatin landscape. (**a**) pYSTAT3 interacts with and recruits chromatin remodelers, and thereby promotes changes in chromatin compaction. (**b**) uSTAT5 and pYSTAT5 interact with different chromatin remodelers, thereby promoting chromatin changes associated with euchromatin (green arrows) or heterochromatin (red arrows) formation.

In the case of STAT3, acetylation or methylation at different residues leads to different activity and functionality of the protein (Figure 2a) [12]. For example, acetylation of STAT3 by CBP/p300 on lysine 685 in the C-terminal domain increases the DNA binding ability of STAT3 [58]. On the other hand, methylation of phosphorylated, promoter-bound STAT3 on lysine 140 by SET9 reduces its transcriptional activity on a subset of target genes [59], whereas dimethylation on lysine 49 by EZH2 is required for the expression of IL-6-dependent genes [60]. It was also shown that STAT3 binds to the promoter of the tyrosine phosphatase *SHP-1* and recruits DNMT1 and HDAC1 to silence its transcription in cutaneous T-cell lymphoma (CTCL) and in ALK^+ ALCL cell lines [57]. In regulatory T-cells, STAT3 was found to cooperate with FoxP3 and HAT1 to induce expression of IL-10 [61].

STAT5 is also known to recruit chromatin remodelers (Figure 2b). One example of such an interaction is co-activation of STAT5 by HAT nuclear receptor coactivator 1 (NCoA-1). NCoA-1 and STAT5A transiently co-transfected in HEK293T cells were shown to interact with each other by co-immunoprecipitation. This interaction required amino acids 751 to 753 in the STAT5 transactivation domain, which is conserved in both STAT5A and STAT5B [54]. Furthermore, in Ba/F3 cells, STAT5A was shown to interact with HDAC3 and lysine-specific demethylase 1 (LSD1), thereby activating or repressing gene expression [55]. The interaction between STAT5A and LSD1/HDAC3 is mediated by the STAT5A DNA-binding domain, linker and its SH2 domain and HDAC3 can additionally interact with the coiled-coil domain of STAT5A [55]. STAT5 influences not only the acetylation but also the methylation status of its surroundings, for example by recruiting TET1/2 to the *Foxp3* locus. This causes demethylation of the locus and plays an important role in regulatory T-cell differentiation [56].

Mandal et al. showed that during B-cell maturation and B-cell receptor rearrangement, gene regions required for immunoglobulin κ light chain expression are silenced by histone methyltransferase EZH2-STAT5 tetramer interactions (Figure 2b) [62]. This underlines the importance of the STAT5 N-terminal domain and tetramerization during B-cell development or as a mechanism for acute B-cell leukemia initiation or progression.

5. Direct STAT Targeting of the SH2 Domain

Treating cancers with hyperactivated or mutated STAT3 and STAT5 is currently achieved by targeting upstream kinases. However, despite tyrosine kinase inhibitors being significantly superior to classical chemotherapy, their application often causes severe side-effects and development of resistance [63]. Therefore, development of more specific and effective inhibitors that also target downstream components of hyperactivated pathways is desirable to overcome limitations of current strategies. In the following section, we focus specifically on small-molecule inhibitors of the STAT3/5 SH2 domains.

5.1. STAT3 Inhibitors

The first two small-molecule STAT3 inhibitors were fragment-sized compounds discovered by random biochemical and virtual screening. One compound, Stattic, was identified in a high-throughput screen of a diverse chemical library (Figure 3a) [64]. Another anthraquinone-based compound, STA-21 (Figure 3b), was discovered by structure-based virtual screening against the published X-ray structure of STAT3β [65,66]. Later, multiple analogs of STA-21 were reported, such as LLL-3 and LLL-12 (Figure 3c,d) [67,68]. Recently, several different chemotypes have emerged, often consisting of ring systems connected by amide-containing linkers. An important step forward was the identification of the salicylic acid moiety that is an efficient bioisostere of the phosphate group required for STAT-STAT dimer formation. Salicylic acid analogs were described as potent STAT3 inhibitors as exemplified by the inhibitor S31-201 (Figure 3e), as well as its optimized successors, SF-1-066, SF-1-121 and S31-1757 (Figure 3f,g) [69–71].

Virtual screening was useful to find new chemotypes of STAT3 inhibitors. Matsuno et al. and Xu et al. described further double-digit micromolar STAT3 inhibitors, STX-0119 and Cpd30-12 (in cellular assays; Figure 3h,i) [72,73]. Furthermore, a number of natural products (or analogs thereof) and antioxidants have been proposed and identified as potential inhibitors of STATs, most particularly STAT3, displaying even single-digit micromolar inhibitory activities [74–78].

Another noteworthy study reported an in silico fragment-based drug discovery approach, resulting in a single-digit micromolar STAT3 inhibitor, LY5 (in both cell-free and cell-based assays; Figure 3j), targeted towards the SH2 domain [79]. Recently, Zhang et al. identified benzothiazole as a novel scaffold among STAT3 inhibitors, resulting from a virtual screening of more than 200,000 compounds by a multistep protocol. In this study, four compounds were confirmed experimentally, with the benzothiazole-based compound 9 (Figure 3k) displaying a single-digit micromolar IC_{50} value against the IL-6/STAT3 signaling pathway [80]. Two further analogs were discovered by a similarity-based hit expansion. When the number of known STAT3 inhibitors reached a sufficient level to compile a training set for a three-dimensional (3D) pharmacophore-based virtual screening study, Leung et al. screened a small in-house dataset and tested five compounds, out of which one (Cpd1, Figure 3l) was experimentally confirmed in multiple STAT3-related endpoints [81].

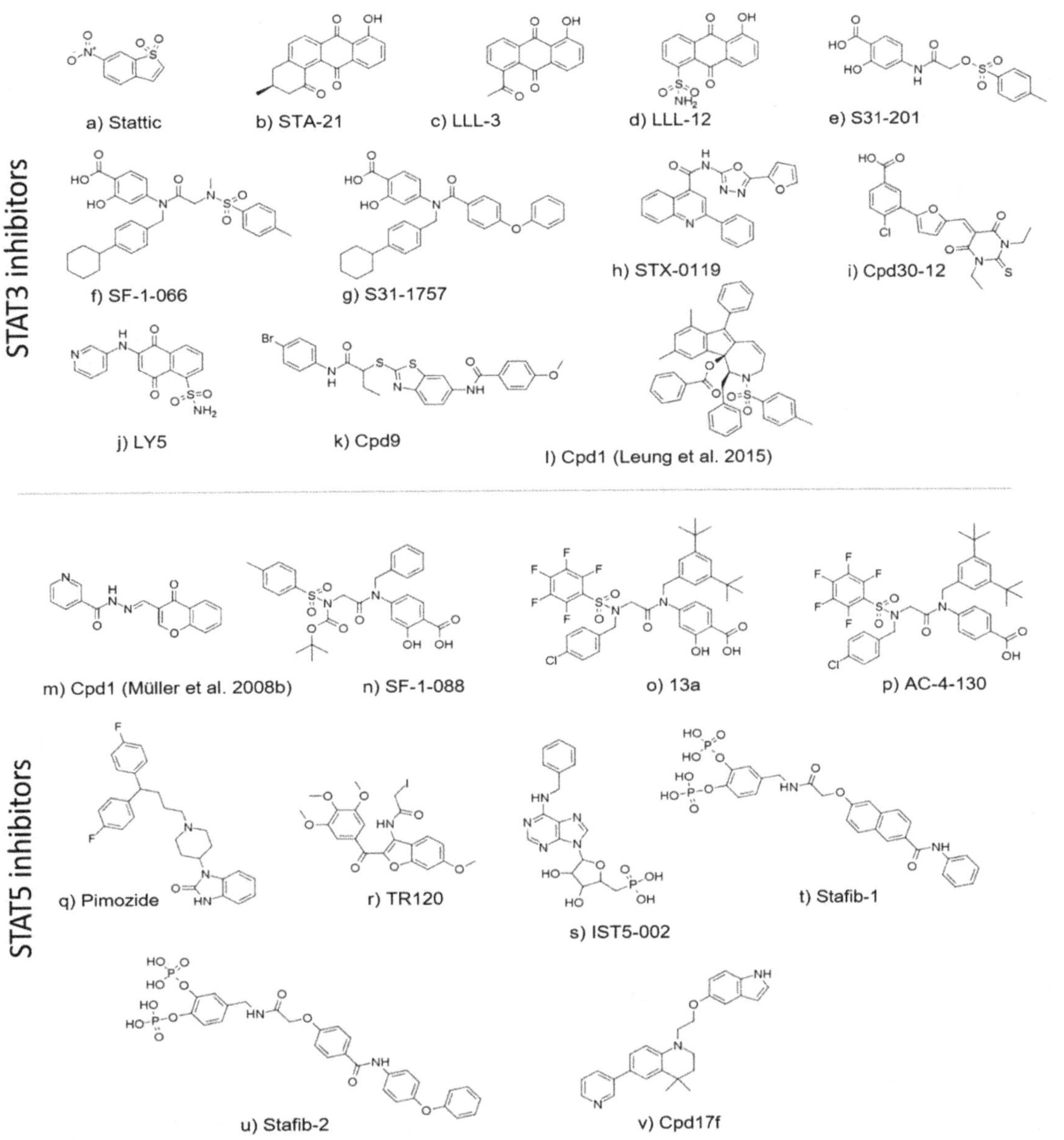

Figure 3. Chemical structures of STAT3 and STAT5 inhibitors (in their order of citation in the main text). Compounds with identical names (Cpd1) are further specified by citations.

The compounds OPB-31121, OPB-51602 and OPB-111077, which are substances from Otsuka Pharmaceuticals, were designed to inhibit STAT3 phosphorylation in cancer cell lines and xenograft models by targeting the STAT3 SH2 domain. Available studies with OPB-51602 indicate induction of STAT3 aggregation in autophagosomes. Additionally, there has been controversy on the activity of OPB-51602 against mitochondrial STAT3. Two of these STAT3 SH2 inhibitors, OPB-31121 and OPB-51602, were already tested in phase I/II clinical trials for solid tumors, non-Hodgkin lymphoma, myeloma and other hematopoietic malignancies [81]. In these studies, the compounds were promising based on a relatively long half-life, suggesting the possibility of a reduced dosing regimen to limit toxic side effects. However, the clinical trials for both lead structure drugs were terminated due to minimal antitumor activity, toxicity issues and poor pharmacokinetics. Another STAT3 inhibitor, OPB-111077, has completed a phase I trial for solid cancers (NCT02250170), and phase I/II trials are recruiting for acute myeloid leukemia (AML) (NCT03197714) and other refractory tumors (NCT03158324) [82,83]. Efficacies of the above-mentioned STAT3 SH2 inhibitors in vitro and in vivo are summarized in Table 1.

Table 1. Small-molecule compounds targeting the STAT3 SH2 domain.

Cpd	Protein-Based		Cell-Based			In Vivo Application Tested	Refs.
	Assay	IC_{50} or Ki [μM]	Cell Line	Readout	IC_{50} [μM]a		
Stattic	pY binding	5.1	HepG2, MDA-MB-231	viability	3.8		[64,84,85]
			RAW264.7	pYSTAT3	s (20)	Osteoclastogenesis in C57/BL6 mice (10 mg/kg)	
			M-SCC-17B, OSC-19, Cal33, UM-SCC-22	viability	2.2–3.5	Head and neck cancer xenograft (50 mg/kg)	
STA-21			Caov-3	reporter assay	s (20)	Psoriatic disease in mouse model and phase I in clinical trial (NCT0104794)	[66,86]
			MDA-MB-435s, MDA-MB-468, MDA-MB-231	DNA binding, viability	s (20)		
LLL-3			U373, MDA-MB-231	DNA binding	s (20)	Xenograft glioblastoma (50 mg/kg)	[68]
			MDA-MB-231	reporter assay	s (20)		
LLL-12			MDA-MB-231, SK-BR-3, PANC-1, HPAC, U87, U373, A549	viability, pYSTAT3, reporter assay	0.16–3.09	Glioblastoma, breast cancer xenograft (2.5, 5 mg/kg) Lung cancer xenograft (20, 10 mg/kg)	[67,87]
S31-201		80	NIH 3T3/v-Src	DNA binding	86	Xenograft breast cancer (5 mg/kg)	[69,71]
			MDA-MB-468, MDA-MB-231	pYSTAT3	s (100)		
			DU145, MDA468, OCI-AML-2	viability	28–112		
SF-1-066	FP	20	NIH 3T3/v-Src	DNA binding	35		[69]
			DU145, MDA468, OCI-AML-2	viability	17–37		
S31-1757	pY binding	13.5	HEK293	CoIP	s (50)		[88]
			MDA-MB-468, A549	pYSTAT3, reporter assay	s (50)		
STX-0119			HeLa	reporter assay	74	Xenograft lymphoma (160 mg/kg)	[73]
			HEK293	FRET-based dimerization	s (50)		
Cpd30-12	pY binding	114	HepG2, MEF/GFP-Stat3α, MDA-MB-468, MDA-MB-231, MBA-MD-435, MCF7	pYSTAT3, nuclear translocation, apoptosis	60		[72]
LY5	FP	2.5	U2OS, RH30, RD2, MDA-MB-231	viability, pYSTAT3	0.52–1.39	Xenograft breast cancer (5 mg/kg)	[79,89]
			UW426, UW288-1, DAOY	pYSTAT3	s (0.5)		
Cpd9			HepG2/STAT3	reporter assay, pYSTAT3	3.57		[80]
			MDA-MB-468	viability	8.83		
Cpd1	FP	~10	HeLa	reporter assay, DNA binding	~10		[81]

[a] s (20): significant effect at 20 μM (or other concentration, as indicated); cpd—compound; FP—fluorescence polarization.

5.2. STAT5 Inhibitors

The first landmark papers on STAT5 SH2 domain inhibitors were published in 2008 by the Berg group. These were driven by the development of a robust high-throughput screening assay for STAT5B inhibitors [90,91]. This facilitated the discovery of chromone-based STAT5B inhibitors as well as a nicotinoyl hydrazine derivative, Cpd1 (Figure 3m), as a selective STAT5B inhibitor (in comparison to STAT1 and STAT3) [91].

Later, four salicylic acid-based compounds (including the single-digit micromolar inhibitor SF-1-088, Figure 3n) were identified by the Gunning group [92]. These hits were optimized to generate the STAT5B inhibitor, 13a, through a structure-guided approach (Figure 3o). Studies with 13a have shown it can effectively reduce pYSTAT5B levels in cellulo, and follow up thermal stability studies showed an inhibitor-induced reduction in STAT5 stability and the potential to block de novo phosphorylation [28,93,94]. Additional studies extended this work to demonstrate AML cell viability inhibition with AC-4-130, a further improved lead compound (Figure 3p) [95].

It is worth noting that in a 2011 study, Nelson et al. identified the neuroleptic drug pimozide as a STAT5 inhibitor (Figure 3q). However, recent studies have linked pimozide with proteolysis upstream of STAT5, rather than direct binding [96]. Nonetheless, the discovery later prompted Rondanin et al. to synthesize and screen a series of pimozide derivatives, two of which have surpassed the cytotoxic potency of pimozide as evaluated against imatinib-resistant BCR-ABL-expressing leukemia cells [97]. In 2016, the same group synthesized and tested 22 iodoacetamide-containing heterocycles for STAT5 inhibition, many of which (including TR120, Figure 3r) were confirmed experimentally in an in vitro cytotoxicity assay, although direct binding to STAT5 was not examined [98].

In 2015, Liao et al. conducted a large scale structure-based virtual screening campaign for STAT5A/B inhibitors [99]. Using a STAT3 based homology model of STAT5, the authors docked ~30 million compounds to the dimerization interface on the SH2 domain [65]. The top 30 hits were evaluated in various cell lines, with IST5-002 (Figure 3s) identified as a lead compound that inhibited STAT5A and STAT5B in the low micromolar range in cellulo. However, the first STAT5A/B gene product-selective inhibitor was developed in the same year, by the Berg group. Stafib-1 (Figure 3t), a catechol type bisphosphate-containing nanomolar STAT5B inhibitor (as evaluated in a fluorescence polarization assay), was identified by structure-based virtual screening against the SH2 domain of a STAT5B model derived from the structure of unphosphorylated STAT5A [30,100]. This compound was recently optimized into the single-digit nanomolar inhibitor Stafib-2 (Figure 3u) using a structure-based approach [101]. Stafib-2, similar to its predecessor, has shown high selectivity for STAT5B compared to other STAT proteins, including STAT5A. The hydrophilicity of the phosphate motifs was reduced by generating a pro-drug precursor, which employs pivaloyloxymethyl esters to conceal the negatively charged phosphate groups and increase cell penetrance. Recently, Natarajan et al. reported Stafia-1, a selective inhibitor for STAT5A, discovered by docking-based screening [102]. Tested applications for STAT5 inhibitors in vivo and in vitro are summarized in Table 2.

Berg et al. also identified nucleotide scaffolds with potentially selective inhibition properties against STAT5B. Although, the IC_{50} values in a fluorescence polarization assay are in the high micro-molar range (STAT5B, IC_{50}[ATP] = 97.4 ± 0.9 μM, IC_{50}[GTP] = 95.5 ± 3.2 μM; STAT5A, IC_{50}[ATP] = 443 ± 34 μM, IC_{50}[GTP] = 311 ± 46 μM), these concentrations are still well below intracellular ATP concentrations (>2 mM). It would be of high interest to validate these findings in cellulo. These results suggest STAT5B may also play a role in directly coupling gene expression to cellular metabolism, and also highlight a potential new targeting strategy using nucleotide-based inhibitor scaffolds [104]. Recently, a novel mechanism of selectively blocking STAT5B activity was proposed through protein-mediated Mannich reactions. The ligand-efficient 4-amino-furazan-3-carboxylic acid molecule (K_d = 420 μM, STAT5B fluorescent polarization assay) was identified from a library of 17,000 compounds. This phosphate-mimetic reacts with 1*H*-tetrazoles in the presence of formaldehyde, and this reaction only proceeds in acidic conditions (pH 5.0). However, the addition of MBP-tagged STAT5B-SH2 domain peptide catalyzed the reaction even at physiological conditions.

Although tetrazoles were not active against STAT5B (>10 mM), the ligation products showed substantial activity, which the authors attribute to super-additive binding interactions. Intracellular physiological concentrations of formaldehyde also emphasize the viability of this molecule as a STAT inhibitor and the utility of bio-catalytic Mannich reactions [105].

Table 2. Small-molecule compounds targeting the STAT5 SH2 domain.

Cpd	Protein-Based		Cell-Based			In Vivo Application Tested	Refs.
	Assay	IC_{50} or K_i [μM][a]	Cell Line	Readout	IC_{50} [μM][a]		
Cpd1	FP	47	K562, Daudi	DNA binding, pYSTAT5	s (100)		[91]
SF-1-088	FP	8.3	K562,MV4-11	viability, pYSTAT5	80–77		[92]
13a			K562	pYSTAT5, viability	s (15)		[28,93,94]
			MV4-11	viability	3.5		
AC-4-130	binding (thermal shift)	s (100)	MV4-11, MOLM-13	viability, reporter assay	1.7–1.9	AML xenograft (25 mg/kg)	[95]
			AML patient samples	viability	1.6–4.9		
Pimozide			KU812, K562	pYSTAT5, viability	s (5)	Approved by FDA as antipsychotic drug	[96]
TR120			K562	viability	0.12		[98]
				apoptosis	0.45		
IST5-002			K562, DU145, PC-3, COS-7	pYSTAT5, reporter assay, DNA binding	s (5)	Prostate cancer xenograft (25, 50, 100 mg/kg)	[99]
				viability	3.5		
Stafib-1	FP	0.044	K562	pYSTAT5	s (3)		[100]
Stafib-2	FP	0.009	K562	pYSTAT5	1.5		[101]
Cpd17f			K562, KU812, KG1a, MV4-11	viability, pYSTAT5	2.6–22.7		[103]

[a] s (100): significant effect at 100 μM (or other concentration, as indicated); cpd—compound; FP—fluorescence polarization.

A study by Juen et al. reported the optimization of the STAT5 inhibitor, Cpd17f (Figure 3v) [103]. Interestingly, the initial hit was originally intended for PPARα/γ inhibition, while the inhibition of STAT5 phosphorylation was an off-target effect [106]. Since the compound did not inhibit PPARs, but showed a considerable inhibition of STAT5 phosphorylation, 18 analogs were synthesized and tested in a cell-based assay. As shown by Brachet-Bottineau et al., in this special issue, Cpd17f inhibits STAT5B protein expression through non-transcriptional mechanisms. However, as with the majority of the aforementioned inhibitors, further confirmatory assays demonstrating the mechanism of action are required. Although multiple studies using molecular modeling or computational dynamics have been insightful in STAT5 inhibitor design, protein-inhibitor complexes characterized with atomic-level resolution, such as through X-ray crystallization, would provide a clearer understanding of target engagement in efficacy and selectivity studies.

Apart from these efforts targeting the SH2 domain of STAT3 or STAT5 molecules, studies have also reported describing approaches to block STAT3/5 DNA binding or the use of antisense RNA interference, discussed further in this special issue with separate overview articles.

6. Conclusions

STAT3 and STAT5 are the key nodes in transcriptional activation downstream of cytokine or kinase action in multiple cancers. This makes them attractive, but challenging targets for drug development. Recent findings expand on a previously rather simplistic understanding of STAT3/5 function as parallel phosphorylated dimers. It has become evident that higher-order conformations of pYSTATs, as well as uSTAT, are involved in chromatin landscape shaping, thereby acting beyond classical transcription factors. This knowledge provides a deeper understanding of their role in cancer biology, which together with various targeting efforts, will open novel therapeutic options.

Acknowledgments: Open Access Funding by the Austrian Science Fund (FWF).

References

1. Wingelhofer, B.; Neubauer, H.A.; Valent, P.; Han, X.; Constantinescu, S.N.; Gunning, P.T.; Müller, M.; Moriggl, R. Implications of STAT3 and STAT5 signaling on gene regulation and chromatin remodeling in hematopoietic cancer. *Leukemia* **2018**, *32*, 1713–1726. [CrossRef] [PubMed]
2. Koromilas, A.E.; Sexl, V. The tumor suppressor function of STAT1 in breast cancer. *JAK-STAT* **2013**, *2*, e23353. [CrossRef] [PubMed]
3. Yu, H.; Jove, R. The stats of cancer—New molecular targets come of age. *Nat. Rev. Cancer* **2004**, *4*, 97–105. [CrossRef]
4. Meissl, K.; Macho-Maschler, S.; Müller, M.; Strobl, B. The good and the bad faces of STAT1 in solid tumours. *Cytokine* **2017**, *89*, 12–20. [CrossRef]
5. Klover, P.J.; Muller, W.J.; Robinson, G.W.; Pfeiffer, R.M.; Yamaji, D.; Hennighausen, L. Loss of STAT1 from Mouse Mammary Epithelium Results in an Increased Neu-Induced Tumor Burden. *Neoplasia* **2010**, *12*, 899–905. [CrossRef]
6. Kovacic, B.; Stoiber, D.; Moriggl, R.; Weisz, E.; Ott, R.G.; Kreibich, R.; Levy, D.E.; Beug, H.; Freissmuth, M.; Sexl, V. STAT1 acts as a tumor promoter for leukemia development. *Cancer Cell* **2006**, *10*, 77–87. [CrossRef]
7. Godfrey, A.L.; Chen, E.; Massie, C.E.; Silber, Y.; Pagano, F.; Bellosillo, B.; Guglielmelli, P.; Harrison, C.N.; Reilly, J.T.; Stegelmann, F.; et al. STAT1 activation in association with *JAK2* exon 12 mutations. *Haematologica* **2016**, *101*, e15. [CrossRef]
8. Prutsch, N.; Gurnhofer, E.; Suske, T.; Liang, H.C.; Schlederer, M.; Roos, S.; Wu, L.C.; Simonitsch-Klupp, I.; Alvarez-Hernandez, A.; Kornauth, C.; et al. Dependency on the TYK2/STAT1/MCL1 axis in anaplastic large cell lymphoma. *Leukemia* **2019**, *33*, 696–709. [CrossRef]
9. Sanda, T.; Tyner, J.W.; Gutierrez, A.; Ngo, V.N.; Glover, J.; Chang, B.H.; Yost, A.; Ma, W.; Fleischman, A.G.; Zhou, W.; et al. TYK2–STAT1–BCL2 Pathway Dependence in T-cell Acute Lymphoblastic Leukemia. *Cancer Discov.* **2013**, *3*, 564. [CrossRef]
10. Furth, P.A. STAT signaling in different breast cancer sub-types. *Mol. Cell. Endocrinol.* **2014**, *382*, 612–615. [CrossRef]
11. Levy, D.E.; Darnell, J.E. STATs: Transcriptional control and biological impact: Signalling. *Nat. Rev. Mol. Cell Biol.* **2002**, *3*, 651–662. [CrossRef] [PubMed]
12. Avalle, L.; Camporeale, A.; Camperi, A.; Poli, V. STAT3 in cancer: A double edged sword. *Cytokine* **2017**, *98*, 42–50. [CrossRef]
13. Bromberg, J.F.; Wrzeszczynska, M.H.; Devgan, G.; Zhao, Y.; Pestell, R.G.; Albanese, C.; Darnell, J.E., Jr. Stat3 as an Oncogene. *Cell* **1999**, *98*, 295–303. [CrossRef]
14. Corvinus, F.M.; Orth, C.; Moriggl, R.; Tsareva, S.A.; Wagner, S.; Pfitzner, E.B.; Baus, D.; Kaufman, R.; Huber, L.A.; Zatloukal, K.; et al. Persistent STAT3 Activation in Colon Cancer Is Associated with Enhanced Cell Proliferation and Tumor Growth. *Neoplasia* **2005**, *7*, 545–555. [CrossRef]
15. Yu, H.; Lee, H.; Herrmann, A.; Buettner, R.; Jove, R. Revisiting STAT3 signalling in cancer: new and unexpected biological functions. *Nat. Rev. Cancer* **2014**, *14*, 736. [CrossRef]
16. Mohanty, S.K.; Yagiz, K.; Pradhan, D.; Luthringer, D.J.; Amin, M.B.; Alkan, S.; Cinar, B. STAT3 and STAT5A are potential therapeutic targets in castration-resistant prostate cancer. *Oncotarget* **2017**, *8*. [CrossRef]

17. Gu, L.; Dagvadorj, A.; Lutz, J.; Leiby, B.; Bonuccelli, G.; Lisanti, M.P.; Addya, S.; Fortina, P.; Dasgupta, A.; Hyslop, T.; et al. Transcription Factor Stat3 Stimulates Metastatic Behavior of Human Prostate Cancer Cells in Vivo, whereas Stat5b Has a Preferential Role in the Promotion of Prostate Cancer Cell Viability and Tumor Growth. *Am. J. Pathol.* **2010**, *176*, 1959–1972. [CrossRef]
18. Boutillon, F.; Pigat, N.; Sackmann Sala, L.; Reyes-Gomez, E.; Moriggl, R.; Guidotti, J.-E.; Goffin, V. STAT5a/b Deficiency Delays, but does not Prevent, Prolactin-Driven Prostate Tumorigenesis in Mice. *Cancers* **2019**, *11*, 929. [CrossRef]
19. Cahu, X.; Constantinescu, S.N. Oncogenic Drivers in Myeloproliferative Neoplasms: From JAK2 to Calreticulin Mutations. *Curr. Hematol. Malig. Rep.* **2015**, *10*, 335–343. [CrossRef]
20. Staerk, J.; Constantinescu, S.N. The JAK-STAT pathway and hematopoietic stem cells from the JAK2 V617F perspective. *JAK-STAT* **2012**, *1*, 184–190. [CrossRef]
21. Warsch, W.; Walz, C.; Sexl, V. JAK of all trades: JAK2-STAT5 as novel therapeutic targets in BCR-ABL1+ chronic myeloid leukemia. *Blood* **2014**, *122*, 2167–2175. [CrossRef] [PubMed]
22. Hoelbl, A.; Kovacic, B.; Kerenyi, M.A.; Simma, O.; Warsch, W.; Cui, Y.; Beug, H.; Hennighausen, L.; Moriggl, R.; Sexl, V. Clarifying the role of Stat5 in lymphoid development and Abelson-induced transformation. *Blood* **2006**, *107*, 4898. [CrossRef]
23. Pham, H.T.T.; Maurer, B.; Prchal-Murphy, M.; Grausenburger, R.; Grundschober, E.; Javaheri, T.; Nivarthi, H.; Boersma, A.; Kolbe, T.; Elabd, M.; et al. STAT5BN642H is a driver mutation for T cell neoplasia. *J. Clin. Invest.* **2018**, *128*, 387–401. [CrossRef] [PubMed]
24. Waldmann, T.A.; Chen, J. Disorders of the JAK/STAT Pathway in T Cell Lymphoma Pathogenesis: Implications for Immunotherapy. *Annu. Rev. Immunol.* **2017**, *35*, 533–550. [CrossRef]
25. Schrader, A.; Crispatzu, G.; Oberbeck, S.; Mayer, P.; Pützer, S.; von Jan, J.; Vasyutina, E.; Warner, K.; Weit, N.; Pflug, N.; et al. Actionable perturbations of damage responses by TCL1/ATM and epigenetic lesions form the basis of T-PLL. *Nat. Commun.* **2018**, *9*, 697. [CrossRef]
26. Koppikar, P.; Bhagwat, N.; Kilpivaara, O.; Manshouri, T.; Adli, M.; Hricik, T.; Liu, F.; Saunders, L.M.; Mullally, A.; Abdel-Wahab, O.; et al. Heterodimeric JAK–STAT activation as a mechanism of persistence to JAK2 inhibitor therapy. *Nature* **2012**, *489*, 155–159. [CrossRef]
27. Berger, A.; Sexl, V.; Valent, P.; Moriggl, R. Inhibition of STAT5: a therapeutic option in BCR-ABL1-driven leukemia. *Oncotarget* **2014**, *5*, 9564–9576. [CrossRef]
28. Cumaraswamy, A.A.; Lewis, A.M.; Geletu, M.; Todic, A.; Diaz, D.B.; Cheng, X.R.; Brown, C.E.; Laister, R.C.; Muench, D.; Kerman, K.; et al. Nanomolar-Potency Small Molecule Inhibitor of STAT5 Protein. *ACS Med. Chem. Lett.* **2014**, *5*, 1202–1206. [CrossRef]
29. Mertens, C.; Zhong, M.; Krishnaraj, R.; Zou, W.; Chen, X.; Darnell, J.E. Dephosphorylation of phosphotyrosine on STAT1 dimers requires extensive spatial reorientation of the monomers facilitated by the N-terminal domain. *Genes Dev.* **2006**, *20*, 3372–3381.
30. Neculai, D.; Neculai, A.M.; Verrier, S.; Straub, K.; Klumpp, K.; Pfitzner, E.; Becker, S. Structure of the Unphosphorylated STAT5a Dimer. *J. Biol. Chem.* **2005**, *280*, 40782–40787. [CrossRef]
31. Fahrenkamp, D.; Li, J.; Ernst, S.; Schmitz-Van de Leur, H.; Chatain, N.; Küster, A.; Koschmieder, S.; Lüscher, B.; Rossetti, G.; Müller-Newen, G. Intramolecular hydrophobic interactions are critical mediators of STAT5 dimerization. *Sci. Rep.* **2016**, *6*, 35454. [CrossRef] [PubMed]
32. Moriggl, R.; Sexl, V.; Kenner, L.; Duntsch, C.; Stangl, K.; Gingras, S.; Hoffmeyer, A.; Bauer, A.; Piekorz, R.; Wang, D.; et al. Stat5 tetramer formation is associated with leukemogenesis. *Cancer Cell* **2005**, *7*, 87–99. [CrossRef]
33. Lin, J.-X.; Du, N.; Li, P.; Kazemian, M.; Gebregiorgis, T.; Spolski, R.; Leonard, W.J. Critical functions for STAT5 tetramers in the maturation and survival of natural killer cells. *Nat. Commun.* **2017**, *8*, 1320. [CrossRef]
34. de Araujo, E.D.; Erdogan, F.; Neubauer, H.A.; Meneksedag-Erol, D.; Manaswiyoungkul, P.; Eram, M.S.; Seo, H.-S.; Qadree, A.K.; Israelian, J.; Orlova, A.; et al. Structural and functional consequences of the STAT5BN642H driver mutation. *Nat. Commun.* **2019**, *10*, 2517. [CrossRef] [PubMed]
35. Park, H.J.; Li, J.; Hannah, R.; Biddie, S.; Leal-Cervantes, A.I.; Kirschner, K.; Flores Santa Cruz, D.; Sexl, V.; Go ttgens, B.; Green, A.R. Cytokine-induced megakaryocytic differentiation is regulated by genome-wide loss of a uSTAT transcriptional program. *EMBO J.* **2016**, *35*, 580–594. [CrossRef] [PubMed]
36. Zhao, Y.; Zeng, C.; Tarasova, N.I.; Chasovskikh, S.; Dritschilo, A.; Timofeeva, O.A. A new role for STAT3 as a regulator of chromatin topology. *Transcription* **2013**, *4*, 227–231. [CrossRef]

37. Kornfeld, J.-W.; Grebien, F.; Kerenyi, M.A.; Friedbichler, K.; Kovacic, B.; Zankl, B.; Hoelbl, A.; Nivarti, H.; Beug, H.; Sexl, V.; et al. The different functions of Stat5 and chromatin alteration through Stat5 proteins. *Front. Biosci. J. Virtual Libr.* **2008**, *13*, 6237–6254. [CrossRef]
38. Li, G.; Wang, Z.; Zhang, Y.; Kang, Z.; Haviernikova, E.; Cui, Y.; Hennighausen, L.; Moriggl, R.; Wang, D.; Tse, W.; et al. STAT5 requires the N-domain to maintain hematopoietic stem cell repopulating function and appropriate lymphoid-myeloid lineage output. *Exp. Hematol.* **2007**, *35*, 1684–1694. [CrossRef]
39. Murphy, T.; Yee, K.W.L. Cytarabine and daunorubicin for the treatment of acute myeloid leukemia. *Expert Opin. Pharmacother.* **2017**, *18*, 1765–1780. [CrossRef]
40. Ota, N.; Brett, T.J.; Murphy, T.L.; Fremont, D.H.; Murphy, K.M. N-domain–dependent nonphosphorylated STAT4 dimers required for cytokine-driven activation. *Nat. Immunol.* **2004**, *5*, 208–215. [CrossRef]
41. Vogt, M.; Domoszlai, T.; Kleshchanok, D.; Lehmann, S.; Schmitt, A.; Poli, V.; Richtering, W.; Muller-Newen, G. The role of the N-terminal domain in dimerization and nucleocytoplasmic shuttling of latent STAT3. *J. Cell Sci.* **2011**, *124*, 900–909. [CrossRef] [PubMed]
42. Zhang, X.; Darnell, J.E. Functional Importance of Stat3 Tetramerization in Activation of the α2-Macroglobulin Gene. *J. Biol. Chem.* **2001**, *276*, 33576–33581. [CrossRef]
43. Hu, T.; Yeh, J.E.; Pinello, L.; Jacob, J.; Chakravarthy, S.; Yuan, G.-C.; Chopra, R.; Frank, D.A. Impact of the N-Terminal Domain of STAT3 in STAT3-Dependent Transcriptional Activity. *Mol. Cell. Biol.* **2015**, *35*, 3284. [CrossRef]
44. Yang, J.; Chatterjee-Kishore, M.; Staugaitis, S.M.; Nguyen, H.; Schlessinger, K.; Levy, D.E.; Stark, G.R. Novel Roles of Unphosphorylated STAT3 in Oncogenesis and Transcriptional Regulation. *Cancer Res.* **2005**, *65*, 939. [PubMed]
45. Pfeffer, S.R.; Fan, M.; Du, Z.; Yang, C.H.; Pfeffer, L.M. Unphosphorylated STAT3 regulates the antiproliferative, antiviral, and gene-inducing actions of type I interferons. *Biochem. Biophys. Res. Commun.* **2017**, *490*, 739–745. [CrossRef]
46. Yang, J.; Liao, X.; Agarwal, M.K.; Barnes, L.; Auron, P.E.; Stark, G.R. Unphosphorylated STAT3 accumulates in response to IL-6 and activates transcription by binding to NFκB. *Genes Dev.* **2007**, *21*, 1396–1408.
47. Timofeeva, O.A.; Tarasova, N.I.; Zhang, X.; Chasovskikh, S.; Cheema, A.K.; Wang, H.; Brown, M.L.; Dritschilo, A. STAT3 suppresses transcription of proapoptotic genes in cancer cells with the involvement of its N-terminal domain. *Proc. Natl. Acad. Sci. USA* **2013**, *110*, 1267–1272. [CrossRef]
48. Lee, J.E.; Yang, Y.-M.; Liang, F.-X.; Gough, D.J.; Levy, D.E.; Sehgal, P.B. Nongenomic STAT5-dependent effects on Golgi apparatus and endoplasmic reticulum structure and function. *Am. J. Physiol. Cell Physiol.* **2011**, *302*, C804–C820. [CrossRef]
49. Hu, X.; Dutta, P.; Tsurumi, A.; Li, J.; Wang, J.; Land, H.; Li, W.X. Unphosphorylated STAT5A stabilizes heterochromatin and suppresses tumor growth. *Proc. Natl. Acad. Sci. USA* **2013**, *110*, 10213–10218. [CrossRef]
50. Engblom, D.; Kornfeld, J.-W.; Schwake, L.; Tronche, F.; Reimann, A.; Beug, H.; Hennighausen, L.; Moriggl, R.; Schutz, G. Direct glucocorticoid receptor-Stat5 interaction in hepatocytes controls body size and maturation-related gene expression. *Genes Dev.* **2007**, *21*, 1157–1162.
51. Freund, P.; Kerenyi, M.A.; Hager, M.; Wagner, T.; Wingelhofer, B.; Pham, H.T.T.; Elabd, M.; Han, X.; Valent, P.; Gouilleux, F.; et al. O-GlcNAcylation of STAT5 controls tyrosine phosphorylation and oncogenic transcription in STAT5-dependent malignancies. *Leukemia* **2017**, *31*, 2132–2142. [CrossRef]
52. Lin, J.-X.; Li, P.; Liu, D.; Jin, H.T.; He, J.; Rasheed, M.A.U.; Rochman, Y.; Wang, L.; Cui, K.; Liu, C.; et al. Critical Role of STAT5 Transcription Factor Tetramerization for Cytokine Responses and Normal Immune Function. *Immunity* **2012**, *36*, 586–599. [CrossRef]
53. Rauth, M.; Freund, P.; Orlova, A.; Grünert, S.; Tasic, N.; Han, X.; Ruan, H.-B.; Neubauer, A.H.; Moriggl, R. Cell Metabolism Control Through O-GlcNAcylation of STAT5: A Full or Empty Fuel Tank Makes a Big Difference for Cancer Cell Growth and Survival. *Int. J. Mol. Sci.* **2019**, *20*, 1028. [CrossRef] [PubMed]
54. Litterst, C.M.; Kliem, S.; Marilley, D.; Pfitzner, E. NCoA-1/SRC-1 Is an Essential Coactivator of STAT5 That Binds to the FDL Motif in the α-Helical Region of the STAT5 Transactivation Domain. *J. Biol. Chem.* **2003**, *278*, 45340–45351. [CrossRef]
55. Nanou, A.; Toumpeki, C.; Lavigne, M.D.; Lazou, V.; Demmers, J.; Paparountas, T.; Thanos, D.; Katsantoni, E. The dual role of LSD1 and HDAC3 in STAT5-dependent transcription is determined by protein interactions, binding affinities, motifs and genomic positions. *Nucleic Acids Res.* **2016**, *45*, 142–154. [CrossRef]

56. Yang, R.; Qu, C.; Zhou, Y.; Konkel, J.E.; Shi, S.; Liu, Y.; Chen, C.; Liu, S.; Liu, D.; Chen, Y.; et al. Hydrogen Sulfide Promotes Tet1- and Tet2-Mediated Foxp3 Demethylation to Drive Regulatory T Cell Differentiation and Maintain Immune Homeostasis. *Immunity* **2015**, *43*, 251–263. [CrossRef]
57. Zhang, Q.; Wang, H.Y.; Marzec, M.; Raghunath, P.N.; Nagasawa, T.; Wasik, M.A. STAT3- and DNA methyltransferase 1-mediated epigenetic silencing of SHP-1 tyrosine phosphatase tumor suppressor gene in malignant T lymphocytes. *Proc. Natl. Acad. Sci. USA* **2005**, *102*, 6948. [CrossRef]
58. Wang, R.; Cherukuri, P.; Luo, J. Activation of Stat3 Sequence-specific DNA Binding and Transcription by p300/CREB-binding Protein-mediated Acetylation. *J. Biol. Chem.* **2005**, *280*, 11528–11534. [CrossRef]
59. Yang, J.; Huang, J.; Dasgupta, M.; Sears, N.; Miyagi, M.; Wang, B.; Chance, M.R.; Chen, X.; Du, Y.; Wang, Y.; et al. Reversible methylation of promoter-bound STAT3 by histone-modifying enzymes. *Proc. Natl. Acad. Sci. USA* **2010**, *107*, 21499. [CrossRef]
60. Dasgupta, M.; Dermawan, J.K.T.; Willard, B.; Stark, G.R. STAT3-driven transcription depends upon the dimethylation of K49 by EZH2. *Proc. Natl. Acad. Sci. USA* **2015**, *112*, 3985. [CrossRef]
61. Hossain, D.M.S.; Panda, A.K.; Manna, A.; Mohanty, S.; Bhattacharjee, P.; Bhattacharyya, S.; Saha, T.; Chakraborty, S.; Kar, R.K.; Das, T.; et al. FoxP3 acts as a cotranscription factor with STAT3 in tumor-induced regulatory T cells. *Immunity* **2013**, *39*, 1057–1069. [CrossRef] [PubMed]
62. Mandal, M.; Powers, S.E.; Maienschein-Cline, M.; Bartom, E.T.; Hamel, K.M.; Kee, B.L.; Dinner, A.R.; Clark, M.R. Epigenetic repression of the Igk locus by STAT5-mediated recruitment of the histone methyltransferase Ezh2. *Nature Immunol.* **2011**, *12*, 1212–1220. [CrossRef] [PubMed]
63. Boumahdi, S.; de Sauvage, F.J. The great escape: tumour cell plasticity in resistance to targeted therapy. *Nat. Rev. Drug Discov.* **2019**. [CrossRef] [PubMed]
64. Schust, J.; Sperl, B.; Hollis, A.; Mayer, T.U.; Berg, T. Stattic: A Small-Molecule Inhibitor of STAT3 Activation and Dimerization. *Chem. Biol.* **2006**, *13*, 1235–1242.
65. Becker, S.; Groner, B.; Müller, C.W. Three-dimensional structure of the Stat3β homodimer bound to DNA. *Nature* **1998**, *394*, 145–151. [CrossRef]
66. Song, H.; Wang, R.; Wang, S.; Lin, J. A low-molecular-weight compound discovered through virtual database screening inhibits Stat3 function in breast cancer cells. *Proc. Natl. Acad. Sci. USA* **2005**, *102*, 4700. [CrossRef]
67. Lin, L.; Hutzen, B.; Li, P.-K.; Ball, S.; Zuo, M.; DeAngelis, S.; Foust, E.; Sobo, M.; Friedman, L.; Bhasin, D.; et al. A novel small molecule, LLL12, inhibits STAT3 phosphorylation and activities and exhibits potent growth-suppressive activity in human cancer cells. *Neoplasia* **2010**, *12*, 39–50. [CrossRef]
68. Fuh, B.; Sobo, M.; Cen, L.; Josiah, D.; Hutzen, B.; Cisek, K.; Bhasin, D.; Regan, N.; Lin, L.; Chan, C.; et al. LLL-3 inhibits STAT3 activity, suppresses glioblastoma cell growth and prolongs survival in a mouse glioblastoma model. *Br. J. Cancer* **2009**, *100*, 106–112. [CrossRef]
69. Fletcher, S.; Singh, J.; Zhang, X.; Yue, P.; Page, B.D.G.; Sharmeen, S.; Shahani, V.M.; Zhao, W.; Schimmer, A.D.; Turkson, J.; et al. Disruption of transcriptionally active Stat3 dimers with non-phosphorylated, salicylic acid-based small molecules: potent in vitro and tumor cell activities. *Chembiochem Eur. J. Chem. Biol.* **2009**, *10*, 1959–1964. [CrossRef]
70. Urlam, M.K.; Pireddu, R.; Ge, Y.; Zhang, X.; Sun, Y.; Lawrence, H.R.; Guida, W.C.; Sebti, S.M.; Lawrence, N.J. Development of new N-Arylbenzamides as STAT3 Dimerization Inhibitors. *MedChemComm* **2013**, *4*, 932–941. [CrossRef]
71. Siddiquee, K.; Zhang, S.; Guida, W.C.; Blaskovich, M.A.; Greedy, B.; Lawrence, H.R.; Yip, M.L.R.; Jove, R.; McLaughlin, M.M.; Lawrence, N.J.; et al. Selective chemical probe inhibitor of Stat3, identified through structure-based virtual screening, induces antitumor activity. *Proc. Natl. Acad. Sci. USA* **2007**, *104*, 7391. [CrossRef] [PubMed]
72. Xu, X.; Kasembeli, M.M.; Jiang, X.; Tweardy, B.J.; Tweardy, D.J. Chemical Probes that Competitively and Selectively Inhibit Stat3 Activation. *PLoS ONE* **2009**, *4*, e4783. [CrossRef] [PubMed]
73. Matsuno, K.; Masuda, Y.; Uehara, Y.; Sato, H.; Muroya, A.; Takahashi, O.; Yokotagawa, T.; Furuya, T.; Okawara, T.; Otsuka, M.; et al. Identification of a New Series of STAT3 Inhibitors by Virtual Screening. *ACS Med. Chem. Lett.* **2010**, *1*, 371–375. [CrossRef] [PubMed]
74. Shin, D.-S.; Kim, H.-N.; Shin, K.D.; Yoon, Y.J.; Kim, S.-J.; Han, D.C.; Kwon, B.-M. Cryptotanshinone Inhibits Constitutive Signal Transducer and Activator of Transcription 3 Function through Blocking the Dimerization in DU145 Prostate Cancer Cells. *Cancer Res.* **2008**, *69*. [CrossRef] [PubMed]

75. Lin, L.; Hutzen, B.; Ball, S.; Foust, E.; Sobo, M.; Deangelis, S.; Pandit, B.; Friedman, L.; Li, C.; Li, P.-K.; et al. New curcumin analogues exhibit enhanced growth-suppressive activity and inhibit AKT and signal transducer and activator of transcription 3 phosphorylation in breast and prostate cancer cells. *Cancer Sci.* **2009**, *100*, 1719–1727. [CrossRef]
76. Amani, H.; Ajami, M.; Nasseri Maleki, S.; Pazoki-Toroudi, H.; Daglia, M.; Tsetegho Sokeng, A.J.; Di Lorenzo, A.; Nabavi, S.F.; Devi, K.P.; Nabavi, S.M. Targeting signal transducers and activators of transcription (STAT) in human cancer by dietary polyphenolic antioxidants. *Biochimie* **2017**, *142*, 63–79. [CrossRef]
77. Li, M.; Yue, G.G.-L.; Song, L.-H.; Huang, M.-B.; Lee, J.K.-M.; Tsui, S.K.-W.; Fung, K.-P.; Tan, N.-H.; Lau, C.B.-S. Natural small molecule bigelovin suppresses orthotopic colorectal tumor growth and inhibits colorectal cancer metastasis via IL6/STAT3 pathway. *Biochem. Pharmacol.* **2018**, *150*, 191–201. [CrossRef]
78. Verdura, S.; Cuyàs, E.; Llorach-Parés, L.; Pérez-Sánchez, A.; Micol, V.; Nonell-Canals, A.; Joven, J.; Valiente, M.; Sánchez-Martínez, M.; Bosch-Barrera, J.; et al. Silibinin is a direct inhibitor of STAT3. *Food Chem. Toxicol.* **2018**, *116*, 161–172. [CrossRef]
79. Yu, W.; Xiao, H.; Lin, J.; Li, C. Discovery of Novel STAT3 Small Molecule Inhibitors via in Silico Site-Directed Fragment-Based Drug Design. *J. Med. Chem.* **2013**, *56*, 4402–4412. [CrossRef]
80. Zhang, M.; Zhu, W.; Li, Y. Discovery of novel inhibitors of signal transducer and activator of transcription 3 (STAT3) signaling pathway by virtual screening. *Eur. J. Med. Chem.* **2013**, *62*, 301–310. [CrossRef]
81. Leung, K.; Liu, L.; Lin, S.; Lu, L.; Zhong, H.; Susanti, D.; Rao, W.; Wang, M.; Ian, W.; Chan, D.S.; et al. Discovery of a small-molecule inhibitor of STAT3 by ligand-based pharmacophore screening. *Methods* **2015**, *71*, 38–43. [CrossRef]
82. Tolcher, A.; Flaherty, K.; Shapiro, G.I.; Berlin, J.; Witzig, T.; Habermann, T.; Bullock, A.; Rock, E.; Elekes, A.; Lin, C.; et al. A First-in-Human Phase I Study of OPB-111077, a Small-Molecule STAT3 and Oxidative Phosphorylation Inhibitor, in Patients with Advanced Cancers. *Oncologist* **2018**, *23*, 658–e72. [CrossRef] [PubMed]
83. Yoo, C.; Kang, J.; Lim, H.Y.; Kim, J.H.; Lee, M.-A.; Lee, K.-H.; Kim, T.-Y.; Ryoo, B.-Y. Phase I Dose-Finding Study of OPB-111077, a Novel STAT3 Inhibitor, in Patients with Advanced Hepatocellular Carcinoma. *Cancer Res. Treat.* **2018**, *51*, 510–518. [CrossRef] [PubMed]
84. Li, C.; Xu, L.; Jian, L.; Yu, R.; Zhao, J.; Sun, L.; Du, G.; Liu, X. Stattic inhibits RANKL-mediated osteoclastogenesis by suppressing activation of STAT3 and NF-κB pathways. *Int. Immunopharmacol.* **2018**, *58*, 136–144. [CrossRef] [PubMed]
85. Adachi, M.; Cui, C.; Dodge, C.T.; Bhayani, M.K.; Lai, S.Y. Targeting STAT3 inhibits growth and enhances radiosensitivity in head and neck squamous cell carcinoma. *Oral Oncol.* **2012**, *48*, 1220–1226. [CrossRef]
86. Miyoshi, K.; Takaishi, M.; Nakajima, K.; Ikeda, M.; Kanda, T.; Tarutani, M.; Iiyama, T.; Asao, N.; DiGiovanni, J.; Sano, S. Stat3 as a Therapeutic Target for the Treatment of Psoriasis: A Clinical Feasibility Study with STA-21, a Stat3 Inhibitor. *J. Investig. Dermatol.* **2011**, *131*, 108–117. [CrossRef]
87. Nie, Y.; Li, Y.; Hu, S. A novel small inhibitor, LLL12, targets STAT3 in non-small cell lung cancer in vitro and in vivo. *Oncol. Lett.* **2018**, *16*, 5349–5354. [CrossRef]
88. Zhang, X.; Sun, Y.; Pireddu, R.; Yang, H.; Urlam, M.K.; Lawrence, H.R.; Guida, W.C.; Lawrence, N.J.; Sebti, S.M. A novel inhibitor of STAT3 homodimerization selectively suppresses STAT3 activity and malignant transformation. *Cancer Res.* **2013**, *73*, 1922–1933. [CrossRef]
89. Xiao, H.; Bid, H.K.; Jou, D.; Wu, X.; Yu, W.; Li, C.; Houghton, P.J.; Lin, J. A Novel Small Molecular STAT3 Inhibitor, LY5, Inhibits Cell Viability, Cell Migration, and Angiogenesis in Medulloblastoma Cells. *J. Biol. Chem.* **2015**, *290*, 3418–3429. [CrossRef]
90. Müller, J.; Schust, J.; Berg, T. A high-throughput assay for signal transducer and activator of transcription 5b based on fluorescence polarization. *Anal. Biochem.* **2008**, *375*, 249–254.
91. Müller, J.; Sperl, B.; Reindl, W.; Kiessling, A.; Berg, T. Discovery of Chromone-Based Inhibitors of the Transcription Factor STAT5. *ChemBioChem* **2008**, *9*, 723–727. [CrossRef] [PubMed]
92. Page, B.D.G.; Khoury, H.; Laister, R.C.; Fletcher, S.; Vellozo, M.; Manzoli, A.; Yue, P.; Turkson, J.; Minden, M.D.; Gunning, P.T. Small Molecule STAT5-SH2 Domain Inhibitors Exhibit Potent Antileukemia Activity. *J. Med. Chem.* **2012**, *55*, 1047–1055. [CrossRef] [PubMed]
93. de Araujo, E.D.; Manaswiyoungkul, P.; Israelian, J.; Park, J.; Yuen, K.; Farhangi, S.; Berger-Becvar, A.; Abu-Jazar, L.; Gunning, P.T. High-throughput thermofluor-based assays for inhibitor screening of STAT SH2 domains. *J. Pharm. Biomed. Anal.* **2017**, *143*, 159–167. [CrossRef] [PubMed]

94. de Araujo, E.D.; Manaswiyoungkul, P.; Erdogan, F.; Qadree, A.K.; Sina, D.; Tin, G.; Toutah, K.; Yuen, K.; Gunning, P.T. A functional in vitro assay for screening inhibitors of STAT5B phosphorylation. *J. Pharm. Biomed. Anal.* **2019**, *162*, 60–65. [CrossRef]
95. Wingelhofer, B.; Maurer, B.; Heyes, E.C.; Cumaraswamy, A.C.; Berger-Becvar, A.; de Araujo, E.D.; Orlova, A.; Freund, P.; Ruge, F.; Park, J.; et al. Pharmacologic inhibition of STAT5 in acute myeloid leukemia. *Leukemia* **2018**, *32*, 1135–1146. [CrossRef]
96. Nelson, E.A.; Walker, S.R.; Weisberg, E.; Bar-natan, M.; Barrett, R.; Gashin, L.B.; Terrell, S.; Klitgaard, J.L.; Santo, L.; Addorio, M.R.; et al. The STAT5 inhibitor pimozide decreases survival of chronic myelogenous leukemia cells resistant to kinase inhibitors. *Blood* **2017**, *117*, 3421–3430. [CrossRef]
97. Rondanin, R.; Simoni, D.; Romagnoli, R.; Baruchello, R.; Marchetti, P.; Costantini, C.; Fochi, S.; Padroni, G.; Grimaudo, S.; Maria, R.; et al. Inhibition of activated STAT5 in Bcr/Abl expressing leukemia cells with new pimozide derivatives. *Bioorg. Med. Chem. Lett.* **2014**, *24*, 4568–4574.
98. Romagnoli, R.; Baraldi, P.G.; Prencipe, F.; Lopez-Cara, C.; Rondanin, R.; Simoni, D.; Hamel, E.; Grimaudo, S.; Pipitone, R.M.; Meli, M.; et al. Novel iodoacetamido benzoheterocyclic derivatives with potent antileukemic activity are inhibitors of STAT5 phosphorylation. *Eur. J. Med. Chem.* **2016**, *108*, 39–52. [CrossRef]
99. Liao, Z.; Gu, L.; Vergalli, J.; Mariani, S.A.; De Dominici, M.; Lokareddy, R.K.; Dagvadorj, A.; Purushottamachar, P.; McCue, P.A.; Trabulsi, E.; et al. Structure-based screen identifies a potent small-molecule inhibitor of Stat5a/b with therapeutic potential for prostate cancer and chronic myeloid leukemia. *Mol. Cancer Ther.* **2015**, *14*, 1777–1794. [CrossRef]
100. Elumalai, N.; Berg, A.; Natarajan, K.; Scharow, A.; Berg, T. Nanomolar Inhibitors of the Transcription Factor STAT5b with High Selectivity over STAT5a. *Angew. Chem. Int. Ed.* **2015**, *54*, 4758–4763. [CrossRef]
101. Elumalai, N.; Berg, A.; Rubner, S.; Blechschmidt, L.; Song, C.; Natarajan, K.; Matysik, J.; Berg, T. Rational development of Stafib-2: a selective, nanomolar inhibitor of the transcription factor STAT5b. *Sci. Rep.* **2017**, *7*, 819. [CrossRef] [PubMed]
102. Natarajan, K.; Müller-Klieser, D.; Rubner, S.; Berg, T. Stafia-1: a STAT5a-selective inhibitor developed via docking-based screening of in silico O-phosphorylated fragments. *Chem. Eur. J.* **2019**, in press. [CrossRef] [PubMed]
103. Juen, L.; Brachet-Botineau, M.; Parmenon, C.; Bourgeais, J.; Hérault, O.; Gouilleux, F.; Viaud-Massuard, M.-C.; Prié, G. New Inhibitor Targeting Signal Transducer and Activator of Transcription 5 (STAT5) Signaling in Myeloid Leukemias. *J. Med. Chem.* **2017**, *60*, 6119–6136. [CrossRef]
104. Berg, A.; Sperl, B.; Berg, T. ATP Inhibits the Transcription Factor STAT5b. *ChemBioChem* **2019**, *20*, 2227–2231. [CrossRef]
105. Wong, E.L.; Nawrotzky, E.; Arkona, C.; Kim, B.G.; Beligny, S.; Wang, X.; Wagner, S.; Lisurek, M.; Carstanjen, D.; Rademann, J. The transcription factor STAT5 catalyzes Mannich ligation reactions yielding inhibitors of leukemic cell proliferation. *Nat. Commun.* **2019**, *10*, 66. [CrossRef]
106. Parmenon, C.; Guillard, J.; Caignard, D.-H.; Hennuyer, N.; Staels, B.; Audinot-Bouchez, V.; Boutin, J.-A.; Dacquet, C.; Ktorza, A.; Viaud-Massuard, M.-C. 4,4-Dimethyl-1,2,3,4-tetrahydroquinoline-based PPARα/γ agonists. Part I: Synthesis and pharmacological evaluation. *Bioorg. Med. Chem. Lett.* **2008**, *18*, 1617–1622.

Permissions

All chapters in this book were first published by MDPI; hereby published with permission under the Creative Commons Attribution License or equivalent. Every chapter published in this book has been scrutinized by our experts. Their significance has been extensively debated. The topics covered herein carry significant findings which will fuel the growth of the discipline. They may even be implemented as practical applications or may be referred to as a beginning point for another development.

The contributors of this book come from diverse backgrounds, making this book a truly international effort. This book will bring forth new frontiers with its revolutionizing research information and detailed analysis of the nascent developments around the world.

We would like to thank all the contributing authors for lending their expertise to make the book truly unique. They have played a crucial role in the development of this book. Without their invaluable contributions this book wouldn't have been possible. They have made vital efforts to compile up to date information on the varied aspects of this subject to make this book a valuable addition to the collection of many professionals and students.

This book was conceptualized with the vision of imparting up-to-date information and advanced data in this field. To ensure the same, a matchless editorial board was set up. Every individual on the board went through rigorous rounds of assessment to prove their worth. After which they invested a large part of their time researching and compiling the most relevant data for our readers.

The editorial board has been involved in producing this book since its inception. They have spent rigorous hours researching and exploring the diverse topics which have resulted in the successful publishing of this book. They have passed on their knowledge of decades through this book. To expedite this challenging task, the publisher supported the team at every step. A small team of assistant editors was also appointed to further simplify the editing procedure and attain best results for the readers.

Apart from the editorial board, the designing team has also invested a significant amount of their time in understanding the subject and creating the most relevant covers. They scrutinized every image to scout for the most suitable representation of the subject and create an appropriate cover for the book.

The publishing team has been an ardent support to the editorial, designing and production team. Their endless efforts to recruit the best for this project, has resulted in the accomplishment of this book. They are a veteran in the field of academics and their pool of knowledge is as vast as their experience in printing. Their expertise and guidance has proved useful at every step. Their uncompromising quality standards have made this book an exceptional effort. Their encouragement from time to time has been an inspiration for everyone.

The publisher and the editorial board hope that this book will prove to be a valuable piece of knowledge for researchers, students, practitioners and scholars across the globe.

List of Contributors

Neele Schumacher and Stefan Rose-John
Biochemical Institute, University of Kiel, 24118 Kiel, Germany

Elvin D. de Araujo and Patrick T. Gunning
Centre for Medicinal Chemistry, University of Toronto at Mississauga, Mississauga, ON L5L 1C6, Canada
Department of Chemical & Physical Sciences, University of Toronto at Mississauga, Mississauga, ON L5L 1C6, Canada

Anna Orlova, Heidi A. Neubauer and Richard Moriggl
Institute of Animal Breeding and Genetics, University of Veterinary Medicine, A-1210 Vienna, Austria

Dávid Bajusz and György M. Keserű
Medicinal Chemistry Research Group, Research Centre for Natural Sciences, H-1117 Budapest, Hungary

Hyuk-Soo Seo and Sirano Dhe-Paganon
Department of Cancer Biology, Dana-Farber Cancer Institute, Department of Biological Chemistry & Molecular Pharmacology, Harvard Medical School, Boston, MA 02115, USA
Department of Biological Chemistry, Department of Biological Chemistry & Molecular Pharmacology, Harvard Medical School, Boston, MA 02115, USA

Grégory Verdeil
Laboratory Regulation of immune dysfunction in cancer, Department of Oncology, University of Lausanne, CH-1066 Epalinges, Switzerland

Toby Lawrence
Aix Marseille University, Centre National de la Recherche Scientifique (CNRS) UMR7280, Institut National de la Santé et de la Recherche Médicale (INSERM) U1104, Centre Immunologie Marseille-Luminy (CIML), Parc Scientifique de Luminy, Case 906, 13288 Marseille CEDEX 09, France
Centre for Inflammation Biology and Cancer Immunology, School of Immunology & Microbial Sciences, Faculty of Life Sciences and Medicine, King's College London, London SE1 1UL, UK

Anne-Marie Schmitt-Verhulst and Nathalie Auphan-Anezin
Aix Marseille University, Centre National de la Recherche Scientifique (CNRS) UMR7280, Institut National de la Santé et de la Recherche Médicale (INSERM) U1104, Centre Immunologie Marseille-Luminy (CIML), Parc Scientifique de Luminy, Case 906, 13288 Marseille CEDEX 09, France

Brigitte M. Pützer
Institute of Experimental Gene Therapy and Cancer Research, Rostock University Medical Center, 18057 Rostock, Germany
Department Life, Light & Matter, University of Rostock, 18059 Rostock, Germany

Stella Logotheti
Institute of Experimental Gene Therapy and Cancer Research, Rostock University Medical Center, 18057 Rostock, Germany

Sebastian Igelmann and Gerardo Ferbeyre
Department of Biochemistry and Molecular Medicine, Université de Montréal, C.P. 6128, Succ. Centre-Ville, Montréal, QC H3C 3J7, Canada
CRCHUM, 900 Saint-Denis St, Montréal, QC H2X 0A9, Canada

Heidi A. Neubauer
Institute of Animal Breeding and Genetics, University of Veterinary Medicine Vienna, Vienna 1210, Austria

Marie Brachet-Botineau, Margaux Deynoux and Frédéric Mazurier
LNOx, GICC, CNRS ERL 7001, University of Tours, 37000 Tours, France

Fabrice Gouilleux
INSERM, ERI-12, Faculté de Pharmacie, Université de Picardie Jules Verne, 80000 Amiens, France
CNRS UMR 6239, GICC, Faculté de Médecine, Université François Rabelais, 37020 Tours, France
LNOx, GICC, CNRS ERL 7001, University of Tours, 37000 Tours, France

Nicolas Vallet
LNOx, GICC, CNRS ERL 7001, University of Tours, 37000 Tours, France
Service d'Hématologie et Thérapie Cellulaire, CHRU de Tours, 37000 Tours, France

Marion Polomski, Ludovic Juen, Marie-Claude Viaud-Massuard and Gildas Prié
IMT, GICC, EA 7501, University of Tours, 37000 Tours, France

Olivier Hérault
LNOx, GICC, CNRS ERL 7001, University of Tours, 37000 Tours, France
Service d'Hematologie Biologique, CHRU de Tours, 37000 Tours, France

Cédric Rébé and François Ghiringhelli
Platform of Transfer in Cancer Biology, Centre Georges François Leclerc, INSERM LNC UMR1231, University of Bourgogne Franche-Comté, F-21000 Dijon, France

Kelsey L. Polak, Noah M. Chernosky, Jacob M. Smigiel and Ilaria Tamagno
Department of Pathology, Case Western Reserve University, School of Medicine, Cleveland, OH 44106, USA

Mark W. Jackson
Department of Pathology, Case Western Reserve University, School of Medicine, Cleveland, OH 44106, USA
Case Comprehensive Cancer Center, CaseWestern Reserve University, School of Medicine, Cleveland, OH 44106, USA

Peter Valent
Ludwig Boltzmann Institute for Hematology and Oncology, Medical University of Vienna, 1090 Vienna, Austria
Department/Hospital for Companion Animals and Horses, University Hospital for Small Animals, Internal Medicine Small Animals, University of Veterinary Medicine Vienna, 1210 Vienna, Austria

Emir Hadzijusufovic
Ludwig Boltzmann Institute for Hematology and Oncology, Medical University of Vienna, 1090 Vienna, Austria
Department/Hospital for Companion Animals and Horses, University Hospital for Small Animals, Internal Medicine Small Animals, University of Veterinary Medicine Vienna, 1210 Vienna, Austria
Department of Internal Medicine I, Division of Hematology & Hemostaseology, Medical University of Vienna, 1090 Vienna, Austria

Alexandra Keller, Florian K. M. Schur and Christoph Kornauth
Department of Internal Medicine I, Division of Hematology & Hemostaseology, Medical University of Vienna, 1090 Vienna, Austria

Daniela Berger, Daniel Ivanov and Yüksel Filik
Ludwig Boltzmann Institute for Hematology and Oncology, Medical University of Vienna, 1090 Vienna, Austria
Department of Internal Medicine I, Division of Hematology & Hemostaseology, Medical University of Vienna, 1090 Vienna, Austria

Georg Greiner, Nadine Witzeneder and Gregor Hoermann
Department of Laboratory Medicine, Medical University of Vienna, 1090 Vienna, Austria

Bettina Wingelhofer
Institute of Animal Breeding and Genetics, University of Veterinary Medicine Vienna, 1210 Vienna, Austria

Emmanuel Pecnard
INSERM, ERI-12, Faculté de Pharmacie, Université de Picardie Jules Verne, 80000 Amiens, France

Harini Nivarthi and Robert Kralovics
Research Center for Molecular Medicine (CeMM), 1090 Vienna, Austria

Leonhard Müllauer
Department of Pathology, Medical University of Vienna, 1090 Vienna, Austria

Gary Tin and Jisung Park
Department of Chemistry, University of Toronto, Toronto, ON M5S 1A1, Canada

Linus Wahnschaffe, Till Braun, Alexandra Schrader and Marco Herling
Department I of Internal Medicine, Center for Integrated Oncology (CIO), Aachen-Bonn-Cologne-Duesseldorf, University of Cologne (UoC), 50937 Cologne, Germany
Excellence Cluster for Cellular Stress Response and Aging-Associated Diseases (CECAD), University of Cologne, 50937 Cologne, Germany
Center for Molecular Medicine Cologne (CMMC), University of Cologne, 50937 Cologne, Germany

Prerana Wagle
Excellence Cluster for Cellular Stress Response and Aging-Associated Diseases (CECAD), University of Cologne, 50937 Cologne, Germany

Sanna Timonen
Hematology Research Unit Helsinki, Helsinki University Hospital Comprehensive Cancer Center, FI-00029 Helsinki, Finland
Translational Immunology Research program and Department of Clinical Chemistry and Hematology, University of Helsinki, FI-00014 Helsinki, Finland
Institute for Molecular Medicine Finland (FIMM), University of Helsinki, FI-00014 Helsinki, Finland

Anil K. Giri and Henrikki Almusa
Institute for Molecular Medicine Finland (FIMM), University of Helsinki, FI-00014 Helsinki, Finland

Patricia Johansson
Department of Hematology, University Hospital Essen, University of Duisburg-Essen, 45147 Essen, Germany

Dorine Bellanger and Marc-Henri Stern
Institut Curie, Centre de Recherche, 75248 Paris, France
French National Institute of Health and Medical Research (INSERM) U830, 75248 Paris, France

Cristina López and Reiner Siebert
Institute for Human Genetics, Christian-Albrechts-University Kiel & University Hospital Schleswig Holstein, 24105 Kiel, Germany
Institute of Human Genetics, Ulm University, Ulm University Medical Center, D-89081 Ulm, Germany

Claudia Haferlach
MLL Munich Leukemia Laboratory, Max-Lebsche-Platz 31, 81377 Munich, Germany

Jan Dürig
Department of Hematology, University Hospital Essen, University of Duisburg-Essen, 45147 Essen, Germany
German Cancer Consortium (DKTK), 69120 Heidelberg, Germany

Tero Aittokallio
Institute for Molecular Medicine Finland (FIMM), University of Helsinki, FI-00014 Helsinki, Finland
Department of Mathematics and Statistics, University of Turku, FI-20014 Turku, Finland

Emma I. Andersson
Hematology Research Unit Helsinki, Department of Hematology, University of Helsinki and Helsinki University Hospital Comprehensive Cancer Center, 00290 Helsinki, Finland
Translational Immunology Research program and Department of Clinical Chemistry and Hematology, University of Helsinki, 00014 Helsinki, Finland
HUSLAB, Laboratory of Genetics, Helsinki University Hospital, 00290 Helsinki, Finland

Oscar Brück and Satu Mustjoki
Hematology Research Unit Helsinki, Department of Hematology, University of Helsinki and Helsinki University Hospital Comprehensive Cancer Center, 00290 Helsinki, Finland
Translational Immunology Research program and Department of Clinical Chemistry and Hematology, University of Helsinki, 00014 Helsinki, Finland

Susanna Mannisto and Sirpa Leppä
Department of Oncology, Comprehensive Cancer Center, Helsinki University Hospital, 00290 Helsinki, Finland

Leena Saikko and Panu E. Kovanen
Department of Pathology, HUSLAB, Helsinki University Central Hospital and University of Helsinki, 00290 Helsinki, Finland

Sonja Lagström and Pekka Ellonen
Institute for Molecular Medicine Finland (FIMM), University of Helsinki, 00014 Helsinki, Finland

Christina Wagner
Institute of Animal Breeding and Genetics, University of Veterinary Medicine, 1210 Vienna, Austria

Index

www.ingramcontent.com/pod-product-compliance
Lightning Source LLC
LaVergne TN
LVHW080927210926
848485LV00004B/743
* 9 7 8 1 6 4 6 4 7 5 2 3 0 *